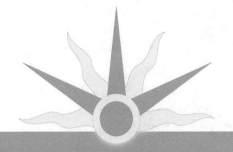

A STUDY GUIDE for the
NCLEX-PN© Exam

6th Edition

Editors

JoAnn Zerwekh, MSN, EdD, RN
President/CEO
Nursing Education Consultants, Inc.
Chandler, AZ

University of Phoenix - Online Campus
Nursing Faculty
Phoenix, AZ

Jo Carol Claborn, MS, RN
Nursing Education Consultants, Inc.

NursingEd

Nursing Education Consultants, Inc.
PO Box 12200
Chandler, AZ 85248

A Study Guide for the NCLEX® PN Exam, 6ᵗʰ ed

ISBN 10: 1-892155-14-1
ISBN-13: 978-1-892155-14-6

© **Copyright 2010 by Nursing Education Consultants, Inc.**

NCLEX and NCLEX –PN® are registered trademarks of the National Council of State Boards of Nursing, Inc.

ISBN-10: 1-892155-14-1
ISBN-13: 978-1-892155-14-6

Project manager: Lindy Nobles
Cover design: Jana Jennings
Printed by: Gingerbread Press, Waxahachie, Texas
Publishing manager: Mike Cull

Printed in the United States of America

Last digit is the print number: 6   5   4   3

Contributors and Reviewers

Joanna G. Barnes, MSN, RN

ADN Program Coordinator
Grayson County College
Denison, Texas

Sharon I. Decker, PhD, ACNS-BC, ANEF, RN

Professor and Director of Clinical Simulations
Covenant Health System Endowed Chair in Simulation and
Nursing Education
Texas Tech University Health Science Center
Lubbock, Texas

Barbara S. Devitt, MSN, RN

Lecturer
Louise Herrington School of Nursing
Baylor University
Dallas, Texas

Ashley Garneau, MS, RN

Nursing Faculty
Gateway Community College
Phoenix, Arizona

Lt. Col. (Ret.) Michael W. Hutton, MSN, RN

Instructor
Blinn College
Bryan, Texas

Susan B. Priest, MSN, CNS, RN

Director, Health and Medical Programs
Continuing Education Workforce Development;
Adjunct Faculty, Associate Degree Nursing
Alvin Community College
Alvin, Texas

Catherine Rosser, EdD, CNA-BC, RN

Undergraduate Program Director
Louise Herrington School of Nursing
Baylor University
Dallas, Texas

Mary Ann Yantis, BS, MS, PhD, RN

Associate Professor of Nursing
Louise Herrington School of Nursing
Baylor University
Dallas, Texas

Preface

This sixth edition of *Illustrated Study Guide for the NCLEX-PN® Exam* continues to provide an up-to-date review book illustrated with graphics, pictures, and cartoon images to enhance your review and retention of critical nursing information. The book contains information specifically designed to assist you in preparing for the National Council Licensure Examination for Practical Nurses (NCLEX-PN®). This text emphasizes the integrated approach to nursing practice that the NCLEX-PN is designed to test. This book's primary purpose is to assist you to thoroughly review facts, principles, and applications of the nursing process. It should alleviate many of the concerns you may have about what, how, and when to study.

We have spent a great deal of time studying the NCLEX-PN test format and have incorporated this information into this book. We have included an explanation and examples of alternate format questions. In our review courses, which we have taught across the country, we have identified specific student needs and correlated this information with the test plan in order to develop this study guide. Study questions are at the end of each chapter for you to check your reading and comprehension. In addition, there are over 1400 test questions available online for practicing your testing skills.

We have designed graphics that highlight important information to make the book more visually appealing:

 TEST ALERT: Identifies important concepts that are reflected on the PN Practice Analysis from the National Council of State Boards of Nursing, Inc.

 NURSING PRIORITY: Assists to distinguish priorities of nursing care and includes both geriatric and pediatric nursing priorities.

 Disease conditions are easily located by this design element.

 Home Care can be found under the Nursing Interventions section.

 Medication information is easily found in chapter appendixes.

 High Alert medications identified by Joint Commission and the Institute for Safe Medication Practices are noted by this symbol.

The comments from our review course participants, as well as extensive faculty reviews on our fifth edition, have helped to shape the development of this sixth edition. We hope this text will prove even more beneficial to nursing faculty, students, and graduate nurses. Thank you for allowing us to be part of your success in nursing.

JoAnn Zerwekh
Jo Carol Claborn

Acknowledgements

We wish to express our appreciation to our children - Ashley Garneau, Tyler Zerwekh, Mike Brown, Kimberley Aultman, and Jaelyn Conway who have watched their mothers write and revise books throughout their childhood and now as adults continue to support our endeavors - for this we are most grateful! To Robert and John, thank you for your tolerance, love, and willingness to continue to share and support us in the midst of our hectic professional lives.

A special note of thanks to CJ Miller, RN, BS, our cartoonist, who has worked with us from the beginning of the *Memory Notebooks of Nursing* and the past few editions of *Nursing Today: Transition & Trends,* and more recently with the *Mosby's Memory Notecard* series. She continues to brighten our day and brings to all of our books, images and cartoons that are so unique.

The revision of a book offers the opportunity to be responsive to nursing faculty and students who have utilized the book. We appreciate their comments and suggestions for the production of this sixth edition. It is our pleasure to express an appreciation to the individuals who assisted us in the technical preparation and production of this sixth edition. Our sincere appreciation to:

Lindy Nobles, our technical assistant, for assisting us in the preparation and typesetting of the manuscript into a working design for publishing.

Jana Jennings, for helping us with the arduous task of putting together detailed tables, boxes, and appendices.

Elaine Nokes, our administrative assistant, who keeps everything organized and running smoothly for our business.

Mike Cull, our publisher at Gingerbread Press, for always coming through for us in all of our printing needs.

Thank you to all!

Contents

Testing Strategies for the NCLEX-PN® Examination

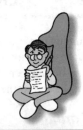

One of the first steps to be being successful on the NCLEX® (National Council Licensure Examination) for practical nursing is to understand how the test is developed. An important step in preparing for the examination is to find out as much as possible about the test; this will help reduce stress and anxiety. During school there were course objectives and faculty class presentations to guide you through the information that would be included on the next examination. In most academic settings, the nursing faculty responsible for teaching a course was also responsible for the development and construction of the course examinations. As you begin to prepare for the NCLEX-PN, it is important to consider who determines the content of the test plan and constructs the questions based on the test plan.

The term practical nurse (PN) is used in this text. There are several states that refer to the practical nurse as a licensed vocational nurse (LVN). There is no difference between these two titles, but the National Council consistently uses the term practical nurse.

The National Council of State Boards of Nursing (NCSBN) is responsible for the development of the content and the construction of questions or items for the NCLEX -PN examination. A practice analysis is conducted by the NCSBN every 3 years to validate the test plan and to determine currency of nursing practice. Content experts are consulted to assist in the creation of the practice analysis. The activity performances and knowledge identified by the content experts are analyzed with consideration given to frequency of performance, impact on client safety, and variety of client care settings. This analysis provides the basis for development of the content to be included in the NCLEX Test Plan.

The content experts are practicing nurses who work with or supervise new graduates in the practice setting. These content experts represent geographical areas across the United States and are selected according to their area of practice; therefore all areas in the practice of practical nursing are addressed in the development of the test plan. Item writers are selected to create questions based on the content identified in the test plan. Item writers are nurses currently licensed in their jurisdiction who are responsible for supervision and teaching of practical nursing students in the clinical area, or who are currently employed in clinical nursing practice working with new graduate practical nurses. An additional panel of practicing nurses reviews all new test items or questions to ensure that each question or item reflects entry level practical nursing practice.

Not only do content experts and item reviewers create new items, they are also involved in the continual review of items in the NCLEX test pool to ensure all items reflect the current practice of practical nursing.[1]

So, what does this all mean? It means that nurses in current practice and nursing faculty work together to identify the content and to develop questions for the NCLEX-PN. The purpose of the examination is to assure the public that each candidate who passes the examination can practice safely and effectively as a newly licensed, entry-level PN.

The NCLEX-PN is used by every U.S. state to determine entry into nursing practice as a PN. Each state is responsible for the testing requirements, retesting procedures, and entry into practice within that state. Each state requires the same competency level or passing standard on the NCLEX; there is no variation in the passing standard from state to state.

TEST PLAN

The test plan is based on research conducted by the NCSBN every 3 years. The purpose of this research is to determine the most important and frequent activities of practical nurses who were successful on the NCLEX and who have been working after successful completion of the NCLEX. The current research indicates that the majority of graduate practical nurses are working in long term care facilities or in hospitals and are caring for clients ages 65 to over 85 years old.[1] Each question will reflect a level of the nursing process or an area of client needs, and each question will be categorized according to a validated level of difficulty. The exam consists of questions that are designed to test the candidate's ability to apply the nursing process and to determine appropriate nursing responses and interventions to provide safe nursing care.

Integrated Processes

Integrated throughout the test plan are principles that are fundamental to the practice of practical nursing.

Nursing Process

The nursing process is a scientific approach to problem solving; it has been a common thread in your nursing curriculum since the beginning of school. There is nothing new about the nursing process on the NCLEX. Data collection, planning, implementation and evaluation are all integral steps in the nursing process. It is important to keep the steps of the nursing process in mind when you are critically evaluating an NCLEX question, data must be obtained and analyzed before an action can be determined. (Box 1-1)

Caring

The interaction of the client and the nurse occurs in an atmosphere of mutual respect and trust. To achieve the desired outcome, the nurse provides hope, support, and compassion to the client.

Communication and Documentation

Events and activities—both verbal and nonverbal—that involve the client, the client's significant others, and the health care team are documented in handwritten or electronic records. These records reflect quality and accountability in the provision of client care. Principles of documentation and provision of client confidentiality are important considerations in any area of nursing practice.

Teaching and Learning

Nurses provide or facilitate knowledge, skills, and attitudes that promote a change in clients' behavior through teaching and learning. Nurses provide education to clients and to their significant others in a variety of settings. [2]

Areas of Client Needs

The National Council Examination Committee has identified four primary areas of client needs, which provide a structure to define nursing actions and competencies across all practice settings and for all clients. These areas reflect an integrated approach to the testing content; no predetermined number of questions or percentage of questions pertain to any particular area of practice (e.g., medical-surgical, pediatric, obstetrical).

Table 1-1 lists the areas of client needs, with the subcategories and the specific weight associated with each subcategory. The range of percentages for each category reflects how important that area is on the test plan. Physiological Adaptation, Basic Care and Comfort, and Coordinated Care are the subcategories with the highest emphasis. [2] When you are studying for the NCLEX, these are concepts that should be identified across the scope of nursing practice. This table has been adapted and summarized; it does not reflect the entire test plan content. The National Council Detailed Test Plan for the NCLEX-PN may be obtained from the NCSBN, Inc. (*www.ncsbn.org*). New information or new practices must be established as a standard of practice across the nation before being included on the NCLEX. Throughout this book are ***TESTING ALERT*** boxes that call your attention to areas of the test plan. Pay attention to these boxes and think about how each concept or principle can apply to different types of clients.

BOX 1-1   KEY WORDS FOR IDENTIFYING THE NURSING PROCESS

The following words are often interchangeable and have the same meaning:

- **Assessment:** collect date, determine, observe, identify findings, recognize changes, notice, detect, find data, gather information, describe status, assess client
- **Planning:** include goals, plan interventions, create plan, generate goals, arrange priorities and interventions, formulate short-term goal or long-term goals, prepare list of client outcomes
- **Implementation:** implement nursing interventions, offer alternatives, teach, give, administer, chart, document, explain, inform, encourage, advise, provide, prepare
- **Evaluation:** evaluate nursing care, question results, monitor findings, repeat assessment, re-establish, consider alternatives, determine changes and response, appraise findings

---

As client conditions or nursing principles are presented, the ***NURSING PRIORITY*** boxes call your attention to critical information regarding a client with a specific condition or situation being presented.

> ✔ ***NURSING PRIORITY:*** *This is critical information to consider in providing safe nursing care for a client with a specific problem.*

Classification of Questions

The majority of questions on the NCLEX are written at the level of application or higher level of cognitive ability. This means a candidate must have the knowledge and understand concepts to be able to apply the nursing process to the client situation presented in the question. NCLEX questions are not fact, recall, or memory-level questions. The questions are based on critical thinking concepts that demonstrate a candidate's ability to make decisions and solve problems. Nurses who have taken the NCLEX have stated that the NCLEX questions were not like any questions they had on nursing school examinations; however, the nursing content and principles needed to determine the answer were provided in their nursing school curriculum. The questions and answers have been thoroughly researched and validated. The standardization of information is important because the NCLEX is administered nationwide to determine entry level into nursing practice. This ensures that regional differences in nursing care will not be a factor in the exam.

All questions presented to a candidate taking the NCLEX-PN have been developed according to the NCLEX-PN Test Plan. The questions have been researched and documented as pertaining to entry-level nursing behaviors. [2,3]

WHAT IS COMPUTER ADAPTIVE TESTING?

Computer adaptive testing provides a method for generating an examination according to each candidate's ability. Each time a candidate answers a question, the computer then selects the next question based on the candidate's answer to the previous question. The examination continues to present test items based on the test plan and provides an opportunity for each candidate to demonstrate competency. The NCLEX-PN is graded in a manner different from the grading of conventional school exams. A candidate's score is not based on the number of questions answered correctly, but rather on the standard of competency as established by the NCSBN. A student's competency level is calculated against the preestablished level of competency.

A test bank of questions is loaded into the candidate's computer at the beginning of the examination. Different candidates receive different sets of questions, but all test banks contain questions that are developed according to the same test plan.

For example, standard precautions are a critical element of the test plan. Many situations and clients can be presented to test this concept: one candidate may have a question based on standard precautions required for a client who is postoperative, someone else, a situation with implications for a newborn, and still someone else, a situation involving an older adult client. All the questions are different, but they are all based on the test plan's critical element of standard precautions.

The candidate will receive new questions based on the response to the previous question. When a question is answered correctly, the next question presented to the candidate may have a higher level of difficulty. A candidate cannot skip questions or go back to previously answered questions. As the examination progresses, it is interactively assembled. As questions are answered correctly, the next question is selected to test another area of the test plan, and it may be at a higher level of difficulty. When a question is answered incorrectly, the computer will select an easier question. This helps to prevent a candidate from being bombarded with very difficult questions and becoming increasingly frustrated. The computer will continue

TABLE 1-1	NCLEX-PN® TEST PLAN - APRIL, 2008 - APRIL, 2011
Safe, Effective Care and Environment	
Coordinated Care (12%-18%)	Management of nursing care—client care assignments, supervision, prioritizing nursing care, and delivery of safe care; maintaining continuity of care, legal and ethical practices; client rights
Safety and Infection Control (8%-14%)	Prevention of errors, accidents, and injury; proper use of restraints and safety devices; implementation of standard precautions; asepsis, ergonomics, handling hazardous materials
Health Promotion and Maintenance (7%-13%)	
Aging process and expected body changes; growth and development and transitions; ante/intra/postpartum, and newborn care; techniques for data collection (physical assessment); disease prevention; principles of learning and teaching; immunizations	
Psychosocial Integrity (8%-14%)	
Mental health and illness concepts; crisis intervention; abuse and neglect; end-of-life care, cultural, religious and spiritual influences on health; grief and loss; therapeutic communication; changes in body image (expected and unexpected); substance abuse.	
Physiological Integrity	
Basic Care and Comfort (11%-17%)	Assistive devices, elimination, mobility, nutrition, hygiene and oral hydration, comfort measures,
Pharmacological and Parenteral Therapies (9%-15%)	Medication administration; adverse effects, expected effects and contraindications for medications
Reduction of Risk Potential (10%-16%)	Perform diagnostic testing; laboratory values – collect specimens, compare data to normal value, reinforce client teaching; perform therapeutic procedures; accurately monitor vital signs; monitor client for potential alteration in body systems (neuro checks, circulatory checks, prenatal complications, immobilization)
Physiological Adaptation (11%-17%)	Alterations in body systems (drainage devices, alterations in blood glucose, wound care, suctioning, identify symptoms of infection, complications of pregnancy/labor/delivery/postpartum, etc); fluid and electrolyte imbalances; medical emergencies, radiation therapy; identify and intervene to unexpected response to therapies (IV, bleeding, infection, etc).

Adapted from the *2008 NCLEX-PN® Detailed Test Plan* (Item writer, item reviewer, nurse educator version), Chicago, 2008, National Council of State Boards of Nursing.

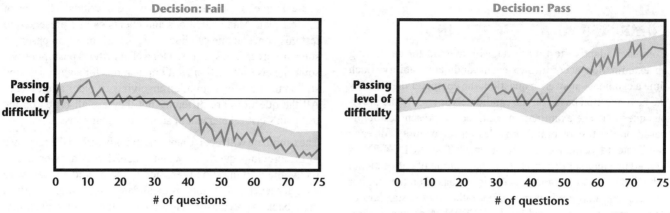

FIGURE 1-1   Plateau to Establish Pass or Fail.

to present questions that are based on the test plan and on the level of ability of the candidate until a level of competency has been established (see Figure 1-1)[3].

TAKING THE NCLEX® EXAMINATION

Application

An application must be submitted to the state board of nursing in the state in which the candidate wants to be licensed. The contact information for the state boards of nursing is available on the National Council website. After the candidate's application and registration fees have been received and approved by the state, the candidate will receive an authorization to test (ATT) from the NCSBN. After the examination fee has been paid, it will not be refunded, regardless of how the candidate registered.[3] The candidate may register for the NCLEX at the NCLEX Candidate website or by regular mail or by telephone. All the contact information is listed in the ATT. The Candidate Bulletin (CB) is available on the National Council website—be sure to print this bulletin for future reference. The CB provides critical information, including addresses and phone numbers for registration and specific details regarding the registration process.

Scheduling the Examination

After a candidate has been declared eligible to take the NCLEX and has received an ATT, the candidate may schedule an examination date. A candidate *must have an ATT* before they can schedule their examination. The CB lists the phone number to call to schedule the examination. Once the ATT has been issued, the state stipulates a period of time within which the candidate must take the examination. This ranges from 60 to 365 days, with the average being 90 days; this period *cannot* be extended. You must test within the validity dates noted on your ATT. The ATT must be presented at the testing site before you can be admitted to take the examination. You are encouraged to call and schedule the appointment to take the examination as soon as possible after receiving the ATT, even if you do not plan to take the test immediately. This will

increase the probability of getting the testing date you want.

Early in the last semester, students should begin planning for when they want to take the examination. Students should plan on taking the examination within 2-6 weeks of graduation. If a review course is considered, then that should be factored into the schedule. The month after graduation is not a good time to plan a vacation or any life-changing events. Complete the NCLEX and then move on with your life. Do not procrastinate about scheduling the examination, the longer after graduation and review course that the examination is taken, the colder the knowledge. Take the examination when the nursing content is most current in your mind and you are still in the testing mode from school.[3]

Pearson Vue is the company that provides the testing facility and computers for the examination. A tutorial on how to use the computer on NCLEX is available at *www.vue.com/nclex/*. Go to the site and review the tutorial. It should be very familiar to you when you see it on NCLEX; this same tutorial will be presented to you at the beginning of your examination.

Testing Center Identification

Photo identification with a signature and the ATT will be required at the testing site. The name printed on the ATT must match the identification presented at the course site. Identification must be in English and cannot be expired. Acceptable forms of identification are a U.S. driver's license, a passport, or a U.S. state-issued identification, or a U.S. military issued identification. At the testing site before testing, each candidate will be digitally fingerprinted, a photo will be taken, and a signature will be required.

Day of the Examination

You should plan on arriving at the center about 30 minutes before scheduled testing time. If you arrive more than 30 minutes late, the scheduled testing time will be canceled and you will have to reapply and repay the examination fee. An erasable note board will be available at your computer terminal. You will not be allowed to take any type of books, personal belongings, hats, coats, blank tablets, or scratch paper into the testing area. A fingerprint scan will be required to reenter the testing area after each break.

Testing

You will have a maximum of 5 hours to complete the examination. After 2 hours of testing, you have an optional 10-minute break; another optional break occurs after $3^1/_2$ hours of testing. If you need a break before that time, notify one of the attendants at the testing center. The computer will automatically signal when a scheduled break begins. All of the break times and the tutorial are considered part of the total 5 hours of testing time.

The examination will stop when one of the following occurs:

1. 85 questions have been answered, and a minimum level of competency has been established; or a lack of minimum competency has been established (see Figure 1-1).

2. The candidate has answered the maximum number of 205 questions.

3. The candidate has been testing for 5 hours, regardless of the number of questions answered.

Each candidate will receive between 85-205 questions. The number of questions on the NCLEX is not indicative of the level of competency. The majority of candidates who complete all 205 questions will have demonstrated a level of minimum competency and therefore pass the NCLEX. A mouse will be used for selecting answers, so candidates should not worry about different computer keyboard function keys. An onscreen calculator will also be available to use for math problems. If any problems occur with the environment or with the equipment, someone will be available to provide assistance.

In each candidate's examination, there will be 25 pretest or unscored items or questions. The statistics on these items will be evaluated in order to determine whether the item is a valid test item to be included in future NCLEX test banks. All of the items that are scored, or counted, on a candidate's examination have been pretested and validated. It is impossible to determine which questions or items are scored items and which are pretest items. It is important to treat each question as a scored item.

The CB from the NCSBN is very important; read it carefully and keep it until the results from NCLEX have been received. This bulletin will provide directions and will answer more of your questions regarding the NCLEX. The CB is available online (from the NCSBN at *www.ncsbn.org* or from Pearson Vue at *www.vue.com/nclex*).

Test Results

Each examination is scored twice, once at the testing center and again at the testing service. The test results are electronically transferred to the state boards of nursing. Test results are *not* available at the testing center, from Pearson Vue, or from the NCSBN. Check the information received from the appro-

priate state board of nursing to determine how and when your results will be available. Test results may be available online. In some states, results may be available within 2 to 3 days; in others, the results will be mailed, which will require a longer notification period. Do *not* call the Pearson Professional Center, NCLEX Candidate Services, the National Council, or the individual state board of nursing for test results. Follow the procedure found in the information from the state board of nursing where the license will be issued.[3]

SUCCESSFUL TEST TAKING ON THE NCLEX® EXAM

> ☀ *TESTING ALERT: Practicing test-taking skills is critical if you are going to be able to effectively use them on the NCLEX. Practice test taking should be a component of your NCLEX preparation.*

Being able to effectively apply test-taking strategies on an examination is almost as important as having the basic knowledge required to answer the questions correctly. Everyone has taken an examination only to find, on review of the exam, that questions were missed because of poor test-taking skills. Nursing education provides the graduate with a comprehensive base of knowledge; how effectively the graduate can *demonstrate* the use of this knowledge will be a major factor in the successful completion of the examination.

The NCLEX-PN is designed to evaluate a minimum level of competency. The purpose of the examination is to determine whether a candidate has the knowledge, skills, and ability required for safe and effective entry-level nursing practice as a practical nurse. Throughout the examination, questions are described as being based on clinical situations common in nursing; uncommon situations are not emphasized. NCLEX questions are not fact, recall, or memory-level questions; they are questions that require critical thinking to determine the correct answer. Critical thinking will require an evaluation and interpretation of client data, an understanding of the client's condition or disease, and the ability to determine the best action that will most effectively meet the client's needs.

Practice testing is an excellent method of studying for the NCLEX. After taking a practice test, use the results to determine whether you need additional review in certain areas or whether you are missing questions because of poor test-taking strategies.

NCLEX® TEST-TAKING STRATEGIES

The NCLEX questions are different from those found on nursing school exams. One of the biggest problems candidates encounter is that there appears to be two or more correct answers. Sometimes a candidate believes that more information is necessary to answer the question. However, the answer must be determined from the information provided; no one will clarify or provide additional information regarding a specific question or content. The strategies described in this section are critical in evaluating and successfully answering NCLEX questions.

- **The NCLEX Hospital:** What a great place to work! In the situations or questions presented on NCLEX, all clients are being cared for in an ideal environment—the NCLEX Hospital. *NCLEX questions are based on textbook practices, not necessarily on the real world.* It must be assumed that clients will respond just as the textbooks indicate they will. Candidates who have a lot of clinical experience may experience problems on the test if they answer questions based on the possibility that there may not be adequate staff or equipment or if they believe the option for the nursing care presented is not "realistic." Nursing care provided on the examination is performed in the NCLEX Hospital, where the nurse has adequate staff, supplies, and anything else required to provide the safest care for the client. This approach is necessary because this is a nationally standardized examination.

- **Calling the Doctor (or anyone else):** Be cautious about passing the responsibility for care of the client to someone else. This is an exam on nursing care; evaluate the question carefully and see what nursing action should to be taken before consulting or calling someone else. This includes the RN supervisor, social worker, respiratory therapist, and hospital chaplain, as well as the doctor. After you have carefully evaluated the question, if the client's condition is such that the nurse cannot do anything to resolve the problem, then calling for assistance may be the best answer. Evaluate situations, is there a nursing action to be taken before contacting someone for assistance. A specific item on the test plan states that the nurse will identify client data that must be reported immediately.[2] It is important to identify critical changes in a client's condition, as well as make a nursing judgment when the client's condition requires reporting to the RN or to the physician.

- **Doctor's Orders:** It should be assumed that a doctor's order is available to provide the nursing care in the options presented in the question. If the question asks for administration of a specific medication for the client's problem, then assume that there is an order for it. If the focus of a question is to determine if a nursing action is a dependent or an independent nursing action, then it will be stated in the stem of the question. For example, the question may request an independent nursing action to provide pain relief for a client.

- **Focus on the Client:** Look for answers that focus on the client. Identify the significant or central person in the question. Most often, this is going to be the client. Wrong choices would be those that focus on maintaining hospital rules and policies, dealing with equipment, or solving the nurse's problems. Evaluate the status of the client first, provide for client safety and then deal with the equipment problems, or concerns. Other questions may ask the nurse to respond to a client's family or significant others. Determine the person to whom the question is directed.

- **Client's Age:** Consider a client to be an adult unless otherwise stated. If the age of a client is important to the question, it will be stated in years or in months. Descriptions such as "elderly adult" and "geriatric client" are not commonly used. These terms have been established as negative descriptors of older clients. The description of such a client may be "older adult," or a specific age may be given.

- **Laboratory Values:** It is important to know normal values for the common laboratory tests. A question may be based on nursing activities regarding a specific lab value, knowledge of lab values or a diagnostic procedure that would indicate a client's condition is getting better or worse. Be able to identify lab values and/or diagnostic procedures that indicate a client's progress or lack of progress. Determine whether specific nursing actions are required based on the abnormal values or diagnostic results. For example, when a client's blood glucose level is 50 mg/mL and he or she is awake and alert, the client will need something to eat, preferably a complex carbohydrate. If a client has a hemoglobin value of 8.5 g/dL, nursing care will involve avoidance of unnecessary physical activities, and the client will need to be kept warm.

- **Positions:** If a specific position for the client appears in the stem of the question, then consider whether the position is for comfort, for treatment, or to prevent a complication. Evaluate the question: What is to be accomplished by placing the client in the position, and why is the position important for this client? Sometimes a client position will appear in the options. Consider whether positioning is important to the care of the client presented. For example, the semi-Fowler's position is very important to a client who is having difficulty breathing, and the supine position or low Fowler's position may provide the most comfort for a client postoperatively. Determine the purpose of a specific client position and then determine whether this is a priority in planning or intervention. See Appendix 3-1 for a further description of positions.

- **Mathematical Computations:** Mathematical computations may include calculations of medication dosages, conversion of units of measurement, as well as calculation of intake and output. You should be able to apply the appropriate formula to the situation. Some of the questions may call for two computations, as in a question in which all items must be converted to one unit of measurement before a dosage is calculated. There will be an on screen calculator, find the "calculator" button when you do the NCLEX Tutorial. The mathematical calculations may be presented in a multiple-choice format or in an alternate format question in which you are asked to fill in the blank. For fill in the blank questions, calculate your answer and then type the answer number into the box provided. The unit of measurement will be provided in the box.

Management of Client Care

As the role of the licensed practical nurse (LPN) has expanded, management of client care has become increasingly important. A large percentage of graduates surveyed on the last job analysis reported they had "charge nurse" responsibilities. The majority of the management responsibilities were in the long term care facilities.[1] LPN's may direct the care of the nursing assistants as well as other LPN's. However, LPNs are under the supervision of a registered nurse. There is a director of nurses, or an administrator that is an RN and is ultimately responsible for nursing care delivered in that facility. Do not panic: pay close attention to what nursing action the question is focusing on and to whom the nurse is assigning the care or nursing activity – is it to another LPN, or is it to a less qualified person?

- **Keep in mind the NCLEX Hospital.** Adequate staff is available to provide safe client care; don't worry about staff shortages. Focus on the needs of the client in the question – the activities on the rest of the unit are not pertinent to answering the question. The only client to consider in each question is the one involved in that question, not the other clients the practical nurse may have been assigned.

- **Identify the most stable client.** The most stable client is the one who has the *most predictable outcome* and is *least likely* to have abrupt changes in condition that would require critical nursing judgments. When determining the stability of clients, Maslow's hierarchy of needs should be considered (see Chapter 2, Figure 2-1). The most stable client is often the one for which nursing activities can be delegated to a nursing assistant.

- **Assign tasks that have specific guidelines.** Those tasks that have specific guidelines that are unchanging and are used in the care of a stable client can often be assigned to the nursing assistant. Bathing, collecting urine samples, feeding, providing personal hygiene, and assisting with ambulation are just a few examples of these activities.

- **Identify your priority client.** The priority client is the one who is most likely to experience problems or ill effects if they are not taken care of first. Priority clients include those with conditions that are unstable and changing, and those who are at an increased risk for developing complications. NCLEX questions may present a typical nursing care assignment and ask which client the nurse would care for first; or a situation with a client may be presented, and you will be asked to select the first nursing action. Review the testing strategies regarding priority questions. It is important to identify the most unstable client, to see him or her first, and then to determine what is necessary to do first for this client.

- **Carefully read the question** and determine which clients are in a changing unstable situation, these are clients that

may require contacting the RN or the physician. This judgment could be tested in a question where the LPN cannot meet the client needs and needs to obtain further assistance and or direction.

- **Client Care Assignments:** Nursing care assignments should take into consideration the caregiver who is educationally prepared, experienced, and most capable of caring for the client. Unlicensed assistive personnel (UAP), patient care attendants (PCA), and/or nursing assistants must be directly supervised in the provision of safe nursing care. Pay close attention to the person to whom the nurse is assigning the care or nursing activity: Is it to another LPN, or is a specific activity (bathing, ambulating, etc.) being delegated to an unlicensed nursing assistant?

Establishing Nursing Priorities

Almost all nurses will agree that the NCLEX has a lot of priority questions. These questions may be worded in a variety of ways:

"What is the priority nursing action?"

"What should the nurse do first?"

"What is the initial nursing action?"

In other words, the NCLEX wants to know if the PN can identify the most important nursing action to be taken in order to provide safe care for the client in the situation presented. This may be found in questions where three of four of the options are correct; however, one of the options or actions needs to be performed before the others. This is where critical thinking is necessary—*think like a nurse!* There are three areas to consider when determining priority nursing actions: Maslow's hierarchy of needs, the nursing process, and client safety.

- **Maslow's Hierarchy of Needs:** And you thought this was just for fundamentals! *Always consider Maslow's hierarchy of needs and remember that physiological needs must come first.* (Figure 3-1) When evaluating options, identify client needs that are physiological and those that are psychosocial. Physiological needs are a higher priority than psychosocial needs. A client's physical needs must be met before considering his or her psychosocial needs. Also remember that the ABCs (airway, breathing, and circulation) are the critical physiological needs because these are at the base of Maslow's pyramid. However, be cautious— don't always select "airway" as the best answer. Sometimes the client does not have an airway problem, so don't read that into the question and give the client an airway problem! If a client is in pain, it is difficult to determine what is contributing to his/her psychosocial problem. Maslow's hierarchy of needs also applies to the client with psychosocial problems – take care of the physiological needs, then focus on the psychosocial needs. (see the section in this chapter regarding answering psychosocial questions).

- **Nursing Process:** The first step in the nursing process for the practical nurse is data collection. When evaluating a question, it is important to determine if the question provides adequate data for the nurse to make a decision regarding nursing interventions. Obtaining more information (data collection) may be the first nursing action. However, do not automatically select an option that involves data collection. If client data are provided in the stem of the question, then it will be important to consider Maslow's hierarchy of needs when planning or selecting the best nursing action or implementation. If a nursing action has been implemented, then the question may focus on evaluating the effectiveness of the nursing action. Read the question carefully and determine what is being asked. (Box 1-1).

- Safety Issues: This may include situations in the hospital, in a long term care facility, or in the client's home environment. The first issue to consider is meeting basic needs of survival: oxygen, nutrition, elimination. Reduction of environmental hazards is also a concern and may include prevention of falls, accidents, and medication errors. Environmental safety also includes the prevention and spread of disease. This may include how to avoid contagious diseases or even activities such as hand hygiene. When you are critically evaluating questions that involve a client's safety and multiple options appear to be correct, determine what activity will be of most benefit to the client.

Example Questions for Management and Priority Setting

The LPN is making assignments on a nursing care unit. What tasks could be assigned to the experienced nursing assistant?

1   Evaluate the skin in the sacral area for a client on bed rest.
2   Report on the quantity and characteristics of a client's urine output.
3   Assist a client to obtain a clean-catch urine specimen
4   Evaluate the tolerance of client on tube feedings.

Answer: Option 3
The nursing assistant can be assigned activities that involve standard, unchanging procedures such as helping to obtain a clean-catch urine specimen from a client. The LPN should evaluate the skin on the sacral area for any evidence of a break in skin integrity. The characteristics of the urine should be evaluated by the LPN, however the nursing assistant can empty and measure the amount of urinary output. Dietary intake for client's who do not have a problem with nutrition can be reported by the nursing assistant, however the LPN needs to determine the tolerance of the tube feedings.

The LPN is in charge of the nursing unit on the afternoon shift in an ambulatory care center. After receiving a hand off report on the clients, who would the nurse evaluate first?

1   A client who had a laparoscopic cholecystectomy, has been in the unit for 4 hours, and is complaining of left shoulder pain.
2   A client who had a prostate biopsy about 6 hours ago and is beginning to complain of perineal discomfort, chills, and feeling flushed.
3   A young adult who complains of being nauseated and refuses to take his first dose of the oral postoperative antibiotic.
4   An older adult who experienced gastric distention and required placement of a nasogastric tube.

Answer: Option 2
The client who is post-biopsy of the prostate should be evaluated first, because he could be developing a sepsis secondary to the biopsy. The client who is postcholecystectomy is experiencing referred shoulder pain, which is common after this procedure. The young adult client and the older adult client can be evaluated after the cholecystectomy client.

The practical nurse is working on a step down nursing telemetry unit. A client tells the nurse he is beginning to have midsternum chest pain. What is the first nursing action?

1   Begin oxygen at 4L/min per nasal cannula.
2   Request the charge nurse evaluate the cardiac rhythm.
3   Auscultate breath sounds and maintain airway.
4   Determine client activities prior to onset of chest pain.

Answer: Option 1
When a client complains of chest pain, oxygen should be started immediately, and then the status of the vital signs should be determined. The client is on a telemetry unit and is experiencing chest pain – this is enough information for a nursing action. Data collection will determine the status of the vital signs and further action can be evaluated. If the vital signs are unstable or if the client is experiencing an untoward dysrhythmia, then oxygen administration would still be the most important first nursing action. Activity prior to the chest pain can be evaluated after the current physical status is determined. Option 3 assumes the client has airway problems, there is no indication in the question stem that airway is a problem.

The LPN received a shift handoff report for a group of assigned clients. Which client should the practical nurse see first?

1   A client who underwent a thoracotomy 3 days ago, his vital signs are stable and he is complaining of chest pain when he coughs.
2   An 85-year-old client who has a fractured hip, she is in Buck's traction and is complaining of pain; she is scheduled for surgery in 4 hours.
3   An adult male client admitted 3 hours ago for dehydration; the vital signs are temperature 99° F, pulse 100 beats/min and irregular, and BP 118/80 mm Hg.

4   A cardiac client whose was admitted 24 hours ago who is beginning to complain of increased chest pain.

Answer: Option 4
The client with cardiac disease is the most unstable and is beginning to exhibit symptoms that could be warning signs of cardiac ischemia. This client needs to be assessed immediately, and the nurse should anticipate administration of sublingual nitroglycerin. After assessment of vital signs, this client's change in condition may need to be reported to the charge nurse and or to the doctor. The client with a thoracotomy may be developing pneumonia secondary to surgery and immobility, but the situation does not require immediate attention. The client with a fractured hip is also not in an unstable situation, even though she is uncomfortable. The client with dehydration is exhibiting symptoms related his dehydration but is not unstable at this time.

A client has returned from abdominal surgery and the nurse is assessing the incisional site. The dressing has some bright red blood on it, and on closer observation the nurse determines a small area of evisceration. What is the best nursing action?

1   Remove the dressing and place a sterile saline soaked dressing on the wound and reinforcement dressing on top.
2   Remove the dressing and with sterile gloves apply very gently pressure to replace exposed bowel.
3   Leave the dressing in place and apply an abdominal pressure dressing to prevent further exposure of the bowel.
4   Remove all of the stained dressing, cleanse the wound area using sterile antiseptic solution and replace the dressing.

Answer: Option 1
The best nursing action is to cover the exposed bowel with sterile saline soaked dressing to prevent drying and tissue damage to the exposed bowel and then the physician should be notified. Option 2 should not be performed, there may be vascular impairment to the bowel below the surface. In option 3 the dressing needs to be replaced with a moist dressing to protect the bowel. In option 4, the wound should not be cleansed as it is not a dirty wound.

Strategies for Evaluating Multiple-Choice Questions

Test-taking strategies are very beneficial during nursing school, as well as on the NCLEX. Start using them on current exams. Implementing testing strategies now will help to increase test scores in school, in addition to being one more step toward success on the NCLEX.

Question Characteristics

The majority of questions on the NCLEX, as well as on nursing school exams, are in a multiple-choice format. This is the type of test question that is the most familiar to candidates.

Stem of the Question

The *stem* presents information or describes a client situation. The part of the stem that asks the question will present a problem or situation. The question may be presented as complete or an incomplete sentence. One of the options presented will most correctly answer the question or complete the sentence. (Figure 1-2)

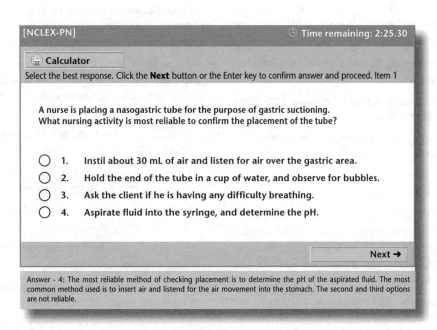

Figure 1-2   Multiple-choice question.

Options

There are four options from which to choose an answer.

- Three options are distracters; they are designed to create a distraction from the correct answer.

- One option correctly answers the question asked in the stem.

- There is only one correct response; no partial credit is given for another answer.

Specific Strategies and Examples of Multiple-Choice Questions

1. **Read the question carefully before ever looking at or considering the options.** If you glance through the options before understanding the question, you may pick up key words that will affect the way you perceive the question. Make sure you understand the question and do not formulate an opinion about the answer before you have read and understand the question. On a paper-and-pencil test, cover the answers with your hand or a note card. If you practice this strategy before taking the NCLEX, you will be able to focus on the question without physically covering the answers when taking a test on the computer.

2. **Do not read extra meaning into the question.** The question is asking for specific information; if it appears to be simple "common sense," then assume it is simple. Do not look for a hidden meaning in a question. Avoid asking yourself "what if . . . ?" or the client might..." Don't make the client any sicker then he or she already is!

Example: A bronchoscopy was performed on a client at 7:00 am. The client returns to his room, and the nurse plans to assist him with his morning care. The client refuses the morning care. What is the best nursing action regarding the morning care for this client?

1. Perform all of his morning care to prevent him from becoming short of breath.

2. Avoid morning care and continue to monitor vital signs and assess swallowing reflexes.

3. Postpone the morning care until client is more comfortable and can participate.

4. Cancel all of the morning care because it is not necessary to perform it after a bronchoscopy.

The correct answer is #3. The question is asking for a nursing judgment regarding morning care. Do not read into the question and make it more difficult by trying to put in information relating to respiratory care, such as checking for gag and swallowing reflexes.

3. **Read the stem correctly.** Make sure you understand exactly what information the question is asking. Determine whether the question is stated in a positive (true) or negative (false) format.

Watch for words that provide direction to the question. A positive or true stem may include the following: "indicates the client understands," "the best nursing action is," "the preoperative teaching would include," or "the best nursing assignment is." Also watch for words in the stem that have a negative meaning so that the question is asking for a response that is not accurate or is false. Phrases such as "is contraindicated," "the client should avoid," "indicate the client does not understand," "does not occur," and "indicates [medication, equipment, nursing action] is not working" are negative indicators. The question is asking for information that is not accurate or actions the nurse would not take. The following words or phrases change the direction of the question: except, never, avoid, least, contraindicated, would not occur. It may help to rephrase the question in your own words to better understand what information is being requested.

Example: The nurse is discussing body mechanics with a client who has had back surgery. What nursing observations would indicate the client *did not understand* the principles discussed? The client:

1. Bends at the knees to pick up an object from the floor.

2. Carries the object close to his body.

3. Places his feet apart when bending to pick up an object.

4. Bends from the waist to pick up an object on the floor.

The correct answer is #4 Rephrase the question: I need to identify what the client is doing wrong regarding body mechanics. Bending from the waist does not represent good body mechanics; the client should bend with the knees (squatting), not from the waist. All other options represent good body mechanics.

4. Pay attention to **where the client is in their disease process or condition.** Examples of this are terms such as "immediately postoperatively," "the first postoperative day," and "experienced a myocardial infarction this morning."

Example: A client had a cardiac catheterization through the left femoral artery. During the first few hours after the cardiac catheterization procedure, which nursing action would be most important?

Rewording: What is the **most important** nursing care in the **first few hours** after a cardiac catheterization?

1. Check his temperature every 2 hours and monitor catheter insertion site for inflammation.

2. Elevate the head of his bed 90 degrees and keep affected extremity straight.

3. Evaluate his blood pressure and respiratory status every 15 minutes for 4-6 hours.

4. Check his pedal and femoral pulses every 15 minutes for first hour, and then every 30 minutes.

The correct answer is #4. The phrase, "during the first few hours after the procedure," is important in answering this question correctly. The danger of hemorrhage and hematoma at the puncture site is greatest during this time. The question also asks for the most important nursing care. Option 3, it is important to evaluate vital signs, but does not require them to be done every 15 minute for 4-6 hours if client is stable. Option 4 is critical in the first few hours following a cardiac catheterization.

5. **Before considering the options, think about the characteristics of the condition and critical nursing concepts.** What are the nursing priorities in caring for a client with this condition/procedure/medication/problem?

Example: A woman who is 3 days postpartum returns to the clinic with complaints of soreness and fullness in her breasts and states that she wants to stop breast-feeding her infant until her breasts feel better. What is the best nursing response?

This is a positive question. The answer will be a true statement. Think about breast-feeding and the common discomforts and problems the client encounters. Don't look at the options yet. Think, "Is it normal to have fullness and soreness in the breasts during the first 3 days of lactation, and what happens if she stops breast-feeding the infant?" Now evaluate the options:

1. Show the client how to apply a breast binder to decrease the discomfort and the production of milk.

2. Tell the client that breast fullness may be a sign of infection and she will not be able to continue breast-feeding.

3. Suggest to the client that she decrease her fluid intake for the next 24 hours to temporarily suppress lactation.

4. Explain to the client that the breast discomfort is normal and that the infant's sucking will promote the flow of milk.

In this question, option #4 is correct. Initially, breast soreness may occur for about 2 to 3 minutes at the beginning of each feeding until the let-down reflex is established. Options 1, 2, and 3 would decrease her milk production; the question did not state that she wanted to quit breast-feeding permanently.

6. **Identify the step in the nursing process being tested.** Remember, you must have adequate client data before you move through the steps of the nursing process. Is there adequate information presented in the stem of the question to determine appropriate nursing planning or intervention? Is the correct nursing action to obtain further assessment data? Look for key words that can assist you in determining what type of information is being requested.

Example: An 85-year-old client is a resident in a long-term care facility. The nurse assigned to the client for morning care observes numerous bruises and abrasions in various stages of healing on the client's back and torso. The nurse from the previous shift explains that the client fell down.

What is the best nursing action?

1. Review the chart for details regarding the client's fall.

2. Cover the abrasions with a protective dressing. .

3. Notify the supervisor regarding the possibility of an abusive situation.

4. Further evaluate the client to determine presence of other injuries.

The correct answer is #4, to determine or assess the extent of injuries. The stem of the question did not present adequate information with which to make a nursing judgment, and the client's physiological needs are the priority. Option 1 does not immediately alleviate any client problem or provide any assistance to the client. Options 2 and 3 relate to nursing actions that may be done after the immediate injuries and needs have been assessed. Focus on the client; priority setting and physiological needs must be addressed first.

7. **Confused at this point? What if, after reading the question, you do not know what the question is even asking?** Take a deep breath, reread the question, and ask yourself, "What is the main topic of the question?" Now read the option choices, not to eliminate options or select a correct answer, but to get a clue as to the direction of the question. It might be helpful to read the options from the bottom up (start with option 4, rather than option 1) to help your brain focus on the options.

Example: The nurse is caring for a client who is scheduled for a thoracotomy at noon. The nurse is evaluating the client at 10am. Which client finding would be most important for the practical nurse to report to the nursing supervisor?

Is the question asking for problems regarding the surgical preparation, or the current status of the client's conditions, or maybe even preoperative teaching? Check out the options.

1. Vital signs are: pulse rate 100 beats/min, respirations 20 breaths/minute, oral temperature 99° F.

2. Surgical consent form is not signed and on the chart.

3. The client states that he is anxious about the surgery.

4. Lab reports indicate the hemoglobin level is 12.5g/dl and the hematocrit level is 36%.

After checking the options, it appears the question is asking for the preoperative or surgical preparation of the client. Now that you have determined what you need to identify, you can begin the process of elimination of the options until you have found the correct answer. *The correct option is #2.* The surgical consent should be on the chart and the client should not be given any preoperative narcotics before the consent form is signed. This needs to be taken care of immediately. The vital signs are within acceptable limits (option 1), anxiety is normal before surgery (option 3), and the hemoglobin and hematocrit levels are within normal limits (option 4). This is a preoperative question that could be asked in any surgical client situation.

8. **Don't focus on predicting a right answer!** Frequently, the answer you anticipate is not going to be an option! Keep in mind the characteristics and concepts of nursing care for a client with the condition or problem in the situation presented. Eliminate options: every time you eliminate an option, you increase your chance of selecting a correct answer. If all of the options are plausible, then rank the options. The first one is the highest priority, and the fourth one is the lowest priority. Which one is the first action or answers the question?

Example: A client has an ulcer (2 in × 2 in) on the calf of his right leg. The area around the ulcer is inflamed, and the ulcer is draining purulent fluid. The vital signs are pulse, 114 beats/min; respiration, 22 breaths/min; temperature, 101° F. Which order will the nurse implement first?

Reword the question: The client has an infection in the ulcer on his leg. His temperature is elevated, and so is his pulse; this is a normal response to infection. Of the orders listed here, what nursing action will I need to do first?

1. Penicillin V potassium (**Pen Vee K**) 500mg, PO, every 6   hours.

2. Blood cultures × 2, 20 minutes apart and drawn from different venipuncture sites.

3. Polysporin (**Bacitracin**) ointment topically to leg ulcer three times a day.

4. Acetaminophen (**Tylenol**), 650mg suppository, every 4 hours for temperature above 101.8° F.

Rank the options:

1st—Option 2; blood cultures must be obtained prior to antibiotic.

2nd—Option 1 needs to done after the blood cultures have been drawn.

3rd—Option 4 will not produce any immediate response or assistance in treating the problem, although it will make the client more comfortable.

4th—Option 3 will help to reduce the infection, but the priority is to obtain the culture and then for the antibiotic to be started.

Here is another approach to the options:

Consider option 1—This is an antibiotic that will begin to fight the infection.

Consider option 2—This is important to do to identify the causative bacteria. This is more important now than option 1; eliminate option 1.

Consider option 3—This is treating the infection topically. It will cause a decrease in the surface bacteria, but the blood cultures are still a priority. Eliminate this option because both options 1 and 2 are more important.

Consider option 4—This is treating the symptoms rather than the cause of the problem, which is not as important as option 1 or option 2; eliminate it.

All of these options are feasible for treating this client; however, obtaining the blood culture is the most important (*option 2*). If you had approached this question with a specific answer in mind (give an antibiotic), you would have found that answer; however, it would have been wrong.

9. **Evaluate all of the options in a systematic manner.** After you understand the question, read all options carefully. Remember, distracters are designed to be plausible to the situation and thus to "distract" you from the correct answer. All the options may be correct, but only one will be the best answer.

Example: A client has just returned to his room from the recovery room after a lumbar laminectomy with a spinal fusion. The client's vital signs are stable. In considering possible complications the client might experience in the next few hours, what nursing action is most important?

1. Monitor vital signs every 4 hours.

2. Assess breath sounds every 2 hours.

3. Evaluate every 2 hours for urinary retention.

4. Check when he last had a bowel movement.

All of these options are plausible for the situation. However, consider that this is the client's operative day, he is currently stable, and the question is asking for complications he might encounter in the next few hours after lumbar laminectomy. Options 1 and 4 are not appropriate at this period of postoperative recovery; vital signs should be checked more often, and constipation can be more effectively addressed at a later time—eliminate these from consideration. Option 2 would be appropriate if respiratory problems were anticipated; however, there is no indication of respiratory compromise. (Remember, don't always select airway-related answers.) *The correct answer is #3*, because urinary retention is a common problem related to restrictions on mobility, pain medication as well as anesthesia in the immediate postoperative period after a lumbar laminectomy.

10. **As you read the options, eliminate those that you know are not correct.** Consider each option as true or false. This will help narrow the field of choice. When you select an answer or eliminate an option, you should have a specific reason for doing so. Correctly eliminating options will increase your chances of selecting the correct answer.

Example: The nurse is performing a urinary catheterization on a female client. When cleansing the labia, the nurse should:

1. Cleanse the inner labia and then cleans the outer labia.

2. Cleanse the perineum from back to front with a cotton ball.

3. Use each cotton ball only one time.

4. Inspect the vaginal opening for blood.

Systematically evaluate the options:

Option 1 – no, the outer labia should be cleansed before the inner labia.

Option 2 – no, cleansing should be performed from front to back.

Option 3 – yes, each cotton ball should only be used one time, and then discarded.

Option 4 – no, it does not affect the procedure even if the client is menstruating.

After a systematic evaluation of the options, *option #3* is the correct answer. Always evaluate every option; do not stop with what you think is the first correct answer.

11. **Identify similarities in the options.** Frequently, the options will contain similar information, and sometimes you can eliminate similar options. If three options are similar, the different one may be the correct answer. When two of the options are very similar and one of those options is not any better than the other, both of them are probably wrong, so start looking for another answer. Sometimes three of the options have very similar characteristics; the option that is different may be the correct answer.

Example: The nurse is assisting a client to identify foods that would meet the requirements for a high-protein, low-residue diet. Which foods would represent correct choices for this diet?

1. Roast beef, slice of white bread.
2. Fried chicken, green peas.
3. Broiled fish, green beans.
4. Cottage cheese, tomatoes.

Options 1, 2, and 3 all contain a meat or fish that would be needed for a high-protein diet; therefore option 4 can be eliminated. Options 2, 3, and 4 all contain a vegetable that has a skin, making these high-residue choices. The *correct answer is option #1*, for both high-protein and low-residue qualities. Note that the NCLEX will not focus on dishes that contain a mixture of foods in which you would need to know the recipe to answer correctly. Also, unless specified, do not attribute special characteristics to a food; if a food has a special characteristic, it will be stated (e.g., "low sodium" soup or "low fat" yogurt).

12. Identify words in the options that are "qualifiers." Every, none, all, always, never, and only are examples of words that have no exceptions. Options containing these words are frequently incorrect. Seldom in health care is anything absolute with no exceptions; thus you can often eliminate these options. In some situations the qualifiers can be correct, especially when a principle or policy is described. For example, the nurse always establishes positive client identification before administering medications. This would be a correct statement. Carefully evaluate qualifiers; they are clues to the correct answer.

Example: The nurse is obtaining a specimen from a client's

incisional area for a wound culture and sensitivity. What client information will the sensitivity part of the procedure reflect?

1. Presence and characteristics of all bacteria present in the client's wound
2. Which antibiotics will effectively treat the bacteria present
3. Differentiation of the bacteria and viruses present in the wound
4. All the treatments to which the bacteria are responsive

Options 1 and 4 contain the word "all." If you did not know the answer, you could eliminate options 1 and 4. Identifying all the bacteria and all the treatments is not feasible from a culture and sensitivity. This would give you a 50% chance of finding *the right answer, which is option #2.*

13. Select the most comprehensive answer. All of the options may be correct, but one option may include the other three options or need to be considered first.

Example: The nurse is planning to teach a client with diabetes about his condition. Before the nurse provides instruction, what is most important to evaluate? The client's:

1. Required dietary modifications.
2. Understanding of the exchange list.
3. Ability to administer insulin.
4. Present understanding of diabetes.

Options 1, 2, and 3 are certainly important considerations in diabetic education. However, they cannot be initiated until the nurse evaluates the client's knowledge of his or her disease state. When two options appear to say the same thing, only in different words, then look for another answer; that is, eliminate the options that you know are incorrect. Options 1 and 2 both refer to the client's understanding of nutrition.

14. **Some questions may have options that contain several items to consider.** After you are sure you understand what information the question is requesting, evaluate each part of the option. Is the option appropriate to what the question is asking? If an option contains one incorrect item, the entire option is incorrect. All of the items must be correct if that option is to be the correct answer to the question.

Example: The practical nurse is preparing a client's 8am medications. The client has the following medications ordered: digoxin (**Lanoxin**) 0.125mg, PO; furosemide (**Lasix**) 20mg, PO, captopril (**Capoten**) 25mg, PO. The client's current vital signs are: blood pressure 110/86, pulse 78, respirations 18, and temperature 99° F orally. What would be the best nursing action?

1. Administer all of the medications, chart them as given, and document the client's apical heart rate.
2. Hold the digoxin and the captopril; recheck the heart rate and blood pressure in 30 minutes.

3. Hold the captopril, administer the other medications and notify the nursing supervisor.

4. Hold the furosemide until the intake and output can be evaluated, administer all other medications.

In the methodical evaluation of the items in the options, you can eliminate items. Option 2: there is no reason to hold the digoxin or the captopril. Option 3, there is not reason to hold the captopril or to notify the nursing supervisor. Option 4, there is no reason to hold the furosemide. Therefore, *option #1 is correct*.

15. **After you have selected an answer, reread the question**. Does the answer you chose give the information the question is asking for? Sometimes the options are correct but do not answer the question.

Example: A client is 88 years old and has previously been alert, oriented, and active. The nursing assistant reports that on awakening this morning, the client was disoriented and confused. What initial action would the nurse take to determine the possible cause of this change in the client's behavior?

1. Review the history for any previous episodes of this type of behavior.

2. Call the health care provider and discuss the changes in the client's behavior.

3. Do a thorough neurological evaluation to evaluate the specific changes in behavior.

4. Evaluate for the presence of a urinary tract infection and for adequate hydration.

Option #4 is the only answer that supplies what the question asked for ("determine the possible cause of this change"). The most common cause of a sudden change in the behavior of a geriatric client is a significant physiological change, often an infection (commonly in the urinary tract), dehydration, or hypoxia. Options 1 and 3 relate more to the gradual behavior changes seen in the progression of dementia and do nothing "to determine the possible cause. . ." Option 2 also does not provide any assistance in determining the cause of the behavior change; further nursing assessment needs to be conducted before calling for assistance.

Alternate Format Questions

In an effort to improve and more effectively assess the entry-level nurse, the NCSBN has introduced "alternate format questions" to the examination. These questions were included on the NCLEX beginning in April 2003. There is no established percentage of alternate format items a candidate will receive. The alternate format questions that have been previously validated are placed in the test item pools and are randomly selected to meet the items on the test plan and the established level of difficulty. The NCSBN has not specified a number of alternate format questions that will be included in a candidate's test bank. A candidate should expect several alternate format questions. It is important to consider that there will be 25 pretest or unscored items in the first 85 questions on every candidate's examination. Within those 25 items, there may be several unscored alternate format items. It is important to answer all the questions to the very best of your ability because you do not know which questions are scored items and which are unscored items.[3,4]

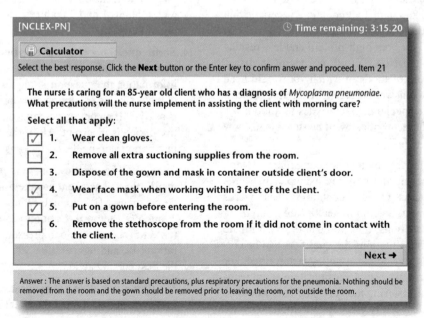

Figure 1-3   Alternate format question—multiple response.

The alternate format questions should not have any impact on what or how you study. The content on the alternate format questions is from the same test plan as the other questions. The test-taking strategies are essentially the same with minor modifications. In other words, there is no reason to be alarmed about the alternate format questions; they are testing the same information, just in a different type of question.

Multiple-Response Items

Multiple-response items require you to select all of the options that apply to the question. The items have more than four options from which to select and will clearly state "Select all that apply." Using the mouse, you will select each item to be included in the answer – consider each item, make a decision if it is to be included in the correct answer or not. You must select all the answers that are correct to the question, if you do not select all of the correct options that apply to the question, the answer will be considered wrong.

Testing Strategy: Think about the question presented in Figure 1-3. Standard plus droplet precautions will be used for this client. What is added to standard precautions when droplet precautions are included? Go through all of the options and decide which options are true and are something the nurse should do; then select all of the true options that apply to this client.

> *Answer: Options 1, 4, and 5. In option 1, yes (true), the nurse is going to provide morning care and have direct contact with the client; therefore gloves should be worn. Option 2, no (false), the suctioning supplies should be left in the room. Option 3, no (false), the gown and mask are disposed of in the client's room. Option 4, yes*

> *(true), a mask is necessary if the nurse is to come within 3 feet of the client, which the nurse can expect to do when providing or assisting with morning care. Option 5, yes, (true), a gown should be worn because the nurse is going to be close to and have direct contact with the client. Option 6, no (false), the stethoscope should not be taken into the client's room; if it is taken into the room, it should be left in the room.*

Fill-in-the-Blank

Fill-in-the-blank questions are frequently presented for medication dosage calculations, or intake and output calculations—just to name a few (Figure 1-4). A drop-down calculator is provided on the computer screen. With calculation questions, the final unit of measurement will always be provided. Only the number will be placed in the answer box. Check the items necessary to make this calculation. For example, is it necessary to make conversions from cups to ounces or to milliliters? Make sure all of the units of measure needed in the final answer are in the same system of measurement.

Memorize the formulas necessary to calculate the drug dosages and conversions. The number of decimal places to be included in the answer will be indicated in the question. Do not round any numbers until you have the final answer. You should not enter any other characters except those necessary to form a number.[3] To calculate the correct answer on the question in Figure 1-5: ½ cup broth is 120mL, 1 cup gelatin is 240mL, 200mL of water and 950mL of IV fluid for a total intake of 1510mL.

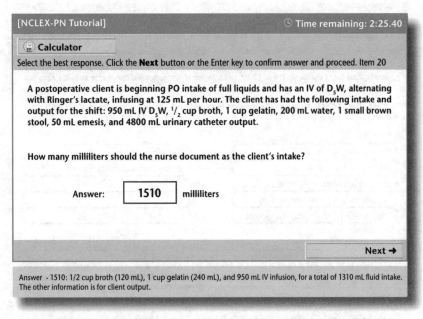

Figure 1-4   Alternate format question—fill-in-the-blank.

Hot Spot Questions

In a hot spot question, you will be presented with a graphic and asked to identify a specific item, area, or location on the graphic. Look at Figure 1-5. Identify the area on the graphic and then you would click on it with the mouse.

Answer: The "hot spot" (in this case, the correct area to assess the apical heart rate) is at the PMI, or point of maximum impulse, which is located at the fifth intercostal space, just to the left of the sternal border. In this situation, you would place the mouse over the area and click on that area.

Drag and Drop

In a drag-and-drop question, several steps or actions are listed, and you will need to place them in a correct sequence (Figure 1-6). All of the options will be used, but you must place them in the correct order. The first thing to do is to decide in what order you want to place the options or rank the actions. After you have determined your answer, click on the option you want to place first, "drag" that option over, and place it in the first box. Then select the option you want to place second, drag that option over, and place it in the next box. Continue this process until you have used all of the options present. Practice by considering how you would answer the question in Figure 1-6.

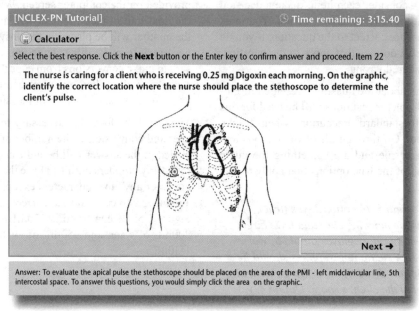

Figure 1-5 Alternate format question—hot spot.

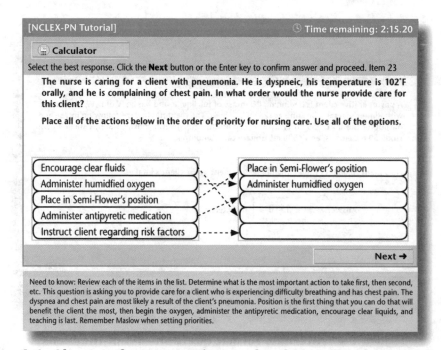

Figure 1-6 Alternate format question—ordered response (drag and drop).

Answer: The client should be placed in a semi-Fowler's position before oxygen administration is started; an antipyretic medication should then be given. This action addresses current needs. Next, encourage intake of clear liquids to decrease viscosity of secretions. Finally, provide instruction regarding risk factors (psychosocial need).

Chart or Exhibit Items

In this type of question, a client situation or problem and client information are provided in a chart or an exhibit (Figures 1-7 through 1-10). First, read the information presented and understand what information the question is asking for. Then click on the tabs within the exhibit to find the information needed to answer the question. There may be several tabs to click on, check the information included within each tab and determine if it is pertinent to the situation.

The question is asking you to identify what would be the best pain medication to administer to this client. On reviewing the information, you will find that all answers are feasible. Check the tabs or exhibit information. Check the nurses notes, the medication administration record (MAR) and the doctor's orders. What you should find within these tabs is that the client received morphine 10 mg IM at 11:00 am; became lethargic and slept for the next 5 hours. He received hydrocodone PO at 4:00 pm and was comfortable for the next 4 hours. The doctor's orders are current for both the IM and the PO medication for pain.

Answer: 4. Give the hydrocodone, PO, for pain at this time. It is preferable to give a client a PO pain medication than a parenteral pain medication. The hydrocodone provided effective pain relief for 4 hours when it was administered the last time, and the doctor's order is current.

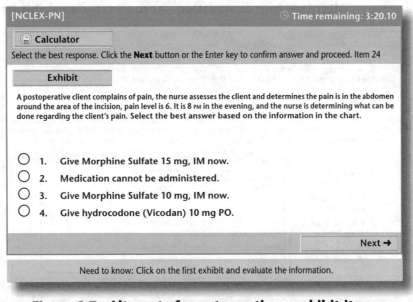

Figure 1-7   Alternate format question—exhibit item.

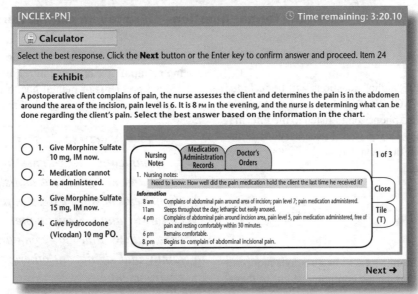

Figure 1-8   Alternate format question—first tab on exhibit item.

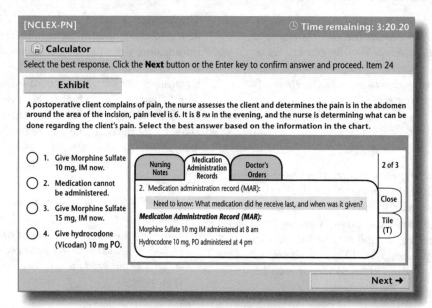

Figure 1-9   Alternate format question—second tab on exhibit item.

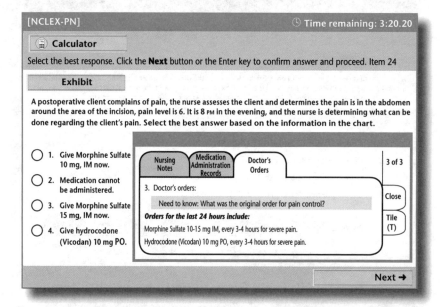

Figure 1-10   Alternate format question—third tab on exhibit item.

Audio Questions

Beginning in April, 2010, "audio" questions will be included in the test banks for the NCLEX-PN. The screen will tell the candidate to place the head phones on to listen to the information. The information may be replayed if necessary. After listening to the information, the candidate will select an answer from the options presented.

Therapeutic Nursing Process: Principles of Communication

Throughout the examination there will be questions requiring use of the principles of therapeutic communication. In thera-peutic communication questions, do not assume the client is being manipulative or is in control of how he or she feels. Psychosocial problems or mental health problems are most often not under the conscious control of the client.

> *TESTING ALERT: Use therapeutic communication techniques to provide support to client and the family; establish a trusting nurse-client relationship; assess psychosocial, spiritual, cultural and occupational factors affecting care; allow time to communicate with client/family and significant others; provide therapeutic environment.*

- **Situations requiring use of therapeutic communication are not always centered around a psychiatric client.** Frequently, these questions are centered on the client experiencing stress and anxiety. There may be questions relating to therapeutic communication in the care of clients experiencing stress, anxiety related to a specific client situation, or a change in body image as a result of physiological problems.

- **Look for responses that focus on the concerns of the client.** Do not focus on the concerns of the nurse, hospital, or physician. Determine whether the client is the central focus of the question or whether the question pertains to a spouse or significant other.

- **Watch for responses that are open-ended and encourage the client to express how he or she feels.** Clients frequently experience difficulty in expressing their feelings. Focus on responses that encourage a client to describe how he or she feels. These are frequently open-ended statements made by the nurse.

- **Eliminate responses that are not honest and direct.** In order to build trust and promote a positive relationship, it is important to be honest with the client. Options that include telling the client "don't worry," or "everything is going to be all right," or "your doctor knows best" will most likely be wrong answers.

- **Look for responses that indicate an acceptance of the client.** Regardless of whether you agree with the client's views or moral values, it is important to respect his or her views and beliefs. Carefully evaluate responses that involve telling clients what they *should* or *should not* be doing, these are often wrong answers (e.g., telling an alcoholic that she should quit drinking or telling a depressed client that he should not feel that way).

- **Be careful about responses that give opinions or advice on the client's situation.** Do not assume an authoritarian position. You should not insist that the client follow your advice (e.g., quit drinking, exercise more, quit smoking).

- **Look for responses that reflect, restate, or paraphrase feelings the client expressed. Do not tell the client how he or she should or should not feel.** Look for responses that encourage the client to describe how he or she feels—responses that reflect, restate, or paraphrase feelings the client expresses. An option such as "You should not feel that way" would be a wrong answer; it would be better to ask "How did that make you feel?"

- **Do not ask "why" a client feels the way he or she does.** If a client understood why he or she felt a certain way, the client would most likely be able to do something about it. The most common answer when a nurse asks a client why he or she feels a certain way is "I don't know," which does provide any information.

- **Do not use coercion to achieve a desired response.** Do not tell clients that they can't have their lunch until they get out of bed or bribe children to take their medicine with a promise of candy.

- **See examples of therapeutic and nontherapeutic communication in Chapter 6 (Table 6-1).**

TIPS FOR TEST-TAKING SUCCESS

- **Do not indiscriminately change answers.** On a paper-and-pencil test, if you go back and change an answer, you should have a specific reason for doing so. Sometimes you do remember information and realize you answered the question incorrectly. However, students often "talk themselves out" of the correct answer and change it to the incorrect one. The good news - you cannot go back to previously answered questions on the NCLEX. Before leaving the question, review the strategies you used to answer the question. When you press the enter bar, or select Next, another question will be presented and you cannot go back to the previous question.

- **Watch your timing. Do not spend too much time on one question.** It is very important to evaluate your timing on practice exams. This will help you be more comfortable with timing on computer testing. The NCLEX will allow you a total of 5 hours to complete the examination. When you are taking a practice test, plan to spend about a minute on each question. Some questions you will answer quickly; others may take some time. Do not spend more than 2 minutes deliberating the answer to a question. If you do not have a good direction for the right answer in 2 minutes, then you probably don't know the answer. Eliminate all of the options you can, pick the best one, and move on. (Remember, you are not supposed to know *all* of the right answers.)

- **The NCLEX is a nursing competency examination, and the correct answer will focus on nursing knowledge and the provision of nursing care.** Medical management or identifying a diagnosis based on symptoms are not the focus of the examination.

- **Eliminate distracters that assume the client "would not understand" or would be ignorant of the situation and those distracters that indicate the nurse needs to protect clients from worry.** For example, "The client should not be told she has cancer because it would upset her too much" would most likely be an incorrect answer.

- **There is no pattern of correct answers.** The exam is compiled by a computer, and the position of the correct answers is selected at random. There is no validity in the rumor to select option 3 when you are guessing.

STUDY HABITS

Study Effectively

1. **Use memory aids, mindmapping, and mnemonics.** Memory aids and mind mapping are tools that assist you in drawing associations from other ideas with the use of visual images (Figure 1-11). Mnemonics are words, phrases, or other techniques that help you remember information. Images, pictures, and mnemonics will stay with you longer than written text information.

2. **Develop 3 × 5 cards with critical information.** Do not overload the card; put a statement or question on one side and answers or follow-up information on the other side. For example, on one side you might write "low potassium," and on the other side you would list the relevant values. Another card might say "nursing care for hypokalemia" on the front, and on the back, you could list the nursing care. These cards are much easier for you to carry than a load of books or class notes. When you have developed and studied your set of cards with priority information, trade them with friends, and see what they have put on their cards. Sets of cards can be used whenever you have only 15 to 20 minutes of study time. Take 20 cards with you to soccer practice, the doctor's office, or anywhere you are going where you will to have to sit and wait for a few minutes. This is quick, easy, and a very effective way to study.

3. **Review class notes the next day.** A very effective study habit to develop during school is to review your class notes the day after the class. Set aside about an hour on the day after the class and spend about 30 to 45 minutes reviewing the notes from class. Do the notes make sense to you, or are you unclear on the meaning of some of the areas? Correlate the notes and the visuals the instructor presented with the information in the textbook. It is important to take the time now to understand the information presented the previous day because it is fresher in your mind and you are more receptive to learning.

4. **Plan your study time when you are most receptive to learning.** Do not wait until the end of the day when you have finished everything else. It is difficult to get up at 6:00 am, work all day, deal with family activities, and finally decide at 10:30pm that you are just too tired to study. You may feel guilty that you were not able to study for the intended 2 hours that evening. Schedule your study time – it may be easier for you to study for 2 hours prior to leaving school than it will be to study for 2 hours when you get home.

5. **Set a schedule and let everyone know the schedule.** For example, when you set aside 1 hour for review on the day after your class, make sure everyone knows this is your study time. Do not expect your family to leave you alone while you study; this is frequently too much to ask, especially of children or a spouse. Go to the library, nursing school, or someone's house where there are no disturbances.

PERITONITIS "HOT BELLY"

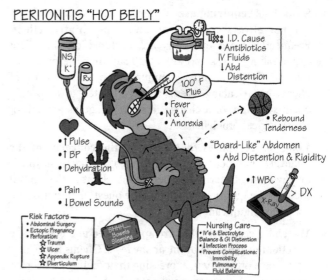

FIGURE 1-11 Peritonitis: "Hot Belly." (From Zerwekh J, Claborn J, Miller CJ: *Memory notebook of nursing, vol 1,* ed 4, Ingram, 2008, Nursing Education Consultants.)

6. **Start planning your NCLEX preparation at the beginning of your last semester in school or 2 to 3 months before you will take the NCLEX.** Do not wait until the week before the exam to start preparing. Even if you were an A student, you still need to review. Information that was presented at the beginning of school, last year, or even last semester may not be current in your knowledge base.

Set a Study Goal

1. Decide on a study method.

2. Divide the review material into segments.

3. Prioritize the segments; review first the areas in which you feel you are deficient or weak. Leave those areas you are the most comfortable with and most knowledgeable about for last.

4. Practice testing, or an end of the semester assessment exam will assist you to identify areas in which you need additional review.

5. Establish a realistic schedule and follow it. Planning for 8 hours of studying on your day off does not work. Instead, plan for 2 to 4 hours each day (in 20- to 30-minute chunks of time) and maybe 3 to 4 hours on your days off. Let everyone know when you are planning on studying and how important it is for you to study.

6. Plan on achieving your study goal several days before the examination.

Group Study

1. Limit the group to four or five people.

2. Group members should be mature and serious about studying.

3. The group should agree on the planned study schedule.

4. If the group makes you anxious or you do not feel it meets your study needs, do not continue to participate.

5. Group study is very effective with the right mix of participants.

Testing Practice

1. Include testing practice in your schedule.

2. Structure your practice testing.

   - Select a group of questions, plan for about 1 minute per question for practicing testing. After answering the questions, review the correct answers and focus on what and why you missed questions. Set aside 10 questions and answer them in 10 minutes; then review the answer and rationale for the questions. This will allow you to focus on testing strategies and not break your train of thought by checking the right answers.

   - Evaluate your comfortable pace for answering questions; this will keep you on target with your timing as you practice answering test questions. Initially, it may take you longer to answer questions when you have to think about testing strategies. Practicing testing strategies will help you improve your testing time.

   - Do not answer a question and then stop to look up the correct answer. Answer all of the questions in the section you have set aside; then review the correct answers. This will reinforce your test-taking strategies and your test timing.

3. Try to answer the questions as if you were taking the real exam.

4. Use the testing strategies and practice on the questions included at the end of each chapter in the book and with the online questions.

5. Evaluate your practice exams for problem areas.

   - Test-taking skills: Did you know the material but answer the question incorrectly? In this case, a test-taking strategy can be applied; go back and review the strategies. Can you identify what strategy you should have used to identify the correct answer? By becoming aware of your test-taking habits, you will become more aware of the strategies you need to implement and you can begin to practice them more effectively.

   - Knowledge base: You did not know the material. Make a note of these areas and see whether the content begins to show trends or clusters of information in areas you need to study/review. Refer to an NCLEX Review book for further information, if you still do not understand the concept or information, go to your nursing textbooks.

6. Evaluate the questions you answered incorrectly. Review the rationale for the right answer and understand why you missed it.

7. Reuse the questions at a later point to review the information again.

8. A test bank of questions is available online, check your book for the code to access these questions. The more questions you practice answering, the more effectively you will be able to implement test-taking strategies.

DECREASE ANXIETY

Your activities on the day of the examination can influence your level of anxiety. By carefully planning ahead, you can eliminate some anxiety-provoking situations.

1. Review the NCLEX tutorial at the Pearson Vue website -www.vue.com/nclex/ or at the National Council website – *www.NCSBN.org*. The same tutorial is on both sites and will be your orientation to the computer and the testing process. It should seem like an old friend when you see it.

2. Visit the examination site before the day of the exam. Consider travel time, parking, and time to get to the designated area. Get an early start to allow extra time; you need to arrive at the site 30 minutes before your scheduled testing time.

3. If you have to travel some distance to the examination site, try to spend the night in the immediate vicinity. Don't cram four or five people in one room. Everyone needs his or her own bed!

4. Do something pleasant the evening before the examination. This is not the time to cram.

5. Anxiety is contagious. If those around you are extremely anxious, avoid contact with them before the examination.

6. Carefully consider whether you want to go to the testing site with anyone else. If your companion finishes before you do, will it put increased pressure on you to hurry up and finish? You don't need any additional pressures on the day of the exam or while you are taking it.

7. Your meal before the test should be a light, healthy one. Do not go into NCLEX on an empty stomach. Avoid eating highly spiced or different foods. This is not the time for a gastrointestinal upset.

8. Wear comfortable clothes. This is not a good time to wear tight clothing or new shoes.

9. Wear clothing of moderate weight. It is difficult to control the temperature to keep everyone comfortable. Wear layers of clothes that can be removed if you get too warm.

10. Wear soft-soled shoes; this decreases the noise in the testing area.

11. Make sure you have the ATT papers and photo ID that are required to gain admission to the examination site.

12. Do not take study material to the examination site. You are not allowed to take it into the testing area, and it is too late to study.

13. Do not panic when you encounter a clinical situation you have not heard of or a situation that increases your anxiety. Take a deep breath, close your eyes, and take a "mini" vacation to one of your very favorite places. Give yourself about 30 to 45 seconds and then return to the question. You may have gained a different perspective. Use good test-taking strategies, select an answer, and move on.

14. Reaffirm to yourself that you know the material. This is not the time for self-defeating behavior or negative self-talk. YOU WILL PASS!! Build your confidence by visualizing yourself in 6 months as an PN working in the area you desire. Create that mental picture of where you want to be and who you want to be—an LPN or LVN. Use your past successes to bring positive energy and "vibes" to your NCLEX exam. WE KNOW YOU CAN DO IT!

REFERENCES

1. Smith J, Crawford L: *Report of findings from the 2006 LPN/VN Practice Analysis Linking the NCLEX PN Examination to Practice, NCSBN research brief,* vol 28, March 2007, Chicago, 2007, National Council of State Boards of Nursing.

2. Wendt A, Kenny L, Stasko, J: *2008 NCLEX PN Detailed Test Plan* (Item writer, item reviewer, nurse educator version), Chicago, 2008, National Council of State Boards of Nursing.

3. *2009 NCLEX Examination Candidate Bulletin.* Chicago, National Council of State Boards of Nursing. Available at: http://www.ncsbn.org. Accessed April, 2009.

4. *Fast facts about alternate item formats and the NCLEX examination.* National Council of State Boards of Nursing, Available at: http://www.ncsbn.org.

Health Implications Across the Life Span

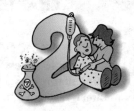

LONG-TERM CARE

✳   **Long-term care includes those services provided in institutional settings, such as a nursing home, rehabilitation center, or adult day care program, after the acute phase of the illness has passed. It often involves restorative care for clients with chronic health care problems.**

A.   Types of long-term care facilities.
1.   Nursing home: Provides services ranging from maintenance to restorative care with skilled nursing and use of certified nursing assistants (CNAs), licensed practical nurses (LPNs), and registered nurses (RNs).
2.   Adult day care home: Client lives at home during the evening and overnight hours and spends the day in a facility that provides a range of care from skilled nursing to restorative care.
3.   Hospice care: Care is provided in both the home and inpatient care settings; funded by Medicare for the terminally ill older adult, with other programs available for other age groups.
a.   Does not institute life support by extraordinary means.
b.   Emphasis on pain control for client and support of family members through the end-of-life process.
4.   Respite care: This is a type of short-term care for the primary caregiver (often a family member) to give caregiver a break from the daily responsibilities of taking care of the long-term client.
5.   Rehabilitation center: This is a facility that provides multiple services for the client and family to make adjustments to daily living.
6.   Home care: Nursing care is provided in the home to clients who do not need hospitalization, but do need additional assistance with medical problems.
7.   Adult housing or assisted living centers: These are places where clients can live independently, but under minimal supervision; meals and other services are offered to the residents.

Rehabilitation

✳   **Rehabilitation is the restoration of an individual to his/her optimal level of functioning. This includes physical, mental, social, vocational, and economic parameters.**
A.   Rehabilitation: term used when an individual has lost functional ability due to illness or injury.
B.   Habilitation: term used to refer to congenital problems or deficiencies.

Goals of Rehabilitation

In order for the rehabilitation client to achieve the highest level of productivity, the rehabilitation process must begin when the condition becomes evident, or when the disease is diagnosed.
1.   Prevent deformities and complications.
a.   Maintain function and prevent deterioration of unaffected organs or areas.
b.   Prevent further injury to affected area or organ.
c.   Prevent or reduce complications of immobility.
2.   Assist client to perform activities of daily living (ADLs) with minimal or no assistance, depending on level of disability.
Examples of ADLs: Eating, dressing, bathing.
3.   Assist client with independent activities of daily living (IADLs).
Examples of IADLs: Shopping for groceries, paying bills, lawn care.
4.   Promote continuity of care when the client is discharged or transferred.

Psychological Responses to Disability

Not every client will progress through all stages of grief in an orderly fashion. Clients will fluctuate between emotional crises.
A.   Initial responses of confusion, disorganization, and denial represent a state of internal conflict. Conflict is precipitated by:
1.   Forced dependency.
2.   Loss of self-esteem.
3.   Threat to personal and family integrity.
B.   A period of depression may occur as the client mourns for the lost body function or activity.
C.   An anger stage may occur as the client projects blame and hostility on family and health care providers.
D.   Adaptation and adjustment will occur as the client begins to redirect his or her energy toward coping with the disability.
E.   New situations (e.g., going home from hospital, new job) may precipitate emotional outbursts and trauma.
F.   Some clients will refuse to accept their disability and will not put forth any effort to adapt to everyday living.

23

CARE OF THE CHRONICALLY ILL CLIENT

* **A chronic illness may be defined as an illness or condition that is present for more than 3 months in a year and interferes with daily function and lifestyle.**

Nursing Considerations

A. Client may remain free from symptoms, but must remain in contact with health care provider in order to maintain optimal level of wellness.

B. The condition of the client and the level of the disease will have a variable impact on the client's lifestyle and coping strategies.

C. The majority of clients with extended health care needs are suffering from at least two chronic health conditions. These conditions may or may not be interrelated.

D. The focus of care for the chronically ill client is on assisting the client to control his/her disease and manage his/her lifestyle. This is true of the pediatric chronically ill client as well as the adult client.
   1. Prevention and management of medical crises.
   2. Control of disease symptoms, which may focus on pain control and comfort measures.
   3. Implementation of the prescribed therapeutic regimens.
   4. Psychosocial implications and adjustment of lifestyle; frequently requires dealing with social isolation.
   5. Adjustments of lifestyle as disease and/or condition changes.
   6. Financial strain to pay for medical care and supplies.
   7. Coping with strain on marriage and on family structure.

E. The majority of clients with chronic health care needs are over 65 years of age. The feeling of powerlessness is not uncommon in the older adult.

Nursing Considerations in the Chronically Ill Pediatric Client

The diagnosis of a child's chronic illness is a major situational crisis in the family. Support systems, perception of the problem, and coping mechanisms will ultimately determine the resolution of the crisis.

A. Focus care on the child's developmental age rather than the chronological age. Emphasis should be made on the child's strengths rather than on the child's disabilities.

B. Promote the child's maximal level of growth and development. The current trend is to return the child to the academic environment of the child's peer group. A variety of supplemental programs are being developed in the school systems to meet the needs of these children.

C. Assess the family response to the child's illness and evaluate for parental overprotection. Overprotection by the parents prevents the child from developing self-esteem, independence, and self-control over disease and activities of daily living. The practical nurse should observe for the following parental characteristics:
   1. Shows inconsistency with discipline; for example, discipline often differs from that of the other children in the family.
   2. Attempts to protect the child from every discomfort, both physical and psychosocial; for example, frequently restricts play with peers for fear of injury and/or rejection by peers.
   3. Makes decisions for the child without involving the child.
   4. Does not allow the child the opportunity to learn self-care; frequently afraid the child cannot handle the requirements for self-care, for example, encouraging and assisting the diabetic child to become responsible for administration of own insulin.
   5. Continues to do things for the child, even when the child is capable of performing tasks for self.
   6. Shows self-sacrifice and isolation of family from social interactions.

GROWTH AND DEVELOPMENT

A. Normal growth and development progress in a steady, predictable pattern across the life span.
   1. Development progresses in a cephalocaudal (head to tail) manner.
   2. Development progresses from proximal to distal, with a progression from gross to fine motor skills.

B. The developmental age of a client is important to consider in the implementation of nursing care.
   1. Nurses need to be aware of the major developmental milestones.
   2. Nursing care is planned around the client's developmental level, not his or her chronological age.

> ***TEST ALERT: Provide care appropriate to developmental level (e.g., newborn, child, older adult), especially for the adult and older adult.***

C. Physical development is described in Table 2-1.

Dietary Considerations throughout the Life Span

Infant

A. Growth.
   1. Birth weight doubles in 4 months.
   2. Birth weight triples at 1 year.
   3. Infant gains only another 4 to 6 lb until 2 years old.

   Example: Birth weight 7 lb; at 4 months infant should weigh 14 lb; another 7 lb will be added in the next 8 months.

TABLE 2-1	GROWTH AND DEVELOPMENT	
Birth-4 months	Consistently gains weight (5-7 oz per week) Posterior fontanel closes Responds to sounds and begins vocalizing Gains head control → lifts chest → rolls over one way Smiles responsively → smiles when spoken to	Teething may begin Coordination progresses from jerky movement to grasping objects Provide toys that increase hand-eye coordination
4-9 months	Doubles birth weight (gains 3-5 oz per week) Teething begins with lower incisors Sits with support; begins crawling Turns over in both directions Laughs aloud	Reaches for objects and grasps them Begins "stranger anxiety" Begins vocalizing with single consonants Provide brightly colored toys that are easy to grasp Enjoys noisemakers and mirrors; plays pat-a-cake
9-12 months	Birth weight triples Head and chest circumferences are equal Anterior fontanel begins to close Teething: has 6-8 teeth Sits alone → moves from prone to sitting position Crawling → pulling up → walks holding on to furniture	May stand alone Has developed crude to fine pincer grasp Transfers objects from one hand to another Recognizes own name Enjoys playing alone (solitary) Explores objects by putting them in mouth
Toddler (12-24 months)	50% of height at 2 years Exaggerated lumbar curve Mobile: walks, runs, jumps Walks up and down stairs, one foot at a time Begins using eating utensils Obeys simple commands Begins to develop vocabulary	Speech becomes understandable Thumb sucking may be at peak Solitary play at 12 months; parallel play at 18 months Beginning to develop bladder and bowel control Attention-seeking behavior: temper tantrums Enjoys activities that provide mobility: riding vehicles, wagons, pull toys
Preschool (3-5 years)	Birth length doubles at 4 years Coordination continues to improve Rides tricycle, throws a ball Walks up and down stairs with alternating feet	Begins to demonstrate self-care abilities Knows own name Good verbalization: talks about activities Plays "dress up"; plays with cars, dolls, grooming aids
School-age (6-10 years)	Growth spurts begin Increasingly active Very concerned with body image Need for conformity: rules and rituals	Increasing importance of peer groups Plays with groups of same sex Competes for attention
Adolescence (11-17 years)	Beginning and completing puberty Girls mature earlier than boys Very conscious of changes in body Rapid growth	Moves from concrete to abstract thinking Increased independence Strong peer group association Increased interest in opposite sex
Young adult (18-30 years)	Physical maturity Full mental capacity Assumes responsibility for own learning Adult relationship with parents	Launches career Selects a mate, begins own family Begins involvement in community
Adult (30-60 years)	Physiological processes begin slow decline Cognitive skills peak Creativity at maximum Increase in community involvement Increase in concern for future of society	Family tasks Assist children to responsible adulthood Role reversal with aging parents Defines role of grandparenting
Older adult (60+ years)	Decline of physiological status Demineralization of bones ↓ Cardiac output ↓ Respiratory vital capacity ↓ Glomerular filtration rate ↓ Serum albumin ↓ Glucose tolerance	Maintains reasoning ability and abstract thinking Restructure in family roles Retirement Reorganization of activities Continues with community involvement and politics

4. Newborn will lose weight for the first few days following birth, but should not lose more than 10% of the birth weight or take longer than 10 to 14 days to regain it.
5. Newborn has a higher fluid requirement in relation to body size than an adult.
B. Diet.
1. Ideal food is breast milk, because it is nutritionally superior to alternatives.
2. Cereal is usually the first solid food, given at 4 to 6 months; rice cereal is easily digested and less likely to cause an allergic reaction.
3. Order of introduction of food is cereal, then vegetables or strained fruits with meat being last.
4. Before adding another food item, wait 4 to 7 days to ensure no allergic or adverse reaction has occurred due to previously added food item.
5. Maintain infant on formula or breast milk until 12 months old, may need iron supplement after 6 months if on formula.

✔ **PEDIATRIC PRIORITY:** *Infants should not be given honey until after their first birthday.*

C. Nursing implications.
1. Newborns cannot swallow voluntarily until 10 to 12 weeks of age.
2. Extrusion reflex (pushing food out of mouth with tongue) lasts until 4 months.
3. Usual progression of food texture is strained to mashed to minced to chopped to cut table foods.
4. Increase the use of small-sized finger foods as pincer grasp develops (9 months).
5. Texture of food becomes increasingly important from 6 months to 1 year, but the food must be easily dissolved (e.g., crackers or zwieback).

✔ **PEDIATRIC PRIORITY:** *Raw carrots, celery, popcorn, nuts and hard candies should not be given until the toddler stage due to problem with choking.*

Toddler

A. Growth.
1. Steady increases in growth.
2. Legs grow more rapidly than the trunk.
B. Diet.
1. Needs 16 oz of milk daily; more than 24 oz can lead to milk anemia (peak incidence at 18 months).
2. Milk intake should not exceed 800 to 1000 mL daily in toddlers and young children in order to prevent refusal of other foods.
3. Fruit snacks should be given rather than fruit juices.

4. Prefers finger foods (e.g., bananas, green beans, crackers).
5. Tends to refuse casseroles, salads, and mixed dishes.
C. Nursing implications.
1. Struggle for autonomy may be manifested by refusal of food, mealtime negativism, and ritualism.
2. Bribery and rewards for eating should be avoided.
3. Do not mix food on plate.

Preschooler

A. Growth.
1. Growth rate slows and appetite decreases.
2. Activity level and nutrient requirements remain high.
B. Diet.
1. Food jags are common; may refuse to eat anything except one food at each meal.
2. Continues to refuse casseroles and mixed food items.
3. Finger foods remain popular.
C. Nursing implications.
1. Should not be forced to eat all food on plate. If sufficient amounts are not eaten during mealtimes, then eliminate snacks.
2. Recognize that refusing to eat is a way to attract attention.

School-Age Child

A. Growth.
1. Growth is slow and steady.
2. Food intake gradually increases while energy needs per unit of body weight decline.
3. There is a yearly gain of 3 to 5 kg in weight and 6 cm in height, ending with a growth spurt in puberty.
B. Diet.
1. Food intake is more varied.
2. Enjoys most foods, with vegetables being least favorite.
C. Nursing implications.
1. After-school snacks are popular; encourage fruits, raw vegetable sticks, and peanut butter sandwiches.
2. Child learns good table manners from imitating parents.
3. Promote good health habits (e.g., regular exercise; weight control is a balance between physical activity and food intake); encourage routine dental checkups for dental caries.

Adolescent

A. Growth.
1. Rapid growth rates and maturation changes make adolescents vulnerable to nutritional deficiencies.

2. Girl's peak growth occurs between 10 and 13 years of age.
3. Boy's peak growth occurs between 11 and 14 years of age. Energy needs are highest in boys between 15 and 18 years of age, when muscle mass is developing.

B. Diet.
  1. Diets in general are deficient in calcium and vitamin C.
  2. Out of 10 girls, 6 eat only two thirds of the nutrients required. Girls tend to be deficient in iron, while boys tend to be deficient in thiamine.

Adult

A. Growth.
  1. For ages 20 to 80, body fat in proportion to body weight increases 35%.
  2. For ages 20 to 80, plasma volume decreases by 8%.
  3. For ages 20 to 80, lean body mass and total body water decrease by 17%.

B. Diet.
  1. Energy requirements decrease with age. *Example: 55-year-old man requires 2400 kcal; at age 76 requires only 2050 kcal. Example: 55-year-old woman requires 1800 kcal; at age 76 only requires 1600 kcal.*
  2. Improved financial status during middle adulthood increases intake of rich foods and frequency of dining out.
  3. Obesity gradually becomes a problem as a sedentary lifestyle develops.

C. Nursing implications.
  1. Encourage adherence to a prudent diet pattern.
  2. Promote a regular exercise program.
  3. Reduce sodium intake to 3 to 6 g daily.
  4. Maintain serum cholesterol level at or below 200 mg/dl, with high-density lipoprotein (HDL) level above 35 mg/dl.

> **TEST ALERT: Provide care that meets the special needs of the older client** (Box 2-1).

Older Adult

A. Diet.
  1. Encourage a diet high in fiber, iron, vitamin C, and thiamine with adequate sources of calcium.
  2. If confined to bed rest, the older adult requires an increased fluid intake as high as 3 L/day to promote good renal function, providing there are no fluid restrictions (e.g., heart failure).

 OLDER ADULT PRIORITY: *The older adult may intentionally restrict fluids because of nocturia or stress incontinence.*

3. Monitor renal function, protein may be limited if renal function is compromised.

B. Nursing implications.
  1. Income is usually fixed; may have less money to spend on food.
  2. Food shopping and transportation may be a problem because of physical disability.
  3. Alteration in taste and reduced digestive function occurs.
  4. Often needs to wear dentures.
  5. Constipation is a chronic problem; encourage fluid intake and high-fiber diet.
  6. Loneliness and depression are often associated with poor appetite.

> **OLDER ADULT PRIORITY:** *Usually it takes more time for an older person to eat and early satiety is reached. Encourage frequent small feedings rather than three meals a day. May need additional liquid supplements.*

Nutritional Evaluation

A. Determine nutritional needs.
B. Examine client profile: age, sex, height, weight, socio-economic status, culture.
C. Determine nutritional status: food habits; observe for physical signs indicative of nutritional status.
D. Determine disease or pathophysiological process.
E. Be alert to high-risk clients: overweight; underweight; surgery of GI tract; problems with ingestion, digestion, or absorption; and clients on intravenous (IV) therapy for 10 days or more.

BOX 2-1	OLDER ADULT CARE FOCUS
	Age-Related Factors Influencing Older Adult Care

- Frequent absence of social and financial support
  Examples: Disease and/or loss of spouse, inadequate income from pension
- Presence of significant concurrent illness
  Examples: Dementia, chronic obstructive disease, congestive heart failure, depression, diabetes
- Altered pain perception
  Example: Increased incidence of referred pain
- Impaired homeostatic mechanisms
  Examples: Increased problems with dehydration, incontinence, impaired defecation, altered immune status
- Impaired mobility
  Examples: Dependence on walkers, need for assistance with bed transferring, change in use of transportation, presence of Parkinsonism or degenerative joint disease
- Increased frequency of adverse reactions to drugs
- Impaired equilibrium, resulting in falls

Diet Therapy for High-Level Wellness

A. MyPyramid (Figure 2-1).
B. Prudent diet.
  1. Increased amounts of fruits, vegetables, and grains.
  2. Reduced amounts of animal fats, cholesterol, refined sugar, salt, and alcohol.
  3. Adaptations to the MyPyramid Plan (see Figure 2-1).
    a. Meat: increase amounts of fish, chicken, turkey, and veal; also increase use of legumes, nuts, and seeds as a source of protein; limit egg yolks to two or three weekly, including those used in cooking.
    b. Milk: use low-fat dairy products.
    c. Fruits and vegetables: increase total intake.
    d. Grains, breads, and cereals: select whole-grain products and eat at least 3 oz every day.

Therapeutic Meal Plans

❋ **A therapeutic meal plan or prescription diet is a modification of an individual's normal nutritional needs based on the pathophysiological disease process** (Table 2-2).

> *TEST ALERT: Collect data on client's nutrition or hydration status; identify client's ability to eat (chew, swallow); provide for nutritional needs by encouraging client to eat, feeding client, or assisting with menu.*

COMMUNICABLE DISEASES

> *TEST ALERT: Understand communicable diseases and modes of organism transmission (airborne, droplet, contact); apply principles of infection control.*

A. Incubation period: time from exposure to the pathogen until clinical symptoms occur.
B. Communicability: period of time in which an infected person is most likely to pass the pathogens to another person.
C. Prodromal period: begins with early manifestations of the disease or infection and continues until there are overt clinical symptoms characteristic of the disease.
D. Vaccinations for health care workers (Table 2-3).

 ## Varicella (Chicken Pox)

Characteristics

A. Herpes virus: varicella zoster; highly contagious, usually occurs in children under 15 years of age.
B. Maculopapular rash with vesicular scabs in multiple stages of healing.

C. Incubation period: 14 to 16 days.
D. Transmission: contact, airborne.
E. Communicability: 1 day before lesions appear to time when all lesions have formed crusts.

Data Collection

A. Prodromal: low-grade fever, malaise.
B. Acute phase: red maculopapular rash.
C. New crops of vesicles continue to form for 3 to 5 days, spreading from trunk to extremities.
D. Rash appears profusely on the trunk; begins as macule and progresses to papule, vesicle and then crusts. All three stages are usually present in varying degrees at one time; pruritus.
E. Complications: secondary infection may lead to sepsis, abscess, cellulitis, or pneumonia.

Health Care Interventions

A. Preventive: varicella immunization (see Figure 2-2, Figure 2-3).
B. Skin care to decrease itching.
  1. Topical antihistamines, antipruritics, calamine lotion.
  2. Cool baths.
C. Keep child's fingernails short; apply mittens if necessary.
D. Isolate affected child from other children until vesicles have crusted.
E. Provide quiet activities to keep child occupied to lessen pruritus and prevent scratching.
F. Avoid use of aspirin.
G. Check with health care provider before administering vaccine to immunocompromised clients. Vaccine should not be given to pregnant women.

 ## Parotitis (Mumps)

Characteristics

A. An acute viral disease characterized by tenderness and swelling of one or both of the parotid glands and/or the other salivary glands.
B. Incubation period: 14 to 21 days.
C. Transmission: direct contact and droplet.
D. Communicability: immediately before and after swelling begins.

Data Collection

A. Prodromal: headache, fever, malaise.
B. Acute phase: Swelling of salivary glands (peaks in 3 days), leading to difficulty in swallowing, earache.
C. Complications.
  1. Postinfectious encephalitis.
  2. Sensorineural deafness.
  3. Orchitis, epididymitis.

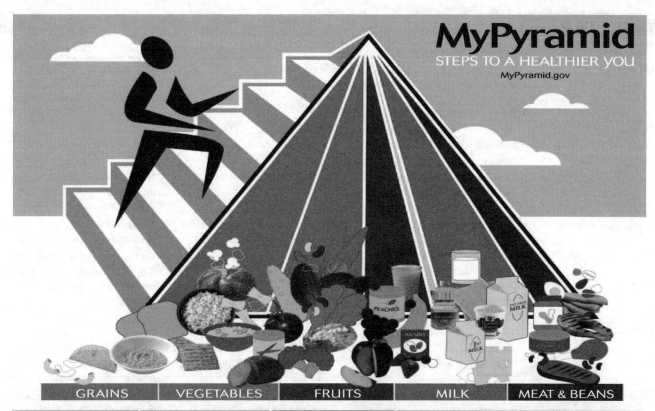

MyPyramid
STEPS TO A HEALTHIER YOU
MyPyramid.gov

GRAINS	VEGETABLES	FRUITS	MILK	MEAT & BEANS

GRAINS	VEGETABLES	FRUITS	MILK	MEAT & BEANS
Make half your grains whole	Vary your veggies	Focus on fruits	Get your calcium-rich foods	Go lean with protein
Eat at least 3 oz. of whole-grain cereals, breads, crackers, rice, or pasta every day 1 oz. is about 1 slice of bread, about 1 cup of breakfast cereal, or ½ cup of cooked rice, cereal, or pasta	Eat more dark-green veggies like broccoli, spinach, and other dark leafy greens Eat more orange vegetables like carrots and sweetpotatoes Eat more dry beans and peas like pinto beans, kidney beans, and lentils	Eat a variety of fruit Choose fresh, frozen, canned, or dried fruit Go easy on fruit juices	Go low-fat or fat-free when you choose milk, yogurt, and other milk products If you don't or can't consume milk, choose lactose-free products or other calcium sources such as fortified foods and beverages	Choose low-fat or lean meats and poultry Bake it, broil it, or grill it Vary your protein routine — choose more fish, beans, peas, nuts, and seeds

For a 2,000-calorie diet, you need the amounts below from each food group. To find the amounts that are right for you, go to MyPyramid.gov.

Eat 6 oz. every day	Eat 2½ cups every day	Eat 2 cups every day	Get 3 cups every day; for kids aged 2 to 8, it's 2	Eat 5½ oz. every day

Find your balance between food and physical activity
- Be sure to stay within your daily calorie needs.
- Be physically active for at least 30 minutes most days of the week.
- About 60 minutes a day of physical activity may be needed to prevent weight gain.
- For sustaining weight loss, at least 60 to 90 minutes a day of physical activity may be required.
- Children and teenagers should be physically active for 60 minutes every day, or most days.

Know the limits on fats, sugars, and salt (sodium)
- Make most of your fat sources from fish, nuts, and vegetable oils.
- Limit solid fats like butter, margarine, shortening, and lard, as well as foods that contain these.
- Check the Nutrition Facts label to keep saturated fats, *trans* fats, and sodium low.
- Choose food and beverages low in added sugars. Added sugars contribute calories with few, if any, nutrients.

MyPyramid.gov
STEPS TO A HEALTHIER YOU

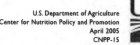
U.S. Department of Agriculture
Center for Nutrition Policy and Promotion
April 2005
CNPP-15

USDA

USDA is an equal opportunity provider and employer.

FIGURE 2-1 MyPyramid. *(From United States Department of Agriculture, Center for Nutrition Policy and Promotion, April 2005. Retrieved from http://www.mypyramid.gov/downloads/MiniPoster.pdf _)*

TABLE 2-2	THERAPEUTIC MEAL PLANS		
Diet	*Purpose/Use*	*Foods Allowed*	*Foods Restricted*
Clear liquid	To begin introduction of food after removal of NG tube, after GI surgery. Prior to GI diagnostics.	Liquids that are clear	Milk products, juice with pulp, any solid food; anything that is not liquid at room temperature
Full liquid	To begin introduction of food; used after removal of NG tube or after GI surgery	Any food that is liquid at room temperature	Any solid food
Soft diet	To progress diet as tolerated; food should be easy to chew and swallow	Soft, tender foods easy to swallow and digest	Highly seasoned foods, whole grains, fruits, vegetables, nuts, fried foods
Mechanical soft diet	To assist clients who cannot chew effectively	Soft foods that are easy to chew and swallow	Tough foods that are difficult to chew and swallow
Bland diet	To eliminate foods irritating to the digestive system; used in clients after GI surgery and those with peptic ulcer disease and GI inflammatory problems	Milk, custards, refined cereals, creamed soups, potatoes (baked or broiled); all foods are white; no bright-colored food	Highly seasoned or strong-flavored foods; tea, colas, coffee, fruits, whole grains, raw fruit, most vegetables
Low-residue diet	To decrease fiber or stool in GI tract; acute episodes of enteritis, diarrhea; before and/or after GI surgery	Clear liquids, meats, fats, eggs, refined cereals, white bread, peeled white potatoes, small amount of milk	Cheeses; whole grains; raw fruits and vegetables; high-carbohydrate foods, which are usually high in residue and fiber
High-residue diet	To prevent constipation and prevent acute diverticulitis	Raw fruits and vegetables; whole grains; high-carbohydrate foods, which are high in residue and fiber	Indigestible fibers: celery, whole corn; seeds such as sesame and poppy; foods with small seeds
Lactose-free diet	To prevent GI effects of lactose intolerance	Nonmilk products, yogurt	Milk and milk products, processed foods that may have dried milk as filler
PKU diet	To control intake of phenylalanine, an essential acid; affected children cannot metabolize it	Specially prepared infant formula if infant is not breast-fed, vegetables, fruits, juices, some cereals, and breads; may allow 20-30 mg of phenylalanine per kilogram of body weight to fulfill normal growth needs	Most high-protein foods, including meat and dairy products, are significantly reduced
Low-fat/low-cholesterol diet	To prevent gall bladder spasms, clients with increased cholesterol levels, or problems with malabsorption of fat (cystic fibrosis)	Low-fat or fat-free milk, fruits, vegetables, breads, cereals, reduced amounts of red meat	Egg yolks, whole milk, fried foods, processed cheese, shrimp, avocados, pastries, butter
Low-sodium diet	To reduce sodium intake to decrease retention of fluids, especially in clients with cardiac disease or hypertension	Salt-free preparations, fresh fruits, vegetables with no added salt	Processed foods, smoked or salted meats, prepared foods, frozen and canned vegetables, breads and pastries
High-potassium diet	To replace lost potassium in clients taking diuretics and/or digitalis	Dried fruits, fruit juices, fresh fruits (e.g., bananas, apricots, grapefruit, oranges, and tomatoes)	No specific restrictions
Renal diet	Control potassium, sodium, and protein levels in clients with renal problems	High biological protein (limited intake): eggs, milk, meat; decreased sodium products and decreased potassium (cabbage, peas, cucumbers are low in potassium)	High-potassium foods (dried fruits), high-sodium foods (processed foods), salt substitutes with high-potassium content
Low-purine diet	To decrease serum levels of uric acid; prescribed for clients with gout and high levels of uric acid	Vegetables, fruits, cereals, eggs, fat-free milk, cottage cheese	Glandular meats, fish, poultry, nuts, beans, oatmeal, whole wheat, cauliflower

GI, Gastrointestinal; *NG*, nasogastric; *PKU*, phenylketonuria.

Health Care Interventions

A. Preventive: measles, mumps, and rubella (MMR) immunization (see Figure 2-2, Figure 2-3). MMR vaccine should not be given to pregnant or severely immunocompromised clients.
B. Bed rest until swelling subsides.
C. Fluids and soft, bland food.
D. Orchitis: warm or cold packs; light support to scrotum.
E. Cool compresses applied to swollen neck area.

Rubeola (Measles, Hard Measles, Red Measles)

Characteristics

A. An acute viral disease characterized by fever and a rash.
B. Incubation: 10 to 20 days.
C. Transmission: direct contact with respiratory droplet.
D. Communicability: 4 days before rash to 5 days after rash appears.

Data Collection

A. Prodromal: fever, malaise, cold-like symptoms.
B. Koplik's spots: small, irregular red spots noticed on the buccal mucosa opposite the molars; usually appear 2 days before rash.
C. Acute phase: begins 3 to 4 days after prodromal symptoms; maculopapular rash begins on face and gradually spreads downward from head to feet.
D. Photophobia, conjunctivitis, and bronchitis.
E. Complications: otitis media, pneumonia, laryngotracheitis, and encephalitis.

Health Care Interventions

A. Preventive: MMR immunization (see Figure 2-2, Figure 2-3). MMR should not be given to pregnant or severely immunocompromised clients.
B. Bed rest until fever subsides, acetaminophen or ibuprofen for fever control.
C. Dim lights to decrease photophobia.
D. Tepid baths and lotion to relieve itching.
E. Encourage intake of fluids to maintain hydration; temperature may spike 2 to 3 days after rash appears.

Rubella (German Measles, Three-Day Measles)

Characteristics

A. An acute, mild systemic viral disease that produces a distinctive 3-day rash and lymphadenopathy.
B. Incubation: 14 to 21 days.
C. Transmission: nasopharyngeal secretions, direct contact.
D. Communicability: from up to 7 days before rash until 5 days after rash.

Data Collection

A. Prodromal: low-grade fever, headache, malaise, and symptoms of a cold.
B. Rash first appears on face and spreads down to neck, arms, trunk, and then legs.
C. Diagnostics: persistent rubella antibody titer of 1:8 usually indicates immunity.
D. Complications: can have teratogenic effects on fetus.

TABLE 2-3	CENTERS FOR DISEASE CONTROL (CDC) AND PREVENTION HEALTH CARE PERSONNEL (HCP) VACCINE RECOMMENDATIONS
Vaccine	**Recommendations in brief**
Hepatitis B	Give 3-dose series (dose #1 now, #2 in 1 month, #3 approximately 5 months after #2). Give IM. Obtain anti-HBs serologic testing 1–2 months after dose #3.
Influenza	Give 1 dose of influenza vaccine annually. Give inactivated injectable influenza vaccine intramuscularly or live attenuated influenza vaccine (LAIV) intranasally.
MMR	For healthcare personnel (HCP) born in 1957 or later without serologic evidence of immunity or prior vaccination, give 2 doses of MMR, 4 weeks apart. For HCP born prior to 1957, see below. Give SC.
Varicella (chickenpox)	For HCP who have no serologic proof of immunity, prior vaccination, or history of varicella disease, give 2 doses of varicella vaccine, 4 weeks apart. Give SC.
Tetanus, diphtheria, pertussis	Give all HCP a Td booster dose every 10 years, following the completion of the primary 3-dose series. Give a 1-time dose of Tdap to all HCP younger than age 65 years with direct patient contact. Give IM.
Meningococcal	Give 1 dose to microbiologists who are routinely exposed to isolates of *N. meningitidis*.

Hepatitis A, typhoid, and polio vaccines are not routinely recommended for HCP who may have on-the-job exposure to fecal material.

From Centers for Disease Control and Prevention: *Healthcare personnel vaccine recommendations, Atlanta,* 2009, Center for Disease Control and Prevention. Retrieved October, 2009, from *http://www.immunize.org/catg.d/p2017.pdf.* For recent updates and a full explanation of footnotes, refer to the Centers for Disease and Prevention Web site at *www.cdc.gov.*

Recommended Immunization Schedule for Persons Aged 0 Through 6 Years—United States • 2009
For those who fall behind or start late, see the catch-up schedule

Vaccine ▼ Age ►	Birth	1 month	2 months	4 months	6 months	12 months	15 months	18 months	19–23 months	2–3 years	4–6 years
Hepatitis B[1]	HepB	HepB	see footnote 1			HepB					
Rotavirus[2]			RV	RV	RV[2]						
Diphtheria, Tetanus, Pertussis[3]			DTaP	DTaP	DTaP	see footnote 3	DTaP				DTaP
Haemophilus influenzae type b[4]			Hib	Hib	Hib[4]	Hib					
Pneumococcal[5]			PCV	PCV	PCV	PCV				PPSV	
Inactivated Poliovirus			IPV	IPV		IPV					IPV
Influenza[6]						Influenza (Yearly)					
Measles, Mumps, Rubella[7]						MMR		see footnote 7			MMR
Varicella[8]						Varicella		see footnote 8			Varicella
Hepatitis A[9]						HepA (2 doses)				HepA Series	
Meningococcal[10]										MCV	

Range of recommended ages

Certain high-risk groups

This schedule indicates the recommended ages for routine administration of currently licensed vaccines, as of December 1, 2008, for children aged 0 through 6 years. Any dose not administered at the recommended age should be administered at a subsequent visit, when indicated and feasible. Licensed combination vaccines may be used whenever any component of the combination is indicated and other components are not contraindicated and if approved by the Food and Drug Administration for that dose of the series. Providers should consult the relevant Advisory Committee on Immunization Practices statement for detailed recommendations, including high-risk conditions: http://www.cdc.gov/vaccines/pubs/acip-list.htm. Clinically significant adverse events that follow immunization should be reported to the Vaccine Adverse Event Reporting System (VAERS). Guidance about how to obtain and complete a VAERS form is available at http://www.vaers.hhs.gov or by telephone, 800-822-7967.

FIGURE 2-2 **Recommended Immunization Schedule for Persons Aged 0-6 Years, 2009.** For recent updates and a full explanation of footnotes, refer to the Centers for Disease Control and Prevention website, *http://www.cdc.gov/vaccines/recs/schedules/child-schedule.htm#printable. (From Centers for Disease Control and Prevention, Advisory Committee on Immunization Practices [ACIP], United States, 2009. Retrieved from www.cdc.gov.)*

Health Care Interventions

A. Primarily symptomatic; bed rest until fever subsides.

B. Preventive: MMR immunization (see Figure 2-2, Figure 2-3). MMR should not be given to severely immunosuppressed clients.

C. Pregnant women should avoid contact with children who have rubella. If not immunized before pregnancy, vaccination should not be given until completion of pregnancy.

Roseola Infantum (Exanthema Subitum)

Characteristics

A. A common, acute benign viral infection, usually occurring in infants and young children (ages 6 months to 3 years), characterized by sudden onset of a high temperature, followed by a rash.

B. Incubation period: usually 5 to 15 days.

C. Transmission: unknown, generally limited to children ages 6 months to 3 years.

D. Communicability: unknown.

Data Collection

A. Sudden onset of high fever.

B. As fever drops, a maculopapular, nonpruritic rash appears abruptly; rash blanches or fades under pressure and disappears in 1 to 2 days.

C. Complications: febrile seizures.

Health Care Interventions

A. Symptomatic: provide tepid baths, offer fluids frequently, keep child cool.

B. Acetaminophen and/or ibuprofen for fever control.

Diphtheria

A. An infection caused by *Corynebacterium diphtheriae.*

B. Incubation period: 3 to 6 days.

C. Transmission: direct contact, contaminated articles (fomites).

D. Communicability: variable, usually 2 weeks, but may be longer

E. Smooth, white or gray membrane over tonsillar region; hoarseness and potential airway obstruction.

F. Preventive: diphtheria, tetanus, and pertussis (DTaP) immunization (see Figure 2-2, Figure 2-3) beginning at 2-4 months of age.

Pertussis (Whooping Cough)

A. An acute inflammation of the respiratory tract caused by *Bordetella pertussis*; is most severe in children under 2 years of age.

B. Incubation period: 6 to 20 days; average, 7 days.

C. Transmission: air droplet, communicability is greatest before onset of paroxysms of coughing.

D. Prevention: DTaP immunization. (see Figure 2-2, Figure 2-3)

Tetanus (Lockjaw)

A. An acute, very serious, potentially fatal disease characterized by painful muscle spasms and convulsions caused by the anaerobic gram-positive bacillus *Clostridium tetani.*

B. Incubation period: generally from 2 days to 2 months; average is 10 days.

C. Transmission: through a puncture wound that is contaminated by soil, dust, or excreta that contain Clostridium tetani or by way of burns and minor wounds (e.g., infection of the umbilicus of a newborn).

D. Prevention
    1. Careful cleansing and debridement of wounds.
    2. Immunization: DTaP (Figure 2-2); adult tetanus toxoid (Td) every 10 years (see Figure 2-3).
    3. Encourage all clients to maintain current immunization.

Poliomyelitis

A. An acute, contagious disease affecting the central nervous system.

B. Incubation period: 5 to 35 days; average, 7 to 14 days.

C. Transmission: fecal-oral or pharyngeal-oropharyngeal contact.

D. Communicability: virus in throat for 1 week after onset; in feces, intermittently for 4 to 6 weeks.

E. Preventive: inactivated polio virus vaccine (IPV), (see Figure 2-2, Figure 2-3).

Scarlet Fever (Scarlatina)

A. Group A beta-hemolytic streptococcal infection that often follows acute streptopharyngitis.

B. Incubation period: 1 to 7 days; average, 3 days.

C. Transmission: direct contact or droplet of nasopharyngeal secretions.

D. Communicability: variable, approximately 10 days.

E. Sudden onset of high fever and tachycardia, "strawberry" tongue.

F. Diagnostics: history of a recent streptococcal infection, positive antistreptolysin-O (ASO) titer, and a throat culture positive for *group A beta-hemolytic streptococci.*

G. Complications: otitis media, tonsillar abscess, glomerulonephritis.

H. Health Care Implications
    1. Administration of a full course of penicillin (or erythromycin in penicillin-sensitive clients).
    2. Encourage intake of fluids to prevent dehydration during febrile phase.

Recommended Adult Immunization Schedule
UNITED STATES - 2009
Note: These recommendations *must* be read with the footnotes that follow containing number of doses, intervals between doses, and other important information.

Recommended adult immunization schedule, by vaccine and age group

VACCINE ▼ AGE GROUP ▶	19–26 years	27–49 years	50–59 years	60–64 years	≥65 years
Tetanus, diphtheria, pertussis (Td/Tdap)[1,*]	Substitute 1-time dose of Tdap for Td booster; then boost with Td every 10 yrs				Td booster every 10 yrs
Human papillomavirus (HPV)[2,*]	3 doses (females)				
Varicella[3,*]	2 doses				
Zoster[4]				1 dose	
Measles, mumps, rubella (MMR)[5,*]	1 or 2 doses		1 dose		
Influenza[6,*]	1 dose annually				
Pneumococcal (polysaccharide)[7,8]	1 or 2 doses				1 dose
Hepatitis A[9,*]	2 doses				
Hepatitis B[10,*]	3 doses				
Meningococcal[11,*]	1 or more doses				

*Covered by the Vaccine Injury Compensation Program.

For all persons in this category who meet the age requirements and who lack evidence of immunity (e.g., lack documentation of vaccination or have no evidence of prior infection)

Recommended if some other risk factor is present (e.g., on the basis of medical, occupational, lifestyle, or other indications)

No recommendation

Report all clinically significant postvaccination reactions to the Vaccine Adverse Event Reporting System (VAERS). Reporting forms and instructions on filing a VAERS report are available at www.vaers.hhs.gov or by telephone, 800-822-7967.

Information on how to file a Vaccine Injury Compensation Program claim is available at www.hrsa.gov/vaccinecompensation or by telephone, 800-338-2382. To file a claim for vaccine injury, contact the U.S. Court of Federal Claims, 717 Madison Place, N.W., Washington, D.C. 20005; telephone, 202-357-6400.

Additional information about the vaccines in this schedule, extent of available data, and contraindications for vaccination is also available at www.cdc.gov/vaccines or from the CDC-INFO Contact Center at 800-CDC-INFO (800-232-4636) in English and Spanish, 24 hours a day, 7 days a week.

Use of trade names and commercial sources is for identification only and does not imply endorsement by the U.S. Department of Health and Human Services.

FIGURE 2-3 Recommended Adult Immunization Schedule, 2009. For recent updates and a full explanation of footnotes, refer to the Centers for Disease Control and Prevention website, *http://www.cdc.gov/vaccines/recs/schedules/adult-schedule.htm#print. (From Centers for Disease Control and Prevention, Advisory Committee on Immunization Practices [ACIP], United States, 2008. Retrieved from www.cdc.gov.)*

Infectious Mononucleosis

A.   An acute, self-limiting infectious disease caused by the Epstein-Barr virus; member of the herpes group of viruses, occurring most often among young persons under 25 years old; often called the "kissing disease."
B.   Incubation period: 30-50 days.
C.   Transmission: direct or indirect contact with oral secretions—intimate contact, sharing same drinking cup, hand to mouth; probably oral pharyngeal route.
D.   Onset of symptoms occurs anytime from 10 days to 6 weeks after exposure; may be acute or insidious; malaise, sore throat, fever with generalized lymphadenopathy.
E.   Diagnostic: a positive heterophil antibody test (titer of 1:160 is considered diagnostic); positive Monospot test result.

CANCER

Characteristics of Cancer

✳   **Cancer must be regarded as a group of disease entities with different causes, manifestations, treatment, and prognoses. The basic disease process begins when normal cells undergo change and begin to reproduce in an abnormal manner.**

Major Dysfunction in the Cell

A.   Cellular proliferation: cancer cells divide in an indiscriminate, unregulated manner.
B.   There is a loss of contact inhibition. The cancer cells have no regard for cellular boundaries; normal cells respect boundaries and do not invade adjacent areas or organs.
C.   Tumors (neoplasm).
   1.   Benign: encapsulated neoplasm that remains localized in the tissue of origin.
      a.   Exerts pressure on surrounding organs.
      b.   Will decrease blood supply to the normal tissue.
   2.   Malignant: nonencapsulated neoplasm that invades surrounding tissue. The stage of the neoplasm determines whether or not metastasis or spread to distant body parts has occurred. There are four primary mechanisms by which the metastasis spreads:
      a.   Vascular system: cancer cells penetrate vessels and circulate until trapped. The cancer cells may penetrate the vessel wall and invade adjacent organs and tissues.
      b.   Lymphatic system: cancer cells penetrate the lymphatic system and are distributed along lymphatic channels.
      c.   Implantation: cancer cells implant into a body organ. Certain cells have an affinity for particular organs and body areas.
      d.   Seeding: a primary tumor sloughs off tumor cells into a body cavity, such as the peritoneal cavity.
D.   Etiology:
   1.   Viruses
   2.   Exposure to carcinogens: sunlight, radiation, tobacco use, or chemical agents can produce toxic effects by altering DNA structure in body sites distant from chemical exposure (e.g., dyes, asbestos)
   3.   Genetic and familial factors
   4.   Hormonal agents: tumor growth is promoted by disturbances in hormonal balance of the body's own (endogenous) hormones or administration of exogenous hormones (e.g., prolonged estrogen replacement, oral contraceptives).

Prevention

A.   Cancer prevention.
   1.   Eat a balanced diet that includes fresh fruits and vegetable, adequate amount of fiber, and a decreased fats and preservatives; avoid smoked and salt-cured foods containing increased nitrates.
   2.   Avoid exposure to know carcinogens—e.g., cigarette smoking and sun exposure.
   3.   Maintain weight in normal range
   4.   Get enough rest and sleep.
   5.   Decreased stress, or perception of stress, improves ability to effectively manage stress.
   6.   Regular exercise, encourage least 30 minutes of moderate to vigorous exercise 5 days a week.
   7.   Limit alcohol use.
B.   Screening guidelines—early detection.
   1.   Pap test: screening should begin within 3 years of becoming sexually active or at age 21; thereafter should be done annually or every 2 years. Age 30, after 3 normal Pap tests, then Pap screening every 3-4 years.
   2.   Digital rectal examination (DRE): DRE with prostate-specific antigen blood test should be offered to men annually beginning at age 50. African-American males and those men with strong family history should begin at age 45.
   3.   Colon: beginning at age 50, all clients should have either a yearly fecal occult blood test or a flexible sigmoidoscopy every 5 years and/or both, depending on the client's risk factors.
   4.   Breast: annual mammogram and clinical breast exam (CBE) for women over 40. Women ages 20-39 should have a CBE every 3 years. Monthly breast self-examination is an option for women in their 20s, but does not replace need for CBE or mammogram.
   5.   Testicular self-examination: monthly from age 20 to 40.

Treatment of Cancer

A. Diagnostic studies.
1. Chest x-ray.
2. Tissue biopsy.
3. Radiologic studies: mammography, ultrasonography.
4. Radioisotopic scans: bone, liver, lung, brain.
5. Spiral computed tomography (CT).
6. Cytology studies (bone marrow aspiration, urine and cerebrospinal fluid analysis, cell washings, Pap smears and bronchial washings).
7. Position emission tomography (PET) scan.
8. Tumor markers.
9. Sigmoidoscopy or colonoscopy examinations—including stool for occult blood.
10. CBC, chemistry profile, liver function tests.
11. Bone marrow examination (if hematolymphoid malignancy is suspected).
B. Biopsy.
1. Used for definitive diagnosis.
2. Needle: tissue samples are obtained by aspiration or with a large-bore needle.
3. Incisional: tumor mass may be too large for removal; this may be done for staging the disease level. Incisional: a scalpel or dermal punch is used to obtain a tissue sample.
4. Excisional: involves removal of the entire tumor.
5. Endoscopic biopsy: direct biopsy through an endoscopy of the area (gastrointestinal, respiratory, genitourinary tracts).

Goals of Cancer Therapy

A. Cure: client will be disease-free and live to normal life expectancy.
B. Control: client's cancer is not cured but controlled by therapy over long periods of time.
C. Palliative: maintain as high a quality of life for the client when cure and control are not possible; neither hastens nor postpones death, but provides relief of symptoms experienced by the dying client.
D. Prophylaxis: provide treatment when no tumor is detectable but when client is known to be at risk for tumor development, spread, or recurrence.

Modalities of Cancer Treatment

A. Surgery: excision of the tumor or extensive resection of tumor and surrounding tissue.
1. Evaluate any adverse effects of previous treatment and their implications for proposed surgery (e.g., poor nutritional status or fibrosis from effects of radiation therapy that may lead to poor wound healing, leukopenia from chemotherapeutic agents).
2. Evaluate extent of disfigurement or debilitation caused by surgery and consider its impact on client (e.g., ostomy formation, amputation).
3. Promote healthful self-image and return to normal lifestyle by recommending cancer support groups and other rehabilitation resources.
B. Chemotherapy: overall goal of chemotherapy is to attack the cancer cell during its most vulnerable stage.
1. Chemotherapy agents are administered in doses large enough to damage or kill cancer cells, but small enough to limit adverse effects to safe and tolerable levels.
2. Nursing implications in chemotherapy (Table 2-4):
    a. Collect data on client for symptoms of bone marrow depression (increased bruising and bleeding, sore throat, fever).
    b. Prevent exposure of client to people with communicable diseases.
    c. Before therapy, establish a baseline regarding intake and output, bowel habits, oral hygiene, psychological status, and family relationships.
    d. Monitor fluid intake and output; maintain adequate hydration to prevent urinary complications.
    e. Client education.
        (1) Client should avoid all over-the-counter (OTC) medications while on chemotherapy.
        (2) If treated on an outpatient basis, client should not alter dosages and should maintain schedule of administration.

> **TEST ALERT: Follow procedures when handling biohazardous materials (such as sharps, radioactive sources, and chemotherapeutic materials).**

C. Radiation therapy.
1. The purpose of radiation therapy is to destroy the rapidly dividing cancer cells. Cells that are reproducing rapidly are more sensitive to the radiation.
    a. Time: client care should be coordinated to allow greatest amount of care to be provided in shortest time frame possible.
    b. Distance: except when giving direct care, attempt to maintain a distance of 6 feet from the source of radiation.
    c. Shield: some institutions provide lead shielding; generally not necessary if time and distance principles are observed.
2. Common side effects of radiation therapy.

> **NURSING PRIORITY: Adverse effects are related to the radiation dose delivered within a specified time, the method of delivery, and the client's overall health status.**

TABLE 2-4	NURSING IMPLICATIONS AND CHEMOTHERAPY
Problem	Nursing Implications

Bone marrow suppression: Thrombocytopenia (decreased platelets)	1. Initiate bleeding precautions and observe for bleeding tendency (bruising, hematuria, bleeding gums, etc). 2. Decrease invasive procedures; minimize injections.
Anemia (decreased hemoglobin)	1. Fatigue is normal with chemotherapy; client should report any significant increase in fatigue. 2. Encourage diet high in protein, calories, and iron; administer iron supplements.
Leukopenia (decreased white cells)	1. Advise health care provider regarding any unexplained temperature elevation above 100° F. 2. Monitor white cell (neutrophil) levels. 3. Protect client from exposure to infections: frequent hand hygiene, location of room, screen visitors, etc. 4. See Goals for Home-Care.
Pulmonary toxicity	1. Monitor for persistent nonproductive cough, fever, exertional dyspnea, and tachypnea. 2. Medications may be cumulative, pulmonary complications may be fatal.
Hyperuricemia (increased serum levels of uric acid)	1. Encourage fluid intake up to 3000 mL daily, if allowed. 2. Assess for involvement of the kidney, ureters, and bladder. 3. Allopurinol (**Zyloprim**) may be used as prevention or as treatment.
Alopecia	1. Encourage client to wear something to cover the scalp (e.g., wig, scarf, turban, hat). 2. Avoid exposure of scalp to sunlight. 3. Do not rub scalp; do not use hair rollers, hair dryers, curlers, or curling irons. 4. Hair usually grows back in 3-4 weeks after chemotherapy; is usually a different texture and color.

Stomatitis (mucositis)	1. Encourage good oral hygiene and frequent oral checks.
	  a. Encourage frequent mouth rinses of saline solution to keep mucous membranes moist.
	  b. Brush teeth with a small, soft toothbrush after every meal and at bedtime.
	  c. Remove dentures to prevent further irritation.
	2. Avoid alcohol, spicy or hot foods; mechanical soft, bland diet may be ordered.
	3. Rinse mouth with antacid solutions or viscous lidocaine for pain control.

GI: anorexia, nausea and vomiting, diarrhea, and constipation	1. Assist client to maintain good nutrition.
	  a. Discuss food preferences with client and dietitian; encourage small, frequent meals.
	  b. Correlate meals with antiemetic medications.
	  c. Encourage family to provide client with favorite foods.
	  d. Increase calories, protein, and iron; encourage supplemental vitamins.
	2. Monitor hydration status and electrolyte imbalances.
	3. Evaluate skin around anal area in the client with diarrhea; prevent excoriation.
	4. May be prone to constipation—maintain high fluid and high fiber intake.
	5. Monitor weight

Tissue irritation, necrosis, ulceration from infusion therapy	1. Monitor infusion site for infiltration, extravasation and for infection. 2. Extra precautions should be taken to prevent extravasation (infusion of chemotherapy medication into subcutaneous tissue): tape securely, assess for blood return, observe for continuous flow of IV.

a. Skin reactions.
   (1) Skin erythema, followed by dry desquamation of the skin in the treatment field.
   (2) Wet desquamation, particularly in areas of skinfolds (breast, perineum, axillary); skin may be blistered.
   (3) Loss of hair on the skin in the treatment field.
   (4) Skin pigmentation and discoloration.
b. Gastrointestinal disturbances are more pronounced when radiation is delivered to area closely associated with the GI tract.
c. Cystitis when radiation source is near to urinary tract.
d. Radiation pneumonitis.

3. Nursing implications for a client with an internal radiation source (implant or sealed source) (Box 2-2):
   a. Private room and bath.
   b. A lead container and tongs should be present in the client's room.
   c. If implant becomes dislodged, it should be picked up with the forceps and returned to the lead container. Notify radiation therapist or officer immediately.
   d. Observe time, distance, and shield precautions.
   e. Examples of this type of radiation therapy include uterine implants, testicular implants, or implants used in head and neck tumors.
   f. Inform all people coming in contact with the client of the specific precautions necessary.
   g. Use badges or radiation monitors for caregivers having direct client contact.
   h. List on the client's chart:
      (1) Type of radiation.
      (2) Time inserted.
      (3) Anticipated removal time.
      (4) Specific precautions for the type of radiation used.

> ✔ **NURSING PRIORITY:** *Check linens, bedpans, and other items for signs of a dislodged implant. Move client away from implant and use tongs to place it in a protective safety lead container, which should be in the client's room. Notify radiation therapy department of any problems.*

4. Nursing implications for the client receiving systemic radiation therapy.
   a. Systemically administered radionuclides (radioisotopes) may cause radioactive body secretions.
   b. May be necessary to have the linens and trash checked for radioactivity before removing them from the room.

Nursing Interventions

❖ Goal: To maintain client at optimal psychosocial level.
A. Encourage verbalization.
B. Assist client to understand disease process and therapeutic regimen.
C. Include family in the care.
D. Assist client to cope with changes in body image due to hair loss.
   1. Encourage client to select a head covering they are comfortable with (e.g., wig, turban, scarf, cap).
   2. Instruct client with regard to hair care.
      a. Use mild protein-based shampoo and conditioner to help prevent hair dryness.
      b. Advise client to shampoo only every 3 to 5 days.
      c. Teach client to pat, not rub, hair dry after shampooing to avoid excessive handling of brittle hair.
      d. Encourage client to avoid excessive brushing to prevent tearing or unnecessary manipulation of hair.
      e. Suggest client sleep on a satin pillowcase to decrease hair tangles and friction.
      f. Discourage use of electric hair dryers, hot rollers or crimpers, hair clips, sprays, dyes, or permanents to prevent further hair damage.
E. Recognize client's emotional outbursts and anger as part of coping process.
F. Encourage measures to maintain ego.
   1. Allow client to participate in own care and decision-making.
   2. Maintain active listening.
   3. Encourage personal lifestyle choices (e.g., clothing, makeup, hobbies).

❖ Goal: To maintain nutrition.
A. Diet: appropriate to age level.
   1. Increase calories; increase protein intake.
   2. Supplement diet with vitamins.
   3. Institute small, frequent feedings.
   4. Increase fluid intake.
   5. Use between-meal supplements.
B. Total parenteral nutrition (see Chapter 13).
C. Prevent and/or decrease complications associated with nutrition.
   1. Anorexia.
   2. Nausea and vomiting.
   3. Stomatitis.
      a. Follow good oral hygiene after each meal and at bedtime.
      b. Observe oral mucosa daily.
      c. Provide nonirritating foods.
      d. Keep mucous membranes moist; encourage fluid intake to prevent dehydration.

❖ Goal: To maintain normal elimination pattern.
A. Provide adequate fluids and fiber in diet to prevent constipation.

BOX 2-2 RADIATION SAFETY PRECAUTIONS AND NURSING IMPLICATIONS

Internal Implant
- Provide private room and bath.
- Plan care so minimal time is spent in the room.
- When prolonged care is required, use a lead shield or wear a lead apron.
- Wear a film badge to measure exposure; do not share badges.
- Mark on the room and in the Kardex that pregnant women, infants, and young children should not come in contact with the client during treatment.
- Check all linens and materials removed from the bed for presence of foreign bodies that could be a source of radioactivity.
- Keep long-handled forceps and lead container in the room of a client with an implant in place.
- Post notice on client's door – visits should be limited to 30 minutes per day and advise them to stay about 6 feet from the client.

External Radiation
- Do not wash off marks placed on client's body for purpose of identifying area for external radiation.
- Skin reactions after radiation therapy may not develop for 10 to 14 days and may not subside until 2 to 4 weeks after treatment.
- Gently cleanse skin with a mild soap; do not remove skin markings.
- Avoid tight-fitting clothing; encourage loose-fitting cotton clothes.
- Avoid direct sunlight on radiation area.
- Avoid exposure of treatment area to all heat and/or cold sources (hot baths, hot water bottles, ice packs)
- Do not apply any perfumed or medicated lotions or creams.
- Advise client to avoid swimming during treatment period; chemicals can irritate the skin.
- Do not use tape, adhesive bandages, cosmetics, lotions, perfumes, powders, or deodorants on the skin in the treatment field.
- Closely monitor skin condition on area where x-ray treatment is directed.

B. Prevent and/or decrease complications of diarrhea.
  1. Antidiarrheal medications.
  2. Low-residue, high-protein, bland diet.
  3. Evaluate fluid status.
  4. Prevent anal irritation.
    a. Thorough cleansing of rectal area with mild soap and water.
    b. Avoid irritation of the rectal area.
    c. Use ointments and sprays to decrease discomfort and promote healing.

C. Prevent urinary tract infections, primarily cystitis.
  1. Maintain adequate fluid intake: 3000 mL/day.
  2. Frequently assess for symptoms of cystitis (see Chapter 18).
  3. Avoid bladder catheterization if possible.
D. Minimize embarrassment of incontinence and provide appropriate hygiene measures.

❖ Goal: To prevent and/or decrease infectious process.
A. Carefully assess for temperature elevations greater than 100° F orally.
B. Administer antibiotics.
C. Maintain good personal hygiene.
D. Child should be isolated from communicable diseases, especially chickenpox.
E. Frequently assess for potential infectious processes – urinary tract, upper respiratory tract.
F. Do not clean bird cages or cat litter boxes.
G. Cook or peel fruits and vegetables.

✔ **NURSING PRIORITY:** *Implement measures to protect the immunocompromised client.*

❖ Goal: To prevent and/or decrease hematological complications (see Chapter 9).
A. Observe for bleeding problems associated with bone marrow depression.
  1. Increased bruising.
  2. Bleeding gums.
  3. Hematuria.
  4. Anemia (decreased hemoglobin levels).
  5. Nosebleed (epistaxis).
  6. Presence of blood in the stool.

✔ **NURSING PRIORITY:** *Advise client to use electric razor and a soft-bristle toothbrush, and avoid dental flossing if gums are bleeding.*

B. Anemia.
  1. Maintain adequate rest; encourage client to pace activities to avoid fatigue.
  2. *Assess respiratory and cardiac systems and report changes to RN.*
  3. Encourage a diet high in protein, vitamins, and iron.
❖ Goal: To maintain activity level.
A. Encourage daily activities appropriate to developmental level.
B. Assist client to evaluate activity patterns and encourage periods of rest.
C. Avoid fatigue.
❖ Goal: To relieve pain (see Chapter 3).
A. Evaluate client's and family's response to pain.
B. Evaluate characteristics of pain.

C. Promote general comfort, identify and implement non-pharmacologic approaches to pain relief (positioning, imagery, hypnosis, etc.).

D. Administer medications for pain relief.

❖ Goal: To recognize complications specific to radiation and chemotherapy.

A. Alopecia.

B. Hemorrhagic problems.

C. Gastrointestinal distress.

D. Bone marrow depression (myelosuppression).

E. Skin reactions.

F. Decreased immune response.

Home Care

❖ Goal: To effectively manage pain to provide client optimal rest and pain relief.

A. Assist client to identify provoking and alleviating factors and adjust environment accordingly.

B. Assist client with nonpharmacologic pain therapies (Chapter 3).

C. Layer pain management strategies as needed; medicate with narcotic and non-narcotic analgesics as necessary.

D. Assess effectiveness of therapies and medications and modify as necessary.

❖ Goal: To decrease or limit exposure to infection.

A. Limit number of people having direct contact with the client.

B. Good oral hygiene: regular flossing if there is no bleeding problem and no tissue irritation; soft toothbrush; avoid irritating foods.

C. Client should avoid coming in direct contact with animal excreta (cat litter boxes, bird cages, etc).

D. Teach client to take his or her temperature daily and report temperature over 100° F (38° C).

E. Use antipyretics cautiously because they tend to mask infection.

G. Teach client about radiation-induced skin reactions and provide nursing care for these skin reactions (Box 2-2).

1. Moisturize skin 3 to 4 times a day with nonperfumed, nonmedicated cream or lotion.

2. If moist desquamation occurs, cleanse gently with normal saline solution; area should be gently patted dry or air-dried; expose areas to air for 10 to 15 minutes three times a day.

3. Avoid use of perfumes, deodorants, powders, and cosmetics to affected area.

4. Wear loose-fitting cotton clothing; avoid swimming.

5. If dry desquamation is present, apply lotion that is not perfumed, not medicated, and does not contain alcohol.

H. Teach client importance of frequent handwashing.

❖ Goal: To maintain optimum psychosocial function

A. Provide opportunities for client to express feelings, concerns, and fears.

B. Encourage activity; one of the best activities is walking for about 30 minutes at a rate that is comfortable.

Study Questions: Health Implications Across the Life Span

1. The nurse finds the client's radiation implant in the bed. What is the best nursing action?
   1 Using tongs, replace it in the lead container in the room.
   2 Immediately evacuate the client and all others from the room.
   3 Wearing gloves, replace the implant into the body cavity.
   4 Call radiation control to pick up the implant.

2. What immunizations will be given to an infant within the first 6 months?
   1 Varicella, diphtheria, polio, hepatitis B.
   2 Diphtheria, pertussis, tetanus, hepatitis B, polio.
   3 Polio, measles, mumps, rubella, diphtheria, tetanus.
   4 Varicella, measles, mumps, rubella, diphtheria.

3. The mother of a newborn asks when she can begin to give her infant solid food. What is the best response?
   1 Begin cereals at 3 months; then begin fruits at 6 months.

2 Start fruits as the first solids at 6 months, then vegetables.
   3 Fruits can be started at 3 months, followed by cereal.
   4 Cereals are started at 4-6 months, followed by fruit or vegetables.

4. A mother arrives at the office with her 9-month-old infant for a well-baby check. What observation would cause the most concern?
   1 Cannot sit alone without support.
   2 Shows no interest in walking.
   3 Anterior fontanel remains open.
   4 Does not respond to name.

5. The nurse understands that the major difference between benign tumors and malignant tumor is that malignant tumors:
   1 Are encapsulated and immovable.
   2 Grow at a faster rate.
   3 Invade adjacent tissue and metastasize.
   4 Cause death while benign ones do not.

6. The nurse understands that there are general adverse effects of antineoplastic drugs. Select all that apply:
    _____ 1 Peripheral edema.
    _____ 2 Anorexia.
    _____ 3 Stomatitis.
    _____ 4 Increase in urine specific gravity.
    _____ 5 Alopecia.
    _____ 6 Nausea.

7. What is important to teach a client regarding self-care during radiation therapy?
    1 Remove skin dye tattoos between treatments
    2 Avoid exposure to the sun and do not remove dye markers
    3 Reduce carbohydrate and protein intake during treatments.
    4 Decrease fluid intake and increase carbohydrate intake after treatment.

8. A client on chemotherapy therapy is experiencing nausea and vomiting. What is the best nursing action?
    1 Give antiemetics and monitor hydration.
    2 Administer oral care and assess for mouth lesions.
    3 Decrease fluid intake and monitor renal function.
    4 Record daily weight and encourage small meals.

9. At what age does a child begin to discriminate between the mother's face and a stranger's face?
    1 One month
    2 Six weeks
    3 Four months
    4 Thirty weeks

10. A client is receiving chemotherapy for lung cancer. The nurse understands that the mediation can cause renal damage. What is an important nursing action?
    1 Encourage fluids to increase the acidity of urine.
    2 Monitor daily weight and daily intake and output.
    3 Decrease fluids to reduce edema formation.
    4 Monitor urinalysis for presence of bacteria.

11. A client is on furosemide (Lasix) for his heart condition. What foods would the nurse encourage the client to eat?
    1 Breads and fortified cereals.
    2 Dried fruits and juices.
    3 Leafy green vegetables
    4 Lean red mean and whole grains.

12. A client arrives in the emergency department with a penetrating wound he received while working chopping trees. What is an important nursing action?
    1 Cleanse the wound with antibacterial solution
    2 Administer gamma globulin intramuscularly
    3 Anticipate notifying poison control for plant toxicology.
    4 Determine when client received last tetanus injection.

Answers and rationales to these questions are in the section at the end of the book titled Chapter Study Questions: Answers and Rationales.

Nursing Concepts

A. Maslow's hierarchy of basic human needs.
   1. Human behavior is motivated by a system of needs.
   2. Clients will focus or attempt to satisfy needs at the base of the pyramid before focusing on those higher up (Figure 3-1).
   3. Human needs are *universal*; however, some may be modified by cultural influence.
   4. The nursing process is always concerned with physiological needs first; then progresses to teaching, decreasing anxiety, etc. This is also true for the client with psychosocial needs; the client's physiological needs must be met before progressing to the next level.

> ✓ *NURSING PRIORITY: Pay attention to Maslow's hierarchy of needs when answering test questions related to setting priorities. The physiological needs at the base of the pyramid must be satisfied first in order to focus on other needs—and remember that oxygenation is always the first physiological need or priority.*

STEPS OF THE NURSING PROCESS

* **The categories of the nursing process and the activities in each category vary somewhat according to nursing authors. The nursing process as presented here correlates with the categories of the NCLEX-PN.**

Data Collection

A. Collecting data.
   1. Objective data are nursing observations.
Example: Client weighs 125 lb; 50 mL of green drainage via the nasogastric tube.
   2. Subjective data are information given by the client.
Example: "My side hurts; I am scared about surgery."
   3. Client data are collected using three skills.
   a. Observation: what can be seen.
Example: Is the client awake or asleep; is the client obese or underweight; is the client smiling or frowning?
   b. Auscultation: what can be heard.
Example: Is the client laughing; are there breath sounds present; do you hear hyperactive bowel sounds?
   c. Palpation: what can be felt.
Example: Is the client's skin warm and dry; does the client have a pedal pulse; is the client's abdomen soft?

Planning

A. Assign priority to the nursing care activities.
B. Specify goals reflecting desired outcome of nursing care.
   1. Develop short-term and long-term goals.
   2. Identify nursing interventions for goal attainment.
   3. Establish outcome criteria.
C. Develop the written nursing care plan.
   1. Involve client and family in all aspects of planning.
   2. Keep care plan current and flexible.

Implementing

A. Initiate and carry out planned nursing activities.
B. Coordinate activities of client and family members along with health team members.
C. Document client's responses to nursing actions.

Evaluating

A. Collect objective and subjective data and determine if goals were achieved.
B. Identify and make revisions to the nursing care plan.

Maslow's Hiearchy of Basic Human Needs

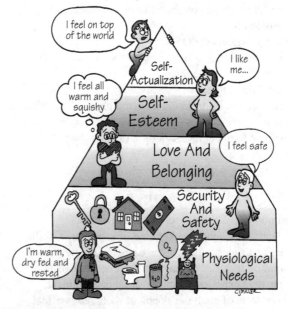

FIGURE 3-1 **Maslow's hierarchy of needs.** (From Zerwekh J, Claborn J, Miller CJ: *Memory notebook of nursing, vol 1*, ed 4, Ingram, 2008, Nursing Education Consultants.)

HEALTH ASSESSMENT

Health History

 TEST ALERT: Collect baseline physical data on admission.

✳ **The health history is a primary source of client information. The source of the information can be the client, relatives, friends, old records, or any combination of these. A predetermined format should be used as a guide for the interview.**

A. Demographic data.
1. Name, address, phone number, age, sex, marital status.
2. Race, religion, usual source of medical care.

B. Chief complaint/reason for visit.
1. Chief complaint (CC) is main reason client sought health care.
2. CC is recorded in client's own words.

Example: "I have been vomiting blood since this morning."

C. History of the present illness.
1. Chronological narrative story of the history of the present state of health.
2. Includes relevant family history.

D. Past history.
1. Childhood diseases.
2. Immunizations.
3. Allergies.
4. Hospitalizations and serious illnesses.
5. Accidents and injuries.
6. Medications.
7. Prenatal, labor and delivery, or neonatal history (recorded for all children under age 5 and older children with a congenital or developmental problem).

E. Review of systems (ROS).
1. Is a verbal listing from head to toe of the client's overall state of health.
2. Contains subjective data given by the client; does not contain information from the physical examination. Specific assessment data for each body system can be found at the beginning of each chapter.

HEALTH TEACHING

Principles of Client Education

A. Common characteristics of the adult learner.
1. The adult client's background of experience, skills, and attitudes will form the basis for any new information received. Frequently the client has had no positive experiences in a hospital environment.
2. The level of adult development will greatly affect the client's readiness to learn. If a client is in a mid-life transition, it may be very difficult to learn new attitudes and skills that threaten self-image.

Example: A man in his early 40s may have difficulty accepting any education regarding his colostomy.

B. Factors contributing to the teaching-learning process.
1. Readiness to learn.
a. The client must feel the material is relevant to his/her health, and must be willing to put forth the effort to learn.
b. The client must have the mental capacity to learn, as well as the physical ability to perform the skills.
c. The client must have physical and safety needs met before focusing on learning. If a client exerts all of his/her energy to cope with the physical stress, then he/she has little energy for learning.
d. Comfort.
(1) Physical comfort: discomforts (such as pain, nausea, hunger, need to void) are distractors to the learning process.
(2) Psychological comfort: anger, frustrations, fear, and guilt severely hamper the learning process.
e. Before the teaching-learning process can begin, the client and the nurse need to discuss and agree on specific long-term and short-term goals. The nurse must carefully evaluate the client's knowledge of the problem.

C. Factors relating to the presentation.
1. State the specific objective of each teaching session: exactly what the client is to gain.
2. Use vocabulary and terminology appropriate to the client's understanding and to his or her developmental level. Use correct terms for body parts.
3. Try to stimulate as many senses as possible. Use charts, handouts, and pieces of equipment when appropriate.
4. Repetition is an integral part of learning. Be ready to repeat the material or to have the client repeat the skill until he/she does it correctly and becomes comfortable with the skill.
5. The more active the client is in the process, the better he/she will retain the information.
6. Plan short sessions; do not overwhelm the client with too much information at one time.
7. When appropriate, actively involve the family and significant others.
8. Be generous with positive reinforcement.

D. Pediatric factors influencing the learning process.
1. Intellectual development moves from the concrete to the abstract.
2. The nurse needs to assess the developmental level of the child before planning the educational approach.
a. Preschool client.
(1) The preschool child frequently experiences fears of body injury. Explanations should be simple.

(2) Separation anxiety is a problem in this age group; include parents in teaching session.

(3) The preschool child is aware of the physical and mechanical causes of problems he/she can see; the child is unaware of physical and mechanical forces that he/she cannot see.

b. School-age client.

(1) Benefits from tours, drawings, anatomical dolls.

(2) Learns well from role-playing and puppets.

(3) Needs to include parents in teaching session for reinforcement and to maintain consistency.

c. Adolescent client.

(1) Needs to be as independent as possible in management of health problem.

(2) Needs assistance in coping with loss of independence and self-direction.

(3) Educational programs need to help adolescent deal with changes in body image and in maintaining ego.

E. Older adult client.

1. Determine the older adult client's functional losses (i.e., hearing or vision impairment, memory loss).

2. Identify social support to aid the older adult; this often increases compliance with information being taught.

3. Determine hearing and visual acuity and make adjustments to leaning process.

4. Determine if the client is experiencing any confusion or disorientation. Ask client to include family member in teaching activity.

BASIC NURSING SKILLS

Hygienic Nursing Measures

 TEST ALERT: Assist with activities of daily living.

A. Beds and comfort measures.

1. Avoid shaking linens.

2. Hold all soiled linens away from your uniform.

3. Mattresses.

a. Alternating pressure mattress.

(1) Provides a continuous shift of pressure by alternating inflation and deflation of air or water every 2 to 5 minutes.

(2) Used to prevent development of or to treat pressure ulcers.

b. Eggcrate mattress.

(1) Foam rubber mattress with projections that look like an eggcrate.

(2) Placed on top of a regular mattress.

(3) Used to prevent pressure areas from developing in a bedridden client.

B. Bathing.

1. Types of bath.

a. Bed bath.

b. Partial bath.

c. Shower.

d. Therapeutic bath: sitz bath or medicated bath.

2. Nursing implications.

a. Room should be kept warm, bath should begin with clean areas and progress to dirty areas.

b. To prevent dry skin, irritation, and infection, carefully rinse all surface areas and dry them.

c. Keep client warm by using a bath blanket and controlling room temperature.

d. Ensure quiet and privacy.

e. Moisturize skin with lotion.

> ✔ **NURSING PRIORITY:** *Clients who are receiving external radiation therapy should not be bathed with soap over the area of the radiation, which will be marked. Lotions and powders should not be used on the area.*

3. Levels of personal care.

a. Complete care: Client requires total assistance from nurse because client is able to do little or nothing without assistance.

b. Partial care: Client performs as much of his or her own care as possible; nurse usually completes remaining care.

c. PM care (bedtime or hour of sleep): Is provided to prepare client for a relaxing, uninterrupted period of sleep; includes oral care, possible partial bathing, skin care, soothing back massage, straightening or changing the bed linen, and offering the bedpan or urinal.

C. Oral hygiene.

1. Includes care of the client's teeth or dentures, gums, tongue, and lips.

2. When providing oral care to unconscious client, turn the client's head to the side to prevent aspiration.

D. Hair care.

1. Newborn infants need scalp scrubbed daily to prevent cradle cap.

2. Adolescents usually require more frequent shampooing because of increase in oily secretions.

3. Older adult clients will need to shampoo less often.

Body Alignment and Range of Motion (ROM)

A. Characteristics of correct body alignment in bed.

1. Head up with eyes looking straight forward.

2. Neck and back straight.

3. Arms relaxed and supported at sides.

4. Legs parallel to hips with knees slightly flexed.

5. Feet separated and parallel to the legs with the toes pointed upward and slightly outward.

BOX 3-1   STERILE TECHNIQUE: PROCEDURES AND GUIDELINES

Procedures Requiring Sterile Technique
- Surgical procedures in the operating room (e.g., transurethral prostatectomy [TURP], appendectomy).
- Biopsies in the operating room, treatment room, or client's room.
- Catheterizations of the heart, bladder, or other body cavities.
- Injections: intramuscular (IM), subcutaneous (subQ), intradermal.
- Infusions: IV, instillations or infusions of medication or radioactive isotopes into body cavities.
- Dressing changes:
  - Usually, first postoperative dressing change done by using sterile technique.
  - Dressings over catheters inserted into body cavities (e.g., Hickman catheter, subclavian lines, dialysis access sites).
  - Dressings of clients with burns, immunological disorders, and skin grafts.

Guidelines for Sterile Field
- Never turn your back on a sterile field.
- Avoid talking.
- Keep all sterile objects within view (e.g., below waist is not within sterile field).
- Moisture will carry bacteria across/through a cloth or paper barrier.
- Transfer of objects from sterile to contaminated (not sterile) = contaminated.
- Do not reach across a sterile field.

B. Range of motion (ROM).
1. Active ROM.
   a. Client performs exercise without assistance.
   b. Used for client who independently performs activities of daily living (ADLs), but for some reason is immobilized or limited regarding activity.
   c. Goal is muscle strengthening, as well as maintenance and prevention of muscle atrophy.
2. Passive ROM.
   a. Client cannot actively move.
   b. Cannot contract muscles; therefore muscle strengthening cannot be accomplished.
   c. Goal is to maintain joint flexibility and prevent contractures.
C. Principles of ROM exercises.
1. Stretch muscles by moving the body part; avoid movement to the point of discomfort.
2. Perform ROM at least twice daily on immobile clients, with a minimum of four to five repetitions of each exercise.
3. Always support extremity above and below the joint when doing passive ROM on extremities.
4. Involve the client in planning the exercise program.

 TEST ALERT: Provide for mobility needs – ambulation, range of motion, repositioning.

Asepsis

A. Medical asepsis.
1. Designed to reduce the number of pathogens in an area and decrease the likelihood of their transfer (e.g., hand hygiene).

✔ **NURSING PRIORITY:** Proper hand hygiene is one of the most important procedures for the prevention of infection.

2. Often referred to as clean technique.
3. Administering oral medications, giving enemas, providing tube feedings, and practicing daily hygiene are all carried out with the clean technique.
B. Surgical asepsis.
1. Designed to not just simply reduce the number of pathogens but to make the object free of all microorganisms.
2. Also known as sterile technique.
3. Surgical asepsis is implemented for sterile procedures, such as changing sterile dressings, completing sterile catheterizations, and performing surgical procedures in the operating room (Box 3-1).

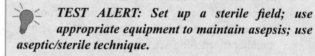 **TEST ALERT: Set up a sterile field; use appropriate equipment to maintain asepsis; use aseptic/sterile technique.**

Postmortem Care

A. Determine whether there are any tissues or organs to be donated.
B. Consult with the nursing supervisor to determine whether the client's death needs to be reported and or if the client's death necessitates an autopsy.
1. Death resulting from an accident, homicide, or suicide.
2. Unattended death; death occurring at a workplace or during incarceration.
C. Perform postmortem care as soon as possible.
1. Determine whether family wants to participate in post mortem care.
2. Unless client is to have an autopsy, remove all equipment according to facility policy.
3. Cleanse the body and cover with a clean sheet. Place a pillow under the head and leave the arms on the outside of the sheet. Deodorize room if necessary.
4. Offer the family an opportunity to be with the client. Provide privacy in an unrushed atmosphere.

5. Return all personal belongings to the family. Document what items were taken and by whom.
6. Attach identifying name tag to the body and to the shroud. Shroud the body according to facility policy.

> ✔ *NURSING PRIORITY: Make sure there is correct identification attached to the body before allowing the body to be removed from the nursing unit.*

Wound Care

✳ **A wound is a disruption in normal tissue caused by traumatic injury; also may be surgically created.**
A. Nursing goals.
   1. Promote healing.
   2. Prevent further damage.
   3. Prevent infection.
B. Wound healing is affected by:
   1. Nutritional status.
      a. Adequate calories and protein are necessary for tissue healing.
      b. The obese client is at increased risk for poor wound healing.
   2. Excessive wound drainage: impairs tissue regeneration and will harbor bacteria.
   3. Aging: slowing of tissue regeneration.
   4. Infection: prolongs inflammation and delays wound granulation.
   5. Location and approximation of wound edges.
   6. Circulation to the wound.
C. Characteristics of wound healing.
   1. Black wounds.
      a. Necrotic devitalized tissue; high risk for infection.
      b. Frequently require sharp or surgical debridement of tissue for healing to occur.
   2. Yellow wounds.
      a. Contain devitalized tissue; require cleaning for healing to occur.
      b. Mechanical debridement requires irrigations and dressing changes. A 19G intravenous (IV) catheter on a 30mL syringe provides safe pressure for irrigation and removal of devitalized tissue.
      c. Wet-to-dry dressings, wet-to-moist dressings, wound packing, and enzymatic debridement may be used to cleanse yellow wounds.
      d. Hydrocolloidal dressings to retain moisture.
   3. Red wounds.
      a. Require protection of fragile granulation tissue.
      b. Topical antibiotic ointment and nonadhering dressings may be used on shallow wounds.
      c. Wounds should be kept moist (moisture-retention dressings, hydrogel dressing); dry dressings will damage the new granulation tissue.

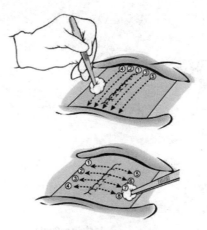

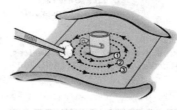

FIGURE 3-2 **Wound cleansing.** (From deWit, S. *Fundamental skills and concepts for nursing,* ed 3, St Louis, 2009, Saunders Elsevier.)

D. Process of wound healing.
   1. Primary intention: wound edges approximated and closed (surgical incision).
   2. Secondary intention: wound left open to heal from the inside out with the formation of granulation tissue.
E. Nursing interventions.

> ✔ *NURSING PRIORITY: When cleansing an area, always start at the cleanest area and work away from that area. Never return to an area you have previously cleaned. Discard the cleansing swab after each horizontal or vertical stroke.*

   1. Cleansing of wound. (Figure 3-2)
      a. Horizontal wound: cleansed from center of incision outward, then laterally.
      b. Vertical wound: cleansed from top to bottom, then laterally.
      c. Drain or a stab wound: cleansed in a circular motion.
   2. Wound irrigations: commonly used for large open wounds that are healing by secondary intention.
      a. Direct the solution from the top to the bottom of the wound, and from clean to contaminated areas.
      b. Irrigation solution should be warmed to promote comfort.
      c. Position client to promote gravity drainage from wound.
   3. Drains are inserted into an open wound to prevent the accumulation of secretions and exudate. (Figure 3-3).
      a. Penrose drain: soft flexible drain inserted into wound.

WOUND DRAIN AND SUCTION DEVICES

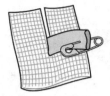

A, Penrose drain.

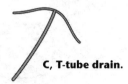

C, T-tube drain.

B, Hemovac drainage system.

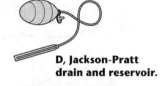

D, Jackson-Pratt drain and reservoir.

FIGURE 3-3   **Medical – Wound drain and suction devices.** (From deWit, S, *Surgical Nursing: Concepts and Practice,* St Louis, 2009, Saunders Elsevier.)

> ✔ ***NURSING PRIORITY:*** *Avoid pooling of excessive drainage under saturated dressing; this can lead to skin irritation and infection.*

     (1) A safety pin or clip may be inserted through the Penrose drain to prevent it from slipping further back into the wound.
     (2) Frequent dressing changes are preferable to reinforcing the same dressing.
   b. Jackson-Pratt catheter or drainage system: Bulb must be compressed to allow air to escape and then is recapped to maintain suction.
   c. Hemovac: Evacuator must be compressed at least every 4 hours to provide suction; be sure to empty drainage from pouring spout.
  4. Wet-to-dry dressings.
   a. Purpose is to trap necrotic tissue in the dressing as it dries.
   b. Dressing should be moist when applied and allowed to dry for 4 to 6 hours.
   c. When dressing is changed, the packed dressing should be gently removed along with absorbed drainage and nonviable tissue. Do not soak packing before removal; this will decrease the removal of nonviable tissue.

> ✔ ***NURSING PRIORITY:*** *When performing wet to dry dressing change, wring out excessive moisture from dressings. The dressings should be thick and wet enough to dry between dressing changes.*

  5. Montgomery straps: used when frequent dressing changes are needed; help to prevent skin irritation that could occur with tape removal.

  6. Elasticized abdominal binders assist to prevent tension on the suture line, especially beneficial in obese clients. (Figure 3-4)
  7. Obtain a specimen of wound drainage.
   a. Gently roll a sterile swab in the purulent drainage.
   b. Obtain wound specimen before any medication or antimicrobial agent has been applied to wound area or administered to client.

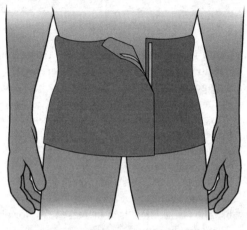

FIGURE 3-4   **Abdominal binding.** (From deWit, S. *Fundamental skills and concepts for nursing,* ed 3, St Louis, 2009, Saunders Elsevier.)

> ***TEST ALERT: Perform wound care and/or dressing change.***

Heat and Cold Applications

A. Heat applications.
  1. Purpose of heat application is to soften exudate and increase blood supply to promote healing.
  2. Unless a physician orders continuous heat applications, treatment time is usually 20 to 30 minutes.
  3. Caution client regarding hot baths and vasodilating effect that may cause postural hypotension.
  4. Moist heat penetrates deeper than dry heat.
  5. Do not use heat on an area that is being treated with radiation, is bleeding, has been injured within the last 24 hours, or has decreased sensation.
  6. Types of heat application.
   a. Moist heat pack.
   b. Pad that circulates warmed water to distribute dry heat to body parts. Cover the source to protect the skin.
   c. Heat lamp or heat cradle.
   d. Sitz bath, use clean water, not water the client has used for bathing.
B. Nursing intervention – heat application.
  1. Take vital signs before, during, and after heat application, if heat is applied to a large area.
  2. Unless an order is for continuous heat applications, treatment time is usually 20 minutes.

3. Closely observe skin under area of heat application.
4. Do not allow client to adjust temperature settings.
C. Cold applications.
1. Ice bag, ice collar, or ice glove.
2. Cold compress or cold pack.
3. Hypothermia blanket.
4. Reduces edema, swelling and pain if applied immediately after an injury.
5. May be used to decrease temperature.
D. Nursing intervention – cold application
1. Frequently check the temperature of a client with a hypothermia blanket for treatment of a fever.

 TEST ALERT: Provide cooling measure for elevated temperature.

2. Remove the cold pack if:
   a. There is mottling, or redness of skin.
   b. Client complains of burning pain or numbness.
3. Prevent chilling.
4. Do not use cold applications on areas of decreased circulation, open wounds, or area treated with radiation therapy.

✔ *NURSING PRIORITY: Do not use hot or cold applications with conditions of impaired circulation (e.g., peripheral vascular disease or diabetes).*

Specimen Collection

 TEST ALERT: Collect specimens for diagnostic testing.

A. General principles.
1. Use sterile equipment to obtain specimen and prevent contamination from outside sources.
2. Use the correct container for each specimen: Preservatives, anticoagulants, or chemicals may be required.
3. Always observe standard precautions when obtaining specimens, keep outside of container clean to prevent contamination in transfer to the laboratory.
4. Properly label the specimen. Collect the correct amount at the correct time.
B. Types of specimen.
1. Urine (see Appendix 18-3).
2. Stool (see Appendix 13-13).
3. Sputum: throat or nasopharyngeal (see Appendix 10-8).
4. Blood.
5. Wound specimen.

TABLE 3-1	NORMAL VITAL SIGNS
NEONATE	
Respiration	30-60 breaths/min
Pulse	120-140 beats/min
CHILD 2 TO 4 YEARS	
Respiration	24-32 breaths/min
Pulse	90-130 beats/min
CHILD 6 TO 10 YEARS	
Respiration	15-26 breaths/min
Pulse	70-110 beats/min
Blood pressure	90/40-110/60 mm Hg
ADULT	
Respiration	12-18 breaths/min
Pulse	60-100 beats/min
Blood pressure	100/60-120/80 mm Hg

✔ *NURSING PRIORITY: Know the range of normal values for vital signs at different age levels. This is critical for identifying changes in a client's status as well as for determining specific criteria for medication administration.*

Vital Signs

 TEST ALERT: Take client vital signs; compare changes in vital signs to client's baseline; notify supervisor or health care provider for change in client status.

A. Normal values (Table 3-1).
B. Assessment.
1. Respirations.
   a. Evaluate an infant's respiratory pattern before stimulation.
   b. Check thoracic cavity for symmetrical excursion.
   c. Breath sounds are best evaluated with client in sitting position.
2. Pulse rate.
   a. Irregular radial pulse (weak volume or low rate) should be assessed by taking an apical pulse rate reading for 1 full minute.
   b. Apical pulse is auscultated at the fifth intercostal space at the midclavicular line (point of maximal intensity, PMI).
   c. Apical-radial pulse is determined by two people counting both the apical and the radial pulse rates at the same time. This provides information about pulse deficit, which is the difference in the two values.
   d. A weak peripheral pulse may be evaluated by a Doppler ultrasound.
   e. Check apical pulse in neonates, infants, small children and in adult clients with irregular pulse.

3. Temperature.
   a. Temperature is affected by mouth breathing and temperature of oral intake.
   b. Oral temperature is taken unless otherwise indicated.
4. Blood pressure (BP) assessment (Box 3-2).

> ✔ *NURSING PRIORITY: Know the range of normal values for vitas signs at different levels. This is critical for identifying changes in a client's status as well as for determining criteria for medication administration.*

IMMOBILITY *Most highly tested!*

✱ **Immobility is the therapeutic or unavoidable restriction of a client's physical activity.**

A. Causes of restricted movement.
   1. Spinal cord or neurological injury.
   2. Presence of severe pain: arthritis, surgery, or injury.
B. Therapeutic reasons for restricted movement.
   1. To decrease pain.
   2. To immobilize a wound.
   3. To limit exercise and activity (e.g., clients with cardiac problems).
   4. To reduce effects of gravity on edema, varicosities.

Adverse Physical Effects of Immobility

The primary nursing goal in the care of the immobilized client is the prevention of complications. This is achieved by initiating nursing activities to prevent complications and by careful assessment of major organ systems for specific data indicating the effects of immobility.

A. Cardiovascular system.
   1. Physical effects.
      a. Orthostatic hypotension (drop in blood pressure [BP] upon standing).
      b. Decrease in ability of the heart to maintain output.
      c. Venous stasis.
      d. Increase in cardiac workload.
   2. Nursing implications.
      a. Position body to enhance circulation.
      b. Change position frequently.
      c. Use passive and active range of motion.
      d. Begin activity gradually; allow client to sit before standing.
B. Respiratory system.
   1. Physical effects.
      a. Decrease in thoracic excursion.
      b. Decrease in O_2/CO_2 exchange.
      c. Increase in pulmonary infections.
      d. Increase in collection of fluids in the lung.
   2. Nursing implications.
      a. Elevate head of bed.
      b. Maintain adequate hydration.
      c. Have client turn, cough, and deep breathe every 2 hours.

BOX 3-2 BLOOD PRESSURE ASSESSMENT

Procedure

Client should be in a sitting position without legs crossed. The inflatable cuff is wrapped snuggly around the upper half of the arm. The cuff is inflated 20 to 30 mm Hg above the point at which radial pulsation disappears. As the cuff is deflated, a sound is produced within the brachial artery just below the cuff and is audible with the stethoscope. The sounds (Korotkoff sounds) coincide with each pulse beat. Usually, when the cuff pressure is below diastolic, the sounds will cease or become muffled.

> ✔ *NURSING PRIORITY: It is important to ascertain and record when the sounds become muffled. If there is any doubt, the blood pressure (BP) may be recorded as a tripartite pressure (120/70/50 mm Hg), implying that the sound became muffled at 70 mm Hg and disappeared at 50 mm Hg.*

Nursing Implications

Size of cuff should be 20% wider than the diameter of the limb. If the cuff is too large (e.g., on a child's arm), the BP obtained will be substantially lower than the true BP. If the cuff is too small (e.g., on an obese person's arm), the BP obtained will be higher than the true BP. The difference in BP between the right and left arms is normally 5 to 10 mm Hg.

   d. Promote increase in activity as soon as possible; have client sit up in chair at bedside.
   e. Assess pulmonary secretions for infection.

> ✔ *NURSING PRIORITY: Encourage mobility to facilitate improvement in respiratory status, to assist in removal of secretions, to prevent pressure areas on the skin, prevent constipation, and prevent contractures.*

C. Urinary system.
   1. Physical effects.
      a. Urinary stasis.
      b. Increased calcium in urine may precipitate stone formation.
      c. Urinary tract infections.
   2. Nursing implications.
      a. Have client sit up to void, if possible.
      b. Increase fluid intake.
      c. Decrease calcium intake.
      d. Assess for urinary retention and urinary tract infection.
D. Musculoskeletal system.
   1. Physical effects.
      a. Demineralization of bones: decrease in bone strength.

PHYSIOLOGIC FACTORS

Organic origin
Integrity of nervous system,
    including endogenous opioids
Concomitant physical influences
    (stress, fatigue)
Age
Type of pain
Location
Intensity
Duration
Frequency
Quality
Threshold
Tolerance
Genetics

AFFECTIVE FACTORS

Distress of pain
Depression
Mood
Anxiety, fear, worry

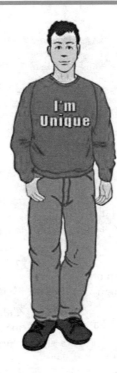

I'm Unique

PSYCHOSOCIAL INFLUENCES

Family and occupational roles
Personal beliefs
Spiritual belief system
Cultural/societal influences
Sexual identity and
    stereotypes
Demographic factors

COGNITIVE

Past experience
Meaning of pain
    experience
Attention paid to
    sensation/distraction
Expectations
Coping mechanisms
Knowledge
Values/attitudes
Communication skills

FIGURE 3-5   Considerations of the Pain Experience. (From: Black J, Hawks, J: *Medical Surgical Nursing: Clinical management for positive outcome,* ed 7, 2005, Philadelphia, Saunders.)

b. Muscle weakness and atrophy, paralytic ileus.
c. Loss of motion in joints leads to fibrosis and contractures.
2. Nursing implications.
  a. Perform range of motion exercises.
  b. Encourage active contraction and relaxation of large muscle groups.
  c. Position body to maintain proper alignment.
  d. Encourage daily weight bearing (standing at bedside) when possible.
E. Gastrointestinal system.
  1. Physical effects.
    a. Anorexia.
    b. Ineffective movement of feces through colon that leads to constipation.
    c. Diarrhea secondary to impaction.
  2. Nursing implications.
    a. Establish bowel program; for example, defecate every other day or three times a week.
    b. Encourage diet with adequate protein, bulk, and liquids.
    c. Check for impaction.
F. Integumentary system.
  1. Physical effects.
    a. Decrease in tissue perfusion leading to pressure ulcer.
    b. Decrease in sensation in an area of increased pressure.
  2. Nursing implications.
    a. Maintain cleanliness.

b. Promote circulation through frequent positioning changes.
c. Protect bony prominences when turning.
d. Prevent pressure areas from tight clothing, cast, or braces.
e. Perform frequent visual inspection of pressure areas.

 TEST ALERT: *Provide for mobility needs; maintain skin integrity; identify signs and symptoms of venous insufficiency.*

PAIN

* **Pain is a complex, universal experience.**
    Pain is a sensory perceptual experience
    Pain is a totally subjective personal experience
    Pain is an early warning sign; its presence triggers awareness that something is wrong in the body (Figure 3-5).
A. Types of Pain
  1. Acute pain: has an identifiable cause; is protective; short, predictable duration (lasting less than 3 months); it frequently has an immediate onset and is reversible or controllable with treatment. Most often has an identifiable source such as post operative pain that disappears as the wound heals.
  2. Chronic pain: lasts more than 6 months; continual or persistent and recurrent. Pain may not go away; periods of decreased and increased pain. Origin of pain may not be known.

BOX 3-3	MNEMONIC TO EVALUATE PAIN

P: Provoking or palliative factors
Q: Quality
R: Region
S: Severity
T: Timing

3. Referred pain: pain that does not occur at the point of injury. For example, pain related to myocardial ischemia may be felt in the left arm or shoulder; cholecystitis may be felt as shoulder pain.
4. Phantom pain: pain that follows the amputation of a body part; may be described as throbbing, cramping, or burning in the body part amputated.
5. Pretended pain (malingering): client expresses that there is pain when actually has no pain.
6. Psychogenic pain: pain due to emotional factors rather than physiological dysfunction.
B. Pain Assessment (Box 3-3).
  1. Pattern of pain.
    a. Pain onset and duration: when it started, precipitating causes, and how long it lasts.
    b. Breakthrough pain: transient; may be moderate to severe and occurs beyond current analgesic treatment; usually rapid onset and very intense.
  2. Area of pain.
    a. Ask the client to identify the pain site.
    b. Pain may be referred from the precipitating site to another location—shoulder pain with cholecystitis, left arm pain with MI.
    c. Sciatica pain follows a nerve pathway of the sciatic nerve, generally down the back of the thigh and inside the leg.
    d. Intensity of pain: use a pain or rating scale to help the client communicate the pain intensity.

BOX 3-4	ASSESSING THE HARMFUL EFFECTS OF PAIN

Acute Pain	**Chronic Pain**
Disturbs sleep	Fatigue
Appetite decreases	Weight gain
Fluid intake decreases	Poor concentration
Nausea and vomiting	Job loss
	Divorce
	Depression

✔ *NURSING PRIORITY: The nurse should administer pain medication to clients experiencing acute pain without fear of addicting the client to the medication.*

TEST ALERT: Validate pain utilizing a rating scale.

3. Type of pain -sharp, burning, throbbing, cramping.
4. Determine any activities and situations that precipitate or increase the level of the pain—movement, ambulation, coughing.
5. Client responses to pain.
  a. Increased blood pressure, pulse, and respirations.
  b. Diaphoresis, increased muscle tension, nausea and vomiting.
6. Client's interpretation and meaning of the pain experience.
7. Harmful effects of pain. (Box 3-4)

Cultural Implications of Pain

A. Cultural beliefs and values affect how a client responds to pain.
B. Nurses frequently assume that their own cultural implications of pain and the ways they deal with pain are the same as those of the client.
C. Assess attitudes and beliefs that may affect effective treatment of the pain. Some clients may believe that taking pain medications will cause "addiction"; other clients may believe that complaining of pain is a sign of weakness.
D. Avoid stereotyping clients by assuming a specific culture will or will not exhibit more or less pain.
E. Nursing considerations of pain control associated with a client's culture:
  1. Identify what the pain means to the client; for example, a woman in labor will perceive pain differently than a client who experiences pain as an indication of advanced disease.
  2. Identify cultural implications regarding how a client responds to or expresses pain; some clients moan and complain loudly while others may be very quiet and stoic.
  3. Individualize pain control based on the client's response to pain.
  4. Establish communication methods for the client to express level of pain and adequacy of pain control (e.g., pain scales, FACES scale, pictures, images).
  5. Expression of pain is subjective; accept client's perception and expression of pain, and facilitate nursing care to meet client's cultural needs in providing pain control.

TEST ALERT: Recognize cultural diversity in client's perception of and response to pain.

Noninvasive Pain Relief Measures

A. Nursing intervention for pain relief (nonpharmacological).
1. Change positions frequently and support body parts.
2. Encourage early ambulation after surgery.
3. Elevate swollen body parts.
4. Check drainage tubes to ensure that they are not stretched, kinked, or pulled.
5. Provide cutaneous stimulation through pressure, massage, bathing, and heat or cold therapy to promote relaxation.

> ✔ **NURSING PRIORITY:** *Low levels of anxiety or pain are easier to reduce or control than are higher levels; pain relief measures should be used before pain becomes severe.*

B. Relaxation techniques.
1. Relaxed muscles result in decreased pain level.
2. Typical relaxation exercises focus on deep breathing and alternate tensing and relaxing of various body parts in a systematic manner.
3. Meditation: focuses attention away from pain.
4. Rhythmic breathing: method of relaxation and distraction by focusing on the breath.
5. Music may assist in relaxation.
C. Guided imagery.
1. Creative visualization is the therapeutic use of images from one's imagination to focus away from pain sensation by emphasizing pleasant memories and experiences.
2. Often combined with relaxation and biofeedback.
D. Hypnosis is also used to produce a state of altered consciousness that is characterized by extreme responsiveness to suggestion.
E. Biofeedback: provides client with information about changes in body functions of which client is usually unaware (e.g., blood pressure, pulse rate).
F. Transcutaneous electric nerve stimulation (TENS).
1. Delivers an electrical current through electrodes applied to the skin surface of the painful region or to a peripheral nerve.
2. Identify trigger points (areas that are extremely sensitive when stimulated) and place electrodes.
3. Instruct client to adjust TENS unit intensity until it creates a pleasant sensation and relieves the pain.
G. Acupuncture: most common complementary therapy to decrease pain.
1. Requires insertion of thin metal needles into the body at designated points to relieve pain.
2. Is effective in pain management, as well as nausea and vomiting associated with postoperative and chemotherapy.
3. Encourage client to review the credentials of the practitioner, who should have a master's degree in oriental medicine and be registered to practice in the state.

> 💡 **TEST ALERT:** *Identify client need for PRN medications; provide nonpharmacological measures for pain relief; use an alternative/complimentary nursing actions in providing pain control (e.g., imagery, massage, repositioning).*

Medications for Pain Relief

A. Administer as-needed (PRN) analgesic medications (see Appendix 3-2: Analgesics).
1. Steps in administering PRN medications.
    a. Assess client to determine source and quality and characteristics of pain.
    b. Check client's chart.
        (1) Last medication received and route of administration.
        (2) The time administered.
        (3) Client's response to medication
    c. Check current order for pain medication.
    d. Select appropriate medication.
        (1) Use nonopioid analgesics for mild to moderate pain.
        (2) Avoid combinations of opioids for older adults.
        (3) IV medications act more rapidly for acute pain relief.
        (4) Avoid IM injections in older adults.
        (5) Sustained-release and extended-release oral medications work well for chronic pain management and will provide pain management over a longer period of time.

> ✔ **NURSING PRIORITY:** *Use a preventive approach in alleviating pain by administering narcotics before the pain occurs (if it can be predicted), or at least before it reaches severe intensity. This is particularly important in regard to care of the new postoperative client.*

    e. Document pain intervention.
    f. Decrease stimuli in room and determine other factors influencing discomfort.
    g. At 15- and 30-minute intervals, assess client's response to pain intervention and document nursing actions.
B. Types of medications.
1. Narcotic analgesics are used for relieving severe pain.
    *Example: Morphine, codeine, hydromorphone (**Dilaudid**), meperidine (**Demerol**), oxycodone (**Percodan**).*
2. Nonnarcotic analgesics act at peripheral sites to reduce pain.
    *Example: Propoxyphene (**Darvon**),*
3. Potentiating drugs are used to intensify the action of the narcotic agent.
    *Example: Promethazine (**Phenergan**), hydroxyzine (**Vistaril, Atarax**), diazepam (**Valium**).*

4. Nonsteroidal anti-inflammatory drugs have analgesic, anti-inflammatory, and antipyretic properties. *Example: Acetylsalicylic acid (ASA) or aspirin, acetaminophen (**Tylenol**), ibuprofen (**Motrin, Advil**), naproxen (**Naprosyn**).*

C. Patient-controlled analgesia (PCA).
 1. Client controls delivery of pain medication via a PCA pump.
 2. A common order is for 1 to 4 mg of morphine every 10 minutes until pain is relieved with a lockout dose of 10mg per hour.
 3. Check for parameters for bolus dose of medication.
    a. Should be available for episodes of increased pain (dressing changes, chest tube insertion, etc).
    b. For the client who goes to sleep and awakens with severe pain unrelieved by PCA.
    c. For cancer clients who experience breakthrough pain.
 4. Advantages of PCA.
    a. More effective pain control.
    b. Decreased client anxiety, client controls pain more effectively.
    c. Increased client independence.
    d. Decreased level of sedation.
    e. Client tends to use less narcotic.
 5. Instruct any family member or significant others not to administer medication (document that you have done this). Explain that PCA works on the principle that when the client is uncomfortable, he or she will use the PCA.

> ✔ **NURSING PRIORITY:** *Fear of addiction is often major concerns of clients (and their families) who are receiving pain medications. The nurse should administer PRN pain medication to clients experiencing acute pain without the fear of addicting the client to the medication.*

D. Palliative Pain Relief
 1. The prevention or relief of pain when a cure for the client's illness is not feasible.

> 💡 **TEST ALERT:** *Palliative/comfort care: assess client for nonverbal signs of pain/discomfort. Assess, intervene, and educate client/family about pain management.*

 2. Administer analgesics based on client's level of pain; medication is increased as client's pain increases.
 3. Pain medication is frequently administered on an around-the-clock schedule rather than a PRN schedule to maintain therapeutic levels of medication. Pain medication is administered in the absence of pain.

4. A nurse's or client's fear that the client will become dependent on, addicted to, or tolerant to medication is inappropriate in the provision of pain control in palliative care.
5. Breakthrough pain frequently occurs in clients with cancer; pain may occur spontaneously, may be precipitated by coughing, may occur at any time during the dosing interval, or may occur toward the end of the dose.
6. Fear that opioids will hasten death is unsubstantiated, even in clients at the very end of life. It is important that nurses provide adequate pain relief for the terminally ill client.

> ✔ **OLDER ADULT PRIORITY:** *Analgesics tend to last longer and there is an increased risk for side effects and toxic effects in the older client.*

E. Evaluation of Pain Control
 1. Identify client behavior response before the intervention and compare with response following the intervention.
 2. Based on assessment of pain prior to medication, determine if pain has been resolved.
 3. Chart client response to pain medication.

END-OF-LIFE CARE

A. Provide psychosocial support to client and family.

> 💡 **TEST ALERT: Provide care and support to clients and families at end-of-life; identify client's end-of-life needs and ability to cope with end of life interventions.**

 1. Assist family to identify resources for decisions about treatment and to prepare advance directives.
 2. Assist client to identify and to contact spiritual advisors.
 3. Respond quickly to call lights, check on client often, this helps to keep the client from feeling abandoned or isolated.
 4. Encourage family to participate in care assisting with food, hygiene measures, physical contact.
B. Assist client to understand implications of resuscitation and associated terms.

> ✔ **NURSING PRIORITY:** *It is important that clients understand that full comfort and physical assistance will continue to be provided regardless of their choice to be resuscitated or not. Respect client choices for palliative care.*

 1. Allow natural death (AND), and or do not resuscitate (DNR): maintain comfort measures, hygiene and pain control; order must be written on chart.

2. Full code: full CPR and resuscitation actions.
3. Hospice care or palliative care
   a. Does not refer to a place, but rather to a concept of care that provides support for the client who is dying.
   b. Care may be provided in long-term care facility, hospital, or at home.
   c. Criteria for hospice care includes the client's desire for the service and a physician's statement that the client will probably not survive beyond the next 6 months (the allowed time frame is somewhat flexible since actual amount of time cannot be predicted).

Physical Management of Symptoms

A. Physical symptoms of impending death.
   1. Sensory.
      a. Hearing is usually the last sense to disappear – always consider the unconscious client can hear.
      b. Taste, smell are diminished.
      c. Vision is often blurred, blink reflex may be absent.
   2. Integumentary: skin is often cool and clammy; mottling occurs on extremities; cyanosis occurs around mouth and nose and on nail beds.
   3. Respiratory
      a. Respirations become shallow and irregular; Cheyne-Stokes—periods of apnea alternating with deep rapid breathing.
      b. Increased mucus in upper airway causing gurgling, noisy respirations.
      c. Inability to cough or clear airway.
   4. Cardiovascular.
      a. Heart rate may vary from a regular, increased rate to a slowing and irregular heartbeat before death.
      b. Decreased blood pressure and tissue perfusion.
   5. Elimination.
      a. Urinary: output decreases, incontinence occurs.
      b. Bowel: monitor for constipation; bowel incontinence may occur.
   6. Musculoskeletal.
      a. Gradual loss of ability to move, loss of facial muscle tone.
      b. Difficulty speaking, unaware of body position.
   7. Neurological.
      a. Decreased level of consciousness.
      b. Decreased reflexes: gag, cough, swallow.
B. Nursing interventions.
   1. Provide palliative pain management—the prevention or relief of pain when a cure for the client's illness is not feasible.
      a. Pain medication is frequently administered on an around-the-clock schedule to maintain therapeutic levels of medication; do not delay or deny pain relief measures to a dying client.

b. Moderate to large amounts of opioids may be required to maintain client's comfort.
c. Administer analgesics based on client's level of pain; medication is increased as client's pain increases.
d. Adjuvant medications to increase effectiveness of analgesics—antiemetics, antidepressants, corticosteroids.
e. A nurse's or family's fear that the client will become dependent on, addicted to, or tolerant to pain the medication is inappropriate in provision of pain control in palliative care.
   2. Dehydration: maintain oral hygiene; do not force the client to eat or drink. The option to withhold artificial nutrition or hydration should be made by the client in the advance directive, or by the person designated in advance directive.
   3. Respiratory distress: elevate the head of the bed, offer oxygen, provide medications to decrease apprehension.
   4. Elimination.
      a. Utilize incontinence pads, prevent skin irritation, follow facility protocol for indwelling catheters.
      b. Monitor bowel function, assess for impaction, promote normal function within client limitations.
   5. Anorexia, nausea and vomiting.
      a. Assess for precipitating cause and administer medications to decrease nausea.
      b. Offer small, frequent meals, but do not focus on client's need to eat.
   6. Determine client's personal preferences and cultural implications regarding death. Provide family care regarding cultural needs.

PERIOPERATIVE CARE

Surgical procedures, whether planned or an emergency intervention, represent a crisis in a client's life. However minor, surgical procedures always carry some degree of risk, physical discomfort, and financial stress.
A. Perioperative refers to the entire operative experience (preoperative, intraoperative, and postoperative care).
B. Preoperative phase: the period of time before the surgical procedure.
   1. Assessment and correction of physiological and psychological problems that may increase the client's risk factors.
   2. Client teaching regarding the surgery.
   3. Client teaching regarding postoperative care and activities.
C. Intraoperative phase: the period of time the client is in the operating room.
D. Postoperative phase: this period begins with the admission of the client to the postanesthesia care unit (PACU) and includes the remainder of the client's hospitalization and recovery period.

Preoperative Care

 TEST ALERT: *Perform care for client before and after surgical procedure.*

A. Client profile.
   1. Age: The older adult and the infant have more difficulty maintaining homeostasis than do the adult and child. The older adult is more likely to have chronic health problems complicating surgery (Box 3-5).
   2. Weight: Obesity predisposes the client to postoperative complications of infection and wound dehiscence. Fatty tissue is more susceptible to the infectious process.
   3. Preoperative interview.
      a. Chronic health problems and previous surgical procedures.
      b. Past and current drug therapy, including over-the-counter (OTC) medications.

✔ **NURSING PRIORITY:** *Evaluate client's current medications, be sure to include OTC medications as well as any alternative medications (herbal remedies).*

   c. History of drug allergies and dietary restrictions.
   d. Client's perception of his or her illness and impending surgery.
   e. Client's level of orientation and any visual or auditory problems that would hinder communication.
   f. Discomfort or symptoms client is currently experiencing.
   g. Religious affiliation.
   h. Family or significant others.
   4. Psychosocial needs: Fear of the unknown is the primary cause of preoperative anxiety in the mentally stable client. The surgical experience is unique to each client and represents a time of crisis.
   5. Check routine laboratory studies – may vary according to client's diagnosis, values should be available to surgical team.
      a. Complete blood count (CBC), blood type.
      b. Clotting studies (PT, PTT, INR, see Appendix 11-1).
      c. Urinalysis.
      d. Chest x-ray – especially for older adults
      e. Serum electrolytes, serum creatinine and blood urea nitrogen (see Appendix 18-1).
      f. Electrocardiogram (ECG) - generally for clients over 40 years or unless otherwise indicated.

BOX 3-5 | OLDER ADULT CARE FOCUS
Preoperative and Postoperative Considerations

Older adult clients are at increased risk for developing postoperative complications because of the decreased response of the immune system (which delays healing) as well as the increased incidence of chronic disease.
- *Cardiovascular*: decreased cardiac output and peripheral circulation, arrhythmias are more frequent and can lead to a decreased cardiac output. There is an increased incidence of arteriosclerosis and atherosclerosis which can lead to hypertension.
- *Respiratory*: decreased vital capacity, reduced oxygen exchange, and decreased cough reflex can lead to an increased risk for atelectasis, pneumonia, and aspiration.
- *Renal*: decreased renal function can lead to fluid overload, dehydration, and electrolyte imbalance.
- *Musculoskeletal*: increased incidence of arthritis and osteoporosis lead to an increased risk of falls and decreased mobility.
- *Sensory*: decreased visual acuity and hearing affect the client's reaction time and can lead to safety problems associated with falls and injuries.

Poor nutritional status which can affect healing as well as postoperative recovery.
The older client may require repeated explanation, clarification, and positive reassurance.

 TEST ALERT: *Provide care that meets the special needs of the older adult client.*

TEST ALERT: *Anticipate questions regarding basic pre and postoperative nursing care as well as questions that apply to a specific surgical condition or procedure. Nursing implications for specific surgical procedures may be found under the major systems in the care of the medical-surgical client.*

B. Preoperative teaching: The goal is to decrease the client's anxiety and to prevent postoperative complications.
   1. Evaluate the client's current understanding of his/her illness and of the anticipated surgical intervention.
   2. Use terminology the client will understand.
   3. Do not overwhelm the client with too much information at one time; allow adequate time for client questions.
   4. Involve the client's significant others in the preoperative teaching.
   5. Preoperative teaching content.
      a. Deep breathing and coughing exercises.
      b. Turning and extremity exercises.
      c. Pain medication policy, for example, PRN, PCA.

d. Adjunct equipment used for breathing: incentive spirometry, nebulizer, O_2 mask.

e. Explanation of NPO policy if indicated.

C. Physical preparation.

1. Skin preparation.

a. The operative site and the surrounding area should be cleaned either by the client or by specific cleansing of the site by a member of the surgical team.

b. Shaving the operative area is no longer recommended to be done by nursing staff; if area is to be shaved it should be done in the preoperative holding area or in the operating room.

2. Food and fluids are restricted for approximately 6 hours preoperatively.

3. Enemas or some type of gastrointestinal cleansing is usually administered the evening before surgery involving the GI tract, pelvic area, or retroperitoneal area. This assists to prevent fecal contamination in the peritoneal cavity. Take safety precautions with older adult client, bowel preparation can be exhausting.

4. Promote sleep and rest: After the preoperative procedures are completed, the client generally receives a sleeping medication to promote rest. Common medications used are barbiturates.

D. Informed Consent

1. The physician is responsible for having the consent form signed. It must be signed before sedation is given. The surgeon should give the client a full explanation of the procedure, including complications, alternatives, and risks involved.

2. The client's informed consent record (permit) must be signed by the physician, the client, and a witness; the witness is frequently the staff nurse.

> ✔ **NURSING PRIORITY:** *The informed consent record (permit) must be signed before the client receives the preoperative medication.*

3. The signed consent record (permit) is part of the permanent chart record and must accompany the client to the operating room.

Day of Surgery

A. Nursing responsibilities.

1. Have client follow routine hygiene care or shower with an antiseptic solution or bactericidal soap.

2. Review client's regularly scheduled medications and determine if any medications are to be held on the day of surgery, or if all medications should be given.

3. Record vital signs within 1 hour of client being transported to surgery.

4. Secure and/or remove valuables according to hospital policy; wedding bands may be taped on finger.

5. Facility may require the client to remove fingernail polish or artificial nail from at least one finger.

6. Most often dentures and removable bridge work are removed to prevent breakage, aspiration or airway obstruction. Check young children for the presence of loose teeth.

7. Remove contact lens, prosthetic devices, glasses, hairpieces and give them to the client's family. Remove any metal hairpins or clips.

8. Check client's identification for first and last name, date of birth, physician, and hospital number.

9. Identify family and significant others who will be waiting for information regarding client's progress.

10. Check the chart for completeness regarding laboratory reports, signed consent form, significant client observations, history and physical records.

11. Make sure the surgical team is aware of advanced directives, or any religious beliefs that could impact surgery (blood transfusions).

B. Preoperative medications (see Appendix 3-3).

1. Purpose.

a. Decrease anxiety and provide sedation.

2. Nursing responsibilities.

a. Ask client to void before administration of medication.

b. Obtain baseline vital signs.

c. Medication is usually administered about an hour before surgery. Many institutions are administering the medication in the operative suite so the client can participate in the "time out" process for identification of operative site.

d. Raise the side rails and instruct the client not to get out of bed.

e. Remove dentures and partial plates.

f. Observe for desired response as well as undesirable side effects of medication.

g. Maintain quiet environment before being transported to the operating room.

h. Allow parent to accompany child as far as possible.

C. The "time out" is the protocol for preventing wrong site, wrong procedure, wrong person surgery; it must occur in the location where the procedure is performed. All members of the surgical team are involved in the positive identification of the client, the name of the intended procedure, and the site of the procedure.

D. Nursing considerations for spinal anesthesia.

1. Client will not be able to feel any sensation below level of anesthesia.

2. Vasodilation below level of anesthesia may precipitate hypotension.

3. Client may experience postanesthesia headache ("spinal" headache).

4. Client may remain awake throughout procedure.

5. May be used in major surgical procedures below the level of the diaphragm.

E. Conscious sedation: the administration of an IV medication to produce sedation, analgesia, and amnesia.
 1. Characteristics.
  a. Client can respond to commands, maintains protective reflexes, and does not need assistance to maintain airway.
  b. Amnesia most often occurs after the procedure.
  c. Slurred speech and nystagmus indicate the end of conscious sedation
 2. Nursing implications.
  a. Client is assessed continuously; vital signs are recorded every 5 to 15 minutes.
  b. Monitor level of consciousness; client should not be unconscious, but relaxed and comfortable.
  c. Client should respond to physical and verbal stimuli; protective airway reflexes remain intact.
  d. Potential complications include loss of gag reflex, aspiration, hypoxia, hypercapnia, and cardiopulmonary depression.
  e. Does not require extensive recovery time following surgery.

Immediate Postoperative Recovery

A. Admission of client to recovery area.
 1. Obtain baseline assessment.
  a. Vital signs.
  b. Status of respirations.
  c. General color.
  d. Type and amount of fluid infusing.
  e. Special equipment.
  f. Dressings.
 2. Notify supervisor or surgeon regarding any deterioration of client's condition during the postoperative recovery period.

Nursing Interventions

Goal: To maintain and support respiratory function.
A. Leave airway in place until pharyngeal reflex (gag reflex) has returned.
B. Position client to maintain ventilation and prevent aspiration.
C. Encourage coughing and deep breathing.
D. Administer humidified oxygen as necessary.
E. Report significant changes in respiratory status.
F. Listen to the chest for a decrease in breath sounds. Notify supervisor or PCP if there are significant changes in respiratory status.
G. Monitor status and changes in pulse oximetry.

❖ Goal: To maintain cardiovascular stability.
A. Check vital signs every 15 minutes until stable; compare with preoperative vital signs.
B. Report blood pressure measurement that is continually dropping 5 to 10 mm Hg with each reading.
C. Report consistently increasing bradycardia or tachycardia.
D. Evaluate quality of pulse and presence of irregular pulse.
❖ Goal: To maintain adequate fluid status.
A. Monitor rate of IV infusion.
B. Measure urine output if bladder catheter is present (minimum of 30 mL per hour for an adult).
C. Evaluate for bladder distention if there is no catheter.
D. Observe amount and character of drainage on dressings or drainage in collecting containers.
E. Assess amount and character of gastric drainage if nasogastric tube is in place.
F. Nausea and vomiting may occur as client is recovering from anesthesia.
❖ Goal: To maintain incisional areas.
A. Evaluate amount and character of drainage from incision and drains.
B. Check and record status of Hemovac, Jackson-Pratt, or any other wound drains.
❖ Goal: To maintain psychological equilibrium.
A. Speak to client frequently in calm, unhurried manner.
B. Continually orient client.
C. Maintain quiet, restful atmosphere.
D. Promote comfort by maintaining proper body alignment.
E. Explain all procedures, even if client is not fully awake.
F. Remember that in the anesthetized client, the sense of hearing is the last to be lost and the first to return.
❖ Goal: Client meets criteria to return to room.
A. Vital signs are stable and within normal limits.
B. Client is awake and reflexes have returned.
C. Dressings are intact with no evidence of excessive drainage.
D. Client can maintain a patent airway without assistance.

General Postoperative Care

❖ Goal: To maintain cardiovascular function and tissue perfusion.
A. Monitor vital signs, usually every 4 hours, after full recovery.
B. Evaluate skin color and nail beds for paleness and cyanosis.
C. Assess client's tolerance to increasing activity.
D. Encourage early activity and ambulation.
E. Monitor for circulatory complications of immobility.

TABLE 3-2 · COMMON POSTOPERATIVE COMPLICATIONS

COMPLICATION	SIGNS AND SYMPTOMS	NURSING INTERVENTION
Atelectasis - a collapse of a portion of the lung producing an airless state in the alveoli. (Chapter 10)	Dyspnea, decreased or absent breath sounds over affected area, asymmetrical chest expansion, hypoxia.	Position client on unaffected side. Maintain humidification, oxygen (see Chapter 15). Administer narcotics cautiously if client is at increased risk. *Prevention*: assist client to turn, cough, and deep breath; provide adequate hydration; encourage ambulation, prevent abdominal distention.
Pulmonary emboli (PE) movement of a thrombus into the pulmonary artery. (Chapter 10)	Chest pain, dyspnea, tachycardia, increased anxiety, decreased pulse oximetry, decreased blood pressure.	Notify RN immediately of any chest pain or difficulty breathing in clients at increased risk. Place client in semi-Fowlers position and begin oxygen. Maintain bed rest. Remain with client in respiratory distress *Prevention*: Encourage ambulation as soon as possible, position client to prevent venous stasis.
Pneumonia – an acute inflammatory process where alveoli fill with fluid. (Chapter 10)	Fever, shallow respirations, wet breath sounds, cough productive of thick yellow mucus, may progress to hypoxia.	Maintain client in low or semi-Fowlers, monitor pulse oximetry levels. Humidified oxygen and maintain good hydration. *Prevention*: cough and deep breath, encourage incentive spirometry. Older adult clients are at increased risk; encourage postoperative activity as soon as possible.
Shock - a decrease in cardiac output due to loss of circulating blood volume. (Chapter 11)	Decreasing blood pressure, weak pulse, restless, confusion, oliguria.	Anticipate RN will initiate IV access if not present, maintain NPO and bed rest. Position client supine. Prevent hypoxia and monitor vital signs. (see Chapter 11). *Prevention*: closely monitor drains and incisions for bleeding, identify clients at increased risk.
Wound infection - an infection of the surgical incision area.	Poor wound healing, redness, tenderness, fever, tachycardia, leukocytosis, purulent drainage.	Culture incision to determine organism. Evaluate progress of wound healing. *Prevention*: identify high-risk clients; maintain sterile technique with dressing changes; good hand hygiene.
Wound dehiscence	Unintentional opening of the surgical incision.	Evaluate for bleeding; maintain bed rest and or position client to prevent further pressure at incision site. *Prevention*: identify clients at increased risk for stress on incision and poor healing; assist client to splint incision when coughing; use abdominal binders. *Notify RN or surgeon.*
Wound evisceration	Protrusion of a loop of bowel through the surgical wound.	Cover bowel with sterile saline soaked dressing. Do not attempt to replace loop of bowel. *Notify RN or surgeon*; client will most likely return to surgery for further exploration.

 TEST ALERT: *Monitor wounds for signs and symptoms of infection.*

Continued

TABLE 3-2   COMMON POSTOPERATIVE COMPLICATIONS—cont'd.

COMPLICATION	SIGNS AND SYMPTOMS	NURSING INTERVENTION
Urinary retention	Inability to void 8 hours after surgery; bladder may be palpable; voiding small amounts, dribbling	Determine amount of fluid intake and when to anticipate client to void—generally within 8 hr. Palpate suprapubic area to evaluate for bladder distention. Assist client into normal voiding position if possible, run tap water, provide privacy. Catheterize only if necessary. *Prevention*: Determine preoperative risks: medications, length of surgery, history of prostate problems.
Gastric dilation	Nausea, vomiting, abdominal distention, decreased bowel sounds.	Clients with abdominal or bowel surgery are at increased risk. Position client in semi-Fowlers to decrease risk of aspiration. Maintain client NPO. *Prevention*: Older adult clients are at increased risk; and clients with abdominal or bowel surgery are at increased risk; encourage activity as soon as possible; carefully monitor analgesics.
Paralytic ileus - caused by decreased peristalsis, or intestinal obstruction, leading to gastric distention.		*Prevention*: same as for gastric distention. Maintain nasogastric tube suction and NPO status. If NG tube is not present, may begin early feeding of clear liquids to increase intestinal motility. Evaluate for distention, status of bowel sounds and abdominal discomfort. Monitor for possible compromised respirations.

IV, Intravenous; *NPO*, nothing by mouth; *NG*, nasogastric

❖   Goal: To maintain respiratory function.
A.   Have client turn, cough, and deep breathe every 2 hours.
B.   Encourage use of incentive spirometry to promote deep breathing.
C.   Maintain adequate hydration to keep mucus secretions thinned and easily mobilized.
D.   Encourage early ambulation.
E.   Evaluate sputum for presence of infection.
❖   Goal: To maintain adequate nutrition and elimination.
A.   Assess for return of bowel sounds and normal peristalsis.
B.   Assess the client with a nasogastric tube for return of peristalsis.
C.   Encourage fluids after client demonstrates tolerance to fluids.
D.   Assess client's tolerance of oral (PO) fluids; usually begin with clear liquids.
E.   Diet is usually progressive as client's condition and appetite indicate.
F.   Record bowel movements; normal bowel function should return as evidenced by normal bowel movement on the second or third postoperative day (provided the client is eating).
G.   Assess urinary output.

1.   Client should void 8 to 10 hours after surgery.
2.   If bladder catheter is present, client should average at least 30 mL per hour.
3.   Promote voiding by allowing client to stand or use bedside commode, if not contraindicated.
4.   Avoid catheterization if possible.
❖   Goal: To maintain fluid balance.
A.   Monitor IV infusions for correct fluid and rate of infusion.
B.   Assess for adequate hydration.
    1.   Moist mucous membranes.
    2.   Adequate urine output with normal specific gravity.
    3.   Good skin turgor.
    4.   Stable vital signs.
    5.   Alert and oriented.
C.   Assess character and amount of gastric drainage through the nasogastric tube.
❖   Goal: To promote comfort.
A.   Anticipate pain; assess and administer appropriate analgesics.
B.   Administer antiemetic for nausea and vomiting.
C.   Maintain good hygiene (e.g., clean dressings, clean gown).
D.   Change client's position every 2 hours.
E.   Allow for periods of rest after administration of analgesics.

> ✔ **NURSING PRIORITY:** *In addition to the pain and discomfort associated with a surgical procedure, it is important to assess other possible sources of discomfort, such as full bladder, occluded catheter or tube, gas accumulation, IV infiltration, or compromised circulation due to position/pressure.*

Postoperative Complications – see Table 3-2

DISASTER PLANNING

> 💡 **TEST ALERT:** *Participate in preparation for internal and external disasters – participating in safety drills, identifying safety manager, locating Material Safety Data Sheet (MSDS).*

A. Fire
 1. Immediately return to your unit if a fire code is called.
 2. If fire is localized (in one room or area), remove the clients from the immediate area.
 3. If clients on your unit are not in immediate danger, close all of the doors to the client's rooms and to the unit.
 4. If you need to evacuate your unit because of an immediate danger to staff and clients, evacuate clients in this order to provide for the most rapid removal of the most clients in a short period of time:
     a. First: Ambulatory clients are first because they can move the quickest and you can remove more clients quickly.
     b. Second: Clients in wheelchairs or walkers or clients that need assistance are next to be evacuated.
     c. Third: Clients that require the most assistance, for example, ventilator clients or those who are totally bed ridden, are the next to be evacuated.
 5. Know the types of fire extinguishers:
     a. Class A: water or solution for paper or linen fires.
     b. Class B: foam extinguisher for grease, chemical, or electrical fires.
     c. Class C: multipurpose for paper, linen, or electrical fires.
 6. Using a fire extinguisher—remember **PASS**:
     Pull the pin.
     Aim at the base of the fire.
     Squeeze the trigger.
     Sweep from side to side.
B. Response acronym: **RACE**
     Rescue—remove all clients in immediate danger.
     Alert—initiate the alarm.
     Confine—close all doors and windows; turn off oxygen valves and electrical equipment.
     Extinguish—use the appropriate extinguisher for type of fire.

LEGAL IMPLICATIONS

Responsibility for Practice

A. Individual liability.
 1. Every nurse is liable for his or her own conduct.
 2. Liability may be shared by another person or group (e.g., the doctor, another nurse, or the hospital), but it cannot be removed by the statements or actions of another.
 3. If an RN is not available, the practical nurse may not carry out functions that are recognized to be outside the scope of practice of a practical nurse.

> 💡 **TEST ALERT:** *Identify your professional practice limitations (refuse to perform tasks outside your scope of practice); report a health care provider's unsafe practice.*

B. Unethical nursing care.
 1. Medication errors that are made and not reported/corrected.
 2. Physical and verbal client abuse.
 3. Providing care while under the influence of alcohol or drugs.
 4. Breach of client confidentiality.
 5. Jeopardizing a client's well-being by withholding care or treatment.
 6. Providing care outside the protocol for safe, ethical nursing practice according to the individual state nurse practice act.
 7. The practical/vocational nurse should follow the line of authority within the institution for reporting an incident.
C. Standard of care: The legal concept of a fictional, reasonable, prudent individual of the same education and profession against which another professional's performance is judged.
 1. Statement of nursing standards.
     a. Practice acts, and rules and regulations.
     b. Joint Commission (JC).
     c. Policy and procedures' manuals.
     d. Prior court decisions.
 2. Used to determine when a breach of duty has occurred.
D. Good Samaritan laws: enacted by individual states with the purpose of protecting health care providers who assist at accidents and emergencies.
 1. Care provided in good faith.
 2. Care must be gratuitous; no compensation is received for the care rendered.
 3. Care provided should not be negligent.
 4. Know the status in your state.

Legal Considerations

A. Negligence: Unintentional harm to another that occurs through failure to act in a reasonable and prudent manner.

B. Malpractice: Unprofessional nursing practice that fails to meet the proper standard of care.

C. Invasion of privacy: Protection of constitutional right to be free from undesired publicity and exposure to public view.
1. Proper covering of physical body.
2. Medical records.
   a. Release with signed client consent form.
   b. Release for medical "need to know" limited to caregivers only.
3. Belongings must be protected and may not be searched without specific authorization. A client's list of belongings should be explained to and signed by the client.
4. Conversations confidential; in some states protected by specific statute.
5. Photographs and viewing of procedures require consent of client.
6. Control of visitor access to client and client information.
7. Reporting laws are an exception – some information is required by law to be reported.

 TEST ALERT: Follow regulation/policy for reporting specific issues (abuse/neglect, gunshot wound, or communicable disease, etc.)

   a. Communicable diseases.
   b. Injuries or deaths that are, or could be, caused by physical violence (gunshot and knife wounds).
   c. Client abuse - children and older adult.
   d. Others defined by state statute.
8. Rights may be waived by the client but never by medical personnel.
9. Nurses are obligated to maintain confidentiality of client's health information in accordance with the Health Insurance Portability and Accountability Act (HIPAA) of 1996.

D. Valid consent (informed consent).

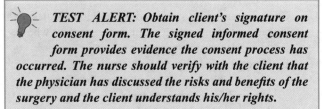 **TEST ALERT: Obtain client's signature on consent form. The signed informed consent form provides evidence the consent process has occurred. The nurse should verify with the client that the physician has discussed the risks and benefits of the surgery and the client understands his/her rights.**

1. Timely: Some states or institutions have specific time restrictions on when consents are signed.
2. Written: This is required for all invasive procedures.

3. Witnessed signature: Do not sign an informed consent as a witness unless you know client has all information and understands the information necessary to an informed decision.
4. Procedure specified in terms the client can understand.
5. Client understanding of significant risks of procedure.
6. Signed while client is free from mind-altering drugs or conditions.
7. Withdrawal of consent can be written or verbal and may occur at any time before the procedure.

E. Orders: doctors/primary health care provider.

 TEST ALERT: Evaluate appropriateness of an order.

1. Question any order that is not clearly written and understood.
2. Each medication order should contain the correct medication name, the route of administration, the dosage amount, and the time of administration.
3. Single-dose orders are for a medication to be given one time.
4. "Stat" orders: procedure or medication should be given/carried out immediately; new orders should be scanned initially to determine if any "stat" orders are present.
5. The nurse is responsible for questioning any medication order if the order is not clear.

Protective Procedures

A. Documentation: written record of events surrounding client's hospital stay.
1. Protects client by promoting good communication among health care providers.
2. Provides evidence in court of care given.
   a. Courts will not assume care is given unless it is recorded.
   b. Demonstrates meeting of standard of care.

B. How to document (Box 3-6).
1. Use the agency format correctly.
2. Complete all portions of format.
   a. Use opinions only in assessment portion of charting, never in areas requiring factual data.
   b. Complete an honest record of events.
      (1) Do not alter record at any time.
      (2) Record all events, even unusual events, factually.
      (3) Give all appropriate information about each note (e.g., status of incision: presence of and type of drainage, inflammation of area, foul odor, and type of dressing if any).
      (4) Explain omissions in care.
3. Time, date, and sign all entries.

4. Do not skip lines; do not leave any blank spaces for other people to chart (paper charts).
5. Correct errors properly.
   a. Draw a straight line through error; date and initial.
      (a) No white-out on error.
      (b) No obliteration or erasure of error.
      (c) No recopying of page to omit note.
   b. Add omitted information by an "addendum" or "late entry"; give date and time of original note as well as date and time of addendum.
6. Use meaningful, specific language, do not use words you do not understand or unacceptable abbreviations.
C. Incident reports.

 TEST ALERT: Report incidents/events/irregular occurrences according to facility guidelines.

1. Only the person directly involved in the incident should document the facts in the report.
2. Do not complete an incident report for someone else.
3. Document the facts.
   a. Do not draw conclusions or speculate on who caused or who was responsible for the incident.
   b. Do not state opinions or make judgments.
4. Report does not replace the documentation of the incident in the chart.
5. Do not document any reference to the incident report in the chart; the same factual information filed on the incident report should be included on the chart.
6. Failure to complete an incident report could be considered a cover-up.
7. Complete an incident report for any unusual occurrence or an event in which client or family safety was compromised. Follow the line of authority within the institution for reporting an incident.
D. Know your limits.

 TEST ALERT: Recognize task/assignments you are not prepared to perform and seek assistance.

1. Physical-emotional: be aware of fatigue and exhaustion and compensate for them.
2. Practice competency.
   a. Do not perform procedures without adequate preparation, knowledge, and experience. Request supervision if you are unsure of your skills.
   b. Report unsafe practices to your supervisor.
   c. Do not allow anyone to talk you into doing something you are not sure of by letting him or her agree to take the liability or telling you that you should do it.

BOX 3-6   GUIDELINES FOR EFFECTIVE DOCUMENTATION

- All entries should be accurate and as objective as possibe.
- Make corrections appropriately and according to agency or hospital policies. Do not obliterate any information that is written on the paper chart.
- If there is information that should have been charted and was not, make a "late entry," indicating the time the charting actually occurred and the specific time the charting reflects. Example: 10/13/09. 10:00 a.m. late entry, charting to reflect 10/12/09.
- All identified client problems, nursing actions taken, and client responses should be noted. Do not describe a client problem and leave it without including nursing actions taken and the client's response.
- Be as objective as possible in charting. Rather then charting "The client tolerated the procedure well," chart the specific parameters checked to determine that conclusion. A chart entry worded "ambulated, tolerated well" would be more effective if charted "ambulated complete length of hall, no shortness of breath noted, pulse rate at 98, respirations at 22."
- Each page of the paper chart or each computer entry should contain the current date and time. Each time information is entered on a new page, make sure it reflects the current time of charting.
- Document who saw the client and what measures were initiated. Particularly note when the doctors visited; if you had to call a doctor because of a problem, record the doctor's response. If orders were received, be sure they are signed according to policy. This is especially important if you had to make several calls to the doctor.
- Make sure your notes on the paper chart are legible and clearly reflect the information you intended. It is a good idea to read over your nurse's notes from the previous day to see whether they still make sense and accurately portray the status of the client. If the notes do not make sense to you the next day, imagine how difficult it would be to decipher the information at a later date, or in court.
- Charting by exception may be available on electronic charts, as well as paper charts. In this case, the nurse may be required to document only significant findings or exceptions. It is important that exception notes are entered and provide a clear picture of the client's care or status.
- Do not give your computer password or ID to anyone, and do not chart for any other health care person.
- If charting by computer in the client's room, make sure the nursing or medical record has been closed before leaving the room.

Adapted from Irvin, Judy: Legal issues. In Zerwekh J, Claborn J, editors: *Nursing today: Transitions and trends,* ed 6, St. Louis, 2009, Saunders.

E. Client identification—The Joint Commission requirements:
    1. Two identifiers are required; for example, the hospital identification number and the client's name on the armband. Physicians name and client's date of birth are commonly on identification armbands.
    2. If client does not have an armband, then the individual's stated name would be one identifier; the client's date of birth, social security number, address, or phone number could serve as the second identifier.
    3. Client's current photograph or visual recognition may be used as one identifier in long-term care facilities, home care settings, or behavioral care facilities. For short-term clients, facilities with unstable staffing, and/or high-risk medications, the two-identifier requirement is necessary.
    4. The client does not have to state his or her name as an identifier.

> ✔ **NURSING PRIORITY:** *Always check client identification according to the Joint Commission guidelines.*

Specific Situations at Risk

A. Physical injury to the client.
    1. Inappropriate side rail use.
    2. Inadequate supervision during ambulation.
    3. Obstacle or dangers on floor or in path of client.
    4. Improper transportation
B. Improper use of index restraints - may be physical or chemical restraints and are used only to protect the physical safety of the client and others.
    1. Use of a restraint on a client requires a physician's order for:
        a. Type and location of restraint.
        b. Type of behavior for which restraint is to be used.
        c. Time frame that the order for the restraint covers.
    2. In an emergency situation, physical restraints may be used without a doctor's order for a very limited period of time.
    3. Safe nursing practice for the care of a client in restraints includes:
        a. Check restrained client every 30 minutes and provide for physiological needs.
        b. Remove restraints and provide range of motion every 2 hours.
        c. Document the time of each check and the neurovascular status of client's extremities.
        d. Remove restraints as soon as possible.
        e. Secure restraints to the bed frame, not to the side rails.
        f. Discuss with family the rationale for and purpose of restraints.
        g. Investigate all alternatives to restraints: family involvement, methods to increase client orientation, scheduled toileting activities.

B. Medication errors (see Chapter 4).
    1. Follow the seven rights of medication administration to protect the client.
    2. Have a basic knowledge of medications administered.
        a. Reason client is receiving the medication.
        b. Major side effects of medication.
        c. Anticipated client response to medication.
    3. Never administer a medication without a complete order.
    4. *Notify the supervisor or RN if there is an obvious contraindication to the administration of a medication.*
C. Administration of narcotics
    1. Never sign out for a narcotic you do not personally administer.
    2. Do not sign as a witness for narcotic wasting unless you actually observe the wasting.
    3. Always have another licensed person witness and co-sign whenever it is necessary to waste a narcotic.
D. Telephone and other verbal orders (Box 3-7).

> **TEST ALERT: Take a verbal or phone order; transcribe a physician's order.**

1. Practical nurses must be aware of the policies and procedures of the institution regarding telephone orders. Some institutions do not allow the PN to take doctor's orders. The practical nurse is legally obligated to follow the policy of the employing institution.
2. Write down the telephone order and read it back; receive confirmation that the order is correct.
3. Do not take verbal orders with the physician present when it is not an urgent situation.
4. Orders left on voice mail are not acceptable; the nurse must call the health care provider to obtain the order directly.

5. Verbal orders left with patients or family members are not acceptable; the nurse must call the health care provider and obtain the order directly.
6. Obtain needed signature promptly for telephone orders.
D. Changes in client's condition.

> ✔ **NUIRSING PRIORITY:** *Identify and report significant changes in client condition.*

1. *Notify appropriate individuals of changes – RN, unit supervisor, physician, or other health care provider.*
2. Follow the chain of command if there is failure to provide appropriate care after notification of significant change in client condition.
3. Document changes and events surrounding the change in the client's status.
4. The practical nurse is responsible for evaluating clients, and obtaining assistance, or notifying appropriate individuals of the change in client condition.
5. Follow up on assessments of client problems and what nursing action was taken to resolve the problem. For example, the nurse may very carefully document the events surrounding a client's fall, but it is also critical to follow up on what was done to provide care and to protect the client after the fall.
E. Hand-off (shift) report: purpose is to provide accurate information and safe quality care throughout the client's hospitalization.
1. Use an interactive communication method understandable for all interdisciplinary teams— **SBAR**:
   Situation—What is happening at the present time?
   Background—What are the circumstances leading up to this situation?
   Assessment—What do I think the problem is?
   Recommendation—What should we do to correct the problem?
2. The oncoming nurse is responsible for the nursing care required on his or her shift.
   a. Status of IVs and amount of fluid to count.
   b. Any abnormal conditions (vital signs, pain, special treatments).
   c. Status of client with regard to diagnosis. For examples, cardiac client—presence or absence of chest pain and dysrhythmias; surgical client—voiding, incision status; orthopedic client—circulation distal to cast or traction.
   d. Psychosocial status of the client.

> **TEST ALERT:** *Provide and receive report on assigned clients.*

Legal Documents

A. Client's medical record or chart.
B. Advance medical directive (AD): a written document regarding a client's desires for provision of medical care if that person is unable to make his or her own choices or decisions.
   a. Living will (natural death act): a written document describing the client's wishes and special instructions regarding life support measures in the event that the client is incapacitated.
   b. Medical power of attorney for health care.
      (1) Identifies the person designated by the client to ensure that previously agreed ADs are carried out according to the client's direction.
      (2) Identifies the person designated to make health care decisions for the client if the client is incapacitated.
   c. ADs may be changed or revoked by the client at any time.

> **TEST ALERT:** *Provide information about advance directives (AD).*

C. Do not resuscitate (DNR) orders.
   1. Written by the physician based on the client's written medical directives.
   2. Nurses are obligated to respect and observe the DNR order.
   3. Health care personnel should be advised of the DNR order.

MANAGEMENT OF HEALTH CARE WORKERS

A. Delegation is transferring to a competent individual the authority to perform a selected nursing task in a selected situation, the process for doing the work. The nurse retains accountability for the delegation, most often delegation is the role of the RN.
B. Assignment describes the distribution of work that each staff member is to accomplish in a given time. To assign is to direct an individual to do activities within an authorized scope of practice.
C. Supervision is the provision of guidance or direction, oversight, evaluation and follow-up by the licensed nurse for the accomplishment of a nursing task delegated to nursing assistive personnel. (NCSBN, 2004).
D. Role of the practical nurse (PN) in supervision
   1. The PN should ensure the unlicensed assistive personal (UAP) understands the assigned task, and the UAP should acknowledge to the PN that he/she understands the directions.
   2. The PN should make periodic checks to determine that the UAP is performing the tasks as directed.

3. If the UAP does not carry out the tasks correctly, the PN should correct the action in a timely professional manner. If the problem is not resolved, the RN should be notified.
4. The PN should assign tasks to the UAP that are clearly defined, are within the expected expertise of the UAP, and have very specific guidelines: for example, bathing, ambulating, client hygiene.

 TEST ALERT: Make client care or related task assignment.

E. Prioritizing client care assignments.
1. Identify the most ill or unstable client of your assigned clients – evaluate and care for that client first.
2. Physiological needs are the priority – education and communication needs can usually wait until the physiological needs are met.
3. Initially review the assigned client list – consider the report received on each client. Determine which client needs immediate physical assistance in order to maintain safety. (Review priority setting in Chapter 1).

 TEST ALERT: Organize and prioritize care of assigned group of clients.

Study Questions: Concepts of Nursing Management

1. Bed rest is frequently prescribed for clients who have had a brain accident or stroke until their condition stabilizes. How can the nurse avoid potential problems?
   1 Insert an indwelling catheter
   2 Help the client bathe two times daily
   3 Place the client on a circulating air mattress
   4 Develop an activity schedule with the client

2. The nurse begins charting on a client's paper chart and after entering data discovers it has been written on the wrong chart. What is the best way to correct this error?
   1 White-out the wrong information and write over it.
   2 Recopy the page with the error so that the chart will be neat.
   3 Draw a straight line through the error, initial, and date.
   4 Obliterate the error so that it will not be confusing.

3. A client is nauseated and has vomited a large amount of foul smelling dark green bile fluid twice in the past hour. What is the best nursing action?
   1 Position the client in a supine position and maintain bed rest.
   2 Place client on nothing by mouth (NPO) status and notify the supervisor.
   3 Encourage clear liquids to help settle the stomach.
   4 Ambulate client to stimulate development of peristalsis.

4. The nurse enters the client's room and discovers the client on the floor beside the bed. The side rails are up, and the client is confused and disoriented. What information would be included in the nurse's documentation in the incident report?
   1 Upon entering the room, I discovered the client on the floor at the side of the bed; the side rails were up.
   2 The client fell out of the bed after the nursing assistant had explained to him the importance of not getting up.
   3 The client was confused and apparently tried to climb out over the side rails of the bed.
   4 Evidently the previous nurse did not check on the client to see that he was confused, and he fell out of bed.

5. The older adult client is being discharged with a prescription for hydrocodone (**Vicodin**) for pain control. What information will the nurse include when discussing with the client the possible adverse effects of the medication?
   1 Increase intake of bulk and fiber to prevent constipation.
   2 The pain control can be increased by taking an additional acetaminophen 500 mg.
   3 Return to the clinic for serum lab studies to determine toxicity levels.
   4 Increased bruising may occur because of changes in the skin.

6. The nurse is explaining to the client the importance of voiding prior to surgery. What would the nurse include in this explanation?
   1 It is important to have an accurate account of I&O for that day.
   2 Voiding before surgery will reduce the risk of bladder pain during surgery.
   3 Voiding prior to surgery will promote the physiological safety during surgery.
   4 Prior to surgery it is important to void to decrease the possibility of infection.

7. The nurse has been assigned an 86-year-old client who has suffered a stroke. The client is not oriented to person, place, or time and is pulling at his IV catheter and trying to climb out of the bed. The nurse has applied a vest restraint and bilateral soft wrist restraints. Which of the following nursing actions would be appropriate? Select all that apply:
   ____ 1 Provide for nutrition and elimination needs every 2 hours.
   ____ 2 Obtain a physician order every shift for continuation of restraints.
   ____ 3 Secure the restraints to the side rails of the bed.
   ____ 4 Tie the restraints in quick release knots.
   ____ 5 Assess and document behaviors that require continued use of restraints.

8. What potential problem should the practical nurse anticipate when too much strain is placed on the suture line?
   1 Thrombosis.
   2 Infection.
   3 Evisceration.
   4 Dehiscence.

9. Postoperative pain and cancer pain may be considered predictable. How can the nurse increase the effectiveness of the analgesics?
   1 Give them PRN.
   2 Administer once a day.
   3 Plan around-the-clock dosing.
   4 Administer twice a day.

10. A wound is left open after surgery and allowed to heal from the inside to the outside. This describes what type of healing?
    1 First intention.
    2 Second intention.
    3 Primary healing.
    4 Superficial healing.

11. A client has experienced a dehiscence and the nurse places the client on bed rest. What is the purpose of bed rest for this client?
    1 To decrease oxygen consumption.
    2 To increase the healing of the site.
    3 To prevent development of pneumonia.
    4 To prevent the occurrence of evisceration.

12. The nurse is caring for an immobilized client. What nursing measure is used to prevent the complications of atelectasis and pneumonia?
    1 Turn, cough, and deep breathe.
    2 Range of motion exercises.
    3 Clear liquid diet with frequent suctioning of secretions.
    4 Bed rest with frequent vital sign measurements.

13. Before a surgical procedure, the nurse asks a client to sign an informed consent form. What is important for the nurse to validate before the client signs this form?
    1 The physician has discussed the surgery with the client.
    2 The client understands the postoperative nursing care.
    3 The physician has discussed the possible complications.
    4 The client understands the surgery and the risks involved.

14. Older adult clients are considered high risk for respiratory problems based on problems of immobility and aging changes. What are these changes related to?
    1 Decreased lung expansion and reduced breathing capacity.
    2 Increased breathing and lung capacity.
    3 Poor posture and decreased size of chest cavity.
    4 Increased lung size and decreased tidal volume.

15. With the client in the prone position, which bony prominences would the nurse identify as being most susceptible to skin breakdown?
    1 Sacrum and elbows.
    2 Shoulder area and trochanter.
    3 Anterior iliac spines and patellae.
    4 Trochanter.

Answers and rationales to these questions are in the section at the end of the book titled Chapter Study Questions: Answers and Rationales.

Appendix 3-1 POSITIONING AND BODY MECHANICS

POSITION	PLACEMENT	USE
Fowler's	Head of bed at 45- to 60-degree angle; hips flexed	The height may be determined by client preference or tolerance; frequently used for client with respiratory compromise.
Semi-Fowler's	Head of bed at 30- to 45-degree angle; hips flexed	Cardiac, respiratory, neurosurgical conditions, or client comfort.
Low Fowler's	Head of bed at 15- to 30-degree angle; hips may or may not be flexed	Postoperative and clients with GI problems; used for client comfort.
Lateral (side-lying)	Head of bed lowered; pillows under arm and legs and behind back; flex knee of anterior side	For client comfort; increases uterine and renal perfusion in pregnancy and prevents supine vena cava syndrome during labor.
Semi-prone (Sims')	Head of bed lowered; client placed on side with dependent shoulder lifted out and lying partially on abdomen; place pillow under flexed arm and under upper flexed knees	Prevents pressure areas, used for comfort
Lithotomy	On back with thigh flexed against abdomen and legs supported by stirrups.	For gynecological examination and surgical procedures in the perineal area.
Prone	Head of bed flat, client on abdomen, head turned to side	Used to promote drainage after oral surgery or tonsillectomy; used to prevent contractures in clients with above-the-knee amputation. Position will protect infant with imperforate anus, or spina bifida.
Supine	Bed in flat position, small pillow under head	For client comfort.

 TEST ALERT: *Position client to prevent complications after tests, treatments, or procedures.*

BODY MECHANICS—PREVENTION OF INJURY

Manual lifting of a client should be avoided. If it is necessary to manually lift most or all of the client's weight, obtain lift equipment and ask for adequate assistance.

Body mechanics:
1. Avoid twisting your body; keep your head and neck aligned with your spine.
2. Flex your knees and place your feet wide apart for good base of support.
3. Position yourself close to the bed or close to the client.
4. Use arms and legs to assist in lifting client, not your back.
5. Use pull sheet or slide board to move client to side of bed and/or to move up in bed.

 TEST ALERT: *Use transfer assistance device (roller, client lifts).*

✔ Key Points: Assisting the Client to Move Up in Bed
• Lower the head of the bed so that it is flat or as low as the client can tolerate; raise the bed frame to a position that does not require leaning.
• If more than one person is needed for assistance, obtain a lifting device.
• Determine the client's strong side and have him or her assist with the move.
• Instruct the client to bend legs, put feet flat on bed, and push.
• With 2 people, use a draw sheet or a lift sheet.
• Never pull a client up in bed by his arms or by putting pressure under his arms.

✔ Key Points: Logrolling the Client
• Spinal immobilization—use a team approach.
• Maintain proper client alignment on head and back areas while turning.
• Before moving patient, place a pillow between client's knees.
• Move client in one coordinated movement, using a turn/lift sheet.

Continued

Appendix 3-1   POSITIONING AND BODY MECHANICS—cont'd.

✔ Key Points: Moving from Bed to Chair
- Move client to the side of the bed (bed wheels locked), closest to the edge where the client will be getting up, place a chair with arms at bedside.
- Plan on assisting client to get out of bed on his strongest side.
- Raise head of bed, assist client to side of the bed.
- Move client to edge of bed and place your hands under client's legs and shift his weight forward, pivot the client's body so he is sitting position and his feet are flat on the floor.
- Have client reach across chair and grasp the arm of the chair.
- Stabilize client by positioning your foot at the outside edge of client's foot.
- Pivot client into chair using your leg muscles instead of your back muscles.
- Assist client to move back and up in the chair for better position.

 TEST ALERT: Maintain correct body alignment.

Tips for Moving and Positioning Clients
- Use a turn sheet to provide more support for client.
- Encourage client to assist in move by using the side rails and strong side of his or her body.
- No-lift policy: use lift equipment and assistance whenever a client requires most of his weight to be supported or lifted by someone.
- Use trochanter roll made from bath blankets to align the client's hips to prevent external rotation when in the supine position.
- Use folded towels, blankets, or small pillows to position client's hands and arms to prevent dependent edema.

Appendix 3-2   ANALGESICS

General Nursing Implications
- Assess client for pain parameters: blood pressure, pulse, and respiratory status before and periodically after administration.
- Use a scale to determine level of pain.
- For more effective analgesic effect, administer medication before pain is severe.
- Older or debilitated clients may require decreased dosage.

Medications	Side Effects	Nursing Implications
NARCOTIC ANALGESICS: Bind to receptors in the central nervous system (CNS), altering the perception of and emotional response to pain. Controlled substances (Schedule II).		
STRONG OPIOID ANALGESICS		
Morphine sulfate: PO, subQ, IM, IV, epidural analgesia	Respiratory depression Orthostatic hypotension Sedation, dizziness, lightheadedness, Increased tendency for seizures	1. Morphine is most commonly used for PCA. 2. Demerol: Not commonly used for control of chronic pain due to neurotoxic effect; use with caution in children and older adult clients because of increased risk for toxicity and seizures.
Meperidine (**Demerol**): PO, subQ, IM	Constipation Tolerance, physical and psychological dependence	3. All opioids: Use with caution in clients who have respiratory compromise.
Fentanyl (**Fentanyl, Sublimaze, Duragesic**): IM, IV, PO, transdermal	May decrease awareness of bladder stimuli	4. Pediatric implications: Medication dosage is calculated according to body surface area and weight.

 NURSING PRIORITY: *Advise clients using fentanyl patches not to expose patch to heat (hot tub, heating pad) since this will accelerate the release of the fentanyl.*

OLDER ADULT PRIORITY: *Prevent problems with constipation, monitor respiratory status.*

5. Assess voiding and encourage client to void every 4 hours.
6. Requires documentation as indicated by Controlled Substance Act.
7. Instruct client to change position slowly to minimize orthostatic hypotension.

Continued

Appendix 3-2 ANALGESICS—cont'd.

Medications	Side Effects	Nursing Implications

MODERATE TO STRONG OPIOID ANALGESICS

Codeine: PO, subQ Hydromorphone (**Dilaudid**): PO, subQ, IM, IV, suppository Oxycodone (**Percodan**, combination with ibuprofen; **Percocet, Tylox** combinations with acetaminophen; **OxyContin**): PO Hydrocodone (**Vicodin, Lorcet** combinations with acetaminophen; **Vicoprofen**, combination with ibuprofen): PO	Sedation, euphoria, respiratory depression, constipation, urinary retention, cough suppression ✓ *NURSING PRIORITY: Help client to identify OTC medications that contain acetaminophen or ibuprofen – increased risk of overdose if taken in addition to combination opiod analgesics.*	1. Usually administered by mouth. 2. Codeine is an extremely effective cough suppressant. 3. Do not confuse hydromorphone with morphine. 4. Warn patient to avoid activities requiring alertness until effects of drug are known. 5. Medications are often in various strength combinations with acetaminophen and/or ibuprofen.

MODERATE OPIOIDS

Butorphanol (**Stadol**): IM, IV, nasal spray Nalbuphine (**Nubain**): subQ, IV, IM	Dizziness, drowsiness	1. Monitor client for effective pain control. 2. Abrupt withdrawal after prolonged use may produce symptoms of withdrawal.

NARCOTIC ANTAGONIST - Antagonists competitively block the effects of narcotics without producing analgesic.

Naloxone (**Narcan**): IV, IM, subQ	Hypotension, hypertension, dysrhythmias. ✓ *NURSING PRIORITY: Pain will return when Narcan is administered.*	1. Assess respiratory status, blood pressure, pulse, and level of consciousness until narcotic wears off. Repeat doses may be necessary if effect of narcotic outlasts the effect of the narcotic antagonist. 2. Remember that narcotic antagonists reverse analgesia along with respiratory depression. Titrate dose accordingly and monitor pain level. 3. *Uses*: Used to reverse CNS and respiratory depression in narcotic overdose. 4. *Contraindications and precautions*: Use with caution in narcotic-dependent patients; may cause severe withdrawal symptoms.

CDC, Centers for Disease Control and Prevention; *CNS*, central nervous system; *IM*, intramuscularly; *IV*, intravenously; *PCA*, patient-controlled analgesia; *PO*, by mouth (orally); *subQ*, subcutaneously.

Pharmacology

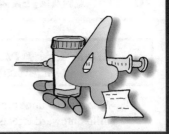

GENERAL CONCEPTS OF PHARMACOLOGY

✻   No medication has a single action; all medications have the potential to alter more that one body function. For example, aspirin may be given for anti-inflammatory action for arthritis, or for antiplatelet action to prevent strokes.

> ✓ *NURSING PRIORITY: Many medications have several actions that are desirable. Carefully evaluate the question to determine the desired response of the medication for the specific client situation.*

A. Desired action: the desired, predictable response for which the medication is administered.
B. Side effects (drug reaction): the undesirable or unwanted response; frequently predictable.
C. Unpredictable response: the unusual response to a medication.
   1. Idiosyncratic reaction: an individual, unexpected response to a medication.
   2. Allergic reaction: may or may not occur with the initial dose of medication; occurs with subsequent doses because it requires that the immune system respond with the production of antibodies in order to trigger the allergic reaction.
D. The Drug Amendments of 1962 made it mandatory that each medication have one official name.
   1. Generic name (nonproprietary): the official designated name that the medication is listed under in official publications.
   2. Chemical name: designates the specific chemical composition of the medication.
   3. Trade name (proprietary name, brand name): the name designated and registered by a specific manufacturer.

> 💡 *TEST ALERT: Typically, the medications on the NCLEX-PN examination will be identified with both the generic and trade name—for example: diazepam (Valium).*

E. Pharmacokinetic process: Consists of four phases - absorption, distribution, metabolism, or excretion, acting together to determine the concentration of a drug at its site of action.

1. Absorption: The movement of the drug from the site of administration into the blood.
   a. Drug absorption can be altered by the increase or decrease in gastric emptying, by changing the gastric pH, or by forming drug complexes.
   b. Administration affects absorption, for example subcutaneous injection vs oral administration.
2. Distribution: The movement of the drug through the body. Drug metabolism and excretion as well as cardiac output will affect the distribution of a drug.
3. Metabolism: the alteration of the drug structure, the alterations occur in the liver with excretion by the kidney.
4. Excretion: Changes in liver and renal function as well as changes in cardiac output will affect the excretion of a drug.

> ✓ *OLDER ADULT PRIORITY: Creatinine clearance is a more effective indication of renal function that serum creatinine in older adults.*

F. Potential for Abuse: Controlled Substances Act, 1970, defines rules for the manufacture and distribution of drugs that are considered to have a potential for abuse.
   1. 5 Categories of medications: Schedules I, II, III, IV, V—potential for abuse decreases with each category, medications in Schedule V have lowest potential for abuse.
   2. Schedule I drugs are highly addictive (e.g., heroin) and are not used in therapeutic administration of medications, Schedule V drugs (e.g., diphenoxylate hydrochloride [**Lomotil**]) have the lowest potential for abuse.

Drug Actions

A. *Desired action:* the desired, predictable response for which the medication is administered.
B. *Adverse drug reactions (ADR):* an undesirable drug effect, ranging from mild untoward effects to severe responses.

✔ *OLDER ADULT PRIORITY: ADRs are 7 times more common in older adults than in young adults.*

1. *Side effects:* undesirable drug effects, ranging from mild untoward effects to severe responses that occur at normal drug dosages.
2. *Toxicity:* drug reactions that primarily occur as a result of receiving an excessive dose (e.g., medication error, poisoning); can also include severe reactions (anaphylaxis) that occur regardless of the dose.
3. *Allergic reactions:* drug reaction that occurs as a result of prior sensitization and results in an immune response. Intensity can range from very mild to very severe (anaphylaxis).
4. *Idiosyncratic effect:* an uncommon drug response.

C. *Tolerance:* an increased dose is required to maintain expected drug response. For example, when a client with chronic pain may requires higher doses of an analgesic to achieve pain relief.
D. *Dependence:* an expected response to repeated use of a drug, resulting in physical signs and symptoms of withdrawal when the serum drug level decreases suddenly. For example, when a client abruptly stops taking a strong opioid agonist (methadone) and develops symptoms of withdrawal.
E. *Addiction:* the continued use of a psychoactive substance regardless of physical, psychologic, or social harm.

Drug Interactions

A. An altered or modified action or effect of a drug as a result of interaction with one or more drugs. It is not an adverse drug reaction or drug toxicity.
B. Drug incompatibility: a chemical or physical reaction that occurs between two or more drugs outside the body.

💡 *TEST ALERT: Assess client for actual or potential side effects and adverse effects of medications; identify symptoms/evidence of allergic reactions to medications; implement procedures to counteract adverse effects of medications; evaluate and document client response to actions taken to counteract side effects and adverse effects of medications.*

C. Potentiation effect (synergistic effect): if two or more drugs are given together and this increases the therapeutic effects, it is beneficial; if it increases adverse effects, it may be detrimental. For example, a diuretic and a beta blocker may be given together for hypertension.
D. Antagonistic or inhibitory effect: if two or more drugs are given together, one may inhibit the effect of the other; this may be beneficial or detrimental. For example, naloxone (**Narcan**) may be given to suppress the effects of morphine.

E. Drug incompatibility: a chemical or physical reaction that occurs when two or more drugs are combined in vitro (outside the body).
F. Breast-feeding: advise women who are lactating to always advise their health care provider; medications may be excreted in breast milk.

💡 *TEST ALERT: Use critical thinking skills when considering the effects and/or outcomes of medications; identify any contraindications to administration of a prescribed or OTC medication.*

G. Food and Drug Administration pregnancy risk categories (Table 4-1).

Herbal Supplements

A. Use of herbs to treat health problems is the most common form of alternative medicine, which can be defined as treatment practices that are not widely accepted or practiced by mainstream clinicians in a given culture.
B. The word *natural* is not synonymous with *safe!* Remember, poison ivy and tobacco are natural, too.
C. Some commonly used medicinal herbs (Table 4-2).

✔ *NURSING PRIORITY: Unlike conventional drugs, herbal and other dietary supplements can be marketed without any proof of safety or efficacy. Dietary supplements are not regulated by the FDA.*

MEDICATION ADMINISTRATION

✔ *NURSING PRIORITY: The nurse's responsibility in administering medication is influenced by three primary factors: nursing guidelines for safe medication administration, pharmacological implications of the medication, and the legal aspects of medication administration.*

Nursing Responsibilities in Medication Administration

A. Follow the "7 Rights" of medication administration.
1. Right medication.
2. Right dosage.
3. Right route of administration.
4. Right time.
5. Right client.
6. Right charting (documentation).
7. Right technique

 💡 *TEST ALERT: Administer medications according to the "7 Rights" of medication administration.*

Table 4-1	FOOD AND DRUG ADMINISTRATION PREGNANCY RISK CATEGORIES

Category	*Description*
A	***Remote Risk of Fetal Harm:*** Adequate and well-controlled studies in pregnant women have not shown an increased risk of fetal abnormalities.
B	***Slightly More Risk Than A:*** Animal studies have revealed no evidence of harm to the fetus; however, there are no adequate and well-controlled studies in pregnant women. *or* Animal studies have shown an adverse effect, but adequate and well-controlled studies in pregnant women have failed to demonstrate a risk to the fetus.
C	***Greater Risk Than B:*** Animal studies have shown an adverse effect, and there are no adequate and well-controlled studies in pregnant women. No animal studies have been conducted, and there are no adequate and well-controlled studies in pregnant women.
D	***Proven Risk of Fetal Harm:*** Studies—adequate well-controlled or observational—in pregnant women have demonstrated a risk to the fetus. However, the benefits of therapy may outweigh the potential risk.
X	***Proven Risk of Fetal Harm:*** Studies—adequate well-controlled or observational—in animals or pregnant women have demonstrated positive evidence of fetal abnormalities. The use of the product is contraindicated in women who are or may become pregnant.

Modified from Lehne RA: *Pharmacology for nursing care*, ed 6, St. Louis, 2007, Saunders; and Meadows M: Pregnancy and drug dilemma, *FDA Consumer Magazine*, May-June 2001. Available at www.fda.gov/fdac/features/2001/301_preg.html.

Table 4-2	COMMONLY USED MEDICINAL HERBS

Medicinal Herb	**Drug Interactions**
Black cohosh is a popular treatment for acute symptoms of menopause and premenstrual syndrome (PMS). Minor side effect of upset stomach may occur.	May potentiate hypotensive effects of antihypertensive drugs, as well as hypoglycemic action of insulin and oral hypoglycemics.
Feverfew for treatment of migraine, fever; stimulates menstruation and suppresses inflammation.	May suppress platelet aggregation and increase risk for bleeding in clients on anticoagulant medications (aspirin, warfarin, heparin).
Garlic reduces levels of triglycerides and cholesterol and decreases formation of atherosclerotic plaque.	Increases risk for bleeding in clients taking antiplatelet drugs (aspirin) or anticoagulants (warfarin, heparin).
Ginger root used for nausea and vomiting caused by motion sickness and perhaps nausea caused by chemotherapy.	Increases risk for bleeding in clients taking antiplatelet drugs (aspirin) or anticoagulants (warfarin, heparin).
Ginkgo biloba is used for increased circulation, memory, clear thinking, and impotence. May cause stomach upset and dose-related headache.	Increases risk for bleeding in clients taking antiplatelet drugs (aspirin) or anticoagulants (warfarin, heparin).
Goldenseal is used for bacterial, fungal, and protozoal infections of mucous membranes in the respiratory, gastrointestinal, and genitourinary tracts. Also used to treat inflammation of the gallbladder. Well tolerated but toxic in high doses.	Contraindicated in pregnancy.
Kava is used to relieve anxiety, promote sleep, and relax muscles. Long-term use and high doses cause CNS depression, skin problems, and liver damage.	Intensifies the effects of CNS depressants. Should not be taken with alcohol.
Ma huang (ephedra) reduces appetite, increases energy, and relieves bronchospasms. Increases blood pressure and heart rate. Potentially dangerous to the cardiovascular system with long-term use or in high doses.	Potentiates the effects of CNS stimulants; can counteract the effects of antihypertensive drugs. May cause hypertensive crisis if taken with MAO inhibitors.
St John's wort is used for depression. Potential interactions with other drugs.	May interfere with oral contraceptives; reduced anticoagulation in clients taking warfarin; decreased effectiveness of cyclosporine. Caution in use with antidepressants.
Saw palmetto is used to relieve urinary symptoms related to benign prostatic hypertrophy (BPH) and is well tolerated. May cause a false-negative result on PSA test.	Avoid use in pregnancy. Should not use with finasteride (**Proscar**) in treatment of BPH.

B. A nurse should administer *only* those medications that he or she has prepared.
C. Be familiar with medication.
1. General reason the client is receiving the medication.
2. Common side effects.
3. Average dose or range of safe doses.
4. Any specific safety precautions before administration (e.g., check apical pulse rate for digitalis; check clotting time for heparin).
D. Document medication against physician's or PCP's orders according to institution policy.
E. Evaluate client's overall condition and assess for changes that may indicate the medication should not be given (e.g., morphine would be contraindicated in a client who has increased intracranial pressure).
F. Use appropriate aseptic technique in preparing and administering medication.
G. Do not leave medications at the client's bedside without a doctor's order to do so.
H. If client is to administer his or her own medication, review the correct method of administration (e.g., eye drops) with the client.
I. Nursing implications for administering medication to an older adult client (Box 4-1).
J. Factors affecting dose – response relationships (Box 4-2).

 TEST ALERT: Maintain current, accurate medication list.

Nurse's Legal Responsibilities in Administration of Medication

A. The nurse administers a medication only by order of a doctor or PCP and according to the provisions of the specific institution.
B. The nurse should not automatically carry out an order if the dosage is outside the normal range or if the route of administration is not appropriate; the nurse should consult the nursing supervisor or PCP.
C. The nurse is legally responsible for the medication he/she administers, even when the medication is administered according to a physician's order.
D. The nurse is responsible for evaluating the client before and after the administration of a PRN medication.
E. The nurse must administer the medication according to the nursing responsibilities previously discussed.
F. The medication should be charted as soon as possible after administration.
G. When taking verbal orders over the phone, carefully repeat all the orders to verify they are correct (Box 3-7).
H. Medication errors:
1. If an error is found in a physician's or PCP's medication order, it is the nurse's responsibility to question the order.

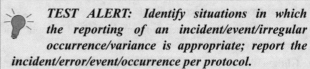
BOX 4-1   Medication Implications for Older Adult Clients

Avoiding adverse drug reactions.
• Obtain a complete drug history that includes over-the-counter drugs and herbs.
• Monitor client responses and drug levels
• Keep dosing regime as simple as possible, use daily dosing when possible rather than twice a day.
• Emphasize to clients the importance of disposing of medications they are no longer taking.

Promoting compliance
• Intentional underdosing (by clients) is the most common reason for nonadherence to drug regimen.
• Provide written instructions to clients regarding medication administration, as well as why they are taking the medication.
• Ask the pharmacist to label drug containers with large type.
• Provide drug containers that can be opened easily.
• Encourage clients to use a system to record or track their drug doses (calendar, pill organizer).
• Determine whether clients can afford their medications.

2. *Always report medication errors to the nursing supervisor or PCP immediately.*
3. It is the nurse's responsibility to carefully assess the client for effects of the erroneous medication.
4. Medication errors should be documented both in an incident report (see Chapter 3) and on the client's chart.

 TEST ALERT: Identify situations in which the reporting of an incident/event/irregular occurrence/variance is appropriate; report the incident/error/event/occurrence per protocol.

I. **High-Alert Medications**.
1. The Joint Commission (TJC) and the Institute for Safe Medication Practices (ISMP) have identified specific medications for which errors could have devastating effects on clients.
2. These medications are identified within the medication tables throughout this book.
3. TJC requires:
a. Institution or facility to develop processes to manage **High-Alert Medications**.
b. A specific process of communication among health careworkers to reconcile medications. This includes a process for reconciling the list of medications during transfer, at discharge, and after major procedures.
4. Nursing Implications for **High-Alert Medications** (Box 4-3).

BOX 4-2 Factors influencing dose-response relationships

- Age: Infants and older adults are generally more sensitive to medications.
- Presence of disease process, specifically kidney and liver problems.
- Method of administration – IV is much more rapid than PO.
- Adequate cardiac output.
- Emotional factors: Clients are more likely to respond to a medication in a positive manner if they have confidence in their treatment and anticipate the therapeutic effects.

Methods of Medication Administration

Note: This section on medications should not be used as a procedure guideline. The purpose is to point out specific characteristics of each method. All medications should be administered according to previously discussed nursing responsibilities in medication administration.

> **TEST ALERT:** *Administer and document medications given by common routes (e.g. oral, topical), administer and document medications given by parenteral routes (intravenous, intramuscular, subcutaneous), and determine the need for administration of PRN medications.*

A. Oral medication.
  1. Assess level of consciousness and ability to follow directions.
  2. Evaluate swallow reflex.

B. Topical medications.
  1. Skin application: evaluate condition of the skin in the area where medication is to be applied; rotate sites to prevent irritation.
  2. Sublingual: allow medication to dissolve under the tongue; client should not chew or swallow.
  3. Nasal: position client to allow nose drops or spray to enter nares directly without contaminating the eyes. Position should foster the movement of the medication to the affected area.
  4. Eyes: medication must be specifically indicated for ophthalmic use.
    a. Instill 1 or 2 drops in the middle of the lower conjunctival sac.
    b. Do not allow tip of applicator to come in contact with the eye.
    c. Do not drop medication directly on the cornea.
    d. Direct client to close his or her eyes gently to distribute the medication.
    e. Make sure you administer the correct medication in the correct eye.
  5. Ears: medication is instilled into the auditory canal.
    a. Position client with affected ear upward.
    b. Children under 3 years: pull pinna down and backward.
    c. Older children and adults: pull pinna up and backward.
    d. Administer solution at room temperature.
    e. Keep client in the same position for appropriate time to prevent medication from coming out.
  6. Suppositories.
    a. Rectal: absorption of medication from rectal mucosa is slower and less predictable than that of medications administered systemically.
      (1) Frequently given for constipation or for nausea and vomiting.
      (2) May be preferred route for infant.

Box 4-3 NURSING IMPLICATIONS FOR HIGH-ALERT MEDICATIONS

- Maintain good communication and locate easily found information regarding the administration of pain medications to prevent overdose, for example, use a visual pain scale. Store narcotics in individual client areas rather than as floor stock.
- Do not store together medications that have the same type of measurements. For example, heparin and insulin are both administered in units.
- Use only accepted abbreviations (See Appendices 4-2, 4-3, 4-4).
- Establish a check system for high alert medications or for calculations, one nurse would prepare the medication and another nurse check it.
- Infusion pump rates and concentrations must have an independent check system.
- Identify medications that have similar names and use caution in administering them. For example, hydromorphone (**Dilaudid**) and morphine; potassium phosphate and potassium chloride; methyldopa (**Aldomet**) with levodopa or L-dopa.
- Premixed solutions and standardized concentrations (potassium chloride, sodium chloride or normal saline) should be available on the nursing unit; decrease the premixing and calculation of medications on the nursing unit.
- Do not store vials or containers of saline in concentrations above 9% on the nursing unit.
- Use single-dose vials when possible.

b. Vaginal: absorption across vaginal mucous membranes.
 (1) Insert suppository about 3 to 4 inches into vagina; maintain supine position after insertion.
 (2) Should not douche unless advised to do so; maintain good perineal hygiene.
C. Transdermal medication: medication is stored in a patch or is measured on a dose-determined applicator placed on the skin; absorption occurs through the skin.
 1. Provides more consistent blood levels and avoids gastrointestinal problems.
 2. Patch sites should be rotated. Old patch should be removed and area should be cleansed after use.
 3. Do not apply a topical patch or apply medication over an inflamed area.
 4. Do not allow transdermal medications to come in contact with your skin, because medication could be absorbed.
 5. Patch must come in contact with client's skin; excessive body hair may need to be removed. Do not shave the area; use scissors to clip hair from area.
D. Inhalation medication: medication is in an aerosol or powder form and is inhaled and absorbed throughout the respiratory tract (see Chapter 10).
 1. Place client in semi-Fowler's position.
 2. Check instructions for use of an inhaler and make sure client understands.
E. Parenteral medications: administration of medications by some method of injection
 1. Injection routes (Figure 4-1)
 2. Selection of a syringe: select a syringe and type of needle that is appropriate for the type of parenteral medication to be administered.
 3. Intradermal injection: administered just below the skin surface.
 a. Use a syringe with appropriate calibrations because amount is very small in volume (0.01 to 0.1 mL).
 b. Use a tuberculin or 1-mL syringe with a small-gauge (25-or 27-gauge) needle, $\frac{3}{8}$ to $\frac{5}{8}$ inch long.
 c. Select area where skin is thin (e.g., inner surface of forearm, middle of back).
 d. Insert needle bevel edge up at a 5- to 15-degree angle.
 e. Frequently used for tuberculin testing, administration of local anesthetic, allergy testing.
 4. Subcutaneous injection: medication is injected into fatty tissue, just below the dermis.
 a. Medication should be small in volume (0.5 to 1 mL) and nonirritating.
 b. Areas on outer surface of upper arm, anterior surface of the thigh, and the abdomen are frequent sites.
 c. Use a 25-gauge needle that is $\frac{5}{8}$ inches long and insert at a 45-degree angle; or a 25-gauge needle that is $\frac{1}{2}$ inch long and insert at a 90-degree angle.

5. Intramuscular injection: injection of medication into the muscle.
 a. The amount of medication is usually 0.5 to 3.0 mL.
 b. Appropriate sites.
 (1) Deltoid (Figure 4-2)
 (2) Vastus lateralis muscles (Figure 4-4), ventrogluteal (Figure 4-3)
 c. Use a 1-inch to $1\frac{1}{2}$-inch needle; gauge of needle depends on viscosity of medication; insert needle at 90-degree angle.
 (1) For oil-based or viscous medications use an 18- to 22-gauge needle.
 (2) For less viscous medications use a 20- to 22-gauge needle.
 d. Aspirate when needle is in place; if no blood returns, administer medication at a rate of 1 mL every 10 seconds.
 e. Z-track technique is used to prevent medication from leaking back through the needle track and irritating or staining subcutaneous tissue.
 (1) After medication is drawn up, change the needle.
 (2) Pull skin over to one side at the injection site.
 (3) Inject medication into taut skin at site selected.
 (4) Remove the needle and release the skin. As the stretched skin returns to its original position, the needle track is sealed.
 (5) The preferable site is the ventrogluteal area.
 f. Intramuscular injections in children.
 (1) Vastus lateralis (see Figure 4-4) muscle is common site in infants.
 (2) Ventrogluteal (see Figure 4-3) site is the preferred site in children.
 (3) A 22-gauge 1-inch needle is appropriate for an IM injection in most children.
6. IV administration medication administered into the blood.
 a. Administration of large volumes of liquid by infusion.
 b. Administration of irritating medications by piggyback method.

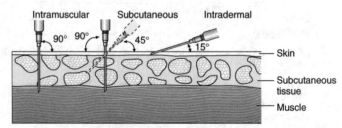

FIGURE 4-1 Injection Routes. Needle insertion angles for intramuscular, subcutaneous, and intradermal injections. (From Lilley L, Harrington S, Snyder J: *Pharmacology and the nursing process, ed 5,* St. Louis, 2007, Mosby.)

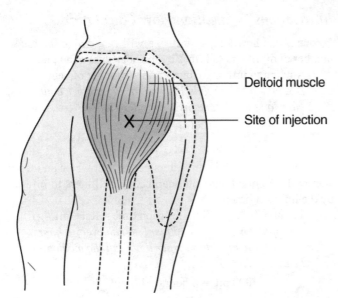

FIGURE 4-2 **Deltoid muscle injection site in the upper arm.** (From Potter P, Perry A: *Fundamentals of nursing, ed 7,* St Louis, 2008, Mosby.)

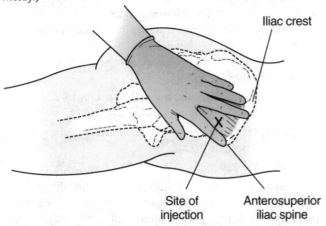

FIGURE 4-3 **Ventrogluteal Intramuscular Injection Site.** Place the palm of your hand over the greater trochanter, with your middle finger pointed toward the iliac crest, your index finger toward the anterosuperior iliac spine, and your thumb toward the client's groin. Administer the injection in the center of the triangle formed by your fingers. (From Lilley L, Harrington S, Snyder J: *Pharmacology and the nursing process, ed 5,* St. Louis, 2007, Mosby.)

    (1) Dilute medication according to directions, usually 25 to 250 mL of a compatible intravenous fluid like normal saline (NS).
    (2) Assess patency of primary infusion.
    (3) Connect medication and adjust flow rate for the time designated, usually 30 to 45 minutes.
    (4) Administration of medications through IV piggyback method enhances the action of the medication.
  c. Retrograde IV administration: medication is mixed with diluent, the port closest to client is clamped and medication is injected into the port and allowed to fill (retrograde) into the IV tubing. The clamp closest to the client is opened and the medication is allowed to infuse at the prescribed flow rate.

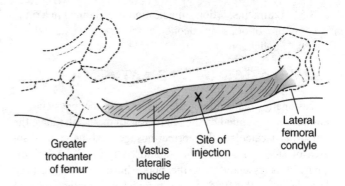

FIGURE 4-4 **Vastus lateralis intramuscular injection site on the right thigh.** Place one hand above the knee and the other hand below the greater trochanter. Locate the midline of both the anterior thigh and the lateral side of the thigh. Give the injection within the rectangular area. (From Lilley L, Harrington S, Snyder J: *Pharmacology and the nursing process, ed 5,* St. Louis, 2007, Mosby.)

  d. Always follow facility guidelines regarding LPN administration of IV piggy back medications.

 TEST ALERT: *Administer IVPB medications, monitor site and flow rate.*

FORMS OF MEDICATION PREPARATIONS

A. Solids.
  1. Capsule: medication is provided in cylindrical gelatin container.
  2. Pills, tablets: medication is pressed into solid form in various shapes and colors.
    a. Enteric-coated: prevents medication from being released in stomach; dissolves in intestine. Do not crush enteric-coated, extended-release (ER), or sustained-release (SR) tablets.
    b. Lozenge: flavored tablet is held in the mouth for slow release of medication.
  3. Suppositories: keep in cool area; will melt at body temperature.
    a. Rectal.
    b. Vaginal.
  4. Ointments: used for external application.
  5. Powders: finely ground medications that are stable only in dry form; frequently mixed with solution before administration.
B. Solutions.
  1. Syrups: medication prepared in an aqueous sugar solution.
  2. Elixirs: solutions containing alcohol, sugar, and water.
  3. Suspensions: finely ground particles of medication dispersed in a liquid; shake all suspensions well before preparing dose (antacids).
  4. Emulsions: medication is dispersed in an oil or fat solution; shake all emulsions well before preparing dose.

5. Liniments, lotions: medication is combined in a mixture of oil, soap, alcohol, water; used for external application.

CALCULATION OF MEDICATION DOSAGES

Occasionally, medications are ordered by the physician in amounts not supplied by the pharmacy. In these situations, the nurse must calculate the correct dosage. Another important area of calculation is in the administration of IV solutions. Thus, it is essential that the nurse have a good working knowledge of the fundamental principles of mathematics to calculate medication dosages correctly.

Oral Medication Calculations

Dose desired ÷ Dose on hand = Amount to give

Example: Order reads to give Keflex 500 mg. Dose on hand is 250-mg capsules.

$$500 \div 250 = 2 \text{ capsules}$$

Dose desired ÷ Dose on hand × Quantity = Amount to give

Example: Order reads to give ampicillin 350 mg. Dose on hand is 250 mg in 5 mL.

$$350 \div 250 \times 5 = x$$

$$350 \div 250 = 1.4$$

$$1.4 \times 5 \text{ mL} = 7 \text{ mL}$$

The problem can also be set up in algebraic proportion:

$$350/x = 250/5 \text{ mL}$$

$$250x = 1750$$

$$x = 7 \text{ mL}$$

Parenteral Medication Calculations

Dose desired ÷ Dose on hand × Quantity of solution = Amount to give

Example: Order reads Gentamycin 60 mg IM. On hand is 80 mg in 1 mL.

$$60 \text{ mg} \div 80 \text{ mg} \times 1 \text{ mL} = x$$

$$60 \div 80 = 0.75$$

$$0.75 \times 1 \text{ mL} = {}^3/_4 \text{ mL or } 0.75 \text{ mL}$$

Set up in algebraic proportion, the equation reads:

$$60 \text{ mg}/x = 80 \text{ mg}/1 \text{ mL}$$

$$60x = 75$$

$$x = 0.75 \text{ mL or } {}^3/_4 \text{ mL}$$

Intravenous Medication Flow Calculation

To determine how long an infusion will run, divide the total number of milliliters to infuse by the hourly infusion rate.

Amount to infuse ÷ Hourly rate = Number of hours

Example: Order reads 1000 mL at 125 mL per hour. How long will it take the 1000 mL to infuse?

$$1000 \div 125 = x$$

$$1000 \div 125 = 8 \text{ hours}$$

To determine the rate in milliliters per hour at which an infusion will run, divide the total number of milliliters to infuse by the infusion time.

Amount to infuse ÷ Total infusion time = Rate (mL/hr)

Example: Order reads 1000 mL to run every 8 hours. At what rate in milliliters per hour will the medication be infused?

$$1000 \text{ mL} \div 8 \text{ hours} = 125 \text{ mL/hr}$$

Calculating drop factors: Check the IV equipment to determine how many drops are delivered in 1 mL. For example purposes, a drop factor of 10 gtt per 1 mL is used. The following are two formulas with which to calculate this factor.

Total mL/Time in min = mL per min × Drop factor = gtt per min

Example: 1000 mL is ordered to infuse in 8 hours. Set drop factor is 10 gtt/mL.

$$1000 \text{ mL} \div 480 \text{ min} = 2.08 \text{ mL/min}$$

$$2.08 \times 10 = 20.8 \text{ or } 21 \text{ gtt/min}$$

Example: 500 mL is ordered to infuse in 2 hours. Set calibration is 10 gtt/mL.

$$500 \text{ mL} \div 120 \text{ min} = 4.16 \times 10 = 41.6 \text{ or } 42 \text{ gtt/min}$$

Determine the number of milliliters per hour and divide by 60 (60 minutes in 1 hour). This equals the number of milliliters per minute. Multiply by set calibration of number of drops per milliliter.

Number of milliliters per hour ÷ 60 = mL/min

Rate (mL/min) × Set calibration = gtt/min

Example: 500 mL is ordered to infuse in 2 hours. Set calibration is 10 gtt/mL (250 mL/hr to infuse).

$$250 \text{ mL} \div 60 = 4.16 \text{ mL/min}$$

$$4.16 \text{ mL} \times 10 = 41.6 \text{ or } 42 \text{ gtt /min}$$

NOTE: *There may be a difference of 2 to 4 gtt when different formulas are used.*

Study Questions: Pharmacology

1. What should the nurse take into consideration when giving medication to an older adult client?
   1 Multiple simultaneous drugs can be dangerous.
   2 The older client metabolizes and excretes medications differently from younger clients.
   3 Medications affect the older client during the early hours of the morning.
   4 Medications have an effect on the respiratory system of the older adult.

2. A client has an order for fluoxetine (**Prozac**) 20 mg in the am and at noon; 10-mg tablets are available. How many tablets will the client receive each day?
   1 8 tablets.
   2 6 tablets.
   3 4 tablets.
   4 3 tablets.

3. A client has been ordered thioridazine (**Mellaril**) elixir 300 mg daily at bedtime. You have Mellaril elixir on the floor at 500 mg/mL. How many milliliters will the client receive?
   1 0.3 mL.
   2 1.3 mL.
   3 0.6 mL.
   4 0.5 mL.

4. Gentamicin (**Garamycin**) 60 mg IM is ordered for a client. Available is a multidose vial with 40 mg/mL. What is the correct amount to give?
   1 1.5 vials.
   2 1.25 vials.
   3 2.0 vials.
   4 1.75 vials.

5. To ensure that the right medication was being given, the first step the nurse would take in preparing to administer the medication would be:
   1 Check the client's ID band.
   2 Read the information insert for directions as to correct administration.
   3 Check the order with the medication administration sheet.
   4 Check the expiration date on the medication.

6. The nurse pours a dose of medication and then finds that the client no longer needs the dose. What action should the nurse take?
   1 Record the dose as taken to keep the count correct.
   2 Charge for the dose because the dose must be paid for.
   3 Record the medication as "not taken" and waste the poured dose.
   4 Pour the medication back into the container.

7. Different medication preparations of drugs are absorbed in the body at different rates of time. Which preparation of a drug absorbs more rapidly?
   1 Ointment applied to the skin.
   2 Liquid medicine given orally.
   3 Oral gelatin capsules.
   4 Enteric-coated tablets.

8. Medications taken orally must undergo a change after contact with body fluids in order to be used by the body. This process is known as:
   1 Concentration.
   2 Elimination.
   3 Transference.
   4 Absorption.

9. The nurse is evaluating information to determine if the client needs a medication. The nurse should first check the:
   1 Client's name.
   2 Expiration date of the drug.
   3 Route of delivery.
   4 Medication administration record.

10. The doctor has indicated that ampicillin and gentamicin are to be given piggyback in the same hour, every 6 hours (12-6-12-6). How would the nurse administer these drugs?
    1 Give both drugs together IV push.
    2 Give each drug separately, flushing between drugs.
    3 Retrograde both drugs into the tubing.
    4 Give one drug every 4 hours and one every 6 hours.

11. Which of the following is correct regarding the administration of an intradermal injection?
    1 It forms a bleb in the dermal area of the skin.
    2 The injection is given at a 40-degree angle.
    3 The injection site is pressed and rubbed in a circular motion.
    4 A 16-gauge needle is used.

12. What is the correct method for administering eye drops to an older adult client?
    1 Drop the medication directly on the cornea.
    2 Instruct the client to rapidly open and close their eye to distribute the medication.
    3 Place the applicator tip on the lower conjunctival sac and instill the drops.
    4 Instill the drops in the lower conjunctival sac.

Answers and rationales to these questions are in the section at the end of the book titled Chapter Study Questions: Answers and Rationales.

Appendix 4-1   CONVERSIONS

Celsius and Fahrenheit
Fahrenheit reading = 9/5 × Celsius reading + 32

Example: Temperature is 50° Celsius
Fahrenheit = 9/5 × 50 + 32
+ 32 = 122° Fahrenheit

Pounds and Grams
1 pound = 454 grams
To convert pounds to grams, multiply the number of pounds by 454.

7.5 × 454 = 3405 g

To convert grams to pounds, divide the number of grams by 454.

Example: An infant weighs 3405 g
3405/454 = 7.5 lb, or 7 lb 8 oz

Appendix 4-2   ABBREVIATIONS AND SYMBOLS

ac	before meals	mL	milliliter
ad lib	as desired	Mg	magnesium
bid	twice daily	mcg	micrograms
c̄	with	N	nitrogen
Ca	calcium	Na	sodium
CBC	complete blood count	NPO	nothing by mouth
Cl	chloridene	OOB	out of bed
et	and	os	mouth
ext	extract	pc	after meals
fl or fld	fluid	po	by mouth
gm	gram	prn	as needed
gt/gtt	drop/drops	q	every
H2O	water	qid	four times a day
H2O2	hydrogen peroxide	q2h	every 2 hours
in	inch	q3h	every 3 hours
K	potassium	s	without
L	liter	ss	one half
lb or #	pound	s̄tat	immediately
liq	liquid	t̄ab	tablet
lytes	electrolytes	tid	three times a day
m	minim	WBC	white blood count/white blood cell

Appendix 4-3	LIST OF "DO NOT USE" ABBREVIATIONS, ACRONYMS, AND SYMBOLS APPROVED BY THE JOINT COMMISSION (TJC)

Abbreviation	Potential Problem	Preferred Term
U (for unit)	Mistaken as zero, four, or cc	Write "unit"
IU (for international unit)	Mistaken as IV (intravenous) or 10 (ten)	Write "international unit"
Q.D., QD, q.d., qd, (Latin abbreviation for once daily) Q.O.D., QOD, q.o.d., qod, (Latin abbreviation for every other day)	Mistaken for each other. The period after the Q can be mistaken for an "I" and the "O" can be mistaken for "I."	Write "daily" and "every other day"
Trailing zero (X.0 mg) Lack of leading zero (.X mg)	Decimal point is missed	Write X mg Write 0.X mg
MS, MSO_4, $MgSO_4$	Can mean morphine sulfate or magnesium sulfate Confused for one another	Write "morphine sulfate" or "magnesium sulfate"

From Joint Commission on Accreditation of Healthcare Organizations: *The Official "Do Not Use" List Updated – March 2009.* Available at www.jointcommission.org/PatientSafety/DoNotUseList/.

Appendix 4-4	ABBREVIATIONS AND SYMBOLS THAT ARE RECOMMENDED BUT NOT YET MANDATED BY THE JOINT COMMISSION (TJC) FOR INCLUSION IN THE OFFICIAL "DO NOT USE" LIST

Abbreviation	Potential Problem	Preferred Term
> (Greater greater than) < (Less less than)	Confused for one another and could be interpreted as the letter "L" or the number "7"	Write "greater than" or "less than"
@ (for the word at) Drug name abbreviations	Mistaken for the number "2" Misinterpreted for another drug due to similar abbreviations	Write "at" Write drug names in full
µg (for microgram)	Mistaken for mg (milligrams) resulting in 1000-fold dosing overdose	Write "mcg" or "microgram"

From Joint Commission on Accreditation of Healthcare Organizations: *The Official "Do Not Use" List Updated – August 2009.* Available at www.jointcommission.org/PatientSafety/DoNotUseList/.

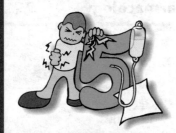

Homeostasis

* **Homeostasis, for the purposes of this chapter, is defined as the mechanism for maintaining a steady state in the body.**

FLUID AND ELECTROLYTES

Physiology

A. Basic concepts of body fluid.
1. Water is a primary body fluid. It is used to transport nutrients as well as to remove waste products.
    a. Infant: 70% to 80% of body weight is water.
    b. Adult: 50% to 60% of body weight is water.
    c. Older adult: 45% to 55% of body weight is water.
2. *Electrolytes:* electrically charged particles; electrolytes found in intracellular fluid and in extracellular fluid are essentially the same; however, the concentrations differ.
3. *Intracellular fluid:* fluid located within the cell wall.
    a. Approximately 40% to 50% of total body fluid.
    b. Potassium is the primary electrolyte.
4. *Extracellular fluid (ECF):* fluid located outside the cell wall.
    a. Approximately 30% to 40% of total body water.
    b. An infant maintains a larger percentage of extra cellular fluids than does an older child or adult.
    c. *Vascular:* circulating plasma volume.
    d. *Interstitial:* fluid surrounding tissue cells.
    e. Sodium is the primary electrolyte.
B. Dynamic transport of fluid and electrolytes.
1. *Diffusion:* movement of molecules from an area of high concentration to an area of low concentration.
2. *Osmosis:* movement of water through a semipermeable membrane from an area of low electrolyte concentration to an area of high concentration; osmotic pressure is the term used to describe osmosis (water goes where the salt is).
3. *Filtration:* movement of water and electrolytes through a semipermeable membrane from an area of high pressure to an area of low pressure; hydrostatic pressure is the term used to describe the force of filtration.
C. Plasma to interstitial fluid shift.
1. *Edema:* accumulation of fluid in interstitial spaces.
2. Hypovolemia may occur as a result of excessive fluid shift into the interstitial spaces, resulting in circulatory collapse.

Fluid Imbalances (ECF)

A. *Fluid deficit:* loss of or failure to replace body fluid.
1. *Sensible fluid loss:* fluid loss of which an individual is aware, such as urine.
2. *Insensible fluid loss:* fluid loss of which an individual is not aware. Approximately 1000 ml of fluid is lost every 24 hours through the skin and lungs in a normal adult.
3. Causes of fluid deficit:
    a. Decrease in or lack of adequate fluid intake.
    b. Loss of body fluid - vomiting, diarrhea, nasogastric suctioning.
4. Clinical manifestations.
    a. Thirst.
    b. Dry skin and dry mucous membranes.
    c. Poor skin turgor
    d. Weight loss.
    e. Urine.
        (1) Less than 30 ml/hr: oliguria.
        (2) Concentrated, dark, foul-smelling.
    f. Postural hypotension.
    g. Increased heart rate.
    h. Poor cerebral perfusion due to decreased blood volume.
        (1) Increased respiratory rate to compensate.
        (2) Restlessness, lethargy, confusion in the older adult client.
        (3) May require supplemental oxygen.
    i. Depressed fontanels in the infant; infants and children may have mottled skin color due to poor tissue perfusion.
5. Laboratory findings:
    a. Increased specific gravity of urine (greater than 1.030)
    b. Increased blood urea nitrogen level (BUN over 25 mg/dl) without increase in creatinine level.
    c. Increased hematocrit: normal ratio of hematocrit (Hct) to hemoglobin (Hgb) is 3:1; for example, if the hemoglobin is 12 g, the hematocrit should be 36%.
    d. Hyperglycemia (blood glucose concentration higher than 120 mg/dl).

> ✔ **NURSING PRIORITY:** *Monitor diagnostic and lab results and modify a client's care based on results.*

B. *Fluid excess:* retention of both water and sodium.
   1. Causes of fluid excess.
      a. Excessive oral fluid intake.
      b. Failure to excrete fluids, as in renal disease and congestive heart failure.
      c. Iatrogenic - fluid increase due to excessive infusion of IV fluids.
      d. Excessive sodium intake.

> **NURSING PRIORITY:** *Sodium is the major electrolyte that affects fluid balance. "Where goes the sodium, so goes the water." Weight gain or loss is most significant indicator of fluid gain or loss.*

   2. Clinical manifestations.
      a. Weight gain.
      b. Presence of pitting edema in lower extremities; sacral edema.
      c. Distended neck veins in semi-Fowler's position
      d. Dyspnea with exertion, wet breath sounds which may precede pulmonary edema.
      e. Bounding pulse, increased pulse rate
      f. Lethargy, dizziness, headache, confusion.
      g. Variable urine volume.
      h. Increased blood pressure.
   3. Laboratory findings:
      a. Decreased urine specific gravity (less than 1.010).
      b. Decreased hematocrit with a loss of the hemoglobin/hematocrit 1:3 ratio (12 g Hgb with a 27% [hemodilution] Hct).

> **TEST ALERT:** *Monitor client's hydration status (I&O, edema, signs and symptoms of dehydration); monitor output (e.g., NG drainage, emesis, stools, urine); adjust intake to improve fluid and electrolyte balance.*

C. Nursing management of client with fluid imbalances.
   1. Data collection.
      a. Evaluate client's history and predisposing factors contributing to the problem.
      b. Evaluate skin turgor.
         (1) Assess skin turgor on the abdomen or the inner thigh in children (unless abdominal distention is present).
         (2) Assess skin turgor on the forehead or sternum in older adult clients.
         (3) Assess skin turgor on the sternum, abdomen, and anterior forearm in adults.
      c. Collect data to determine direction of fluid problem: fluid excess or deficit.
      d. Older adult clients and infants are more sensitive to problem with fluid balance.
      e. Evaluate client's tolerance of fluid imbalance – vital signs, level of consciousness, respiratory status.

   2. Nursing interventions.

> **NURSING PRIORITY:** *Increased urine specific gravity, dark urine, decreased urine output and postural hypotension are very objective clues to fluid deficit.*

      a. Maintain accurate intake and output records.
      b. Obtain accurate daily weights – same scale, same time each day, same amount of clothing (1 L of fluid = 1 Kg [2.2 pounds]).
      c. Evaluate for presence of peripheral edema and sacral edema.
      d. Good skin care.
         (1) Evaluate skin and prevent problems with skin breakdown due to edema or areas of increased pressure.
         (2) Protect skin in areas of edema; prevent excoriation.
         (3) Do not use soap on skin of dehydrated client, cleans gently and apply lubricants to flaky dry skin.
      e. Monitor vital signs and assess client response to correction of the problem (decreased fluid intake, diuretic therapy, or increased fluid intake both PO and IV).
      f. Blood pressure is not a reliable indicator of problems of fluid balance in young children.
      g. Monitor respiratory status, maintain good respiratory hygiene; monitor pulse oximetry for changes in ventilation.
      h. Maintain safety – problems of orthostatic hypotension, confusion, and changes in respirations increase risk of falls.
      i. Monitor sodium intake – encourage decreased sodium diet.
      j. Replace fluid loss
         (1) Unless contraindicated, encourage 2000-3000mL fluid daily in the average adult client.
         (2) If no nausea and vomiting, encourage oral rehydrating solution, offer the client 2-4 ounces of fluid every hour.
      k. Monitor urine output.
         (1) Minimum amount of urine is 30mL per hour or about 720mL daily.
         (2) Check urine specific gravity.
         (3) Monitor BUN, and electrolyte values.
   3. See appendixes on electrolyte imbalances and replacement (Appendixes 5-1 through 5-3).

> **NURSING PRIORITY:** *Daily weight is the most reliable indicator of fluid loss or gain in all clients, regardless of age. Accurate daily weight: same time each day, preferably before breakfast; same scale; same clothing.*

INTRAVENOUS FLUID REPLACEMENT THERAPY

Goals of Fluid Therapy

❖   **Goal:** To maintain adequate fluid balance.
    A.   Client NPO.
    B.   Unable to take fluids by mouth due to disease process.
❖   **Goal:** To correct a fluid or electrolyte deficiency
❖   **Goal:** To maintain nutritional requirements (caloric replacement).
    A.   Nutritional requirements are in excess of the intake, as in burns, extensive surgery.
    B.   Unable to absorb food in small intestine.

> **TEST ALERT:** *Monitor client receiving peripheral IV fluids.*

Intravenous Infusions

A.   Factors influencing rate of fluid administration.
    1.   Type of fluid.
    2.   Age of client.
    3.   Cardiac and renal status.
    4.   Size of the vein and gauge of catheter/needle.
    5.   Client's response to fluids.
B.   Maintain accurate intake and output records.
C.   Average maintenance fluid rate is 2000 to 3000 mL over 24 hours.
D.   Heparin lock.
    1.   Maintain patency of IV access for intermittent administration of medication or fluid.
    2.   May be flushed with a heparin flush solution or saline solution at regular intervals to maintain patency.
    3.   Site may be converted to fluid infusion if necessary.
E.   Intravenous (IV) infusion sites are changed on a regular basis, preferably before inflammation, irritation, or fluid extravasation occurring at the site.
F.   Pediatric considerations - children are very susceptible to rapid fluid shifts resulting in fluid overload. IV solutions of normal saline or percentages of normal saline are frequently used to decrease the possibility of cerebral edema.

> ✔ **NURSING PRIORITY:** *Determine the amount of fluid that has actually been infused and correlate with the rate set on the infusion pump or IV control settings. Monitor IV site and regulate flow rate.*

Indications for Use of Infusion Control Devices

A.   To deliver a medication that requires a precise rate of administration (dopamine, Heparin, aminophylline).

B.   To deliver fluids in controlled amounts to a client very sensitive to volume administered (infants, children, older adult clients, client's with problems managing fluid status).
C.   To deliver IV fluids over a prescribed period of time (1000 mL in 8 hours).

Complications of Intravenous Therapy

Infiltration

A.   *Common causes:* dislodging of the needle by client movement or obstruction of fluid flow, bevel of needle pushed through posterior aspect of vein during insertion, placement of catheter in an area of flexion, needle not taped or anchored properly.
B.   *Signs and symptoms:* edema, blanching of skin, discomfort at site, fluid that is flowing slowly or has stopped, cooler skin temperature. IV solution is much cooler than client's body temperature.
C.   *Preventive nursing management:*
    1.   Use an armboard to stabilize catheter, especially in restless, confused clients, or those with catheters placed in the antecubital fossa area.
    2.   Frequently check for coolness of skin around site.
    3.   Avoid looping tubing below bed level.
    4.   Check IV flow rate at least every 2 hours.
D.   *Nursing interventions:* elevate extremity, apply moist heat to increase fluid absorption; anticipate RN will resite the IV.

Phlebitis

A.   *Common causes:* overuse of a vein, infusion of irritating solutions or medications, catheter in vein for too long a period of time, use of large gauge catheters.
B.   *Signs and symptoms:* tenderness, pain along the course of the vein, edema, redness at insertion site, red streak along course of vein, arm with IV feels warmer than other arm.
C.   *Preventive nursing management:*
    1.   Dilute medications (IV antibiotics) with adequate diluent to provide less irritating solution.
    2.   Infuse at prescribed rate.
    3.   Change IV location site every 72 hours or per facility policy.
D.   *Advise RN if phlebitis occurs and anticipate the catheter will be removed and resited.*
E.   *Nursing interventions:* apply warm compresses to stimulate circulation and promote absorption.

> ✔ **OLDER ADULT PRIORITY:** *(1) Fluids are generally administered at a slower rate due to decreased ability of the heart and kidneys to handle fluids. (2) Older adult clients are prone to circulatory overload. (3) Poor skin turgor is not a reliable indicator of fluid status in the older adult.*

Circulatory Overload

A. *Common causes:* IV is positional and infuses too rapidly, preexisting medical conditions that make client more prone to develop pulmonary edema (more frequent in older adult clients and infants).

B. *Signs and symptoms:* increased blood pressure and central venous pressure (CVP), jugular vein distention with client's head elevated, shortness of breath, increased respirations, wet breath sounds, coughing.

C. *Preventive nursing management:* use infusion control devices to maintain infusion at prescribed rate; closely monitor client at increased risk of problem with fluid excess.

D. *Nursing interventions:* reduce infusion rate to a "keep open" rate; *notify RN and/or health care provider*; position client in semi-Fowler's and begin oxygen.

> ✔ *NURSING PRIORITY: Inspect intravenous site for infiltration and/or extravasation and report to the nursing supervisor or primary care provider (PCP); advise the RN if an IV site is over 72 hours old.*

ACID-BASE BALANCE

Basic Concepts of Acid-Base Balance

A. Terms used to describe acid-base balance.
1. pH: the chemical abbreviation for the negative logarithm of hydrogen ion concentration.
2. CO_2: carbon dioxide.
3. Pco_2: pressure of dissolved carbon dioxide gas in the blood.
4. O_2: oxygen.
5. PO_2: pressure of dissolved oxygen gas in the blood.
6. HCO_3^-: bicarbonate.
7. mm Hg: millimeters of mercury.
8. H^+: hydrogen ion.

B. Normal blood gas values.
1. pH 7.4 (7.35 to 7.45).
2. PO_2: 80 to 100 mm Hg.
3. Pco_2: 35 to 45 mm Hg.
4. HCO_3^-: 22 to 26 milliequivalents (mEq/L).

C. The hydrogen ion (H^+) concentration determines the acidity or alkalinity of a solution. The higher the H^+ concentration; the more acid the solution. The increased H^+ concentration is reflected by a decrease in the pH.

D. Acid-base ratio is determined by sampling arterial blood. This provides a reliable index of overall body function.

E. The body maintains a normal or neutral state of acid-base balance. The stable concentration of H^+ balance is reflected in arterial blood with a relatively constant pH of 7.35 to 7.45.

Regulation of Acid-Base Balance

A. Buffer system: the most rapid-acting of the regulatory systems. The buffer system is activated where there is an excess acid or base present.
1. A buffer is a chemical that helps maintain a normal pH.
2. The buffer system chemicals are paired. The primary buffer chemicals are sodium bicarbonate and carbonic acid. The buffers are capable of absorbing or releasing hydrogen ions as necessary.
3. An effective buffer system depends on normal-functioning respiratory and renal systems.

B. Respiratory system: the second most rapid response in the regulation of acid-base balance. Carbonic acid is transported to the lungs via the veins, where it is converted to carbon dioxide and water, and then excreted.
1. Carbon dioxide is considered an acid substance because it combines with water to form carbonic acid.
2. Increased respirations will decrease carbon dioxide levels, thus decreasing the carbonic acid concentration and resulting in decreased H^+ concentration and an increase in the pH.
3. Decreased respirations will cause a retention of carbon dioxide, increasing the carbonic acid concentrations and resulting in increased H^+ concentration and a decrease in the pH.
4. With excessive acid formation, the respiratory center in the medulla is stimulated, which results in an increase in the depth and rate of respirations. This promotes a decrease in the carbon dioxide levels and attempts to return the pH to a more normal point.
5. With excessive base formation, the respiratory rate slows in order to promote retention of carbon dioxide and decrease the alkalotic state. The Pco_2 levels are influenced only by respiratory system.

C. Renal system: the slower but most effective mechanism of acid-base regulation.
1. The kidneys reabsorb sodium (Na), and produce and conserve sodium bicarbonate ($NaHCO_3$).
2. In acidosis the kidneys will attempt to excrete more H^+.

Alterations in Acid-Base Balance

A. *Respiratory acidosis:* characterized by an excessive retention of carbon dioxide due to hypoventilation.
1. Primary causes: conditions that cause decreased respiratory function.
   a. Head injuries.
   b. Oversedation with sedatives and/or narcotics.
   c. Infection of CNS.
   d. Postoperative anesthesia.
   e. Conditions decrease effective pulmonary function.
     (1) Obstructive pulmonary diseases.

      (2) Pneumonia.
      (3) Cystic fibrosis.
      (4) Atelectasis.
      (5) Occlusion of respiratory passages (asthma).
  2. Clinical manifestations.
    a. Dyspnea on exertion.
    b. Rapid, shallow respirations.
    c. Disorientation, decreased level of consciousness.
    d. Tachycardia, arrhythmias.
    e. Muscle weakness.
  3. Blood gas values.
    a. pH decreases below 7.35.
    b. Pco_2 increases above 45 mm Hg.
    c. HCO_3- may remain within normal limits.
  4. Nursing management.
    a. Use preventive management.
      (1) Have postoperative or immobilized client turn, cough, and deep breathe every 2 hours.
      (2) Decrease use of narcotics as client begins to experience less pain postoperative.
      (3) Maintain adequate hydration.
    b. Position in semi-Fowler's to facilitate breathing.
    c. Thoroughly assess client's pulmonary function.
    d. Try postural drainage and percussion followed by suction to remove excessive pulmonary secretions.
    e. Anticipate use of bronchodilator either systemically or aerosol.
    f. *Report any changes in the client's respiratory status.*

B. *Respiratory alkalosis:* characterized by a low Pco_2 most often due to hyperventilation.
  1. Primary cause of respiratory alkalosis.
    a. Emotional origin (hysteria, fear, apprehension).
    b. Hyperventilation due to disease entity.
    c. CNS problems (encephalitis, increased intracranial pressure).
  2. Clinical manifestations.
    a. Deep, rapid breathing.
    b. Muscle twitching.
    c. Tingling of extremities.
    d. Seizures.
    e. Confusion.
    f. Hyperreflexia.
  3. Blood gas values.
    a. pH increases above 7.45.
    b. Pco_2 decreases below 35 mm Hg.
    c. HCO_3- may remain within normal limits.
  4. Nursing management.
    a. Identify and eliminate (if possible) causative factor.
    b. Evaluate need for sedation.
    c. Use rebreathing devices (mask or paper sack) to increase CO_2 levels.
    d. Remain with client to decrease anxiety levels.

C. Metabolic alkalosis: characterized by an increase in the bicarbonate levels in the serum.
  1. Primary causes.
    a. Diuretic therapy: causes an increase in the loss of H^+ ions, and a decrease in the serum bicarbonate level.
    b. Excessive loss of H^+ ions.
      (1) Prolonged nasogastric suctioning without adequate electrolyte replacement.
      (2) Excessive vomiting resulting in loss of hydrochloric acid and K^+.
  2. Clinical manifestations.
    a. Nausea, vomiting, diarrhea.
    b. Increased irritability, disorientation.
    c. Restlessness.
    d. Muscle twitching.
    e. Shallow, slow respirations.
    f. Arrhythmias.
  3. Blood gas values.
    a. pH increases above 7.45.
    b. Pco_2 normal.
    c. HCO_3- increases above 26 mEq/L.
  4. Nursing management.
    a. Preventive.
      (1) Provide foods high in potassium and chloride for client on diuretics.
      (2) Administer potassium supplement to clients on long-term diuretics.
      (3) Monitor IV solution with replacement electrolytes.
    b. Maintain accurate intake and output records.

D. Metabolic acidosis: characterized by a decrease in bicarbonate level in the serum.
  1. Primary causes (deficit of a base or an increase in acid).
    a. Diabetic acidosis.
    b. Abnormal loss of alkaline substances.
      (1) Deep, prolonged vomiting may precipitate acidosis due to a loss of base products.
      (2) Severe diarrhea and loss of pancreatic secretions may precipitate an acidotic state.
    c. Renal insufficiency: kidney loses ability to retain HCO_3- and to excrete H^+.
    d. Salicylate poisoning due to accumulation of ketone bodies produced as a result of the increased metabolic rate.
  2. Clinical manifestations.
    a. Disorientation.
    b. Deep, rapid respirations (Kussmaul's respirations).
    c. Changes in level of consciousness (drowsiness, stupor, coma).
    d. Muscle twitching.
    e. Arrhythmias.
  3. Blood gas values.
    a. pH decreases below 7.35.
    b. Pco_2 remains normal.
    c. HCO_3- decreases below 22 mEq/L.

4. Nursing management.
   a. Assist in identification of underlying problem.
   b. Maintain accurate intake and output records.
   c. Evaluate client for hydration due to excessive fluid loss.
   d. Support respiratory system.

INFLAMMATION

✱ **Inflammation is the tissue response to localized injury or trauma.**

Basic Concepts of Inflammation

A. Three major categories.
   1. Simple acute.
      a. Occurs most quickly and may leave with no residual damage.
      b. Neutrophils (WBCs) are usually the predominant cell.
   Example: Skin infection, tonsillitis.
   2. Delayed hypersensitivity.
      a. Typical inflammatory response.
      b. Directly caused by an antigen-sensitized lymphocyte reaction.
      c. Develops over time.
   Example: Tuberculin skin testing, subacute bacterial endocarditis (SBE), and organ transplant rejection.
   3. Chronic.
      a. Characterized by pain, redness, and swelling.
      b. Does not subside in 2 weeks, but has a damaging course that lasts for weeks, months, or even years.
      c. Predominant cell types are lymphocytes, plasma cells, and macrophages.
   Example: Rheumatoid arthritis, tuberculosis, chronic glomerulonephritis.
B. Concepts of the inflammatory response.
   1. The movement of blood and fluid into an injured area is necessary to promote healing of the damaged tissue. This is particularly true of a surgical client.
   2. Problems occur when the area of edema impedes tissue perfusion. This is particularly true of edema and swelling with orthopedic injuries (fractured extremities in a cast or traction).

3. Antiinflammatory medications (corticosteroids) may be administered to the client when the swelling is impeding tissue perfusion.
4. Antiinflammatory medications may hamper the healing process and mask the symptoms of an infection.
C. Cardinal signs of inflammation.
   1. Local response (Table 5-1).
   2. Systemic response.
      a. Fever.
      b. Leukocytosis (increased number of neutrophils in circulation).
      c. Malaise.
      d. Nausea and anorexia.
      e. Weight loss.
      f. Increased pulse rate and respiration.

INFECTION

✱ **Infection is the process by which an organism (pathogen, pathogenic agent) invades the host and establishes a parasitic relationship.**

A. Healthcare associated infections (HAIs, nosocomial infections): infections acquired from exposure to pathogens in a hospital setting or health care setting.
B. Iatrogenic infections are HAIs that result from a diagnostic or therapeutic procedure (urinary tract infection from urinary catheterization).
C. Emerging infection is an infectious disease that has increased over past 20 years.
D. Development of multiple drug-resistant organisms (MDRO) has further complicated treatment of infections (they are resistant to antibiotics).

Chain of Transmission

A. Pathogens.
   1. Incubation period: the period of time from exposure to the pathogen until symptoms of infection occur in the host.
   2. A person can be asymptomatic and still transmit a pathogen that will produce an infection in someone else (carrier).
   3. Pathogens vary in how they interact with the host.

TABLE 5-1   CARDINAL SIGNS OF INFLAMMATION

CLINICAL SYMPTOM	PATHOPHYSIOLOGY
Redness	Hyperemia from vasodilation
Heat	Increased metabolism at site and local vasodilation
Pain	Pressure from fluid exudate on adjacent nerve endings, which leads to nerve stimulation; change in local pH
Edema	Fluid shift and accumulation in interstitial spaces
Loss of function	Decreased movement due to swelling and pain

4. Toxigenicity refers to the destructive potential of the toxin that is released by the pathogen.
5. Types of pathogens.
   a. Viruses.
   b. Bacteria: gram-negative and gram-positive.
   c. Fungi.
   d. Chlamydia.
   e. Protozoa.
   f. Mycoplasma.
B. Reservoir.
   1. Environment within which the organism can live and multiply; is provided by some organic substance—human or animal.
   2. Provides essential needs for organism survival.
   3. A carrier provides an environment for the pathogen to grow and multiply, but shows no symptoms of the infection.
C. Exit port.
   1. How the infection leaves the host.
   2. Common ports of exit include feces, secretions, and body fluids.
   3. Understanding port of exit is necessary to prevent transmission of pathogen.
D. Route of transmission.
   1. Method by which the pathogen moves to another host.
   2. Direct transmission is immediate transfer from one host to another, as in sexually transmitted diseases or inhalation of contaminated droplets from respiratory tract infections.
   3. Indirect transmission occurs via an intermediate carrier, for example, mosquitos, contaminated water, or contaminated food.
E. Port of entry into susceptible host.
   1. May enter the host via inhalation, ingestion, through the mucous membranes, or percutaneously.
   2. Whether an infectious disease will occur depends on the defense system of the invaded host.
   3. Biological and personal characteristics of the new host will determine the lines of defense the host will have against the invading pathogen.
F. Control of transmission.
   1. Transmission of a contagious disease can be broken by interfering with any link of the transmission chain.
   2. Treatment is aimed at breaking the transmission chain at the most vulnerable and cost-effective point.
      a. Barrier precautions: gloves, gowns, condoms.
      b. Proper handling of food and water supplies.
      c. Avoidance of high-risk behavior: unsafe sex, IV drug use.
      d. Good hand hygiene technique and good personal hygiene.
   3. Important to consider chain of transmission in order to protect health care workers.

4. Host susceptibility can be greatly reduced through immunizations (see Table 2-3, Figure 2-2).

> 💡 **TEST ALERT:** *Apply principles of infection control (e.g., hand hygiene, isolation, standard precautions, communicable disease reporting). Be able to apply this to clients of all ages and all categories of client care.*

Nursing Interventions

❖ **Goal:** To prevent infection.
A. Hand hygiene is the single most effective mechanism for preventing spread of infection (see Box 5-2).
B. Monitor vital signs: increase in pulse, respiration, and temperature occurring 4 to 5 days after surgery may indicate infectious process.
C. Monitor for Staphylococcus and Pseudomonas pathogens (produce purulent, draining wounds).
D. Maintain aseptic technique in dressing changes and wound irrigations.
E. Maintain standard precautions (see Appendix 5-9).
F. Administer antibiotic medications (see Appendix 5-10).
G. Identify clients at increased risk for infections.
   1. Older adults (Box 5-3).
   2. Immunocompromised clients.
   3. Clients compromised by chronic health care problems.
   4. Poorly nourished clients.
   5. Client with high-risk lifestyle (IV drug use, unprotected sex).
❖ **Goal:** To promote healing.
A. Encourage high fluid intake when client has a fever: 2000-3000 mL daily for adults.
B. Encourage a diet high in protein, carbohydrates, and vitamins—specifically vitamins A, C, and B complex.
C. Immobilize an injured extremity with a cast, splint, or bandage.
D. Administer antipyretic medications (ASA, acetaminophen).

BOX 5-1	SIGNS OF INFECTION

Generalized
- Fever, localized inflammation, joint pain, fatigue, and increased white blood cells

Gastrointestinal Tract
- Diarrhea, nausea, and vomiting

Respiratory Tract
- Purulent sputum, sore throat, chest pain, and congestion

Urinary Tract
- Urgency and frequency, hematuria, purulent discharge, dysuria, and flank pain

E. Identify early signs of infection to facilitate treatment (Box 5-1).
❖ Goal: To decrease pain.
A. Cold packs applied after initial trauma may help decrease swelling and pain.
B. Heat may be used later to promote healing and to localize the inflammatory agents.
C. Elevate the injured area to decrease edema and promote venous return.

> ✔️ *NURSING PRIORITY: Use correct hand hygiene techniques—soap and water or an antimicrobial cleanser.*

BOX 5-2	HAND HYGIENE

Hand hygiene is the most important and most basic action to prevent transmission of infections.

Hand Hygiene With Soap and Water
• Hand washing should be done under flow of water.
• Wet hands and wrists under running water: keep hands and forearms lower than elbows.
• Using antibacterial soap, lather and wash hands using friction for at least 15 seconds.
• Rinse hands thoroughly under running water, keeping hands lower than elbows.
• Do not allow washed hands to touch inside of sink.
• Use soap and water any time the hands are visibly soiled.

Hand Hygiene With Antiseptic Cleanser
• Rub hands together covering all surfaces of the hands and fingers with cleanser.
• Rub hands together until cleanser is dry.
• Use if hands are not visibly soiled.

> ✔️ *NURSING PRIORITY: Hand hygiene must be performed before and after the use of gloves.*

BOX 5-3	OLDER ADULT CARE FOCUS
	INFECTIONS

• May be manifested by changes in behavior: confusion, disorientation.
• May not exhibit fever or pain.
• Closely monitor client response to antibiotics, especially with regard to renal function.
• Maintain adequate hydration.
• Monitor GI function; diarrhea is common with antibiotics.

❖ Goal: To prevent complications.
A. Increase surveillance for clients with decreased white cell counts (leukopenia), or impaired circulation, clients receiving steroids that suppress inflammation or drugs that depress bone marrow as well as clients exposed to a communicable disease.
B. Protect healing wounds from injury that could be caused by pulling or stretching.
C. Identify clients with compromised immune response; they are at high risk for opportunistic infection.

Prevention of Transmission of Infection in the Health Care Setting

A. Maintain standard precautions (see Appendix 5-9), especially good hand hygiene.
B. Consider all blood and body fluids from all clients to be contaminated.
C. Avoid contaminating outside of container when collecting specimens.
D. Do not recap needles and syringes.
E. Cleanse work surface areas with appropriate germicide (household bleach in concentrations of 1:100 to 1:10 is effective).
F. Clean up spills of blood and body fluid immediately. Remove as much of the body fluid as possible, then wash the area with a germicide solution.

Systemic Inflammatory Response Syndrome (SIRS, sepsis)

✳️ **SIRS or sepsis occurs when pathogens enter the blood and are carried throughout the body.**
A. Gram-negative bacteria are most common.
B. Increased risk in clients with urinary catheters, respiratory infections, invasive procedures (arterial lines, CVP, any indwelling line).
C. At-risk clients: older adults, clients with chronic health problems, clients on immunosuppressive therapy and the clients who are malnourished.
D. Clinical manifestations (SIRS and septic shock).
    1. Compromised respiratory function.
       a. Hypoventilation and respiratory acidosis.
       b. Hypoxia and respiratory failure (Chapter 10).
    2. Compromised cardiac function - development of hypotension and tachycardia.
    3. Fever and an elevated white blood cell count.
    4. May rapidly progress to septic shock.

> ✔️ *NURSING PRIORITY: Closely monitor a client with an infection for the development of a septic condition; identifying and reporting the problem are critical to the successful treatment.*

Treatment

A. Prevention of infection.
B. Aggressive treatment of infections.
C. Aggressive pulmonary support.
D. Fluid resuscitation.

Nursing Interventions

❖ **Goal:** To maintain optimal functioning of organs involved.
A. Prevent transmission of infection.
B. Early identification of infectious process – complaints from client that indicate a urinary tract infection, upper respiratory problems, change in level of consciousness.
C. Support cardiac system.
   1. Maintain hydration status.
   2. Monitor blood pressure and tissue perfusion.
   3. Monitor for development of septic shock (Chapter 11).
D. Support respiratory system (Chapter 10).
   1. Prevention of hypoxia.
   2. Monitor for respiratory acidosis.
   3. Good pulmonary hygiene.

Antibiotic-Resistant Infections

A. Strains of bacteria that have developed a resistance to common antibiotics.
   1. Methicillin-resistant *Staphylococcus aureus:* wound, skin and soft tissue, pneumonia.
   2. Vancomycin-resistant *Enterococcus faecalis:* urinary tract infections.
   3. Penicillin resistant *Streptococcus pneumoniae:* pneumonia.
   4. Cephalosporin resistant *Klebsiella pneumoniae:* pneumonia.
B. Transmission.
   1. Most common mode of transmission is from client to client, caused by poor hand hygiene.
   2. Nosocomial infections or healthcare-associated infections (HAIs).

C. Clients at increased risk.
   1. Treatment with multiple antibiotics.
   2. Multiple hospitalizations.
   3. Older adults with chronic conditions.
   4. Immunosuppressed clients.

Treatment

Culture and sensitivity, then administration of antibiotics sensitive to the identified bacteria.

Nursing Interventions

❖ **Goal:** To decrease spread of infection.
A. Routine cultures of health care workers.
B. Identification of clients at increased risk.
C. If there is a draining wound or productive cough droplet and contact precautions are added to standard precautions:
   1. Private room.
   2. Gown and gloves.
   3. Masks are necessary with droplet precautions for a client with a respiratory tract infection.
   4. Teach family importance of gloves and gowns.
D. Most common mode of transmission is via the hands of health care workers; hand washing is critical, even after removal of gloves (Box 5-2).

IMMUNE SYSTEM

Physiology of the Immune System

✳ **The immune system cannot be divided into specific compartments. Immunity includes all physiological mechanisms that enable the body to protect itself against invasion of foreign substances or proteins. An *immunological reaction* is the homeostatic protective response through which the body reorganizes and destroys foreign agents (antigens).**
A. The immune system serves three primary functions.
   1. Defense against infection; protection of the body against invading microorganisms.

TABLE 5-2	ACQUIRED IMMUNITY	
TYPE	**CHARACTERISTICS**	**EXAMPLES**
Active: Antibodies synthesized by body in response to antigen stimulation.	*Natural:* Contact with an antigen through exposure; develops slowly, often lifetime protection.	Recovery from childhood diseases (e.g., chicken pox, measles, mumps).
	Artificial: Immunization with an antigen develops slowly; may provide protection for several years, but "boosters" may be required.	Immunization with live or attenuated vaccines (varicella, IPV, MMR). Toxoid immunization (tetanus toxoid, diphtheria toxoid).
Passive: Antibodies produced in one individual and transferred to another.	*Natural:* Immunity from placenta and colostrum transferred from mother to child; provides immediate temporary protection.	Maternal immunoglobulin in the neonate.
	Artificial: Injection of serum from immune human or animal; short-lived but immediate immunity.	Gamma globulin; injection of animal hyperimmune serum (diphtheria antitoxin, tetanus antitoxin).

2. Maintain homeostasis by removing old cells; the primary organ involved is the spleen.
3. Surveillance of circulating cells with identification and destruction of the abnormal cells.
B. The body recognizes foreign proteins that are not part of the normal constituents of the body. These foreign proteins—antigens—elicit a response from the immune system. The immune system produces antibodies that attack and destroy the invading antigens.

Immunological Responses

A. Properties of the immunological response.
1. *Specificity:* the formation of a specific antibody for each antigen. Antibodies produced against one bacteria will not protect the body from other types of bacteria.
Example: Antibodies against chickenpox will not protect the body against measles.
2. *Memory:* the ability to remember the specific antigen and make the appropriate antibody. Once the body responds to a particular antigen, memory cells are produced. This produces a stronger immune response the next time the body comes in contact with the same antigen.
Example: The body remembers how to make the antibody against the chickenpox virus.
3. *Self-recognition:* the ability of the body to recognize its own proteins and differentiate them from foreign protein. This allows foreign protein to be attacked without injury to the body's own cells.
Example: When the body does not recognize its own cells, the condition is called autoimmunity and can lead to autoimmune diseases or disorders.

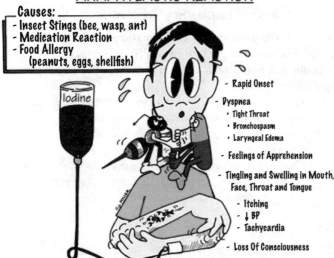

Figure 5-1 Anaphylaxis. (From Zerwekh J, Claborn J, Miller CJ: *Memory Notebook of Nursing*, ed 3, vol 2, Ingram: 2007, Nursing Education Consultants.)

B. Types of specific immunity.
1. Natural immunity: no prior contact with an antigen; may be related to genetic tendency or be species-specific.
2. Acquired immunity: develops either actively or passively (Table 5-2).

Factors Affecting the Immune Response

A. **Age:** An infant's immune system is not fully developed, and in the elderly the immune response is hypoactive.
B. **Metabolism:** Thyroid and adrenal hormone deficiencies decrease the immune response; steroids inhibit the inflammatory response.
C. **Emotional stress:** Stress may precipitate a decrease in the normal production of cells for the immune response.
D. **Hormonal influences:** Females have a greater incidence of autoimmune diseases than do males.
E. **Environment and lifestyle:** Unsanitary living conditions and exposure to pathogens may increase susceptibility to infections.
F. **Nutrition:** Poor nutrition can decrease the overall immune response.

Autoimmune Response

A. When the immune system can no longer recognize normal tissue and begins to destroy healthy tissue, an autoimmune response has occurred. Antibodies (autoantibodies) are then formed against the body's own antigens.
B. Some autoimmune responses are very tissue-specific and only invade that tissue, while another response may cause effects throughout the entire body.
C. Autoimmune response may be systemic or organ-specific.
1. Systemic diseases.
   a. Systemic lupus erythematosus (SLE).
   b. Rheumatoid arthritis.
2. Organ-specific diseases.
   a. Myasthenia Gravis (CNS).
   b. Hyperthyroidism (Graves' disease).
   c. Addison's disease (adrenal glands).
   d. Insulin-dependent diabetes (type 1 diabetes mellitus).

Anaphylactic Reaction

* **Type I occurs in clients who are highly sensitized to a specific allergen—medications, blood products, insect stings. The antigen-antibody response precipitates the release of histamine, causing vasodilatation and increased capillary permeability (Figure 5-1).**

Data Collection

A. Risk Factors.
1. History of exposure to allergen.
   a. Amount of allergen.
   b. Absorption of ingested allergen.

c.   Antibody levels from previous exposure.
2.   The more rapid the onset of symptoms after exposure, the more severe the reaction.
B.   Clinical manifestations—depend on the level of prior sensitivity and the amount of allergen.
1.   Mild to moderate: peripheral tingling/itching (pruritus, urticaria) sensation of warmth, edema of the lips and tongue, nasal congestion, flushing, anxiety.
2.   May rapidly progress to acute anxiety, difficulty breathing (bronchospasm, laryngeal edema), GI cramping, cyanosis, and hypotension; can be fatal.

Diagnostics – *based on symptoms and exposure to allergen.*

Treatment

A.   Mild to moderate reactions—antihistamines and/or epinephrine 0.2 to 0.5 mL (1:1000 solution), administered subcutaneously or intramuscularly (Appendix 5-12).

> ✓ *NURSING PRIORITY: When administering epinephrine, make sure you have the correct concentration of solution. It is most often administered in concentrations of 0.1% or 1:1,000 subcutaneously or IM.*

B.   Oxygen in high concentrations.
C.   IV fluids to maintain circulatory status.
D.   Maintain patent airway—intubation or tracheostomy may be necessary.
E.   Corticosteroids to reduce inflammatory response (see Appendix 5-7).

> 💡 *TEST ALERT: Respond to a life threatening emergency, symptoms progress very rapidly. Emergency treatment should be initiated immediately if anaphylaxis is suspected. Death from an anaphylactic reaction is most often caused by bronchospasm and edema of the airway.*

Nursing Interventions

❖ Goal: To assess clients for predisposition to hypersensitivity reactions.
A.   Evaluate client history regarding reactions to:
1.   Medications, especially penicillin.
2.   Foods (e.g., seafood or iodine, eggs, peanuts).
3.   Insect bites.
4.   Vaccines, especially egg-cultured types.
5.   Blood products (transfusion reaction).
6.   Diagnostic agents (e.g., iodine-based contrast media).

> *TEST ALERT: Check for client allergies.*

B.   Prevention is the priority - always check for allergies when admitting clients and when administering potential allergen (penicillin, iodine based dyes for diagnostics, monitoring blood infusions)
❖ Goal: To maintain adequate ventilation.

> ✓ *NURSING PRIORITY: Airway positioning and mouth-to-mouth resuscitation will not provide adequate ventilation when client has airway edema. An emergency tracheotomy or intubation may be indicated.*

A.   Maintain bed rest; place client in low Fowler's position with the legs elevated.
B.   High oxygen concentrations if airway is compromised.
C.   Anticipate use of airway adjuncts (tracheostomy, endotracheal intubation).
D.   Administration of medications to reverse bronchospasm (albuterol, corticosteroid, epinephrine).
❖ Goal: To restore adequate circulation.
A.   Monitor IV site and rate of IV fluids.
B.   Carefully evaluate client response to fluid replacement – vital signs, urinary output, level of consciousness, breath sounds.
❖ Goal: Client teaching to prevent recurrence.
A.   Once causative agent is identified, instruct client accordingly.
B.   Advise client to wear identification tag or bracelet.
C.   Explain to client that if he or she had any level of allergic reaction previously, the next exposure could be worse (penicillin, insect stings, etc.).

> 💡 *TEST ALERT: Protect immunocompromised clients.*

Systemic Lupus Erythematosus (SLE)

*   **SLE is a multisystem inflammatory autoimmune disorder. SLE is characterized by a diffuse production of autoantibodies that attack and cause damage to body organs and tissue.**
A.   Tissue injury in SLE results from deposition of the immune complexes throughout the body (kidneys, heart, skin, brain, and joints); this activates the inflammatory response.
B.   The severity of symptoms varies greatly throughout the course of the disease; periods of exacerbation and remission occur.

Data Collection

A.   Clinical manifestations
1.   Initially may be nonspecific: weight loss, fatigue, and fever.
2.   Integumentary: characteristic "butterfly" rash over face in about 50% of clients; erythematous rash on

areas of the body exposed to sunlight (photosensitivity); alopecia; dry scaly scalp; palmer erythema.

B. Immune complexes form in the body and cause an inflammatory response in body systems. This inflammation leads to organ dysfunction (e.g., glomerulonephritis, pericarditis and vascular inflammation of small vessels, cerebral inflammation, pleural inflammation).

C. Diagnostics.
1. No specific test is diagnostic; assess configuration of symptoms.
2. Presence of antinuclear antibody (ANA), high levels of anti-DNA, and presence of anti-Smith antibodies are most suggestive of a diagnosis of SLE.
3. C-reactive protein (CRP), erythrocyte sedimentation rate (ESR)—monitor progress of inflammation.

Treatment

SLE has no known cure.
A. Nonsteroidal antiinflammatory medications (see Appendix 5-8).
B. Corticosteroids for exacerbations polyarthritis (see Appendix 5-7).
C. Immunosuppressants

Nursing Interventions

❖ Goal: To prevent exacerbations.
A. Maintain good nutritional status.
B. Avoid exposure to infections.
C. Teach client regarding skin problems and photosensitivity; observe for complications.
D. Teach client personal hygiene to prevent urinary tract infections.
E. Make sure client understands how to take medications.
F. Review with client signs and symptoms of infection; call health care provider (HCP) if fever, chills, anorexia, or worsening of symptoms occurs.
G. Avoid exposure to sunlight; use a heavy sunscreen when exposure is unavoidable.
H. Teach client to contact HCP before participating in any immunization procedures.
❖ Goal: To promote adequate tissue perfusion.
A. Assess for indications of impaired peripheral perfusion—numbness, tingling, and weakness of hands and feet.
B. Prevent injury to extremities—especially fingers.
C. Carefully evaluate fluid status with regard to cardiac output, fluid retention, and weight gain.
❖ Goal: To maintain homeostasis.
A. Effective pain control
1. NSAIDs to control arthritic pain.
2. Nonpharmacologic therapies to supplement analgesics (Chapter 3).
B. Identify problems with fluids and renal function.
C. Monitor for peripheral edema, hypertension, hematuria, decreased output.

D. Monitor for urinary tract infections (glomerulonephritis).
E. Assess for peripheral edema and excess fluid volume.

Acquired Immunodeficiency Syndrome (AIDS)

✳ Occurs as a result of being infected with the human immunodeficiency virus (HIV). Once a client is infected, he or she will harbor the virus for the rest of their life.

Transmission of HIV

A. Blood transmission.
1. Needle-sticks that occur when the client has a high viral load carry a higher risk than those that occur when client is at a low viral load; sharing of contaminated needles accounts for a significant number of transmissions by infected blood.
2. Exposure to an infected client's blood via open wounds or mucous membranes.
3. Transmission via blood transfusions has been greatly reduced with the screening of donated blood.
B. Sexual transmission—most common mode of transmission.
1. Sexual practices, not preferences, place people at increased risk.
2. Risk for infection is greater for the partner who receives the semen during oral, vaginal, or anal sex.
3. Any sexual activity that involves direct contact with vaginal secretions and semen may transmit HIV.
C. Perinatal transmission.
1. Exposure can occur during pregnancy, at the time of delivery, or during the postpartum period through breast milk.
2. 25% of infants born to HIV-positive mothers are infected.
3. Prophylactic antiviral medications during pregnancy can reduce rate of transmission.
D. HIV *cannot* be transmitted by:
1. Hugging, kissing, holding hands, or other nonsexual contact.
2. Inanimate objects (money, doorknobs, bathtubs, toilet seats, etc).
3. Dishes, silverware, or food handled by an infected person.
4. Animals or insects.
5. Tears, saliva, urine, emesis, sputum, feces, or sweat.
F. The viral load in the semen, blood, vaginal secretions, or breast milk is an important variable in the transmission.

> ✓ **NURSING PRIORITY:** *It is essential for the nurse to know the modes of transmission of HIV, activities that do not transmit the virus, and the nursing care to protect yourself, your AIDS client, and other clients under your care.*

Clinical Manifestations

A. The disease progression is highly individualized; the average time between the HIV infection and the development of AIDS is about 11 years, during which the symptoms are frequently vague and nonspecific.

B. CD4$^+$ T helper cells are the regulating cells in the immune system; the level of CD4$^+$ T cells is used to monitor the progression of the virus; normal CD4$^+$ T cell count is at least 800 cells/mm3 of blood.

C. Acute HIV infection.
1. Intense viral replication and dissemination of HIV throughout the body.
2. Symptoms are mild, ranging from no symptoms to flu-like (low fever, fatigue, lymphadenopathy) symptoms.
3. Window of seroconversion: is the time period from when the person is infected with the virus until HIV antibodies can be detected.
4. Average time for seroconversion to occur is 1 to 3 weeks.
5. A client may have vague, nonspecific symptoms for years.
6. During this period, there is a high viral load and the CD4$^+$ T cell count falls, but only temporarily.

B. Early chronic infection—CD4$^+$ T cell count greater than 500 cells/mm3 and low viral load.
1. May be an asymptomatic phase; however, chronic vague symptoms persist.
2. Persistent generalized lymph node enlargement.

C. Intermediate chronic infection—CD4$^+$ T cell count between 200 and 500 cells/mm3 and increased viral load.
1. Exacerbation of symptoms, client begins to experience localized infections, increased lymphadenopathy, and neurologic manifestations.
   a. *Candida* is a common problem—persistent oropharyngeal or vulvovaginal candidiasis.
   b. Hairy oral leukoplakia, which may also be indication of progression of disease.
   c. Shingles, oral or genital herpes lesions.
2. Kaposi's sarcoma.
   a. A cutaneous skin lesion that looks like a bruise; later will turn dark violet or black.
   b. Invades body organs, extremities, skin, and torso.
   c. May become very painful.

> ✔ **NURSING PRIORITY:** *A client who is HIV positive may or may not have AIDS, however a client with AIDS is always HIV positive.*

D. Late chronic infection, or AIDS (acquired immunodeficiency syndrome)—CD4$^+$ T cell count less than 200 cells/mm3 and viral load increases. Diagnosis of AIDS is made when the HIV-positive client develops at least one of the following disease processes.
1. CD4$^+$ T cell count below 200 cells/mm3.
2. AIDS dementia complex.
3. Wasting syndrome caused by HIV.
4. At least one opportunistic cancer—invasive cervical cancer, Kaposi's sarcoma, primary lymphoma of the brain.
5. At least one opportunistic infection—fungal, bacterial, or protozoal infection.

Opportunistic Diseases

A. Diseases and infections that occur in clients with AIDS are called *opportunistic* because they take advantage of the suppressed immune system.
1. The severity of the infection depends on the extent of immunosuppression.
2. Single opportunistic infections are rare; a client usually has multiple infections.

B. Infections may be delayed or prevented by antiretroviral therapy, vaccines (hepatitis B, influenza, and pneumococcal), and disease-specific prevention.

C. *Coccidioides jiroveci* pneumonia, *Pneumocystis jirovecii* pneumonia (previously called *Pneumocystis carinii PCP*).
1. May be caused by a pathogen in the body that is dormant.
2. Is not common in healthy individuals; immune system must be compromised for the infection to occur.
3. Symptoms: fever, night sweats, nonproductive cough, progressive dyspnea.

D. Tuberculosis (see Chapter 10).

E. Kaposi's sarcoma: a bruised, dry-appearing skin lesion; may be present internally as well.

F. Candidiasis of the esophagus, mouth, vagina.

Diagnostics

A. HIV-antibody testing.
1. Enzyme immunoassay testing (EIA): detects the serum antibodies that bind to the HIV antigens. After the acute HIV invasion, an increase in the viral load and a decrease in CD4$^+$ count occur; the client begins to develop antibodies to the HIV. If client has history of recent exposure, retesting is recommended at 3 weeks, 6 weeks, and 3 months.
2. If the EIA test result is positive, then it is repeated; if it remains positive, the Western blot (WB) and immunofluorescence assay (IFA) tests are done to confirm the HIV-positive results.
3. If the EIA is consistently positive and the WB and IFA results are positive, the client is considered to be HIV-antibody positive.

B. Rapid HIV tests—ready in minutes, but results are preliminary and must be confirmed; client needs to return for an antibody-based test (Western blot) 2-4 months later.

C. Serum monitoring after diagnosis.
1. CD4$^+$ T cell counts and plasma assays (HIV RNA viral load).
2. Evaluation for drug resistance.

> ✔ *NURSING PRIORITY: A positive test means the person has HIV, but does not predict the course of the disease. A negative test means that HIV antibodies were not detected; this can occur in the seroconversion window.*

Treatment

A. Medications: antiretroviral therapy (ART) (Appendix 5-11).
   1. Prescribed according to the viral load and the CD4+ T cell counts.
   2. Women should begin ART even if they are pregnant.
   3. Combination drug therapy attacks virus at different stages of replication.
B. Medications will not cure the client, but will decrease the viral replication and slow disease process.
C. Adherence to drug schedules is critical—nonadherence to drug regimen can lead to mutations of the virus and increased virus resistance.

> ✔ *NURSING PRIORITY: Treatment for the AIDS client causes problems in other areas: the high-dose antibiotics and chemotherapy medications will further decrease bone marrow function. The AIDS client on chemotherapy is going to be even further immunocompromised.*

Nursing Interventions

See Nursing Interventions for immunocompromised clients.
❖ **Goal:** To provide and promote client and public education regarding transmission of HIV.

> ✔ *NURSING PRIORITY: Public and client teaching regarding the transmission of the HIV is vital in the control of this disease. The period of time from when the client is infected until the condition is diagnosed is when the majority of new infections are transmitted.*

A. Safe sex.
   1. Maintain monogamous relationships.
   2. Sex with female or male prostitutes is a high-risk activity.
   3. Avoid all direct contact with a partner's mouth, penis, vagina, or rectum if the HIV status of the partner is not known.
   4. Avoid all sexual activities that cause cuts or tears in the vagina, on the penis, or in the rectum.
   5. Males should wear a condom if multiple partners are involved.
   6. If the HIV status of a sexual partner is not known, a condom should always be used during intercourse.

7. Anyone who has been involved in any high-risk sexual activities or who has injected IV recreational drugs should have a blood test to determine presence of the HIV.
B. Needles should not be recapped or shared. Dispose of them in an impenetrable sealed container.

☀ Home Care

A. An employee in a health care setting should advise employer of HIV-positive status.
B. Kitchen and bathroom facilities may be shared, provided that normal sanitary practices are observed.
C. Clean up spills of body fluids or waste immediately with a solution of 1 part bleach to 10 parts water. A bleach solution can be used to disinfect kitchen and bathroom floors, showers, sinks, and toilet bowls.
D. Towels and washcloths should not be shared without laundering.
E. Sanitary napkins, tampons, and any bloody dressings should be wrapped in a plastic bag and placed in a trash container.
F. Needles should not be recapped. Dispose of them in an impenetrable sealed container.
G. Do not donate blood or plasma, body organs, or semen.

📋 Pediatric Acquired Immunodeficiency Syndrome

✳ **The majority of children with AIDS were infected in the perinatal period. Cases related to blood transfusions are relatively rare.**

> ✔ *NURSING PRIORITY: HIV-positive mothers should not breast-feed their infants.*

Data Collection

A. Risk factors.
   1. Pediatric infection from transfused blood is virtually nonexistent.
   2. Sexual activity and IV drug use are the major causes of HIV infection in adolescents.
   3. Infants born to mothers who are HIV-positive account for the majority of children with HIV infection; ART therapy during pregnancy reduces risk for transmission to fetus.
   4. Children rarely have Kaposi's sarcoma; PCP is most common opportunistic infection.
B. Clinical manifestations.
   1. Infants affected during the prenatal period have rapid disease progression.
   2. HIV-positive infants usually have symptoms by 18 to 24 months of age.
   3. Infants diagnosed within the first year of life have a poor prognosis, as do those who develop *Pneumocystis jirovecii pneumonia* (PCP) and progressive encephalopathy.

C. Diagnostics.
   1. EIA and WB for children 18 months or older.
   2. Newborn: polymerase chain reaction (PCR); p24 antigen detection; majority of infants who are HIV-positive can be identified by 3 months of age.
   3. Maternal antibodies to the HIV may persist for up to 18 months.
   4. Positive results on two separate occasions and from separate blood specimens for p24 antigen detection, polymerase chain reaction, and virus culture are required to confirm diagnosis of HIV infection.

Treatment

Treatment for children is essentially the same as that for an adult.

Nursing Interventions Specific to Children

❖ Goal: To maintain homeostasis.
A. Infants and children should receive the standard immunizations against childhood diseases. Measles-mumps-rubella (MMR) and varicella (chicken pox) vaccines may be given if the child is not severely immuno-compromised.
B. Pneumococcal and influenza vaccines are recommended.
C. Nutritional support; high-calorie, high-protein diet.
D. Antifungal medications to prevent fungal infections.
E. Educate adolescents regarding safe sex.

☀ Home Care

A. Teach parent(s) how to care for the child.
   1. How to administer medications and importance of administering medications as scheduled.
   2. Symptoms of complications: PCP, *Candida*, failure to thrive.
   3. Teach parents standard precautions, including proper handling of diapers and avoidance of contact with blood and body fluids.
   4. Help parents deal with child's pain—multiple procedures, infections (abscessed tooth, otitis media).

Nursing Interventions for Immunocompromised Clients

An immunocompromised client does not have the protection of an effective immune system (clients with cancer and on chemotherapy, chronic progressive diseases, HIV).

❖ Goal: To monitor for and/or prevent opportunistic infections.
A. The type, location, and severity of the infection depend on the disease progress and the client's immunosuppressive state.
B. Protect against health care related infections.

C. Observe hospitalized client and/or teach client symptoms of opportunistic infections.
   1. Persistent unexplained fever, night sweats.
   2. Thrush (white spots in the mouth).
   3. Persistent diarrhea and weight loss.
❖ Goal: To maintain ventilation and prevent pulmonary involvement.
A. Frequent assessments for pulmonary changes and hypoxemia.
B. Encourage activities if possible, assess response to activities.
C. Supplemental oxygen.
D. Coughing and deep-breathing exercises.
E. Adequate fluid intake, assess hydration status.

> ✓ **NURSING PRIORITY:** *Clients who have a compromised immune system should not participate in any immunization program until they have checked with their health care provider.*

❖ Goal: To assist client to minimize the effects of neurologic changes.
A. Frequent assessment of neurologic status.
B. Assess for visual changes.
C. Observe for neurologic infections, specifically meningitis.
D. Provide a safe and supportive environment, based on client's neurological status.
   1. Maintain safety in client's room – beds, equipment, cords, etc.
   2. Initiate fall precautions.
   3. Provide frequent reorientation to environment.
❖ Goal: To maintain adequate nutritional intake.
A. Teach as well as provide client a high caloric intake (high-calorie, high-protein diet; nutrition to correct deficiencies).
B. Encourage high-calorie snacks and dietary supplements throughout the day.
C. Encourage client to eat several small meals throughout the day.
D. Avoid foods or beverages that may cause oral, esophageal, or gastric irritation.
❖ Goal: To maintain fluid and electrolyte status.
A. Evaluate daily weight gain and loss.
B. Assess for presence of and effects of chronic diarrhea.
C. Encourage oral rehydrating fluids.
❖ Goal: To prevent formation of pressure ulcers and excoriation of the skin.
A. Wash perineal and anal areas; allow areas to dry thoroughly.
B. Observe bony prominence for adequacy of circulation and development of a pressure ulcer.
C. Do not put any lotions on reddened areas or open lesions.
D. Teach client the importance of frequent changes in position.

E.   Use gel pads, foam mattress pads, and other devices to prevent skin breakdown in pressure prone areas (heels and sacrum).

❖   **Goal:** To assist client to maintain psychologic equilibrium.

A.   Encourage client to express feelings and concerns.

B.   Encourage client to maintain as much independence as possible.

C.   Do not be judgmental regarding client's lifestyle.

D.   Maintain frequent contact with the client.

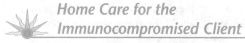

Home Care for the Immunocompromised Client

A.   Maintain personal hygiene and practice standard precautions; wash hands frequently.

B.   Do not share personal items such as toothbrushes, razors, and enema equipment.

C.   Teach client how to prevent infection.
1.   Cook all vegetables and meats, and peel fruit before eating; this eliminates many sources of microorganisms.
2.   Avoid contact with animal waste (e.g., litter boxes, bird cages, or fish); this further decreases contact with microorganisms.
3.   Avoid crowds and people with respiratory tract infections.

D.   Do not get pregnant.

Study Questions: Homeostasis

1.   A client is being started on prednisone (**Deltasone**). What is important to teach the client regarding his medication?
1   Increase fluid intake.
2   Increase dose as needed.
3   Do not discontinue medication abruptly.
4   Do not take medication with food.

2.   The nurse would identify what situation where a client's condition could quickly deteriorate into severe respiratory difficulty and shock?
1   Anaphylaxis.
2   Allergic reaction.
3   Serum sickness.
4   Hay fever.

3.   The nurse is caring for a client who has an autoimmune condition. What would the nurse identify as a physiological principle behind an autoimmune condition?
1   A severe reaction to an allergen can quickly compromise the respiratory status of a client.
2   A body response where the body does not recognize own body tissue.
3   A severe compromise of the body's immune system and inability to fight infection.
4   Antibodies are synthesized in the body as a response to stimulation from a specific antigen.

4.   A client is beginning long-term medication therapy with methylprednisolone (**SoluMedrol**). What is important to teach the client regarding the medication?
1   The medication will decrease the client's inflammatory response and ability to fight infections.
2   The client should return to have anticoagulant blood studies drawn every 3 months.
3   The client should carry a dose of epinephrine (**EpiPen**) in case of an allergic reaction.
4   It will be important for the client to maintain a high fluid intake with supplemental potassium.

5.   A child has received his 3-month series of vaccinations, what type of immunity does this provide?
1   Autoimmune.
2   Natural active immunity.
3   Acquired passive immunity.
4   Acquired active immunity.

6.   A child develops a case of chicken pox. What has developed in the child's immune system as a result of this exposure?
1   Decreased CD4$^+$ T cell count.
2   An autoimmune response.
3   Increased erythrocytes.
4   Presence of antibodies.

7. The nurse is evaluating an older adult client for adequacy of hydration. What would the nurse observe if the client has a fluid volume deficit?
   1   Peripheral edema
   2   Weight gain of 2 pounds in 24 hours.
   3   Dizziness when standing at bedside.
   4   Light color urine in increased amounts.
8. The nurse is evaluating the fluid balance on an older adult client. What is the most accurate measurement to determine changes in a client's fluid balance?
   1   Adequacy of skin turgor.
   2   Daily body weight.
   3   Measure intake and output.
   4   Measure circumference of the legs.
9. The nurse is checking a client's foot for edema and finds barely detectable pitting. What is this level of edema?
   1   4+.
   2   3+.
   3   2+.
   4   1+.
10. What organ system is responsible for the regulation of the fluid and electrolyte balance in the body?
    1   Kidneys.
    2   Heart.
    3   Parathyroid.
    4   Liver.
11. A client has had a fever of 103° F for the past 24 hours. What would be an important nursing action?
    1   Encourage intake of fluids.
    2   Monitor for problem with bradycardia.
    3   Assess lungs for presence of wet breath sounds.
    4   Assess for retention of excess fluids.
12. The nurse observes flushed, dry skin on a client. What would be important for the nurse to further evaluate on this client?
    1   Presence of edema in the lower extremities.
    2   Changes in blood pressure.
    3   Urinary output and concentration.
    4   Presence of upper respiratory infection.
13. The nurse is assessing an older adult client and determines the presence of dry mucous membranes and confusion. The nurse should continue to assess the client for what complication?
    1   Increased blood pressure.
    2   Retention of excess fluid.
    3   Excessive loss of body fluids.
    4   Problems with electrolyte balance.
14. Which client would the nurse identify as being at the greatest risk for having a significant fluid imbalance if their fluid intake was significantly reduced?
    1   46-year-old diabetic adult.
    2   3-week-old infant.
    3   12-year-old underweight teenager.
    4   25-year-old obese adult.

15. The nurse would identify what nursing situation that would require the use of protective eyewear?
    1   When emptying urinals and bedpans.
    2   While administering an IM injection.
    3   While performing direct client care for a client with droplet precautions.
    4   Whenever there is a chance of splashing blood or body fluids.
16. The nurse has been assigned a postoperative client. In report the nurse is told the client is experiencing a problem with respiratory acidosis. What nursing care will be important for this client?
    1   Increase fluid intake.
    2   Provide oxygen via a face mask.
    3   Observe for confusion.
    4   Turn, cough, and deep breathe.
17. What is important for the nurse to teach the HIV-positive client regarding transmission of the human immunodeficiency virus? It is most frequently transmitted:
    1   Via sexual contact with an infected individual.
    2   Through contact with contaminated blood.
    3   From the mother via the placenta at birth.
    4   By sharing a bathroom with an infected individual.
18. In caring for the client who is severely immunosuppressed, what is a priority nursing concern?
    1   Maintaining therapeutic communication.
    2   Preventing opportunistic infections.
    3   Promoting good skin care and wound healing.
    4   Maintaining adequate elimination.
19. A client is taking gentamicin (**Garamycin**). What serious side effect will it be important for the nurse to evaluate for on this client?
    1   Anaphylactic reaction
    2   Gastrointestinal bleeding.
    3   Increased susceptibility to infections.
    4   Decrease in ability to hear.
20. The nurse is performing a dressing change on a client who has a staphylococcus infection in an abdominal incision. What infection control precautions will the nurse implement? Select all that apply:
    ___ 1   Wear clean gloves to remove the old dressing.
    ___ 2   Put on a gown when entering the room.
    ___ 3   Wear a face shield.
    ___ 4   Dispose of the gown and mask in container outside client's door.
    ___ 5   Leave all extra dressing supplies in the room.
    ___ 6   Carefully cleanse the stethoscope and scissors that came in contact with the client.

Answers and rationales to these questions are in the section at the end of the book titled Chapter Study Questions: Answers and Rationales.

Appendix 5-1   POTASSIUM IMBALANCES

NORMAL (K⁺) LEVELS: 3.5-5.0 mEq/L

CAUSES	SYMPTOMS	NURSING IMPLICATIONS

HYPOKALEMIA: Serum K⁺ below 3.5 mEq/L

CAUSES	SYMPTOMS	NURSING IMPLICATIONS

Decreased intake of K⁺
GI loss:
   Vomiting. diarrhea
   Nasogastric suction without
     replacement
Diaphoresis
Diuretics
Diabetics: Insulin and glucose moves
   K⁺ into cell
	Fatigue, muscle weakness, cramps
	Decreased reflexes
	Confusion, drowsiness, fatigue
	Bradycardia, weak irregular pulse
	Decreased bowel sounds.
		1. Identify source of depletion and or increase
		    – maintain good I&O records.
		2. Monitor K+ levels.
		3. Encourage foods high in K+ if deficit is
		    present.
		4. Encourage foods low is K+ if excess is
		    present.
		5. Maintain accurate I&O records.
		6. Evaluate for digitalis toxicity (low serum K⁺
		    potentiates digitalis).
		7. Provide client education regarding diuretics.

HYPERKALEMIA: Serum K⁺ above 5.0 mEq/L

CAUSES	SYMPTOMS	NURSING IMPLICATIONS

Decreased urinary excretion
   Renal failure
Massive tissue injury:
   Burns, trauma
Excessive administration of IV K⁺
Salt substitutes containing
   potassium
	Drowsiness, irritability, anxiety
	Muscle weakness to flaccid paralysis in
	   lower extremities
	Dysrhythmias:
	Bradycardia, ventricular fibrillation,
	   cardiac arrest
	Diarrhea
		See Nursing Implications under Hypokalemia.

Appendix 5-2   POTASSIUM MEDICATIONS

POTASSIUM SUPPLEMENTS

Oral:
   Potassium chloride (**KCl**)
   Sustained release:
   K-Dur, Micro-K, Slow-K
   Potassium gluconate (**Kaon**)
IV: Potassium acetate

1. Sustained-release preparations are better tolerated and more convenient.
2. Oral preparations generally have unpleasant taste and are irritating to GI system; they should be
    administered with a full glass of water or juice.
3. Pediatric implications: make sure child/infant is urinating adequately before beginning
    supplementation.
4. IV K⁺ must be diluted and administered by IV drip. Do not give K⁺ IM or by IV push; may cause
    cardiac arrest.
5. IV K+ solutions are irritating to the vein – notify RN if pain or redness occurs at site.

EXCHANGE RESIN

Sodium polystyrene sulfonate
   (**Kayexalate**):
   PO or rectal retention enema
   (Medication is not absorbed
    systemically.)

1. Laxatives are given to facilitate excretion of the resin.
2. Cleansing enema precedes the Kayexalate retention enema to enhance effectiveness.
3. Monitor serum electrolytes.

Appendix 5-3   SODIUM IMBALANCES

CAUSES	SYMPTOMS	NURSING IMPLICATIONS

NORMAL SERUM SODIUM (NA⁺) LEVELS: 135-145 mEq/L

HYPONATREMIA: Serum Na⁺ below 135 mEq/L (loss of sodium or water excess)

Fluid gain, over hydration (dilutional) Excessive administration of D_5W Excessive fluid intake Increased excretion of sodium Diuretics Adrenal insufficiency	*Hyponatremia from fluid overload:* Bounding pulses, increased blood pressure Edema *Hyponatremia from sodium loss:* CNS problems: confusion, headache, seizures Hypotension Muscle weakness, twitching, cramping Abdominal cramps and diarrhea.	1. Identify source of depletion and or excess. 2. Maintain accurate I&O records, and determine weight daily (best measurement of fluid status). 3. Irrigate nasogastric tubes with normal saline solution to prevent depletion. 4. Seizure and fall precautions. 5. Restrict fluid intake if client has fluid excess.

> ✔ **NURSING PRIORITY:** *Older adult clients and infants are at higher risk because of variations in total body water; carefully monitor clients receiving fluid replacement with D_5W.*

HYPERNATREMIA: Serum Na⁺ above 145 mEq/L (sodium retention or water loss).

Decreased fluid intake Excessive salt intake Excessive water loss: Diarrhea Febrile state Diuretics Increased renal retention Cushing's syndrome	***Fluid excess (Na⁺ retention):*** Symptoms of fluid excess. ***Fluid deficit (hemoconcentration of Na⁺, water loss):*** Symptoms of fluid loss or dehydration.	See Nursing Implications under Hyponatremia.

ADH, Antidiuretic hormone; *BP*, blood pressure; *CNS*, central nervous system; *CVP*, central venous pressure; *D₅W*, 5% dextrose in water; *I&O*, intake and output; *IV*, intravenously; *NPO*, nothing by mouth.

Appendix 5-4   MEDICATIONS TO CORRECT SODIUM IMBALANCE

MEDICATION	NURSING IMPLICATIONS

SODIUM SUPPLEMENTS

Sodium chloride (NaCl, table salt) Saline solutions: 0.9% and 0.45% saline solution for infusion	1. Administer with caution in clients with CHF, renal problems, edema, or hypertension. 2. Determine weight daily; maintain accurate I&O records to evaluate fluid retention. 3. Evaluate serum Na+ levels. 4. Do not store containers of sodium chloride above a concentration of 0.9% (normal saline) on the nursing unit. 5. Diuretics to increase renal excretion of sodium for sodium excess.

CHF, Congestive heart failure; *I&O*, intake and output.

Appendix 5-5   CALCIUM IMBALANCES

CAUSES	SYMPTOMS	NURSING IMPLICATIONS

NORMAL SERUM CALCIUM (CA++) LEVELS: 9-11 mg/dl OR 4-5 mEq/L

HYPOCALCEMIA: Serum Ca++ below 8.6 mg/dl or below 4 mEq/L, or below 3.5 mEq/L in infants

CAUSES	SYMPTOMS	NURSING IMPLICATIONS
Acute pancreatitis Laxative abuse Dietary lack of Ca++ and vitamin D Excessive blood transfusions Excessive IV fluids	Tetany: + Chvostek's sign; + Trousseau's sign (Chapter 8) Neuromuscular irritability Numbness and tingling in extremities or around mouth Laryngeal stridor Seizures Abdominal cramping and distention Dysrhythmias	1. Identify origin of problem – either deficiency or excess. 2. Maintain seizure precautions. 3. Reduce environmental stimuli. 4. Provide client education regarding Ca++ intake and supplemental vitamins.

HYPERCALCEMIA: Serum Ca++ above 10.5 mg/dl or above 5 mEq/L

CAUSES	SYMPTOMS	NURSING IMPLICATIONS
Metastatic malignancy Thiazide diuretics Prolonged immobilization	Anorexia, nausea, constipation CNS depression Decreasing coordination Pathological fractures Dysrhythmias—increases sensitivity to digitalis preparations.	1. Identify origin of increase. 2. Loop diuretics to facilitate removal of serum Ca++ , normal saline fluid replacement. 3. Increase client's fluid intake 3000 to 4000 mL/24 hours. 4. Decrease Ca++ intake. 5. Encourage client mobility. 6. Provide client education regarding supplemental vitamins. 7. Increase fiber intake. 8. Assess client taking digitalis for symptoms of toxicity.

CNS, Central nervous system; *IV*, intravenous.

Appendix 5-6   MEDICATIONS TO CORRECT CALCIUM IMBALANCE

MEDICATION	NURSING IMPLICATIONS
CALCIUM SALTS	
Calcium citrate (**Citracal**): PO Calcium gluconate: IV, PO Calcium carbonate (**TUMS, Rolaids**): PO Loop diuretics may be used to enhance excretion of calcium in treatment of hypercalcemia.	1. May be given in conjunction with vitamin D to enhance absorption. 2. PO supplements are more effective if taken ½-1 hr after meals. 3. Calcium citrate is absorbed more effectively than calcium carbonate. 4. Prevent IV infiltration; Ca++ solutions cause tissue hypoxia and sloughing. 5. Use with caution for client receiving digitalis. 6. Corticosteroids decrease Ca++ absorption. Administer several hours apart.

IV, Intravenous; *PO*, by mouth.

| Appendix 5-7 | ANTIINFLAMMATORY MEDICATIONS | |

General Nursing Implications

- Give oral medications with or after meals to decrease GI irritation and side effects.
- Following therapy, withdrawal from steroids must be done gradually.
- Client should not stop taking medications without directions from health care provider.
- For clients on long-term therapy, increased amounts of corticosteroids will be required during periods of stress such as surgery.
- Decreases client's ability to respond to and fight infection.
- Closely evaluate the client on digitalis preparations and thiazide diuretics for the development of hypokalemia.
- Use with NSAIDs increases risk for intestinal irritation and perforation (Appendix 5-8).
- *Uses:* Inflammatory conditions—respiratory, gastrointestinal, joint inflammation, and skin conditions. Adrenocortical hormone replacement if adrenal glands are insufficient or have been removed. Suppress rejection of transplanted organs.

Medications	Side Effects	Nursing Implications
ADRENOCORTICAL HORMONES *(Corticosteroids, Glucocorticoids):* Suppresses inflammatory response. Suppresses infiltration of area by lymphocytes, further reducing the immune response and inflammation. Used as immunosuppressant for delaying organ rejection. Long-term use will suppresses the function of the adrenal glands.		
Hydrocortisone base (**Cortef**): PO Hydrocortisone sodium succinate (**Solu-Cortef**): IV, IM Dexamethasone (**Decadron**): PO, IV, IM, topical Prednisone (**Deltasone, Meticorten**): PO Methylprednisolone (**Medrol**): PO, IM, IV Methylprednisolone sodium succinate (**Solu-Medrol**): IV	Increased susceptibility to infections (bodywide) GI upset, gastric irritation Osteoporosis Psychological disturbances (depression, euphoria) Hypokalemia Hyperglycemia Hypertension (caused by sodium and water retention) Cushing's syndrome: moon face, buffalo hump, distended abdomen, thin arms and legs, excessive hair growth Cataracts	1. Administer medication before 9:00 a.m. to decrease adrenal cortical suppression. 2. Monitor for psychological changes. 3. Decrease salt intake in diet; encourage high-protein and high-potassium diet. 4. Evaluate weight gain and blood pressure. 5. Topical steroids usually do not provoke physical evidence of absorption. *Teaching:* Take medication in the morning with food. Diet should include adequate K^+ intake and decreased Na^+ intake. Report to health care provider: any early signs of infection; or a weight gain of 5 lb or more in a week. Do not take a live virus vaccine (MMR, varicella) Do not take with aspirin products.

> ✔ **NURSING PRIORITY:** *It is critical that clients on corticosteroids do not stop taking the medications abruptly. This can result in a significant drop in blood pressure and hypoglycemia. Clients should advise all their health care providers if they are on steroids.*

GI, Gastrointestinal; *IM,* intramuscular; *IV,* intravenous; *PO,* by mouth (orally).

Appendix 5-8   NONSTEROIDAL ANTIINFLAMMATORY DRUGS (NSAIDs) AND ACETAMINOPHEN

<u>General Nursing Implications</u>
- Give with a full glass of water, either with food or just after eating.
- Store in childproof containers and out of reach of small children.
- Do not exceed recommended doses.
- Discontinue 1-2 weeks before elective surgery.
- NSAIDs prolong bleeding time by decreasing platelet aggregation; may increase anticoagulant activity of warfarin products.
- Avoid in clients with history of peptic ulcer disease or bleeding problems.
- Acetaminophen may cause renal impairment.
- Do not crush enteric-coated tablets; if available, administer as enteric or buffered tablets.

Uses: <u>Fever:</u> acetaminophen, aspirin, ibuprofen; <u>Inflammation:</u> aspirin, naproxen; <u>Arthritis:</u> aspirin, ibuprofen, naproxen, piroxicam, sulindac; <u>Dysmenorrhea:</u> ibuprofen, naproxen

Medications	Side Effects	Nursing Implications
NONSTEROIDAL ANTIINFLAMMATORY DRUGS (NSAIDS) AND ACETAMINOPHEN: Inhibit the enzyme cyclooxygenase, which is responsible for the synthesis of prostaglandins. Suppresses inflammation, relieves pain, and reduces fever.		
Acetylsalicylic acid (**Aspirin, ASA**): PO	*Salicylism:* skin reactions, redness, rashes, ringing in the ears, GI upset, hyperventilation, sweating, and thirst *Long-term use*: erosive gastritis with bleeding; increases anticoagulant properties of warfarin.	1. Most common agent responsible for accidental poisoning in small children. 2. Associated with Reye's syndrome in children. 3. Assess for bleeding tendencies. 4. Prophylactic use for colon cancer. 5. Prophylactic use for cardiovascular problems due to the antiplatelet aggregation properties.

    NURSING PRIORITY: Aspirin is the only NSAID used to protect against MI and stroke. Advise client that CDC warns against giving aspirin to children or adolescents with a viral infection or influenza.

Medications	Side Effects	Nursing Implications
Ibuprofen (**Motrin, Nuprin, Advil**): PO	Dyspepsia (heartburn, nausea, epigastric distress) Dizziness, rash, dermatitis	1. Do not exceed 3.2 g per day in adults and older adult clients. 2. Avoid taking with aspirin.
Naproxen (**Naprosyn**); Naproxen sodium (**Anaprox, Aleve**): PO	Headache, dyspepsia, dizziness, drowsiness	1. Avoid tasks requiring alertness until response is established. 2. Take with food to decrease GI irritation. 3. Primarily used for pain control.
Acetaminophen (**Tylenol, Datril, Tempra**): PO	Anorexia, nausea, diaphoresis Toxicity: vomiting, RUQ tenderness, elevated liver function tests Antidote: acetylcysteine (Mucomyst, Acetadote)	1. Maximum dose of acetaminophen, 4 g per day. 2. Does not have anti-inflammatory properties. 3. Overdose can cause severe liver injury; client should consult physician if intake of alcoholic beverage is in excess of 3 every day. 4. Has not been conclusively linked to bleeding problems.

    NURSING PRIORITY: Frequently used in combination with OTC medications. Teach client to read labels to prevent overdosing.

Medications	Side Effects	Nursing Implications
Piroxicam (**Feldene**): PO Sulindac (**Clinoril**): PO	Dyspepsia, nausea, dizziness, diarrhea, nephrotoxicity	

GI, Gastrointestinal; PO, by mouth (orally); RUQ, right upper quadrant.

Appendix 5-9   INFECTION CONTROL PROCEDURES

GENERAL INFORMATION

- Many clients with disease-specific isolation precautions require only standard precautions.
- The specific substances covered by standard precautions include blood and all other body fluids, body secretions, and body excretions, even if blood is not visible. Moisture from perspiration (sweat) is an exception.
- Transmission-based precautions are followed, in addition to standard precautions, whenever a client is known or suspected to be infected with contagious pathogens.

STANDARD PRECAUTIONS

1. Practice good hand hygiene (Box 5-2).
   - Hand hygiene with an antiseptic cleanser after removing gloves.
   - Wash hands immediately with soap and water if visibly contaminated with blood or body fluids.
   - Wear gloves if there is a possibility you might come in contact with any body fluid or contaminated surfaces or objects.
2. Change gloves between tasks and procedures on the same client if moving from a contaminated body area (perineal area) to a clean body area. Do not wash gloves for reuse.
3. Wear gloves, gown, eye protection (goggles, glasses) or face shield and a mask during procedures likely to generate droplets of blood or body fluids.
4. Wear a gown when there is risk clothing will come in contact with body fluids. Perform hand hygiene after removing the gown. Do not reuse gowns, even if they are not soiled.
5. Have used client care equipment properly cleaned; discard any single-use items after use.
6. Ensure that hospital procedures for routine care, cleaning, and disinfection of environmental surfaces, beds, bedrails, and bedside equipment are followed.
7. Place contaminated linens in a leak-proof bag; handle contaminated linens in a manner that prevents contamination and transfer of microorganisms.
8. Discard all sharps in puncture resistant container. Do not bend, break, reinsert them into their original sheaths, or handle them unnecessarily. Discard them intact immediately after use.
9. Place clients who pose a risk for transmission to others in a private room. This includes clients who cannot contain secretions/excretions or wound drainage, infants with respiratory or intestinal infections.

RESPIRATORY HYGIENE AND COUGH ETIQUETTE

1. Educate health care personnel regarding measures to contain their own respiratory secretions.
2. Post signs in strategic places regarding covering the mouth and nose when coughing or sneezing; provide non-touch receptacles for disposal of tissue.

SAFE INJECTION PRACTICES

Use single-dose vials for parenteral administration when possible.
1. If multi-dose vials must be used, the needle or cannula and the syringe used to access the vial must be sterile.
2. Do not use the same syringe to administer medications to multiple clients, even if the needle is changed.
3. Do not keep multi-dose vials in the immediate client treatment area.

INFECTION CONTROL FOR LUMBAR PUNCTURES

Wear a surgical mask when placing a catheter or injecting material into the spinal column or subdural space (myelogram, lumbar puncture, spinal or epidural anesthesia).

AIRBORNE PRECAUTIONS (droplet smaller than 5 mcg)

1. Place client in airborne isolation infection room (AIIR) as soon as possible.
2. Personal protection equipment (PPE):
   - Wear respiratory protection (N95 respirator mask approved by the National Institute for Occupational Safety and Health [NIOSH]) when entering the room.
   - Wear gloves, and gown when entering the room, remove prior to leaving room.
3. Limit client transport and client movement out of the room. Health care personnel who are not immune are restricted from entering the client's room.
4. Conditions requiring use of airborne precautions – pulmonary or laryngeal tuberculosis, varicella, rubella and smallpox.

Continued

Appendix 5-9   INFECTION CONTROL PROCEDURES—cont'd.

DROPLET PRECAUTIONS (droplets larger than 5 mcg)

1. Applicable to clients known to be, or suspected of being, infected with pathogens that are transmitted via respiratory droplets (sneezing, coughing, talking).
2. Place the client in a private room whenever possible; may place two clients in the same room if they are infected with the same pathogen.
3. PPE:
   - Wear a mask when entering the client room or examination area.
   - No recommendation regarding routine use of eye protection.
4. Place a mask on the client if transporting in the health care setting.
5. Instruct client and family regarding respiratory hygiene/cough etiquette.
6. Limit movement of the client from the room; if the client must leave the room, have him or her wear a surgical mask.

CONTACT PRECAUTIONS

1. Applicable to clients with diseases easily transmitted by direct contact such as gastrointestinal, respiratory tract, skin, or wound infections and clients colonized with multidrug-resistant bacteria.
2. Place the client in a private room if condition may facilitate transmission—uncontrolled drainage, incontinence. May place two clients infected with same pathogen in the same room.
3. PPE:
   - Wear a gown when entering the client's room; remove gown prior to leaving the room.
   - Wear gloves when entering the client's room. Always change gloves after contact with infected material. Remove gloves before leaving the client's room and perform hand hygiene; do not touch anything in the room as you are leaving.
   - Wear gloves when touching the client's intact skin and surfaces and articles in close proximity to the client.
4. Dedicate use of client care equipment to the single client when possible; if common equipment use is unavoidable, the equipment must be disinfected before use on another client.
5. Limit the transport or movement of the client outside the room; if necessary to move client, ensure that infected or colonized areas of the client's body are contained and covered.
6. Evidence shows that multiple drug-resistant organisms (MDROs) are carried from one person to another via the hands of health care personnel.

PROTECTIVE ENVIRONMENT PRECAUTIONS

1. May be used for clients who are severely immunosuppressed—clients with stem cell transplants, clients with organ transplant, AIDS clients.
2. Place the client in a private room that has positive-pressure air flow and high-efficiency particulate air (HEPA) filtration for incoming air.
3. Wear respiratory protection (N95 respirator mask), gloves, and gown when entering the room.
4. Limit client transport and client movement out of the room.
5. No fresh flowers, fruits, or potted plants allowed in room.

> ***TEST ALERT:** Use critical thinking to ensure standard transmission-based precautions are implemented; prevent environmental spread of infectious diseases.*

Center for Disease Control and Prevention: Standard precautions. In Guidelines for isolation precautions: preventing transmission of infectious agents in health care settings, 2007. www.cdc.gov/ncidod/dhqp/gl_isolation_standard.html

Appendix 5-10	ANTIBIOTIC MEDICATIONS	

General Nursing Implications

- Always assess for antibiotic allergies, especially penicillin allergy, before administration.
- Cultures should be obtained before the administration of the first dose.
- Teach the client to finish the entire prescribed course of medication even though he or she may feel well.
- Schedule IM and IV administration at evenly spaced intervals around the clock.
- Give most oral antibiotic drugs on an empty stomach (1 hour before or 2 hours after meals).
- Take medications with a full glass of water.
- Observe for hypersensitivity:
    - Anaphylaxis—hypotension, respiratory distress, urticaria, angioedema, vomiting, diarrhea
    - Serum sickness—fever, vasculitis, generalized lymphadenopathy, edema of joints, bronchospasm
- Observe for superinfection:
    - Stomatitis—sore mouth, white patches on oral mucosa, black furry tongue, diarrhea
    - Monilial vaginitis—rash in perineal area, itching, vaginal discharge
    - New localized signs and symptoms—redness, heat, edema, pain, drainage, cough
    - Recurrence of systemic signs and symptoms—fever, malaise

Medications	Side Effects	Nursing Implications
PENICILLIN: *Bactericidal:* Interferes with the formation of the bacterial cell wall.		
**Natural penicillins** Penicillin V (**PEN VEE K, Veetids**): PO, IV Aminopenicillins Amoxicillin (**Amoxil**): PO Ampicillin (**Principen, Totacillin**): PO, IM, IV _**Penicillinase-resistant penicillins**_ Cloxacillin (**Tegopen**): PO Nafcillin: IV _**Extended-spectrum penicillin**_ Ticarcillin disodium (**Ticar**): IM, IV Penicillin with beta-lactamase inhibitor Amoxicillin with clavulanic acid (**Augmentin**): PO	Parenteral injection—more hazardous than oral administration. Diarrhea, especially in children. Allergic reactions: skin rashes, joint pain, dermatitis, kidney damage. Anaphylactic reaction (hypersensitivity): decreased BP, increased pulse, respiratory distress, diaphoresis.	1. Observe for allergic reactions and have emergency equipment available. 2. Amoxicillin can be scheduled without regard to meals. 3. Observe client for 30 minutes after IM or IV administration for symptoms of allergic reactions. 4. Clients with beta-hemolytic strep infections should receive penicillin for a minimum of 10 days to prevent development of rheumatic fever or glomerulonephritis. 5. Discard liquid forms of penicillin after 7 days at room temperature and 14 days when refrigerated.
AMINOGLYCOSIDE: *Bactericidal:* Interferes with protein synthesis.		
Gentamicin (**Garamycin**): IM, IV Amikacin (**Amikin**): IM, IV Tobramycin (**Nebcin**): IV, nebulizer Neomycin sulfate (**Neo-Fradin**): PO, IM, topical, ophthalmic	Toxicity: Ototoxicity—hearing loss is irreversible. Nephrotoxicity—albuminuria, casts, oliguria. Skin rash, headache, hypotension, pain, and tenderness at injection site.	1. Monitor serum peak and trough levels to determine toxic levels. 2. Assess for ototoxicity (change in hearing, ringing in the ears, dizziness, or unsteady gait) and nephrotoxicity (monitor BUN and creatinine). 3. Not commonly used for long-term therapy. 4. Encourage PO fluids of 2000-3000 mL of fluid daily. 5. For IV piggyback medications, administer over 30-60 minutes. 6. Neomycin PO may be used to suppress intestinal flora before surgery.

Continued

Appendix 5-10 ANTIBIOTIC MEDICATIONS—cont'd.

CEPHALOSPORINS: *Bactericidal:* Broad-spectrum; interfere with the formation of the bacterial cell wall.

First generation: Cefadroxil (**Duricef, Ultracef**): PO
Cephalexin (**Keflex**): PO
Cefazolin (**Kefzol, Ancef**): IM, IV
Second generation:
Cefuroxime (**Ceftin, Zinacef**): PO, IM, IV
Loracarbef (**Lorabid**): PO
Cefoxitin (**Mefoxin**): IM, IV
Third generation:
Cefixime (**Suprax**): PO
Ceftriaxone (**Rocephin**): IM, IV
Fourth generation:
Cefepime (**Maxipime**): IM, IV

Hypersensitivity—rash, superinfection. GI upset, neutropenia (decreased WBCs), pain at injection site, renal damage seizures.

1. Give oral cephalosporins with food or milk.
2. Administer IM medications deep into the muscle.
3. Should not be given to clients with a known allergy to penicillin.
4. Decrease phlebitis at IV site by diluting IV solutions and administering slowly.
5. There is increasing antibacterial activity from first generation to fourth generation, treatment usually starts with first generation to prevent development of increased resistance.

TETRACYCLINES: *Bacteriostatic:* **Broad-spectrum;** interfere with protein synthesis of infectious organism and thus diminish its growth and reproduction.

Tetracycline (**Sumycin**): PO, IV, IM
Doxycycline (**Vibramycin**): PO, IV
Demeclocycline (**Declomycin**): PO
Minocycline (**Minocin**): PO, IV

PO may cause GI irritation (loose stools, diarrhea), sore throat, photosensitivity.
Diarrhea may indicate severe suprainfection in bowel.
Discoloration of teeth in children up to 8 years old.
Can cause staining of developing teeth in the fetus if taken after fourth month of gestation.

1. Administer on empty stomach; withhold antacids, dairy foods, and foods high in calcium at least 2 hours after PO administration. Do not administer with milk.
2. Can give doxycycline and minocycline with food.
3. Do not give at the same time as iron preparations. Give them as far apart as possible (e.g., 2-3 hours).
4. Advise client to avoid direct or artificial sunlight.
5. If diarrhea occurs, it is important to determine cause.
6. Observe for development of superinfections.

SULFONAMIDES: *Bacteriostatic:* Suppress bacterial growth by inhibiting synthesis of folic acid.

Sulfamethoxazole: PO (available only in combination with trimethoprim)
Sulfisoxazole (**Gantrisin**): PO, IV, IM
Trimethoprim sulfamethoxazole (**TMP-SMZ, Bactrim, Septra**): PO, IV

Blood dyscrasias—hemolytic anemia.
Hypersensitivity—rash, "drug fever," photosensitivity.
Renal dysfunction—crystalluria (irritation and obstruction) (Stevens-Johnson syndrome).

1. Encourage 8-10 glasses of water per day to prevent crystalluria.
2. Contraindicated during pregnancy and for nursing mothers and infants under 2 months of age.
3. Avoid prolonged exposure to sun.

Sulfasalzine (**Azulfidine**): PO

Nausea, vomiting, diarrhea.
Hepatitis, bone marrow suppression.

1. Antiinflammatory properties used to treat irritable bowel (IBS), rheumatoid arthritis.
2. Monitor CBC.
3. Maintain adequate hydration.
4. Urine may turn orange.

MACROLIDES: *Bacteriostatic:* Inhibit protein synthesis.

Erythromycin base (**Erythrocin**): PO,
Azithromycin (**Zithromax**): PO, IV
Clarithromycin (**Biaxin**): PO

Nausea, vomiting, abdominal distress, diarrhea.
Cholestatic hepatitis: abnormal liver function studies, jaundice, fever.

1. Administer with a full glass of water.

Continued

Appendix 5-10 ANTIBIOTIC MEDICATIONS—cont'd.

FLUOROQUINOLONES: *Bactericidal:* Inhibit bacterial DNA.

Ciprofloxacin (**Cipro**): PO, IV Levofloxacin (**Levaquin**): PO, IV	GI: Nausea, vomiting, abdominal distress, diarrhea. CNS: dizziness, headache, confusion Superinfections.	1. Absorption is reduced by milk products, antacids. 2. Administer IV infusions over 60 minutes.

OTHER ANTI-INFECTIVE AGENTS

Metronidazole (**Flagyl**): PO, IV	Nausea, dry mouth, headache. Disulfiram reaction when taken with alcohol: nausea, copious vomiting, flushing, palpitations, headache. May last 30 minutes to an hour.	1. Classified as an antiprotozoal antibiotic; is effective against anaerobic microorganisms. 2. Avoid use with alcohol or products containing alcohol. Will cause a disulfiram reaction.
Vancomycin (**Vancocin**): PO, IV	Ototoxicity, thrombophlebitis at site. Red man syndrome: flushing, rash, pruritus, tachycardia, and hypotension.	1. IV infusions over at least 60 minutes to prevent adverse effects. 2. Serum peak and trough levels are monitored.
Linezolid (**Zyvox**): PO, IV	GI: diarrhea, nausea Myelosuppression—anemia, leukopenia, thrombocytopenia.	1. New class of antibiotics—oxazolidinones. 2. Monitor for blood dyscrasias. 3. Reserved for treatment of infections from MDROs.
Antifungal Nystatin (**Mycostatin**): PO, topical		1. Used for treatment of candidiasis (mouth, esophagus, vagina). 2. Oral treatment encourage client to hold medication in their mouth and "swish" around to provide good contact with all affected areas.

BUN, Blood urea nitrogen; *GI*, gastrointestinal; *IM*, intramuscular; *IV*, intravenous; *PO*, by mouth; *MDRO*, multiple drug resistant organisms.

Appendix 5-11   ANTIRETROVIRAL THERAPY (ART)

General Nursing Implications

- Highly active antiretroviral therapy (HAART) used for treatment of clients with HIV and AIDS.
- Report any sore throat, fever, or other signs of infection to health care provider.
- Very important to administer the medication at the same time each day to maintain consistent blood levels and to decrease drug resistance.
- No vaccines or immunity-conferring agents while client is immunosuppressed.
- Maintain standard precautions, use contact, droplet, and airborne precautions as indicated.
- Medications do not cure AIDS or reduce the risk for transmission.

Medications	Side Effects	Nursing Implications
NONNUCLEOSIDE REVERSE TRANSCRIPTASE INHIBITORS (NNRTIS): All bind directly to the HIV transcriptase and inhibits the enzyme.		
Nevirapine (**Viramune, NVP**): PO	Rash (may be severe—blistering, joint pain, oral lesions), hepatotoxic, hepatitis.	**Viramune:** Monitor LFTs; rash may be so severe that drug is discontinued.
Delavirdine (**Rescriptor, DLV**): PO	Rash (may be severe), hepatoxic, GI symptoms.	**Rescriptor:** Monitor LFTs; rash may be so severe that drug is discontinued.
Efavirenz (**Sustiva, EFV**): PO	Rash, hepatotoxic, teratogenic, CNS symptoms.	**Sustiva:** Monitor LFTs, avoid pregnancy, avoid taking with St. John's wort.
NUCLEOSIDE/NUCLEOTIDE REVERSE TRANSCRIPTASE INHIBITORS (NRTIS): Medications are given with other antiretroviral agents; they are not used alone due to rapid development of resistance.		
Didanosine (**Videx**): PO	Nausea, diarrhea, peripheral neuropathy, liver damage, pancreatitis.	Food decreases absorption; give on empty stomach 30 min before eating or 2 hr after.
Stavudine (**Zerit**): PO	Pancreatitis, lactic acidosis, diarrhea, peripheral neuropathy	Report peripheral neuropathy; do not use in pregnancy.
Zidovudine (**ZDV, Retrovir, AZT, azidothymidine**): PO, IV	Bone marrow suppression, anemia, neutropenia	Maintain upright position to decrease esophageal irritation; monitor levels of anemia and neutropenia.
Lamivudine (**Epivir**): PO	Headache, nausea, malaise/fatigue, diarrhea	St. John's wort may decrease concentration.
Abacavir (**Ziagen**): PO	Hypersensitivity, pulmonary problems.	ETOH increases risk for hypersensitivity reactions; report respiratory changes.
PROTEASE INHIBITORS (PIS): Render the virus immature and noninfectious; are not given alone due to development of increased resistance. **ADVERSE EFFECTS OF ALL PIS:** Fat maldistribution, hyperlipidemia, hyperglycemia, bone loss, hepatotoxic. **SHARED INTERACTIONS:** St John's wort, decreases the effectiveness of PIs.		
Saquinavir (**Fortovase, Invirase**): PO	GI affects, headache	Do not give with grapefruit juice; take with food; check for drug interactions;
Ritonavir (**Norvir**): PO	GI discomfort, perioral paresthesia	Food increases levels; take with food for tolerance.
Indinavir (**Crixivan**): PO	GI discomfort, renal damage	Take 1 hr before or 2 hours after meals.
Nelfinavir (**Viracept**): PO	Diarrhea, rash	Take with food.
Amprenavir (**Agenerase**): PO	N/V, diarrhea, rash	Contraindicated in pregnancy, renal or hepatic failure; high-fat meals decrease absorption.
Lopinavir/ritonavir (**Kaletra**): PO	N/V, diarrhea, increased fatigue	Moderate fat meal increases absorption; take with food.
HIV FUSION INHIBITOR: Blocks entry of HIV into CD4 T cells.		
Enfuvirtide (**Fuzeon, T-20**): subQ	Injection site reaction, bacterial pneumonia, hypersensitivity reactions	Use small-gauge needle to decrease skin reaction; monitor respiratory status.

AIDS, Acquired immunodeficiency syndrome; *GI,* gastrointestinal; *HIV,* human immunodeficiency virus; *IV,* intravenous; *PO,* by mouth (orally); *subQ,* subcutaneous.

Appendix 5-12   MEDICATIONS FOR ALLERGIC REACTIONS

Medications	Side Effects	Nursing Implications
ANTIHISTAMINES: Selectively block histamine receptor sites.		
H1—First Generation		
Diphenhydramine (**Benadryl**): PO, IM, IV Clemastine (**Tavist Allergy**): PO Promethazine (**Phenergan**): PO, IV, IM	Dry mouth, dizziness, blurred vision, urinary retention, constipation, and sedation Children: paradoxical reactions	1. Advise client not to engage in activity that requires mental alertness for safety. 2. Should not take medication with alcohol. 3. Should not be used in clients with asthma.
H1—Second Generation		
Cetirizine (**Zyrtec**): PO Fexofenadine (**Allegra**) PO Loratadine (**Claritin**) PO	Dry mouth and throat Paradoxical reaction in children	1. Second generation is nonsedating. 2. Do not have anticholinergic properties of first generation. 3. Should not be taken with alcohol. 4. Are much more expensive than first generation.
Nasal Sprays		
Fluticasone (**Flonase, Flovent**) Triamcinolone (**Nasacort**)	Nasopharyngeal irritation.	1. Teach client to clear nasal passages before using. 2. Hold spray bottle upright and insert tip into nostril. 3. Used to treat allergic rhinitis.
ADRENERGIC AGONIST: Relaxes smooth muscle of bronchial tree (decreases respiratory distress), cardiac stimulant (increases cardiac rate), produces vasoconstriction (increases blood pressure), drug of choice for anaphylactic reactions.		
Epinephrine (**Adrenalin, EpiPen**): subQ, IV 1%—1:100—oral inhalation 0.1%—1:1,000—subQ, IM 0.01%—1:10,000—IV, intra-cardiac.	Hypertension, dysrhythmias, angina, hyperglycemia Necrosis at IV site if extravasation occurs	1. Clients at risk for anaphylaxis should always carry identification and emergency epinephrine (EpiPen). 2. **EpiPen**—sensitive to extreme heat and light; discard if it is brown in color, has a precipitate, or has passed its expiration date. 3. Advise clients to obtain medical assistance immediately if epinephrine is used. 4. 0.1 to 0.5 mL of 1:1000 dilution subQ or IM is used for mild to moderate reaction. 5. 0.5 mL of 1:10,000 dilution subcutaneously or IV is used for severe reactions and advanced cardiac life support. 6. Drug of choice for severe anaphylactic reactions. 7. Closely monitor pulse rate and blood pressure.

PO, by mouth (orally); *IM*, intramuscular; *IV*, intravenous; *subQ*, subcutaneous.

Psychiatric Nursing Concepts and Care

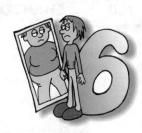

SELF-CONCEPT

A. *Self-concept:* all beliefs, convictions and ideas that constitute an individual's knowledge of himself or herself and influence his or her relationships with others.

B. *Self-esteem:* an individual's personal judgment of his or her own worth obtained by analyzing how well his or her behavior conforms to his or her self-ideal.

> ✔ **NURSING PRIORITY:** *A healthy self-concept, (i.e., positive self-esteem) is essential to psychological well-being; it is universal, (i.e., something everyone wants and needs).*

Data Collection

A. Factors affecting self-esteem.
  1. Parental rejection in early childhood experiences.
  2. Lack of recognition and appreciation by parents as child grows older.
  3. Overpossessiveness, overpermissiveness, and control by one or both parents.
  4. Unrealistic self-ideals or goals.

> ✔ **OLDER ADULT PRIORITY:** *The use of wheelchairs, canes, walkers, hearing aids, or any combination of these will have an impact on the self-esteem of the older client.*

B. Behaviors associated with low self-esteem.
  1. Self-derision and criticism: describes self as stupid, no good, or a born loser.
  2. Self-diminution: minimizes one's ability.
  3. Guilt and worrying.
  4. Postponing decisions and denying pleasure.
  5. Disturbed interpersonal relationships.
  6. Self-destructiveness and boredom.
  7. Polarizing view of life.

> 💡 **TEST ALERT:** *Promoting a positive self-concept is basic to all psychotherapeutic interventions. Look for options that focus on this concept; acknowledging the client as a person is an example.*

Nursing Intervention

A. Promote an open, trusting relationship.
B. Work and expand on whatever ego strength the client possesses.
C. Maximize the client's participation in the therapeutic relationship.
D. Encourage the client to accept his or her own feelings and thoughts.
E. Assist the client to clarify his or her concept of self and relationship with others through appropriate self-disclosure.
F. Explore with client maladaptive thinking patterns such as:
  1. Catastrophizing: thinking that the worst will happen.
  2. Minimizing and maximizing: tendency to minimize the positive and maximize the negative.
  3. Black-and-white thinking: tendency to look at situations in extremes; no middle ground.
  4. Overgeneralization: If something happens once, it will happen again.
  5. Self-reference: tendency to believe that people are particularly aware of their mistakes.
  6. Filtering: selectively taking certain details out of context while neglecting to look at more positive facts.
G. Communicate empathically, not sympathetically, and remind client that he or she has the power to change himself or herself.
H. Encourage client to define and identify problem.
I. Identify irrational beliefs such as:
  a. "I must be loved by everyone."
  b. "I must be competent and not make mistakes."
  c. "My whole life is a disaster if it doesn't turn out exactly as planned."
J. Identify areas of strength by exploring areas such as hobbies, skills, work, school, character traits, personal abilities, etc.

> ✔ **PEDIATRIC PRIORITY:** *If parents assist children to accomplish goals that are important to them, children begin to develop a sense of personal competence and independence.*

K. Explore client's adaptive and maladaptive coping responses.
    1. Determine "pay-offs" for maintaining self-defeating behaviors such as:
        a. Procrastination.
        b. Avoiding risks and commitments.
        c. Retreating from the present situation.
        d. Not accepting responsibility for one's actions.
    2. Identify the disadvantages of the maladaptive coping responses.

> ✔ **NURSING PRIORITY:** *An individual's functional level of overall self-esteem may change markedly from day to day and moment to moment.*

L. Realistic planning.
    1. Assist client to identify alternative solutions.
    2. Encourage creative visualization to enhance self-esteem through goal setting.
    3. Assist client to set realistic goals by encouraging him or her to participate in new experiences.
M. Commitment to action.
    1. Providing an opportunity for client to experience success is essential.
    2. Reinforce strengths, abilities, and skills.

> 💡 **TEST ALERT:** *Assist and reinforce nursing care given by caregivers/family on ways to manage client with behavioral disorders. Promote positive self-esteem and identify strengths of client and family members.*

CULTURAL COMPETENCE

A. Definitions.
    1. Culture: the beliefs, values, and norms of the individual, group, or community that are used in everyday life.
    2. Cultural competence: process whereby the nurse develops cultural awareness, knowledge, and skills to promote effective health care.
    3. Cultural diversity: unique differences in areas such as age, gender, socioeconomic status, religion, race, and ethnicity.
B. Barriers to culturally competent care.
    1. Miscommunication.
    2. Failure to assess for cultural perspective.
    3. Differences in understanding the way in which people function, interact, and behave every day.
    4. Clients use culturally specific language to describe medical symptoms or problems.
        Example: Native Americans may express depression symptoms as "having heart pain or heartbroken." Hispanics may say that their soul is lost because of another's ability to put an "evil eye" on them.

BODY IMAGE

Evaluation of Body Image Alteration

A. Types of body image disturbances.
    1. Changes in body size, shape, and appearance (rapid weight gain or loss, plastic surgery, pregnancy).
    2. Pathological processes causing changes in structure or function of one's body (e.g., Parkinson's disease, cancer, heart disease).
    3. Failure of a body part to function properly (paraplegia or stroke).
    4. Physical changes associated with normal growth and development (puberty, aging process).
    5. Threatening medical or nursing procedures (catheterization, radiation therapy, organ transplantation).
B. Principles.
    1. Body characteristics that have been present from birth or acquired early in life seem to have less emotional significance than those arising later.
    2. Body image changes, handicaps, or changes in body function that occur abruptly are far more traumatic than ones that develop gradually.
    3. The location of a disease or injury greatly affects the emotional response to it; internal diseases are generally less threatening than external diseases (trauma, disfigurement).
    4. Changes in genitals or breasts are perceived as a great threat and reawaken fears about sexuality and virility.

SPECIFIC SITUATIONS OF ALTERED BODY IMAGE AND NURSING INTERVENTION

 Obesity

Data Collection

A. Body weight exceeds 20% above the normal range for age, sex, and height.
B. Feeding behavior is gauged according to external environmental cues (i.e., availability of food, odors, stress) rather than hunger (increased gastrointestinal motility).
C. Increased incidence of diabetes, cardiovascular disease, and poor healing; skinfold thickness greater than 0.2 inches measured with skinfold calipers.
D. Often has symptoms of depression, fatigue, dyspnea, tachycardia, and hypertension.

Nursing Intervention

A. Encourage behavior modification programs.
B. Promote activities and interests not related to food or eating.
C. Identify client's need to eat and relate the need to preceding events or situations.
D. Decrease guilt and anxiety related to being obese.

E. Provide long-range nutritional counseling.
F. Encourage an exercise program.
G. Assess for complications (hypertension, cardiovascular disease).

Stroke

Data Collection

A. Change of body function due to loss of bowel and bladder control, speech, and cognitive skills, as well as loss of motor skills.
B. Disordered orientations in relationship to body and position sense in space; body image boundaries disrupted.

Nursing Intervention

A. Decrease frustration related to speech problems by encouraging speech effort, speaking slowly, and clarifying statements.
B. Do not try to hurry or rush client.
C. Promote reintegration of altered body image caused by paralyzed body part by means of tactile stimulation and verbal reminders of the existing body part.

Amputation

Data Collection

A. Feelings of loss; lowered self-esteem; guilt; helplessness.
B. Depression, passivity, and increased emotional vulnerability.
C. Phantom limb pain in most clients: increased experience if amputation occurs after 4 years of age; almost universal experience after age 8.
D. Phantom limb pain stronger in upper limbs and lasts longer than that in lower limbs.

Nursing Intervention

A. Discussion of phantom limb phenomenon and exploration of client's fears regarding amputation.
B. Acknowledge phantom limb pain; reassure client that this is a normal process.
C. Provide pain medication as needed.

Pregnancy

Data Collection

A. Produces marked changes in a woman's body, resulting in major alterations in body configuration within a short period of time.
B. Second trimester: Woman becomes aware that her body is widening and requires more body space.
C. Third trimester: very much aware of increased size; may feel ambivalent about the changes in her body.

D. Perceives her body as vulnerable, yet as a protective container for the unborn.
E. Mate experiences changed body image and sympathetic symptoms during woman's pregnancy.

Nursing Intervention

A. Explanation and reassurance of the normal physiological changes that are occurring.
B. Provide discussions of alterations in body image for both mates.
C. Encourage verbalization of feelings relating to changed body image.

Cancer

Data Collection

A. Clients with cancer may experience many changes in body image.
B. Removal of sex organs (breasts, uterus) has a significant impact on client's preception of sexuality.
C. Disfiguring head-and-neck surgery has devastating impact on body image, because the face is one of the primary means by which people communicate.
D. Symptoms of depersonalization, loss of self-esteem, and depression may occur.

Nursing Intervention

A. Provide anticipatory guidance to help client cope with crisis of changed body image.
B. Set long-term goals to help client with cancer adjust to physiological and psychological changes.

Enterostomal Surgery

Data Collection

A. Client often shocked at initial sight of ostomy.
B. May experience lowered self-esteem, fear of fecal spillage, alteration in sexual functioning, feelings of disfigurement and rejection.

Nursing Intervention

A. Preoperative explanation by use of drawings, models, or pictures of how stoma will appear.
B. Reassurance that reddish appearance of stoma and large size will diminish in time.
C. Encourage discussion and recognize importance of client talking with a "successful ostomate."

HUMAN SEXUALITY

A. Effect of illness and injury on sexuality.
   1. Depressive episodes often precipitate a decrease in libido.
   2. Sexual preoccupations and overtones may be experienced by the client with psychosis.

3. Certain medications contribute to sexual dysfunction, failure to reach orgasm in women, and impotence or failure to ejaculate in men (e.g., reserpine, phenothiazine, and estrogen use in men decrease libido; while androgen use in women increases libido).
4. Clients with spinal cord injuries may lose sexual functioning.
5. Trauma and disfigurement may precipitate an alteration in sexuality.
B. Effect of the aging process on sexuality.
1. Physiological changes in the woman are frequently caused by decreasing estrogen supply, which results in decreased vaginal lubrication, shrinkage and loss of elasticity in vaginal canal, and decrease in breast size.
2. Physiological changes in the man include a decrease in testosterone, decrease in spermatogenesis, and a longer length of time to achieve erection along with a decrease in the firmness of erection.

CONCEPT OF LOSS

> **TEST ALERT:** *Provide care or support for client and family at end of lie. Assist with coping related to grief or loss.*

Definition

1. Includes both biological and physiological aspects; loss of function (see Chapter 3).
2. Components of loss include death, dying, grief, and mourning.
   a. Death: represents finality, the end of one's biological being.
   b. Dying: the social process of organizing activities that prepare for death; provides others, as well as the client, a way to prepare for the future.
   c. Grief: the sequence of subjective states that follow loss and accompany mourning.
   d. Mourning: the psychological processes that are aroused by the loss of a loved object or person.

Data Collection

A. Characteristic stages.
1. Death and dying (Kübler-Ross, 1969).
   a. Denial and isolation.
   b. Anger.
   c. Bargaining.
   d. Depression.
   e. Acceptance.
2. Grief.
   a. Shock and disbelief.
   b. Developing awareness.
   c. Restitution or resolution of the loss.

Nursing Interventions

❖ Goal: To acknowledge the pain of the loss.
A. Assist the griever to recognize that he/she must yield to the painful process of grief.
B. Explain how grief affects all areas of one's life.
C. Try and view the loss from the griever's perspective.
❖ Goal: To assist the grieving and/or dying client to accept the reality of loss and/or death.
A. Encourage expression and verbalization of feelings with out interruption (i.e., crying, talking).
B. Listen nonjudgmentally with acceptance.
C. Reach out and make contact with client and family; let genuine concern and caring show.
❖ Goal: To provide for spiritual needs of the grieving and/or dying client.
A. Ask clergy to visit.
B. Pray with client and family (if requested to do so), read inspirational literature, play music.
C. Encourage the griever to allow self-respite times from the grieving process.
❖ Goal: To promote adjustment to life and living after the experience of loss.
A. Encourage reinvesting energies into new undertakings and relationships.
B. Promote letting go and moving on.

PSYCHOSOCIAL ASSESSMENT

✳ **Complete data collection assessment includes descriptions of the intellectual functions, behavioral reactions, emotional reactions, dynamic issues of the client relative to adaptive functioning and response to present situations.**

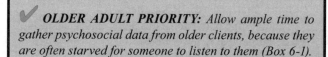

> ✔ **OLDER ADULT PRIORITY:** *Allow ample time to gather psychosocial data from older clients, because they are often starved for someone to listen to them (Box 6-1).*

A. Psychosocial assessment purpose: To obtain data from multiple sources (e.g., client, family, friends, police, mental health personnel) in order to identify patterns of functioning that are healthy, as well as patterns that create problems in the client's everyday life.
B. Psychosocial data to obtain.
1. Chief complaint (CC): main reason client is seeking psychiatric help.
2. History of the presenting illness (HPI): onset and development of symptoms or problems.
3. Past medical history (PMH): previous mental health hospitalizations or treatment; information concerning client's birth, growth and development, illnesses, occupation, marital history, religious practices, use of tobacco, alcohol, or drugs, for example.
4. Family history: Have any immediate family members sought psychiatric treatment or counseling?

OLDER ADULT CARE FOCUS
Aging and Mental Health

- Sensory losses (hearing and vision) can have behavioral changes that can be mistaken for disorientation.
- Financial and physical changes of aging can lead to social isolation.
- Exaggerated personal characteristics occur as a person ages.
- Anxiety, fear, and depression can occur from experiencing multiple losses (death, job changes, relocation from home, loss of independence) and grief, especially if they occur quickly.
- Alcoholism is often found in the older adult.
- Behaviors commonly seen are hopelessness and helplessness, which can lead to suicide.
- To assist coping with life circumstances, encourage reminiscence and life review.

5. Personality profile: client's interests, feelings, mood, and usual leisure or hobby activities.
C. Common client behaviors seen with illness.
   1. Denial: refusal to believe he or she is ill; may result in maladaptive behavior if continues.
   2. Anxiety: may see flight-fight fear response.
   3. Shock: overwhelming feelings and emotion that paralyze client's ability to process information.
   4. Anger: response related to feeling mistreated, injured, or insulted; may escalate to aggression.
   5. Withdrawal: may be a sign of depression; ill person may isolate self from family.

MENTAL STATUS EXAMINATION

✳ **The mental status examination differs from the psychiatric history in that it is used to identify an individual's *present* mental status.**

> **TEST ALERT:** *Identify changes in client's mental status.*

Aspects of the Examination

> ✔ **NURSING PRIORITY:** *Assess level of consciousness, vision, and hearing first (e.g., alert, lethargic, stuporous, or comatose) and ability of the client to comprehend the interview.*

A. Mini Mental State Examination (Folstein, Folstein, and McHugh, 1975).
   1. Widely used common mental status assessment for cognitive function.
   2. Quickly administered – questions related to orientation (person, place and time), registration (repeating items, give client 3 common words and ask them to repeat the words), naming (point to a chair or object and ask client to name it), and reading (ask client to read and follow directions from a simple sentence.
   3. Excludes assessment of mood, abnormal psychological experiences (hallucinations, delusions, illusions), and content and process of thinking.

COPING/DEFENSE/EGO/ MENTAL MECHANISMS

✳ **Specific defense processes used by individuals to relieve or decrease anxieties caused by uncomfortable situations that threaten self-esteem.**

A. Related principles.
   1. The primary functions are to decrease emotional conflicts, provide relief from stress, protect from feelings of inadequacy and worthlessness, prevent awareness of anxiety, and maintain an individual's self-esteem.
   2. Everyone uses defense mechanisms to a certain extent. If used to an extreme degree, defense mechanisms distort reality, interfere with interpersonal relationships, limit one's ability to work productively, and may lead to pathological symptoms.
B. Common defense mechanisms (see Box 6-2).
C. Nursing management.
   1. Accept coping mechanisms.
   2. Discuss alternative coping mechanisms and problem-solving situations.
   3. Assist the client in learning new or alternative coping patterns for a healthier adaptation.
   4. Use techniques to decrease anxiety.

THERAPEUTIC NURSING PROCESS

✳ **Therapeutic interpersonal relationship is the interaction between two persons: the *nurse* promotes goal-directed activities that help to alleviate the discomfort of the *client* by promoting growth and satisfying interpersonal relationships.**

Characteristics

A. Goal-directed.
B. Empathetic understanding.
C. Honest, open communication.
D. Concreteness; avoids vagueness and ambiguity.
E. Acceptance; nonjudgmental attitude.
F. Involves nurse's understanding of self and personal motives and needs.

Phases

A. Initial phase: goal is to *build* trust.
   1. Explore the client's perceptions, thoughts, feelings and actions.
   2. Identify problem.

3. Assess levels of anxiety of self and client.
4. Mutually define specific goals to pursue.
B. Working phase: goal is *to establish objectives* or a working agreement (contract).
   1. Encourage client participation.
   2. Focus on problem-solving techniques; choose between alternate courses of action and practice skills.
   3. Explore thoughts, feelings, and emotions.
   4. Develop constructive coping mechanisms.
   5. Increase independence and self-responsibility.
C. Termination phase: goal is *to evaluate goals* set forth and terminate relationship.
   1. Plan for termination early in formation of relationship (in initial phase).
   2. Discuss client's feelings about termination.
   3. Evaluate client's progress and goal attainment.

✔ ***NURSING PRIORITY:*** *To effectively interview a client, be sure to start with a broad, empathetic statement; explore normal behaviors before discussing maladaptive behaviors; phrase inquiries or questions sensitively to decrease client's anxiety; ask client to clarify vague statements; focus on pressing problems when client begins to ramble; interrupt nonstop talkers as tactfully as possible; express empathy toward client while he or she is expressing feelings.*

THERAPEUTIC NURSE-CLIENT COMMUNICATION TECHNIQUES

A. Planning and goals.
   1. Demonstrate active listening; face-to-face contact.
   2. Demonstrate unconditional positive regard, interest, congruence, respect.
   3. Develop trusting relationship; accept client's behavior and display nonjudgmental, objective attitude.
   4. Be supportive, honest, authentic, and genuine.
   5. Focus on emotional needs and emotionally charged area.
   6. Focus on here-and-now behavior and expression of feelings.
   7. Attempt to understand another point of view.
   8. Develop an awareness of the client's likes and dislikes.
   9. Encourage expression of both positive and negative feelings.
   10. Use broad openings and ask open-ended questions; avoid questions that can be answered by yes or no.
   11. Use reflections of feelings, attitudes, and words.
   12. Explore alternatives rather than answers or solutions.
   13. Focus feedback on *what* is said rather than *why* it is said.
   14. Paraphrase to assist in clarifying client's statements.
   15. Promote sharing of feelings, information, and ideas instead of giving advice.

BOX 6-2 **UNDERSTANDING DEFENSE MECHANISMS**

Name of Defense Mechanism	Definition
Compensation	Attempting to make up for or offset deficiencies, either real or imagined by, concentrating on or developing other abilities
Conversion	Symbolic expression of intrapsychic conflict expressed in physical symptoms
Denial	Blocking out or disowning painful thoughts or feelings
Displacement	Feelings are transferred, redirected, or discharged from the appropriate person or object to a less threatening person or object
Dissociation	Separating and detaching an idea, situation, or relationship from its emotional significance; helps the individual put aside painful feelings and often leads to a temporary alteration of consciousness or identity
Identification	Attempting to pattern or resemble the personality of an admired, idealized person
Introjection	Acceptance of another's values and opinions as one's own
Projection	Attributing one's own unacceptable feelings and thoughts to others
Rationalization	Attempting to justify or modify unacceptable needs and feelings to the ego, in an effort to maintain self-respect and prevent guilt feelings
Reaction Formation	Assuming attitudes and behaviors that one consciously rejects
Regression	Retreating to an earlier, more comfortable level of adjustment
Repression	An involuntary, automatic submerging of painful, unpleasant thoughts and feelings into the *unconscious*
Sublimation	Diversion of unacceptable instinctual drives into personally and socially acceptable areas to help channel forbidden impulses into constructive activities
Suppression	Intentional exclusion of forbidden ideas and anxiety-producing situations from the conscious level; a voluntary forgetting and postponing mechanism
Undoing	Actually or symbolically attempting to erase a previous consciously intolerable experience or action; an attempt to repair feelings and actions that have created guilt and anxiety

💡 ***TEST ALERT:*** *Recognize client's use of defense mechanisms.*

B.   Examples of therapeutic and nontherapeutic communication responses (Table 6-1 and Box 6-3).

> **TEST ALERT:** *Listen to client's concerns and use therapeutic interventions to increase client's understanding of his or her behavior; acknowledge differences between client's views/feelings and the health care provider's views/feelings; establish rapport with client or family.*

INTERVENTION MODALITIES

Crisis Intervention

* **A crisis is a self-limiting situation in which usual problem-solving or decision-making methods are not adequate.**
A.   A crisis offers opportunities for growth and renewal.
B.   Crisis intervention strategy views people as capable of personal growth and able to control their own lives.
C.   Types of crisis intervention strategies.
   1.   Individual crisis counseling.
   2.   Crisis groups.
   3.   Telephone counseling.
D.   Crisis intervention requires support, protection, and enhancement of the client's self-image.

Group Therapy

* **A structured or semi-structured process in which individuals (7 to 12 members is ideal size) are interrelated and interdependent and may share common purposes and norms.**
A.   Emphasis on clear communication to promote effective interaction.
B.   Disturbed perceptions can be corrected through consensual validation.
C.   Socially ineffective behaviors can be modified through peer pressure.

Family Therapy

* **A treatment modality designed to bring about a change in communication and interactive patterns between and among family members.**

> **TEST ALERT:** *Provide emotional support to family, assess dynamics of family interactions, assess family's understanding of illness and emotional reaction, and help family adjust to role changes.*

A.   A family can be viewed as a system that is dynamic. A change or movement in any part of the family system affects all other parts of the system.
B.   Family seeks to maintain a balance or "homeostasis" among various forces that operate within and on it.

> **BOX 6-3   INEFFECTIVE RESPONSES AND BEHAVIORS**
> * Not listening; talking too much
> * Looking too busy
> * Seeming uncomfortable with silence
> * Avoiding sensitive topics
> * Changing the subject
> * Laughing nervously; smiling inappropriately
> * Showing a closed body posture
> * Focusing on personal issues of the nurse
> * Making flippant comments
> * Being defensive or making excuses

C.   Emotional symptoms or problems of an individual may be expression of the emotional symptoms or problems in the family.
D.   Therapeutic approaches involve helping the family members look at themselves in the here and now and recognize the influence of past models on their behavior and expectations.

Milieu

* **A scientifically, planned, purposeful manipulation in the environment aimed at causing changes in the behavior and personality of the client.**

> **TEST ALERT:** *Contribute to maintaining a safe and supportive environment for the client (e.g., therapeutic milieu, structured environment).*

A.   Nurse is viewed as a facilitator and a helper to clients rather than a therapist.
B.   The *therapeutic community* is a very special kind of milieu therapy in which the total social structure of the treatment unit is involved as part of the helping process.
C.   Emphasis is placed on open communication, both within and between staff and client groups.

Mind-Body-Spirit Therapies

* **Alternative therapies different from traditional Western medicine; often influenced by traditional Chinese medicine, which focuses on maintaining unity with nature and balancing our energy systems.**

A.   Acupuncture: movement of energy through meridians of the body to restore energy balance.
B.   Imagery: change reality by creating a different mental picture.
C.   Therapeutic touch: manipulate and direct client's energy through the use of the practitioner's hands and direct energy from the practitioner to the client to enhance healing.

TABLE 6-1	THERAPEUTIC COMMUNICATION

Response	Example
Exploring	"What seems to be the problem?" "Tell me more about..."
Reflecting	Client: "I am really mad at my mother for grounding me." Nurse: "You sound angry."
Focusing	"Give an example of what you mean." "Let's look at this more closely."
Clarifying	"I'm not sure that I understand what you're saying." "Do you mean...?"
Using general leads	"Go on..." "Talk more about..."
Broad opening leads	"Where would you like to begin?" "Talk more about..."
Validating	"Did I understand you to say...?"
Informing	"The time is..." "My name is..."
Accepting	"Yes." "Okay." Nodding, "Uh hmm."
Sharing observations	"You appear anxious. I noticed that you haven't been coming to lunch with the group."
Presenting reality	"I do not hear a noise or see the lights blinking." "I am not Cleopatra; I am your nurse."
Summarizing	"During the past hour we talked about..."
Using silence	Nurse remains silent and waits patiently for the client to begin speaking.

NONTHERAPEUTIC COMMUNICATION

Response	Example
False reassurance	"Don't worry; you will be better in a few weeks." "Don't worry. I had an operation just like it; it was a snap."
Giving advice	"What you should do is..." "If I were you, I would do..."
Rejecting	"I don't like it when you..." "Please, don't ever talk about..."
Belittling	"Everybody feels that way." "Why, you shouldn't feel that way."
Probing	"Tell me more about your relationships with other men."
Overloading	"Hi, I am JoAnn, your student nurse. How old are you? What brought you to the hospital? "How many children do you have? Do you want to fill out your menu right now?"
Underloading	Not giving enough information so that the meaning is clear; withholding information.
Clichés	"Gee, the weather is beautiful outside." "Did you watch that new TV show last night? Everybody's talking about it."

D. Massage: through touch unblocks energy flow and connects client with practitioner.

E. Relaxation: imagery and progressive tensing and relaxing of muscle groups throughout the body.

F. Music therapy and herbal therapy.

G. Transcendental meditation: quiet meditation, focusing on getting beyond the self and becoming one with the universal energy source.

H. Others: exercise, nutrition, prayer, religious practices.

> 💡 **TEST ALERT:** *Assess client's use of alternative/complementary practices; evaluate client's response to alternative therapy.*

Somatic Therapies

A. Restraints (Box 6-4).
1. Mechanical restraints include camisoles, wrist and ankle restraints, and sheet restraints.
2. Chemical restraints include the use of medications – antianxiety or antipsychotic.

> ✔ **NURSING PRIORITY:** *It is important to have a physician's order for applying restraints and to provide for client's biological needs (e.g., hygiene, elimination, nutrition, and method of communication).*

B. Seclusion.
1. Confinement to a room that may be locked. Often, the room is without a mattress or linens, and the client is wearing a hospital gown.
2. There is limited opportunity for communication.

Psychosurgery

❋ **Surgical interruption of selected neural pathways that govern transmission of emotion between the frontal lobes of the cerebral cortex and the thalamus.**

A. Recent resurgence of interest in psychosurgery as knowledge of neuroanatomy and "mapping" the cerebral cortex has become more sophisticated.
B. Area of moral and ethical debate, especially because nerve tissue once damaged cannot regenerate.

Electroconvulsive Therapy

❋ **ECT is an electric shock delivered to the brain through electrodes that are placed on the head. The shock artificially induces a seizure.**

A. Indications.
1. Severe depression; when other treatment modalities are ineffective.
2. Acute schizophrenia (catatonic type).
3. Number of treatments: usually given in a series that varies according to the client's presenting problem and response to therapy; 2 to 3 treatments per week for a total of 6 to 12 treatments. May also use maintenance or continuation of ECT (once per month for 6 to 12 months).
B. Nursing interventions.
1. Assess client's record for routine preoperative-type checklist for information (informed consent).
2. NPO for 6 to 8 hours before treatment.
3. Remove dentures, hairpins, contact lenses, and hearing aids.
4. Administer pre-procedure medication after electrodes are applied and before convulsion occurs.
5. Provide for safety and observe progress of seizure (see Appendix 15-5).
6. Care immediately following treatment.
   a. Provide orientation to time.
   b. Temporary memory loss is usually confusing; explain that this is a common occurrence.
   c. Assess vital signs for 30 minutes to 1 hour after treatment.
   d. Deemphasize preoccupation with ECT; promote involvement in regularly scheduled activities.

Other Therapies

A. Psychodrama: the use of structured and directed dramatization of client's emotional problems and experiences.
B. Activities therapy: a number of vital programs come under this heading, such as music therapy, occupational therapy, art therapy, recreational therapy, ROPES, dance or movement therapy, etc.

BOX 6-4	USE OF RESTRAINTS

- Obtain an order or a consent to apply restraints.
- Selecting a restraint: it should restrict movement as little as possible, be obscure to others, not interfere with the client's treatment, be readily changeable, and be safe for the age of the client (to keep an active child in bed, use a jacket restraint, as opposed to a wrist restraint).
- Secure restraint: check for adequate blood circulation to extremities.
- Pad bony prominences (wrists and ankles) before applying restraint.
- Always tie limb restraint with a knot (e.g., clove hitch) that will not tighten when pulled.
- Never tie ends of restraint to a side rail or to part of fixed bed frame if the bed position is going to be changed.
- Assess restraint every 30 minutes and document.
- Release all restraints every 2 hours and provide ROM and skin care; stay with client when restraint is removed and document.
- Keep in mind the principle of least restriction: restrain the client to the extent necessary to accomplish the restraint's purpose.

TEST ALERT: Apply restraints or other safety devices per protocol (e.g., vests).

ANXIETY

A. Definition.
1. An emotion, a subjective experience.
2. A feeling state that is experienced as vague uneasiness, tension, or apprehension.
3. Occurs when the ego is threatened.
4. Provoked by the unknown; precedes all new experiences.
B. Data collection (Table 6-2).
C. Nursing management (Table 6-3).
D. Specific disorders of anxiety (Table 6-4).

 NURSING PRIORITY: Identify a client's potential for a physical or emotional reaction to a crisis event and use client behavior modification techniques and therapeutic interventions to increase client's understanding of his or her behavior.

Problems Associated with Anxiety

❋ **This group of problems has anxiety as the primary disturbance. In the past, these were grouped together as neuroses. Anxiety can be a predominant disturbance (panic and generalized anxiety), or anxiety is experienced as a person attempts to confront a dreaded situation (phobic disorder) or resist the obsessions and compulsions of an obsessive-compulsive disorder. In general, these are**

TABLE 6-2	ASSESSMENT OF ANXIETY
Physiological	**Psychological**

Physiological	**Psychological**
<u>Sympathetic Responses</u>	<u>Behavioral Responses</u>
Tachycardia	Restlessness
Elevated blood pressure	Agitation
Increased perspiration	Tremors (fine to gross shaking of the body)
Dilated pupils	Startle reaction
Hyperventilation with difficulty breathing	Rapid speech
Cold, clammy skin	Lack of coordination
Dry mouth	Withdrawal
Constipation	
<u>Parasympathetic Responses</u>	<u>Cognitive Responses</u>
Urinary frequency	Impaired attention
Diarrhea	Poor concentration
	Forgetfulness
	Blocking of thought
<u>Related Responses</u>	Decreased perceptual field
Headaches	Decreased productivity
Nausea or vomiting	Confusion
Sleep disturbances	
Muscular tension	
	<u>Affective Responses</u>
	Tension
	Jittery feeling
	Worried
	Apprehension, nervousness
	Irritability
	Dread
	Fear
	Panic
	Fear of impending doom

common responses to emotional problems that are very seldom treated in a psychiatric setting, as the person has no great defect in reality testing nor demonstrates severe antisocial behavior. (Table 6-4)

Interpersonal Withdrawal

* *Interpersonal withdrawal* **is characterized by avoidance of interpersonal contact and a sense of unreality.**

A. Physical withdrawal: Client sits or stands apart from others; may hide, assume a catatonic posture, or (in extreme form) attempt suicide.

B. Verbal withdrawal: avoidance through silence or (in extreme form) mutism; silence may indicate resistance, a pensive moment, or the indication that nothing more is to be said.

Nursing Intervention

A. Avoid punishment of client.

B. Decrease isolation.

C. Invite the client to speak.

D. State the amount of time you are willing to stay with the client whether he or she chooses to speak or not.

E. Change the context of the contact (for example, go for a walk together).

F. Encourage the client to share responsibility for the continuance of the relationship.

Regression

* *Regression* **is retreating to earlier, childish, or less complex patterns of behavior that once brought the client attention or pleasure.**

Nursing Intervention

A. Avoid fostering dependency and childlike attitudes.

B. Be patient and understanding.

C. Confront client directly about his or her plan.

D. Compliment client when he or she does something unusually well or assumes more responsibility.

E. Promote problem solving, reality orientation, and involvement in social activities.

F. Avoid punishment after periods of regression; instead, explore the meaning of the regressive behavior.

G. Regression is a normal occurrence in young children who are hospitalized.

TABLE 6-3 — NURSING MANAGEMENT OF ANXIETY

Level of Anxiety	Assessment	Goal	Nursing Management
Mild	Increased alertness, motivation, and attentiveness.	To assist client to tolerate some anxiety.	1. Help client identify and describe feelings. 2. Help client develop the capacity to tolerate mild anxiety and use it consciously and constructively.
Moderate	Perception narrowed, selective inattention, physical discomforts.	To reduce anxiety; directed toward helping client understand cause of anxiety and new ways of controlling it.	1. Provide outlet for tension, such as walking; crying; working at simple, concrete tasks.
Severe	Behavior becomes automatic; connections between details are not seen; senses are drastically reduced.	To assist in channeling anxiety.	1. Recognize own level of anxiety. 2. Link client's behavior with feelings. 3. Protect defenses and coping mechanisms. 4. Identify and modify anxiety-provoking situations.
Panic	Overwhelmed; inability to function or communicate; potential for bodily harm to self and others; loss of rational thought.	To be supportive and protective.	1. Provide nonstimulating, structured environment. 2. Avoid touching. 3. Stay with client. 4. Medicate client with tranquilizers if necessary.

Anger

* **Anger is the unconscious process used in order to obtain relief from anxiety that is produced by a sense of danger; it involves a sense of powerlessness. Fear of expressing anger is related to fear of rejection.**

Nursing Intervention

A. Have client acknowledge or name feelings.
B. Explore source of personal fear or perceived threat (e.g., illness, disability, disfigurement, or emotional crisis).
C. Encourage verbalization of anxiety.
D. Explore appropriate external expression of feelings.
E. Avoid arguing with client.
F. Acting-out behavior is often an indirect expression of anger; it attracts attention and often represents the feelings the person is experiencing.

✔ **NURSING PRIORITY:** *Nontherapeutic responses to a client's anger are defensiveness, retaliation, condescension, and avoidance.*

Hostility/Aggressiveness

* **Hostility or Aggressiveness is an antagonistic feeling; the client wishes to hurt or humiliate others; the result may be a feeling of inadequacy or self-rejection due to a loss of self-esteem.**

Nursing Intervention

💡 **TEST ALERT:** *Plan interventions to assist client to control aggressive behavior (e.g., contract, behavior modification, set limits).*

A. Prevent aggressive contact by early recognition of increased anxiety.
B. Maintain client contact rather than avoid it.
C. Encourage verbalization of feelings associated with a threat of frustration (helplessness, inadequacy, anger).
D. Reduce environmental stimuli.
E. Avoid reinforcement behavior (e.g., joking, laughing, teasing, and competitive games).
F. Use distraction, or remove the client from the immediate environment to re-establish self-control.
G. Set limits on unacceptable behavior.
H. Protect other clients.

✔ **NURSING PRIORITY:** *When two clients are arguing, engage the dominant client first by using distraction or removing the client from the setting to allow time for de-escalation and processing of the situation.*

Violence

* **Violence is behavior that is a physical assault and risks injury to the self, others, and environment.**

TABLE 6-4	SELECTED ANXIETY DISORDERS	
Problem	**Description**	**Nursing Intervention**
Panic Disorder (with or without agoraphobia): an extreme level of anxiety.	Agoraphobia (fear of being in places or situations; crowds, traveling). May experience shortness of breath, dizziness, diaphoresis, palpitations.	❖ **Goal: To reduce panic level anxiety feelings by reinterpreting the feelings correctly** (see Table 6-3). 1. Anticipate administration of a tricyclic antidepressant. 2. Reduce amount of caffeine in diet.
Phobia: an intense, irrational fear of a specific object, activity, or situation.	Fear of being alone or in public places. Claustrophobia (fear of enclosed spaces). Acrophobia (fear of heights). Social phobia (fear of circumstances that may be humiliating, e.g., speaking in public, eating in restaurants).	❖ **Goal: To reduce phobic behavior.** 1. Do not force client to come in contact with the feared object or source of anxiety. 2. Have client focus on awareness of self. 3. Distract client's attention from phobia.
Obsessive-Compulsive Disorder: unconscious control of anxiety by the use of rituals, thoughts, obsessions, or compulsions.	**Obsessions:** recurrent, persistent ideas, thoughts, or impulses that are not voluntarily produced. *Most common obsessions include thoughts of violence, contamination, and doubt.* **Compulsions:** repetitive, ritualistic behaviors that are performed in a certain fashion to relieve an unbearable amount of tension. *Most common compulsions include hand washing, counting, checking.*	❖ **Goal: To assist in coping with the compulsive behavior.** 1. Accept rituals and avoid punishment or criticism; do not interrupt ritual, because this will increase anxiety. 2. Plan for extra time because of slowness and client's need for perfection. 3. Prevent physical deterioration or harm, and set limits only to prevent harmful acts (such as hand washing excessively that removes the skin from the hand surface). ❖ **Goal: To encourage client to develop different ways of handling anxiety.** 1. Reduce demands on the individual. 2. Convey acceptance of client, regardless of behavior. 3. Encourage alternative activity.
Post-Traumatic Stress Disorder: involves the development of characteristic symptoms after a traumatic psychological event in which the individual is unable to adapt or adjust (e.g., rape, military combat, airplane crashes, torture, or abuse).	Client re-experiences the traumatic event. Client withdraws, becomes isolated, and restricts emotional response. Experiences hyperalertness, insomnia, nightmares, depression, and anxiety.	❖ **Goal: To determine precipitating stress factor in client's reaction.** 1. Reduce and prevent chronic disability. 2. Encourage verbalization of the traumatic event. ❖ **Goal: To maintain personal integrity.** 1. Provide physical, social, or occupational rehabilitation. 2. Somatic therapies are used to decrease anxiety (e.g., anti-anxiety agents, etc.).
Generalized Anxiety Disorder: unrealistic or excessive anxiety and worry about life's circumstances; differs from panic disorder in that it never remits and onset is at early age.	Physical symptoms associated with disorder are restlessness, apprehension, tension, irritability, "free-floating anxiety."	❖ **Goal: To reduce level of anxiety.** 1. Administer anti-anxiety agent. 2. Teach anxiety-reducing techniques. 3. Reduce pressure and anxiety-provoking situations around client. 4. Divert attention from symptoms.

Nursing Intervention

✔ **NURSING PRIORITY:** *Immediate intervention should focus on control and safety, followed by discussion to alleviate guilt and identify alternative behaviors to help prevent future episodes of violence.*

A. Establish eye contact.
   1. Conveys attention and concern.
   2. Elicits more information.
   3. Asks the person to look at you.

> ✔ *OLDER ADULT PRIORITY: Expect some older adult clients to have vision problems; they may not know who you are. Hearing problems occur with the older adult; don't shout or talk rapidly.*

B. Avoid asking, "Why?" Instead ask, "What's bothering you?"
    1. *Why* questions are threatening and decrease self-esteem.
    2. Open-ended questions identify the problem, convey concern, and elicit more information.
C. Speak to client softly, slowly, and with assurance.
D. Give directions clearly and concisely. Tell the patient what you want him or her to do.
E. Encourage client to verbalize feelings.
    1. Give the client an outlet for the physical tension, "Walk with me. Tell me what happened."
    2. Keep the conversation slow. Pace yourself. "Wait, I can't follow that. Tell me what you said."
    3. Listen more than talk.
    4. Let the person walk, move, or pound something to release the tension before you talk.
F. Position yourself near the door.
    1. Don't block the door.
    2. Don't box the client into a corner.
G. Self-protection and protection of other clients are primary concerns.
    1. Never see a potentially violent client alone; call security or other personnel.
    2. Keep a comfortable distance from client; don't intrude on his or her personal space.
        a. With a client experiencing mild or moderate anxiety: sit near, about 2 feet away.
        b. With a client experiencing severe anxiety or panic: stay 4 to 6 feet back (or farther).
    3. Be prepared to move quickly; violent clients act quickly and unpredictably.
    4. Determine that the client has no weapons before approaching him or her.
    5. Be supportive and intervene to increase client's self-esteem.
    6. Be honest; tell the client you are concerned that he or she is out of control, but you are not going to let anyone get hurt.
    7. Stay with the client, but don't touch him or her until you've asked permission and it has been given to you.
H. When client is in control, review and process the situation in order to alleviate client's guilt and to discuss alternatives should client become anxious or angry in the future.

Manipulation/Acting Out

✳ **Manipulation/Acting Out is a type of controlling behavior in which an individual uses others to meet** his or her own needs or to achieve specific goals; often disguises underlying feelings of inadequacy, inferiority, and unworthiness; an attempt to protect against failure or frustration and to gain power over another.

Nursing Intervention

A. Be consistent and firm in the expectations of behavior.
B. Allow some freedom within set limits.
C. Consistently enforce previously set limits.
D. Be alert to client's attempt to intimidate; allow verbal anger.
E. Avoid involvement and intellectualization.
F. Watch carefully for client's use of manipulative patterns; be alert to the many guises in which it may be manifested.
G. Keep staff united, firm, and consistent.
H. Encourage open communication about real needs and feelings.
I. Maintain a sense of authority.
J. Do not accept gifts, favors, flattery, or other forms of manipulation.

Dependence

✳ **Dependence is a behavior pattern characterized by adopting a helpless, powerless stance; a reliance on other people to meet a basic need.**

Nursing Intervention

A. Assess client's abilities and capacities.
B. Set firm and consistent limits on behavior.
C. Provide only help needed.
D. Encourage problem-solving and decision-making skills; emphasize accountability.
E. Avoid making decisions for client or assuming responsibility for client's ability to make decisions.
F. Maintain an attitude of firmness and confidence in client's ability to make decisions.
G. Discourage reliance beyond actual needs.
H. Give positive reinforcements for development of independent, growth-facilitating behavior.
I. Encourage successful participation in social relationships.

Shame

✳ **Shame is the inner sense of being completely diminished or insufficient as a person (e.g., feeling "less than").**

Nursing Intervention

A. Assist client to begin to externalize rather than internalize feelings of shame.
B. Encourage client to share feelings honestly with individuals he or she feels "safe" with.
C. Involve client in "debriefing," which is writing and talking about past shame experiences.

D. Encourage client to make positive self-affirmations and involve himself or herself in creative visualization activities to improve self-concept.

Detachment

✷ **Detachment is characterized by aloofness, superficiality, denial, and intellectualization in interpersonal contact.**

Nursing Intervention

A. Establish awareness of the process of detachment.
B. Explore fears and fantasies inhibiting emotional expression.
C. Encourage verbalization from global generalities to specific personal comments.
D. Provide clarification of client's unclear responses.
E. Emphasize awareness and exploration of feelings.

ABUSE

✷ **Abuse is difficult to define, because the term has been politicized and is not clinical or scientific.**

 TEST ALERT: *Report client abuse to authorities and protect client from injury.*

Types of Abuse

A. **Physical abuse:** nonaccidental, intentional injury inflicted on another person.
B. **Physical neglect:** willing deprivation of essential care needed to sustain basic human needs and to promote growth and development.
C. **Emotional abuse:** use of threats, verbal insults, or other acts of degradation that are intended to be injurious or damaging to another's self-esteem.
D. **Emotional neglect:** absence of a warm, interpersonal atmosphere that is necessary for psychosocial growth, development, and the promotion of positive feelings of self-worth and self-esteem.
E. **Sexual abuse:** lack of comprehension and consent on the part of the individual involved in sexual activities that are either exploitative or physically intimate in nature (e.g., fondling, oral or genital contact, masturbation, unclothing, etc).
F. **Incest:** sexual activity performed between members of a family group.

Intrafamily Abuse and Violence

✷ **Patterns of dysfunctional, violent families can frequently be traced back for several generations. Adult behavior and role models for parenting are influenced by the childhood experiences within the family system.**

TEST ALERT: *Assess dynamics of family interactions; identify risk factors; plan interventions to assist client and family to cope.*

A. The incorporation of violence within the family teaches the children that the use of violence is appropriate. When the children grow up and form their own families, they tend to recreate the same parent-child, husband-wife relationships experienced in their original family.
B. Frequently, the abuser has inappropriate expectations of family members; the abuser may expect perfection and may be obsessed with discipline and control.
C. Family members are confused regarding their roles in the family; parents may be unable to assume adult roles in the family. Adult family members who feel inadequate in their roles may use violence in an attempt to prove themselves and to maintain superiority.
D. Family is usually isolated, both physically and emotionally. The family tends to have few friends and is frequently isolated from the extended family. Family members are ashamed of what is occurring and tend to withdraw from social contacts in fear that the family activities might become known to others.

Characteristics of Abuse: The Perpetrator

A. The person who abuses or the perpetrator.
   1. Perpetrator has an inability to control impulses; explosive temper; low tolerance for frustration.
   2. Possesses greater physical strength than the victim.
   3. Low self-esteem.
   4. Tends to project shortcomings and inadequacies onto others.
   5. Emotional immaturity; decreased capacity to delay satisfaction.
   6. Suspicious of everyone; fear of being exposed; tends to isolate self from family.
   7. High incidence of drug and alcohol abuse.
   8. Often has experienced abuse as a child; has a greater tendency to demonstrate violence in his or her adult relationships.
B. Common similarities between person who abuses and victim.
   1. Poor self-concept and feelings of insecurity.
   2. Feelings of helplessness, powerlessness, and dependence.
   3. Difficulty in handling or inability to handle anger.

Child Abuse

A. Physical child abuse.
   1. Symptoms.
      a. Bruises and welts from being beaten with a belt, strap, stick, or coat hanger or from being slapped repeatedly in the face.
      b. Rope burns from being tied up or beaten with a rope.
      c. Human bite marks.
      d. Burns.
         (1) Burns on the buttocks from being immersed in hot water.

(2) Pattern of burns: round, small burns from cigarettes; patterns that suggest an object was used.

(3) Burns are frequently on the buttocks, in genital area, or on the soles of the feet.

e. Evidence of various fractures in different stages of healing.

f. Internal injuries from being hit repeatedly in the abdomen.

g. Head injuries: skull, facial fractures.

2. Behavior symptoms.

a. Withdrawal from physical contact with adults.

b. Inappropriate response to pain or injury; failure to cry or seek comfort from parents.

c. Infant may stiffen when held; child may stiffen when approached by adult or parent.

d. Very little eye contact with adults.

e. Child may try to protect abusing parent for fear of punishment if abuse is discovered.

3. Parents or caretakers.

a. Conflicting stories regarding accident or injury.

b. Explanation of accident is inconsistent with injuries sustained (fractured skull and broken leg from falling out of bed).

c. Initial complaint is not associated with child's injury (child is brought to the emergency room with complaints of the "flu," and there is evidence of a skull fracture).

d. Exaggerated concern or lack of concern related to level of child's injury.

e. Refusal to allow further tests or additional medical care.

f. Lack of nurturing response to injured or ill child; no cuddling, touching, or comforting child in distress.

g. Repeated visits to various medical emergency facilities.

h. Do not have realistic expectations of the child; do not understand stages of growth and development (severely spanking or beating a 1-year-old for lack of response to toilet training).

Nursing Intervention

❖ Goal: To establish a safe environment.

A. It is important for the nurse to be knowledgeable of the legal responsibilities in regard to state practice acts and child abuse laws.

B. All 50 states have a designated agency that is available on a 24-hour basis for reporting child abuse.

C. All states have mechanism for removing the child from the immediate abusive environment.

Older Adult Abuse

A. Types of older adult abuse (Box 6-5).

B. Typical victim.

BOX 6-5   OLDER ADULT CARE FOCUS
Older Adult Abuse

Types of Older Adult Abuse
- Physical: willful infliction of injury.
- Neglect: withholding goods or services (such as food or attention) to the detriment of the elder's physical or mental health.
- Psychological: withholding affection or imposing social isolation.
- Exploitation: dishonest or inappropriate use of the older person's property, money, or other resources.

Neglect Indicators
- Poor hygiene, nutrition, and skin integrity.
- Contractures.
- Urine burns/excoriation.
- Pressure ulcers.
- Dehydration.

---

1. Woman of advanced age with few social contacts.
2. At least one physical or mental impairment, limiting the person's ability to perform activities of daily living.

C. Assessment of older adult abuse.

1. Symptoms: contusions, abrasions, sprains, burns, bruising, human bite marks, sexual molestation, untreated or previously treated conditions, erratic hair loss from hair pulling, fractures, dislocations, head and face injuries (especially orbital fractures, black eyes, and broken teeth).

2. Behavior: clinging to the abuser, extreme guardedness in the presence of the abuser, wariness of strangers, expression of ambivalence toward family/caregivers, denial of abuse for fear of retaliation, depression, social or physical isolation.

Nursing Intervention

❖ Goal: To assess for older adult abuse.

A. Use a private setting for interviewing victim and perpetrator.

B. The interview must be unbiased, accurate, and appropriately documented.

C. Avoid signs of disapproval that might evoke shame or anger in the older client; be nonjudgmental.

❖ Goal: To establish a safe environment.

A. It is important for the nurse to be knowledgeable of the legal responsibilities in regard to state practice acts and reporting of abuse (see Box 6-6).

B. Client and family teaching in the areas of nutrition, general physical care, etc.

Rape

A. Legal definition of rape (varies from state to state): forced, violent, sexual attack on an individual without his or her consent. Includes sex acts other than forced intercourse as rape; some states do not recognize rape by the husband.

B. Sexual assault is not a means of sexual gratification; it is a violent physical and emotional attack. Men attack women in an attempt to demonstrate their power and dominance; attempt to control, terrify, and degrade the woman.

C. Victims: in all age ranges; highest risk age group is 12 to 20 years old.

D. Majority of rapes are not sudden and impulsive, but they are well-planned.

E. Most women know the rapist; most rape assaults occur between people of the same race.

F. Rape-trauma syndrome – variant of posttraumatic stress disorder; has two phases, an acute phase and a long-term reorganization phase.

Data Collection

A. Women may experience a wide range of emotional responses: rape trauma syndrome symptoms include sleep disturbances, nightmares, loss of appetite, fears, anxiety, phobias, suspicion, disruption in relationships with partner, family, and friends, along with low self-esteem, feelings of worthlessness, self-blame, guilt, and shame.

B. Complete physical assessment: it is important for as much evidence as possible to be obtained.

C. If possible, advise the woman to not "clean up"; the physical evidence may be destroyed. She should go immediately to the emergency department.

Nursing Intervention

❖ **Goal:** To assist the client through the acute phase after the rape experience.

A. Encourage the client to verbalize her feelings regarding the attack.

B. Assist her to set priorities and determine immediate needs.

C. Warm, respectful, accepting response from the nurse; protect the client from becoming overwhelmed and distressed from the initial physical examination and questioning.

D. Discuss need for follow-up care and physical examination regarding possible pregnancy and sexually transmitted disease.

E. Provide information regarding physical and emotional responses to rape.

F. Provide referral information and plan for follow-up contact within the next week.

BOX 6-6	DOCUMENTATION FOR SUSPECTED ABUSE

Procedure

1. Obtain the client's or parent's permission before photographing the victim.
2. Do not make assumptions about the identity of the perpetrator.
3. Chart the exact words used by the client/child to describe the abuser.
4. Record information very objectively; do not record your feelings, assumptions, or opinions of the incident or how it occurred.

History

1. Specify the time, date, and location as described by the client.
2. Report the sequence of events before the abuse/attack.
3. Identify and explain the period of time between the abuse/attack and initiation of medical attention.
4. List other people/children in the immediate vicinity of the abuse/attack.
5. Include quotations from the client.
6. Use objective, specific documentation when recording observations of the client and the person who brought the client to the emergency room.
7. Observe and record the interaction of the child and the parents.

Physical Examination

1. Be very specific in describing the location, size, and shape of bruises and lacerations. If possible, photograph the client to demonstrate the extent of the injuries.
2. If possible, describe the location and extent of injuries on an anatomical diagram.
3. Identify presence of other injuries.
4. Describe the victim's reaction to pain, level of pain, and location of pain.

❖ **Goal:** To assist the client to work through the emotional phases that commonly occur after the initial trauma.

A. Encourage mental health counseling during the first few days after the assault.

B. Assist the client to understand and recognize the period of long-term reorganization that frequently follows a sexual attack.
1. Victim may experience sexual problems.
2. May experience a strong urge to discuss the incident and feelings related to the attack.
3. During the reorganization phase, client should have professional counseling to assist her to positively cope with the situation.

CHILD-RELATED DISORDERS

Cognitive Impairment (Mental Retardation)

❋ **Cognitive impairment, formerly referred to as mental retardation, is associated with developmental disabilities, intellectual deficits, and lack of adapative behaviors.**

Assessment

A. Characteristics.
  1. Irritability, temper tantrums, stereotyped movements.
  2. Multiple neurological abnormalities: dysfunction in vision or hearing or seizure activity.
B. Down Syndrome - is a common chromosomal abnormality characterized by an extra chromosome 21 (trisomy 21); incidence increases with maternal age.
  1. Head: small in size; face has flat profile, sparse hair.
  2. Eyes: inner epicanthal folds; short and sparse eye lashes.
  3. Nose: small and depressed nasal bridge (saddle nose).
  4. Ears: small and sometimes low-set.
  5. Mouth: protruding tongue; high arched palate.
  6. Neck: short and broad; abdomen: protruding.
  7. Genitalia: small penis, cryptorchidism.
  8. Hands: short, stubby fingers; simian crease (transverse palmar crease).
  9. Muscles: hypotonic.
  10. IQ below 70, slow development.

Nursing Intervention

❖ **Goal:** To promote optimal development within a family and community setting.
A. Involve child and parents in early stimulation program.
B. Promote self-care skills.
C. Help parents identify realistic goals for child.
D. Encourage parents to enroll child in special day care programs and education classes.
E. Emphasize to parents that child has same needs of play, discipline, and social interaction as all children.
❖ **Goal:** To promote independence by setting realistic goals.
A. Teach basic skills in simple terms, with steps outlined.
B. Use behavior modification as a method for behavior control.
C. Use the principles of *repetition, reinforcement,* and *routine* when providing information for understanding and learning.
❖ **Goal:** To monitor for complications associated with Down syndrome.
A. Prevent respiratory tract infections by teaching parents about postural drainage and percussion.
B. Encourage use of cool mist vaporizer.
C. Stress importance of changing infant's position frequently.
D. Explain to parents about feeding difficulties; encourage small, frequent feedings; feed solid food by pushing food back inside of mouth; provide foods that will form bulk to prevent constipation.
❖ **Goal:** To prevent Down syndrome.
A. Encourage pregnant women at risk (older than 35 years, family history of Down syndrome, or previous birth of a child with Down syndrome) to consider

amniocentesis before the sixteenth week to rule out Down syndrome.
B. Encourage genetic counseling for couples with a family history of Down's syndrome.

 Eating Disorders

✳ **This group of disorders is characterized by gross disturbances in eating behavior; it includes anorexia nervosa and bulimia nervosa.**

Assessment

A. Anorexia nervosa.
  1. Intense fear of becoming obese.
  2. Need for control and perfectionism.
  3. Disturbance of body image.
  4. Occurs more often in females than males
  5. Weight loss of at least 15% of original body weight.
  6. No known physical illness.
B. Bulimia nervosa.
  1. Recurrent episodes of binge eating.
  2. Awareness that eating pattern is abnormal.
  3. Secretive binge eating and purging behaviors (diuretics, laxatives, excessive exercise).
    a. Russell's sign - bruises or calluses on the thumb or hand caused by trauma from self-induced vomiting.
    b. Erosion of tooth enamel, pharyngitis from vomiting.
  4. Fear of not being able to stop eating voluntarily.
  5. Depressed mood and self-induced vomiting after the eating binges.

Nursing Intervention

❖ **Goal:** To exhibit no signs or symptoms of malnutrition.
A. If client is unable or unwilling to maintain adequate oral intake, a liquid diet may be administered through a nasogastric tube.
B. Explain to client details of behavior modification program.
C. Sit with client during mealtimes for support and to observe amount ingested. A limit (usually 30 minutes) should be imposed on time allotted for meals.
D. Accompany client to bathroom, if self-induced vomiting is suspected.
E. Carefully document intake and output.
F. Do not discuss food or eating with client, once protocol has been established. Do, however, offer support and positive reinforcement for obvious improvements in eating behaviors.
G. Offer support and use nonjudgmental approach with the client.
H. Administer antidepressants as ordered.
❖ **Goal:** To increase self-esteem.
A. Assist client to reexamine negative perceptions of self and to recognize positive attributes.

B. Offer positive reinforcement for independently made decisions influencing client's life.

❖   **Goal:** To identify an eating disorder and rule out a physiological cause.

❖   **Goal:** To recognize complications.

A. Anorexia nervosa – refeeding syndrome can result if system is replenished too quickly leading to cardiovascular collapse.

B. Bulimia nervosa – if syrup of Ipecac is used to induce vomiting and vomiting does not occur, the absorption of the Ipecac can lead to cardiotoxicity and heart failure. Watch for edema and check breath sounds.

 Psychiatric Considerations of Older Adults

✳   **Delirium is a syndrome that usually develops over a short period of time. The constellation of symptoms typically fluctuates and is often reversible and temporary.**

✳   **Dementia is a syndrome characterized by loss of intellectual abilities to such an extent that social and occupational functioning are negatively affected; involves memory, judgment, abstract thought, and changes in personality. Often, the disorders are progressive and follow an irreversible course in which the damage remains permanent (Box 6-7).**

Data Collection

A. Causes of dementia.
1. Alzheimer's disease.
2. Stroke.
3. Parkinson's disease.
4. Injury.
5. Medication therapy.

BOX 6-7   **KEY POINTS: ORGANIC MENTAL SYNDROMES**

- Clients have varying degrees of awareness of the changes that are occurring, which is emotionally painful to them.
- Often, depression is mistaken for the early onset of dementia.
- Dementia disrupts the elderly couple's final stage of family development (generativity, retirement, etc.).
- Dementia interferes with family intergenerational development where adult offspring are unable to rectify past injustices, conflicts, and disappointments with parents.
- Caregiver coping is highly stressful and can be handled with a more positive approach when there is a focus on problem solving and education.
- Clients with Alzheimer's disease (AD) have loss of memory, intellectual functioning, orientation, affective regulation, motor coordination, and personality, with eventual loss of bowel and bladder control to the point of total incapacitation.

B. Alzheimer's disease.
1. More commonly seen in older adult clients.
2. Irreversible.
3. Helpful mnemonic to remember symptoms: JAMCO

    J: Judgment
    A: Affect
    M: Memory
    C: Confusion
    O: Orientation

4. Stages of Alzheimer's disease (Table 6-5).
5. Special concerns.
   a. Recent memory loss. Client can recall events and activities from 10 years ago, but not 10 minutes ago.
   b. Sundown syndrome (sundowning): confused, disoriented behavior that becomes noticeable after the sun goes down and during the night.
   c. Wandering behavior.
     (1) Restlessness and activity-seeking behavior.
     (2) The "stalking of old haunts."
     (3) Disorientation and inability to sustain intentions; the person forgets what she or he set out to do.
   d. Catastrophic reactions: heightened anxiety occurring during interviewing or questioning when a person cannot answer or perform.
   e. Combative behavior.
   f. Delusions and hallucinations.

Nursing Interventions

❖   **Goal:** To maintain adequate nutrition.

A. Reduce distractions while eating, such as television.
B. Encourage snacks.
C. Monitor weight monthly.
D. Encourage family to bring in client's favorite foods.

❖   **Goal:** To provide a quiet, structured environment in order to increase consistency and promote feelings of security.

A. Avoid dependency.
B. Establish routine for activities of daily living.
C. Meet client's physical needs.
D. Do not isolate client from others in the unit.
E. Provide handrails, walkers, and wheelchairs.
F. Do not change schedules suddenly: *routine, reinforcement,* and *repetition* are the key aspects of care.
G. Check for hazards in the environment (rugs on floor); make sure environment is well-lighted; do not move client suddenly into darkness.
H. Provide quiet, nonstimulating environment to decrease hallucinations; avoid furniture and bedding with bright colors and bold patterns.

❖   **Goal:** To promote contact with reality.

A. Make brief and frequent contact.
B. Give feedback and praise whenever possible.
C. Supply stimulation to motivate client to engage in activities.

D. Use concrete ideas in communication.

E. Maintain reality orientation by encouraging reminiscing.

F. Frequently orient client to reality and surroundings. Allow client to have familiar objects around self. Use other items, such as clock, calendar, and daily schedules, to assist in maintaining reality orientation.

G. Use simple explanations and face-to-face interaction when communicating with client. Do not shout message into client's ear.

H. Allow sufficient time for client to complete projects.

I. Reinforce reality-oriented comments and continually orient clients to person, time, place, and date.

J. Use memory joggers: frequent notes, messages on calendars to decrease forgetful incidents.

❖ **Goal:** To manage and minimize wandering behavior.

A. A protective environment is needed for the wanderers as well as room to move about.

B. Bed rails should be avoided (place mattress on floor if necessary).

C. Limit cash in wallet to a few dollars and coins to minimize danger of financial loss.

D. Have client wear a MedicAlert bracelet or necklace that cannot be removed (name, address, telephone number on bracelet or necklace).

E. Place name, address, and phone number on items of

TABLE 6-5	STAGES OF ALZHEIMER'S DISEASE
Stage	**Hallmarks**
Stage 1 **(Mild)** *Forgetfulness*	Shows short-term memory losses; loses things, forgets Memory aids compensate: lists, routine, organization Depression common – worsens symptoms Not diagnosable at this time
Stage 2 **(Moderate)** *Confusion*	Shows progressive memory loss; short-term memory is impaired; memory difficulties interfere with all abilities Withdrawn from social activities Shows declines in instrumental activities of daily living (IADLs), such as money management, legal affairs, transportation, cooking, housekeeping Denial common; fears "losing his or her mind" Depression increasing common; frightened because aware of deficits; covers up for memory loss through confabulation Problems intensified when stressed, fatigued, out of own environment, ill Commonly needs day care or in-home assistance
Stage 3 **(Moderate to Severe)** *Ambulatory dementia*	Shows ADL losses (in order) willingness and ability to bathe, grooming, choosing clothing, dressing, gait and mobility, toileting, communication, reading, and writing skills Shows loss of reasoning ability, safety planning, and verbal communication Frustration common; becomes more withdrawn and self-absorbed Depression resolves as awareness of losses diminishes Has difficulty communicating; shows increasing loss of language skills Shows evidence of reduced stress threshold; institutional care usually needed
Stage 4 **(Late)** *End stage*	Family recognition disappears; does not recognize self in mirror Nonambulatory; shows little purposeful activity; often mute; may scream spontaneously Forgets how to eat, swallow, chew; commonly loses weight; emaciation common Has problems associated with immobility (e.g., pneumonia, pressure ulcers, contractures) Incontinence common; seizures may develop Most certainly institutionalized at this point Return of primitive (infantile) reflexes

From Hall, G.R. (1994). Caring for people with Alzheimer's disease using the conceptual model of progressively lowered stress threshold in the clinical setting. *Nursing Clinics of North America*, 29(1), 129-141, as cited in Varcarolis EM, Carson VB, Shoemaker NC: *Foundations of psychiatric mental health nursing*, page 435.

clothing; attach this information to clothes so that client cannot remove it.

F. Install complex door locks opened by actions demanding thought rather than sheer strength.

G. Implement a buddy system in an institution.

H. Spend extra time with newly admitted clients; provide frequent reassurance, and attend to orientation carefully.

❖ Goal: To promote self-esteem.

A. Client should wear own clothing; no night clothes during daytime hours.

B. Makeup should be available for women.

C. Client should carry purse or wallet; client should have a monthly allowance or a few coins to carry.

D. Use praise whenever possible.

E. Use affection.

F. Let client make choices whenever possible, but offer only two.

❖ Goal: To provide diversion activities that enhance self-esteem.

A. Provide occupational therapy, physical therapy, and recreational therapy that client enjoys.

B. Maintain a flexible schedule and keep client from becoming bored and easily distracted.

C. Recognize specific accomplishments.

D. Encourage family involvement and provide emotional support.

E. Devise methods for assisting client with memory deficit. Examples:
   1. Sign and client picture on door identifying client's room.
   2. Identifying sign on outside of dining room door.
   3. Large clock, with oversized numbers and hands, appropriately placed.
   4. Large calendar, indicating one day at a time, with month, day, and year identified in bold print.

❖ Goal: To administer medication to slow the dementia disease process (Appendix 6-5).

✓ **OLDER ADULT NURSING PRIORITY:** *The 3 Ps for clients with dementia: protecting dignity, preserving functioning, and promoting quality of life.*

Psychophysiological Disorder

❖ **A psychophysiological disorder is a physical illness that is strongly influenced by psychological factors. It was previously called psychosomatic disorder. It is thought that stress and anxiety arouse specific conflicts in an individual, which result in damaging effects on particular organs or organ systems that are under the control of the autonomic nervous system.**

Data Collection

A. Respiratory: hyperventilation syndrome, bronchial asthma.

B. Cardiovascular: essential hypertension, angina, migraine headaches, tachycardia.

C. Gastrointestinal: peptic ulcer disease, ulcerative colitis, colic.

D. Integumentary: dermatitis, pruritus, excessive sweating, atopic dermatitis.

E. Musculoskeletal: cramps, rheumatoid arthritis.

F. Endocrine: diabetes mellitus, sexual dysfunctions, hyperemesis gravidarum, hyperthyroidism.

G. Genital/urinary: amenorrhea, impotence, secondary outbreaks of herpes genitalis type II (HVH II).

Nursing Interventions

Pathophysiology and nursing interventions of the above disorders are discussed in the chapters under the appropriate body system affected.

 Personality Disorders

* **Personality disorders create disruptive lifestyles and are characterized by inflexible and maladapted behaviors. Those with personality disorders clash with society and with cultural norms and are often placed in correctional systems, mental hospitals, and child placement facilities.**

Data Collection

A. Problems are expressed through behavior rather than as physical symptoms of stress.

B. Disruptive lifestyle is deeply ingrained and quite difficult to change; usually related to some form of abnormal behavior or the development of a particular pattern or trait.

C. Often comes in conflict with others.

D. Unable to develop meaningful relationships with others and communicate effectively.

F. Rarely acknowledges that there is a problem.

G. Types: paranoid, schizoid, schizotypic, antisocial, borderline, narcissistic, avoidance, dependent, and passive-aggressive.

Nursing Intervention

❖ Goal: To promote communication and socialization in the paranoid personality.

A. Decrease social isolation.

B. Verbal and nonverbal messages should be clear and consistent.

C. To decrease anxiety, plan several brief contacts, rather than one prolonged contact.

D. Promote trust by following through on commitments.

E. Be open and honest to avoid misinterpretation.

❖ Goal: To convey to the schizoid or schizotypal client the idea that you do not perceive reality the same way as he or she does but are willing to listen, learn, and offer feedback about his or her experiences.

❖ Goal: To promote a positive, therapeutic, interpersonal relationship.

A. Set realistic expectations.

B. Provide a model of mature behavior.

C. Use problem-solving techniques to encourage a client to make changes.

D. Anticipate and deal with depression in a client who gradually acquires enough insight to realize and accept responsibility for his or her behavior.

E. Common sources of frustration for nurses.
   1. Client's immature behavior.
   2. Poor communication skills.

❖   **Goal:** To minimize manipulation and "acting out" behaviors and encourage verbal communication.

A. Set firm, consistent limits without being punitive.

B. Be aware of how client may manipulate other staff members (e.g., playing one against the other or splitting).

C. Promote expression of feelings versus acting out.

D. Promote client's acceptance of responsibility for his or her own actions and a social responsibility to others.

❖   **Goal:** To assist client to manage anxiety.

A. Anticipate client's needs before he or she demands attention.

B. Teach client to express his or her ideas and feelings assertively.

❖   **Goal:** To set realistic limits.

A. Support the client who is gradually making more decisions on his or her own.

B. Offer assistance only when needed.

Alcohol Dependence (Alcoholism)

✳   **Alcoholism is a chronic pattern of pathological alcohol use is characterized by impairment in social or occupational functioning, along with tolerance or withdrawal symptoms.**

Data Collection

A. Risk factors.
   1. History of alcoholism in family.
   2. History of total abstinence.
   3. Broken or disrupted home.
   4. Last or near-last child in a large family.
   5. Heavy smoking.
   6. Cultural groups: Irish, Eskimo, Scandinavian, Native American.

B. General personality characteristics of alcoholics.
   1. Dependent behavior along with resentment of authority.
   2. Demanding and domineering with a low tolerance for frustration.
   3. Dissatisfied with life; tendency toward self-destructive acts, including suicide.
   4. Low self-esteem and poor self-concept.

C. Signs and symptoms of possible alcohol abuse.
   1. Sprains, bruises, and injuries of questionable origin.
   2. Diarrhea and early morning vomiting.
   3. Chronic cough, palpitations, and infections.
   4. Frequent Monday morning illnesses; blackouts (inability to recall events or actions while intoxicated).

D. Alcohol withdrawal syndrome. Consuming one fifth of whiskey daily for 1 month is generally considered sufficient to produce alcohol withdrawal. The withdrawal syndrome develops in heavy drinkers who have increased, decreased, or interrupted the intake of alcohol.
   1. Alcohol withdrawal.
      a. Anorexia, irritability, nausea, and tremulousness.
      b. Insomnia, nightmares, irritability, hyperalertness.
      c. Tachycardia, increased blood pressure, and diaphoresis.
      d. Onset within 8 hours after cessation of drinking (usually 48 to 72 hours); clears up within 5 to 7 days.
   2. Delirium tremens.
      a. Autonomic hyperactivity: tachycardia, sweating, increased blood pressure.
      b. Vivid hallucinations, delusions, confusion.
      c. Coarse, irregular tremor is almost always seen; fever may occur.
      d. Onset within 24 to 72 hours after the last ingestion of alcohol; delirium tremens usually lasts 2 to 3 days.
      e. Convulsions/seizures may occur ("rum fits").
      f. First episode occurs after 5 to 15 years of heavy drinking.
   3. Alcohol hallucinosis.
      a. Auditory hallucinations.
      b. Occurs within 48 hours after heavy drinking episode.
      c. Often includes persecutory delusions.
      d. Client may be suicidal or homicidal.
      e. Spontaneous recovery within 1 week.
      f. Wernicke's encephalopathy.
         (1) an acute, *reversible* neurological disorder.
         (2) triad of symptoms: global confusion, ataxia, and eye movement abnormality (nystagmus).
         (3) occurs primarily in clients with chronic alcoholism; may develop in illnesses that interfere with thiamine (vitamin B1) absorption (e.g., gastric cancer, malabsorption syndrome, regional enteritis).
         (4) treatment: high doses of thiamine; 100 mg, given intramuscularly, usually reverses eye signs within 2 to 3 hours of treatment.

E. Korsakoff's syndrome (alcohol amnesiac disorder).
   1. A chronic, *irreversible* disorder, often following Wernicke's encephalopathy.
   2. Triad of symptoms: memory loss, learning deficit, confabulation (filling in of memory gaps with plausible stories).

G. Other disorders associated with chronic alcoholism: pneumonitis, esophageal varices, cirrhosis, pancreatitis, diabetes (These are discussed in chapters 8, 10, 14 under the appropriate system).

Nursing Intervention

❖ **Goal:** To assess for alcoholism in a client through careful questioning.

A. Identify the alcoholic client in the preoperative period.
  1. Often, alcoholics are undiagnosed at the time of surgery and may go into withdrawal or delirium tremens after the NPO (nothing by mouth) period.
  2. Client usually takes longer to be fully responsive during postoperative period; client is susceptible to severe respiratory complications; client has more difficulty with healing because of poor nutritional state.

❖ **Goal:** To assist in the medical treatment of alcohol withdrawal.

A. Benzodiazepines for agitation (see Appendix 6-1).
B. Thiamine (vitamin B1) to prevent Wernicke's encephalopathy.
C. Magnesium sulfate to increase effectiveness of vitamin B1. It helps reduce postwithdrawal seizures.
D. Anticonvulsant (Phenobarbital) if necessary for seizure control.
E. Encourage use of multivitamins, especially folic acid, B12, and vitamin C.
F. Alpha-adrenergic blockers (clonidine) to decrease withdrawal symptoms.
G. Beta-adrenergic blockers (atenolol, propanolol) to improve vital signs and decrease cravings.
H. Encourage intake of fluids, but do not force.

❖ **Goal:** To provide for the basic needs of rest, comfort, safety, and nutrition.

A. Safety measures, such as bed rest and use of bed rails, may be necessary.
B. *If client is experiencing delirium tremens, stay with client and notify appropriate person.*
C. Have room adequately lit to help reduce confusion and avoid shadows and unclear objects.
D. Monitor vital signs every 1 to 4 hours.
E. Encourage a high-carbohydrate, soft diet.

❖ **Goal:** To recognize complications of alcohol use.

A. Obstetrical implications.
  1. Use of alcohol during pregnancy may lead to fetal alcohol syndrome.
  2. Alcohol withdrawal syndrome may occur in the intrapartal period as early as 12 to 48 hours after the last drink.
  3. Delirium tremens may occur in the postpartum period.
B. Neonatal implications (fetal alcohol syndrome).
  1. Teratogenic effects may be seen along with growth and developmental retardation.
  2. Increased risk for anomalies of the heart, head, face, and extremities.

  3. Withdrawal symptoms can occur shortly after birth and are characterized by tremors, agitation, sweating, and seizure activity.
  4. *Maintain seizure precautions and report any seizure activity.*

C. Medical complications of alcohol abuse.
  1. Trauma-related to falls, burns, hematomas.
  2. Liver disease: cirrhosis, esophageal varices, hepatic coma.
  3. Gastrointestinal disease: gastritis, bleeding ulcers, pancreatitis.
  4. Nutritional disease: malnutrition, anemia caused by iron or vitamin B12 deficiency, thiamine deficiency.
  5. Infections, especially pneumonia.
  6. Neurological disease: polyneuropathy and dementia.

❖ **Goal:** To assist in the long-term rehabilitation of client.

A. Avoid sympathy, because clients tend to rationalize and use dependent, manipulative behavior to seek privileges.
B. Maintain a nonjudgmental attitude.
C. Set behavior limits in a firm but kind manner.
D. Place responsibility for sobriety on client; do not give advice or punish or reprimand client for failures.
E. Provide opportunities to decrease social isolation by encouraging participation in social groups and activities.
F. Encourage client to develop coping mechanisms other than alcohol to deal with stress.
G. Refer clients and family to available community resources.
  1. Alcoholics Anonymous (AA): a self-help group focusing on education, guidance, and the sharing of problems and experiences unique to the individual.
  2. Al-Anon: a self-help support group for the spouses and significant others of the alcoholic.
  3. Alateen: the support group for teenagers with an alcoholic parent.
  4. Adult Children of Alcoholics (ACOA): support group for adult children of alcoholics and dysfunctional individuals.
  5. Families Anonymous: support group for the families whose lives have been affected by the addicted client's behavior.
  6. Codependents Anonymous: support group for codependents who may be alcoholics or drug addicts and for persons who are close to an addict.
H. Promote adherence to prescribed therapeutic regimens.
  1. Disulfiram (**Antabuse**): a drug that produces intense side effects after ingestion of alcohol (severe nausea, vomiting, flushed face, hypotension, and blurred vision).
  2. Aversion therapy: a form of deterrent therapy attempting to induce alcohol rejection behavior by administering alcohol with an emetic.
  3. Naltrexone (**Revia**): opioid antagonist that decreases the craving for alcohol.
  4. Acamprosate (**Campral**): a drug that helps clients abstain from alcohol.

Polydrug Dependence

✳ **Polydrug dependence is the regular use of three or more psychoactive substances over a period of at least 6 months.**

General Concepts

A. Effects of use.
  1. Relieves anxiety.
  2. Overdose can occur.
B. General personality characteristics.
  1. Inability to cope with stress, frustration, or anxiety.
  2. Rebellious, immature, desire for immediate gratification.
  3. Passivity and low self-esteem.
  4. Difficulty forming warm, personal relationships.
  5. Uses defense mechanisms: denial, rationalization, intellectualization.

Data Collection

A. General assessment.
  1. Determine the pattern of drug use.
    a. Which drugs are being used by the client?
    b. When was the last use?
    c. How much does client use and how often?
    d. How long has client been using drugs?
    e. What combination of drugs is being used?
  2. Determine if there are any physical changes present (e.g., needle tracks, swollen nasal mucous membranes, reddened conjunctivae).
B. Narcotic dependence.
  Examples of narcotics: opium, heroin, morphine, meperidine (Demerol), codeine, fentanyl, methadone, OxyContin, oxycodone.
  1. Administration.
    a. Heroin: sniffed, smoked, injected intravenously (mainlining), injected subcutaneously (skin popping).
    b. Other narcotics are usually taken orally or injected.
  2. Symptoms of use.
    a. Drowsiness and decreased blood pressure, pulse, and respiratory rate.
    b. Pinpoint pupils, needle tracks, scarring.
    c. Overdose effects: slow, shallow breathing, clammy skin, convulsions, coma, pulmonary edema, possible death.
  3. Withdrawal symptoms.
    a. Onset of symptoms approximately 8 to 12 hours after the last dose.
    b. Lacrimation, sweating, sneezing, yawning.
    c. Gooseflesh (piloerection), tremor, irritability, anorexia.
    d. Dilated pupils, abdominal cramps, vomiting, involuntary muscle spasms.
    e. Symptoms generally subside within 7 to 10 days.
C. Sedative-hypnotic dependence.

Examples of sedative-hypnotics: barbiturates (Nembutal, Seconal) and the benzodiazepines (Librium, Valium).
  1. Administration: oral or injected.
  2. Symptoms of use.
    a. Alterations in mood, thought, behavior.
    b. Impairment in coordination, judgment.
    c. Signs of intoxication: slurred speech, unsteady gait, decreased attention span or memory.
    d. Barbiturate use: often violent, disruptive, irresponsible behavior.
  3. Withdrawal symptoms.
    a. Insomnia, anxiety, profuse sweating, weakness.
    b. Severe reactions of delirium, grand mal seizures, cardiovascular collapse.
D. Cocaine abuse.
  Example: Cocaine.
  1. Administration: intranasal ("snorting") or by intravenous or subcutaneous injection; also smoked in pipe (free-basing).
  2. Symptoms of use.
    a. Euphoria, grandiosity, and a sense of well-being.
    b. Amphetamine-like or stimulant-like effects such as increased blood pressure, racing of the heart, paranoia, anxiety.
    c. Used regularly, cocaine may disrupt eating and sleeping habits, leading to irritability and decreased concentration.

✔ **NURSING PRIORITY:** *Crack (rock) has been labeled the most addictive drug. It is a potent form of cocaine hydrochloride mixed with baking soda and water, heated (cooked), allowed to harden, and then broken or "cracked" into little pieces and smoked in cigarettes or glass water pipes. Cardiac dysrhythmias, respiratory paralysis, and seizures are some of the dangers associated with crack use.*

  3. Withdrawal symptoms.
    a. Severe craving.
    b. Coming down from a "high" often leads to a severe "letdown," depressed feeling.
    c. Psychological dependence often leads to cocaine becoming a total obsession.
E. Amphetamine dependence.
  Example: dextroamphetamine (Dexedrine).
  1. Administration: oral or injected.
  2. Symptoms of use.
    a. Elation, agitation, hyperactivity, irritability.
    b. Increased pulse, respiration, and blood pressure.
    c. Fine tremor, muscle twitching, and mydriasis (pupillary dilation).
    d. Large doses: convulsions, cardiovascular collapse, respiratory depression, coma, death.
  3. Withdrawal symptoms.
    a. Appear within 2 to 4 days after the last dose.

b. Depression, overwhelming fatigue, suicide attempts.

F. PCP (phencyclidine hydrochloride) abuse.
1. Administration: snorted, smoked, or orally ingested; usually smoked along with marijuana.
2. Symptoms of use.
   a. Euphoria, feeling of numbness, mood changes.
   b. Diaphoresis, eye movement changes (nystagmus), hypertension, catatonic-like stupor with eyes open.
   c. Seizures, shivering, decerebrate posturing, possible death.
   d. Synesthesia (seeing colors when a loud sound occurs).
3. Overdose symptoms ("bad trip"): psychosis, possible death.
   a. User may become violent, destructive, and confused.
   b. Users have been known to go berserk; users may harm themselves and others.
   c. Intoxicating symptoms lighten and worsen over a period of 48 hours.

G. Hallucinogen abuse.
Example: LSD (lisergic acid diethylamide), psilocybin ("magic mushroom"), mescaline (peyote), DMT, MDA.
1. Administration: usually oral, but LSD and mescaline can be injected.
2. Symptoms of use.
   a. Pupillary dilation, tachycardia, sweating.
   b. Visual hallucinations, depersonalization, impaired judgment and mood.
   c. "Flashbacks" and "bad trips."
   d. Usually no signs of withdrawal symptoms after use has been discontinued.

H. Marijuana dependence.
Example: Marijuana, hashish, tetrahydrocannabinol (THC).
1. Administration: oral, sniffed, and smoked.
2. Symptoms of use.
   a. Euphoria, relaxation, tachycardia, and conjunctival congestion.
   b. Paranoid ideation; impaired judgment.
   c. Rarely, panic reactions and psychoses.
   d. Heavy use leads to apathy and general deterioration in all aspects of living.
   e. Overdose effects: flashbacks, bronchitis, personality changes.
3. Withdrawal symptoms.
   a. Anxiety, sleeplessness, sweating.
   b. Lack of appetite, nausea, general malaise.

I. Designer drugs.
Example: Ecstasy, (MDMA [methylenedioxy-methamphetamine], Adam), MTPT (China White).
1. Called *analog drugs* because they retain the properties of controlled drugs (e.g., MTPT is an analog of **Demerol**).

2. Symptoms of use and side effects are similar to those associated with the controlled substance from which they are derived.

Nursing Intervention

❖ **Goal:** To assess the drug use pattern.
❖ **Goal:** To assist in medical treatment during detoxification or withdrawal.
A. Narcotics.
1. Narcotic antagonists, such as naloxone (**Narcan**), nalorphine (**Nalline**), or levallorphan (**Lorfan**), are administered intravenously for narcotic overdose.
2. Withdrawal is managed with rest and nutritional therapy.
B. Depressants.
1. Substitution therapy with a long-acting barbiturate, such as phenobarbital (**Luminal**), may be instituted to decrease withdrawal symptoms.
2. Some physicians prescribe oxazepam (**Serax**) as needed for objective symptoms, gradually decreasing the dosage until the drug is discontinued.
C. Stimulants.
1. Treatment of overdose is geared toward stabilization of vital signs.
2. IV antihypertensives may be used, along with IV diazepam (**Valium**) to control seizures.
3. Oral benzodiazepines (**Librium**) may be administered orally for the first few days while client is "crashing."
D. Hallucinogens and cannabinols.
1. Medications are normally not prescribed for withdrawal from these substances.
2. In the event of overdose, diazepam (**Valium**) or chlordiazepoxide (**Librium**) may be given as needed to decrease agitation.
E. Awareness that gradual withdrawal, detoxification, or dechemicalization is necessary for the client addicted to barbiturates, narcotics, and tranquilizers.
F. Abrupt withdrawal, or quitting "cold turkey," is often dangerous and can be fatal.
G. Maintain a patent airway; have oxygen available.
H. Provide a safe, quiet environment (i.e., remove harmful objects, use side rails).
❖ **Goal:** To decrease problem behaviors of manipulation and "acting out."
A. Set firm, consistent limits.
B. Confront client with manipulative behaviors.
❖ **Goal:** To promote alternative coping methods.
A. Encourage responsibility for own behavior.
B. Encourage the use of hobbies, exercise, or alternative therapies as a means to deal with frustration and anxiety.
❖ **Goal:** To recognize complications of substance abuse.
A. Obstetrical implications.
1. Narcotic addiction.

a. Increased risk of pregnancy-induced hypertension, malpresentation, and third-trimester bleeding.
b. Provide methadone maintenance therapy for the duration of the pregnancy, because withdrawal is not advisable because of the risk to the fetus.
2. Other use of drugs causes increased risk to mother and fetus.
B. Neonatal complications.
1. Withdrawal symptoms depend on type of drug mother used.
2. Restlessness, jitteriness, hyperactive reflexes, high-pitched shrill cry, feeds poorly.
3. Maintain seizure precautions.
4. Administer antiepileptics to treat withdrawal and prevent seizures.
5. Swaddle infant in snug-fitting blanket.
6. Increased risk for congenital malformations and prematurity.
C. Medical implications.
1. Increased risk of hepatitis, malnutrition, and infections in general.
❖ Goal: To assist in the long-term process of drug rehabilitation.
A. Refer client to drug rehabilitation programs.
B. Promote self-help residential programs that foster self-support systems and use ex-addicts as rehabilitation counselors.
C. Methadone maintenance programs.
1. Must be 18 years old and addicted for more than 2 years, with a history of detoxification treatments.
2. Methadone is a synthetic narcotic that appeases desire for opiates.
a. Controlled substance given only under urinary surveillance.
b. Administered orally; prevents opiate withdrawal symptoms.
D. 12-Step self-help groups.
1. Narcotics Anonymous: support group for clients who are addicted to narcotics and other drugs.
2. Nar-Anon: support group for relatives and friends of narcotic addicts.
3. Families Anonymous.

Affective Disorders

* **The major affective disorders are characterized by disturbances of mood.**

Data Collection

A. Bipolar disorder (Figure 6-1).
1. Manic.
a. Onset before the age of 30 years.
b. Mood: elevated, expansive, or irritable.
c. Speech: loud, rapid, difficult to interpret, punning, rhyming, and clanging (using words that

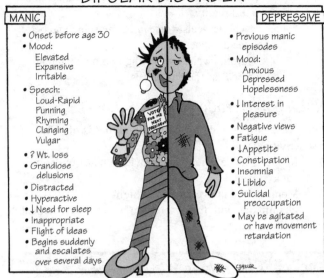

FIGURE 6-1 **Bipolar Affective Disorder.** (From Zerwekh J, Claborn J, Miller CJ: *Memory notebook of nursing, vol 1,* ed 3, Ingram, 2004, Nursing Education Consultants, Inc.)

sound like the meaning rather than the actual word).
d. Cognitive skills: flight of ideas, grandiose delusions, easily distracted.
e. Psychomotor activity: hyperactive, decreased need for sleep, exhibitionistic, vulgar, profane, may make inappropriate sexual advances and be obscene.
f. Course of manic episode: begins suddenly, rapidly escalates over a few days, and ends more abruptly than major depressive episodes.
2. Depressive.
a. Has had one or more manic episodes.
b. Mood: dysphoric, depressive, despairing, loss of interest or pleasure in most usual activities.
c. Cognitive process: negative view of self, world, and of the future; poverty of ideas; crying; and suicidal preoccupation.
d. Psychomotor: may have either agitation or retardation in movements, feelings of fatigue, lack of appetite, constipation, sleeping disturbances (insomnia or early morning wakefulness), and a decrease in libido.
3. Mixed.
a. Involves both manic and depressive episodes, either intermixed or alternating rapidly every few days.
b. Depressive phase symptoms are prominent and last at least a full day.
B. Major depression.
1. May occur at any age.
2. Differentiated as either a single episode or a recurring type.
3. Symptoms the same as those listed under "Bipolar disorder, Depressive."

4. Severity and type of depression vary with the ability to test reality.
   a. Psychotic: feels worse in the morning and better as the day goes on.
   b. Neurotic: wakes up feeling optimistic; mood worsens as the day passes.

Nursing Intervention (Manic Episode)

❖ **Goal:** To provide for basic human needs of safety and rest/activity.

A. Reduce outside stimuli and provide a nonstimulating environment.
B. Monitor food intake: provide a high-calorie, high-vitamin diet with finger foods, to be eaten as the client moves about.

> ✔ **NURSING PRIORITY:** *Physiological needs are the first priority in providing client care. During the manic phase, the client's physical safety is at risk because the hyperactivity may lead to exhaustion, and ultimately, cardiac failure.*

C. Encourage noncompetitive solitary activities such as walking, swimming, or painting.
D. Assist with personal hygiene.
❖ **Goal:** To establish a therapeutic nurse-client relationship.
A. Use firm, consistent, honest approach.
B. Assess client's abilities and involve client in his or her own care planning.
C. Promote problem-solving abilities; recognize that a false sense of independence is often demonstrated by loud, boisterous behavior.
D. Do not focus on or discuss grandiose ideas.
❖ **Goal:** To set limits on behavior.
A. Instructions should be clear and concise.
B. Initiate regularly scheduled contacts to demonstrate acceptance.
C. Maintain some distance between self and client to allow freedom of movement and to prevent feelings of being overpowered.
D. Maintain neutrality and objectivity: Realize that client can be easily provoked by harmless remarks and may demonstrate a furious reaction but calm down very quickly.
E. Use measures to prevent overt aggression (e.g., distraction, recognition of behaviors of increased excitement).
❖ **Goal:** To promote adaptive coping with constructive use of energy.
A. Do not hurry client, because this leads to anxiety and hostile behavior.

> ✔ **NURSING PRIORITY:** *In a hyperactive state, the client is extremely distractible, and responses to even the slightest stimuli are exaggerated.*

B. Provide activities and constructive tasks that channel the agitated behavior (e.g., cleaning game room, going for a walk, gardening, playing catch).
❖ **Goal:** To assist in the medical treatment.
A. Administer lithium (**Lithane** or **Eskalith**).
B. Teach client about lithium medication instructions (see Appendix 6-2).

Nursing Intervention (Depressive Episode)

> ✔ **NURSING PRIORITY:** *Depression and suicidal behaviors may be viewed as anger turned inward on the self. If this anger can be verbalized in a nonthreatening environment, the client may be able to resolve these feelings, regardless of the discomfort involved.*

❖ **Goal:** To assess for suicide potential.
A. Recognition of suicidal intent.
   1. Self-destructive behaviors are viewed as attempts to escape unbearable life situations.
   2. Anxiety and hostility are overwhelmingly present.
   3. There is the presence of ambivalence; living versus self-destructive impulses.
   4. Depression, low self-esteem, and a feeling of hopelessness are critical to evaluate, because suicide attempts are often made when the client feels like giving up.
   5. Assess for *indirect* self-destructive behavior: any activity that is detrimental to the physical well-being of the client in which the potential outcome is death.
      a. Eating disorders: anorexia nervosa, bulimia, obesity, and overeating.
      b. Noncompliance with medical treatment (e.g., diabetic who does not take insulin).
      c. Cigarette smoking, gambling, criminal and socially deviant activities.
      d. Alcohol and drug abuse.
      e. Participation in high-risk sports (e.g., automobile racing and skydiving).
B. Suicide danger signs.
   1. The presence of a suicide plan: specifics relating to method, its lethality, and likelihood for rescue.
   2. Change in established patterns in routines (e.g., giving away of personal items, making a will, and saying good-bye).
   3. Anticipation of failure: loss of a job, preoccupation with physical disease, actual or anticipated loss of a significant other.
   4. Change in behavior, presence of panic, agitation, or calmness; usually, as depression lifts, client has enough energy to act on suicidal feelings.
   5. Hopelessness: feelings of impending doom, futility, and entrapment.
   6. Withdrawal and rejection of help.

C. Clients at risk.
1. Adolescents and older adults; males usually complete the suicide act.
2. Recent stress of a maturational or situational crisis.
3. Clients with chronic or painful illnesses.
4. Previous suicide attempts or suicidal behavior.
5. Withdrawn, depressed, or hallucinating clients.
6. Clients with sexual identity conflicts and those who abuse alcohol and drugs.

❖ **Goal:** To provide for basic human needs of safety and protection from self-destruction.

A. Remove all potentially harmful objects (e.g., belts, sharp objects, matches, lighters, strings, etc.).
B. Maintain a one-to-one relationship and close observation.

> ✔ *NURSING PRIORITY: Be aware of special times when client might be suicidal (e.g., when suddenly cheerful, when there is less staff available, upon arising in the morning, or during a busy routine day).*

C. Have client make a written contract stating he or she will not harm himself or herself, and provide an alternative plan of coping.

❖ **Goal:** To provide for physical needs of nutrition and rest/activity.

A. *Assess for changes in weight (weight loss may indicate deepening depression) and report to nursing supervisor or primary care provider (PCP).*
B. Encourage increased bulk and roughage in diet along with sufficient fluids if client is constipated.

> ✔ *NURSING PRIORITY: Depressed clients are particularly vulnerable to constipation as a result of psychomotor retardation.*

C. Provide for adequate amount of exercise and rest; encourage client not to sleep during the day.
D. Assist with hygiene and personal appearance.

❖ **Goal:** To promote expression of feelings.

A. Encourage expression of angry, guilty, or depressed feelings.
B. Convey a kind, pleasant, interested approach to promote a sense of dignity and self-worth in the client.
C. Support the client in the expression of his or her feelings by allowing the client to respond in his or her own time.
D. Seek out client; initiate frequent contact.
E. Assist with decision making when depression is severe.

❖ **Goal:** To provide for meaningful socialization activities.

> ✔ *NURSING PRIORITY: The depressed client often has impaired decision-making/problem-solving ability and needs structure in his or her life. The nurse must devise a plan of therapeutic activities and provide client with a written time schedule. **Remember:** The client who is moderately depressed feels best early in the day, while later in the day is a better time for the severely depressed individual to participate in activities.*

A. Encourage participation in activities (e.g., plan a work assignment with client to do simple tasks: straightening game room, picking up magazines, etc.).
B. Assess hobbies, sports, or activities client enjoys, and encourage participation.
C. Encourage client to participate in small-group conversation or activity; practice social skills through role playing and psychodrama.
D. Encourage activities that promote a sense of accomplishment and enhance self-esteem.

❖ **Goal:** To assist in medical treatment.

A. Administer antidepressant medication (see Appendix 6-3).
B. Assist in electroconvulsive therapy (ECT) (Box 6-8).

SCHIZOPHRENIC DISORDERS

 Schizophrenia

✳ **Schizophrenia is a maladaptive disturbance characterized by a number of common behaviors involving disorders of thought content, mood, feeling, perception, communication, and interpersonal relationships.**

Prepsychotic Personality Characteristics

A. Aloof and indifferent.
B. Social withdrawal; peculiar behavior.
C. Relatives and friends note a change in personality.
D. Unusual perceptual experiences and disturbed communication patterns.
E. Lack of personal grooming.

Psychodynamics of Maladaptive Disturbances

A. Disturbed thought processes.
1. Confused, chaotic, and disorganized thinking.
2. Communicates in symbolic language in which all symbols have special meaning.
3. Belief that thoughts or wishes can control other people (i.e., magical thinking).
4. Retreats to a fantasy world, rejecting the real world of painful experience while responding to reality in a bizarre or autistic manner.
B. Disturbed affect.
1. Difficulty expressing emotions.
2. Absent, flat, blunted, or inappropriate affect.

BOX 6-8	ELECTROCONVULSIVE THERAPY (ECT)

ECT is an electric shock delivered to the brain through electrodes that are applied to both temples. The shock artificially induces a grand mal seizure.

Indications

1. Severely depressed clients who do not respond to medication.
2. High risk for suicide/starvation.
3. Overwhelming depression with delusions or hallucinations.
4. Number of treatments: usually given in a series that varies according to the client's presenting problem and response to therapy; 2 to 3 treatments per week for a period of 2 to 6 weeks.

Nursing Intervention

- *To prepare client for ECT.*
1. Assess client's record for routine pretreatment checklist for information.
2. Teach client about procedure: what to expect before, during, and after.
3. NPO status for 6 hours before treatment.
4. Remove dentures.
5. Administer pretreatment medication.

- *To provide support and care immediately after treatment.*
1. Provide orientation to time.
2. Temporary memory loss is usually confusing; explain that this is a common occurrence.
3. Assess vital signs for 30 minutes to 1 hour after treatment.
4. Deemphasize preoccupation with ECT; promote involvement in regularly scheduled activities.

- *Long-term goal: To promote and develop a positive self-concept and realistic perception of self.*
1. Encourage problem solving in social relationships; identify problem areas in relationships with others.
2. Acknowledge and encourage statements that reflect positive attributes and/or skills.
3. Reinforce new, alternative coping methods, especially if client uses a new method to handle sad situations and painful feelings.

3. Inappropriate affect makes it difficult to form close relationships.

C. Disturbance in psychomotor behavior.
   1. Display of disorganized, purposeless activity.
   2. Behavior may be uninhibited and bizarre; abnormal posturing (agitated or retardation catatonia); waxy flexibility.
   3. Often appears aloof, disinterested, apathetic, and lacking motivation.

D. Disturbance in perception (Box 6-9).
   1. Hallucinations and delusions; auditory forms are most common.

2. Abnormal bodily sensations and hypersensitivity to sound, sight, and smell.

E. Disturbance in interpersonal relationships.
   1. Establishment of interpersonal relationships is difficult because of inability to communicate clearly and react appropriately.
   2. Difficulty relating to others.
      a. Unable to form close relationships.
      b. Has difficulty trusting others and experiences ambivalence, fear, and dependency.
      c. "Need-fear dilemma": withdraws to protect self from further hurt and consequently experiences lack of warmth, trust, and intimacy.
      d. "As if" phenomenon: feels rejected by others, which leads to increased isolation, perpetuating further feelings of rejection.

Data Collection

A. Four "A's": Eugene Bleuler's classic symptoms.
   1. *Associative looseness:* lack of logical thought progression, resulting in disorganized and chaotic thinking.
   2. *Affect:* Emotion or feeling tone is one of indifference or is flat, blunted, exaggerated, or socially inappropriate.
   3. *Ambivalence:* conflicting, strong feelings (e.g., love and hate) that neutralize each other, leading to psychic immobilization and difficulty in expressing other emotions.
   4. *Autism:* extreme retreat from reality characterized by fantasies, preoccupation with daydreams, and psychotic thought processes of delusion and hallucination.

B. Other characteristics.
   1. Regression: extreme withdrawal and social isolation.
   2. Negativism: doing the opposite of what is asked; typical behavior is to speak to no one and answer no one; used to cover feelings of unworthiness and inadequacy.
   3. Religiosity: excessive religious preoccupation.
   4. Lack of social awareness: crudeness and social insensitivity; neglectful of personal grooming and hygiene.

Nursing Intervention

❖ **Goal:** To build trust.

> **TEST ALERT:** *Building trust is the primary goal for the client with schizophrenia. Maintain a therapeutic milieu; stay with client to promote safety; reducing fear and assisting client to communicate effectively are important nursing care measures.*

BOX 6-9   DISTURBANCES IN PERCEPTION

- Hallucinations: false sensory perception with no basis in reality; can be auditory, olfactory, tactile, visual, and gustatory; auditory most common.
- Delusions: fixed, false beliefs, not corrected by logic; develop as a defense mechanism against intolerable feelings or ideas that cause anxiety.
- Delusions of grandeur: related to feelings of power, fame, splendor, magnificence.
- Delusions of persecution: people are out to harm, injure, or destroy.
- Illusions: misinterpretation of reality (e.g., seeing a mirror image turn into a monster).

 TEST ALERT: Identify behavioral changes associated with mental illness (e.g., hallucinations, delusions).

A. Encourage free expression of feelings (either negative or positive) without fear of rejection, ridicule, or retaliation.
B. Use nonverbal level of communication to demonstrate warmth, concern, and empathy because client often distrusts words.
C. Consistency, reliability, acceptance, and persistence build trust.
D. Allow client to set pace; proceed slowly in planning social contacts.
❖ Goal: To provide a safe and secure environment.
A. Maintain familiar routines. Make sure persons who come in contact with the client are recognizable to the client.
B. Avoid stressful situations or increasing anxiety.
❖ Goal: To clarify and reinforce reality.
A. Involve client in reality-oriented activities.
B. Help client find satisfaction in the external environment and ways of relating to others.
C. Focus on clear communication and the immediate situation.
❖ Goal: To promote and build self-esteem.
A. Encourage simple activities with limited concentration and *no* competition.
B. Provide successful experiences with short-range goals realistic for client's level of functioning.
C. Relieve client of decision-making until he or she is ready.
D. Avoid making demands.
❖ Goal: To encourage independent behavior.
A. Anticipate and accept negativism.
B. Avoid fostering dependency.
C. Encourage client to make his or her own decisions, using positive reinforcement.

❖ Goal: To provide care to meet basic human needs.
A. Determine client's ability to meet responsibilities of daily living.
B. Attend to nutrition, elimination, exercise, hygiene, and signs of physical illness.
❖ Goal: To assist in medical treatment.
A. Administer antipsychotic medications (see Appendix 6-4).
   1. Assist with ECT; may be useful in some instances to modify behavior.
❖ Goal: To deal effectively with withdrawn behavior.
A. Establish a therapeutic one-to-one relationship.
   1. Initiate interaction by seeking out client at every opportunity.
   2. Maintain a nonjudgmental, accepting manner in what is said and done.
   3. Attempt to draw client into a conversation without demanding a response.
B. Promote social skills by helping client feel more secure with other people.
   1. Accept one-sided conversations.
   2. Accept client's negativism without comments.
C. Attend to physical needs of client as necessary.
D. Have client focus on reality.
E. Protect and restrain client from potential destructiveness to self and others.
❖ Goal: To deal effectively with hallucinations.
A. Clarify and reinforce reality.
   1. Help client recognize hallucination as a manifestation of anxiety.
   2. Provide a safe, secure environment.
   3. Avoid denying or arguing with client when he or she is experiencing hallucinations.
   4. Acknowledge client's experience but point out that you do not share the same experience.
   5. Do not give attention to content of hallucinations.
   6. Direct client's attention to real situations, such as singing along with music.
   7. Protect client from injury to self or others when he or she is prompted by "voices" or "visions."

 ## Paranoid Disorders

✲ **Paranoid disorders are maladaptive disorders characterized by delusions, usually persecutory, and extreme suspiciousness.**

Data Collection

A. Extreme suspiciousness and withdrawal from emotional contact with others.
B. Aloof, distant, hypercritical of others.
C. Frequent complaining by letter writing or instigating legal action.
D. Resentment, anger, possible violence.
E. Delusions of grandeur and persecution and hypochondriasis.

F.   Misinterpretation or distortion of reality; may refuse food and medications, insisting that he or she is being poisoned despite evidence to the contrary.

Nursing Intervention

❖   **Goal:** To establish a trusting relationship.

> 💡 **TEST ALERT:** *Use therapeutic interventions to increase client's understanding of behavior. The lack of trust in the paranoid client is often a focus of test questions surrounding the serving of meals or the administration of medications.*

A.   Maintain calm, matter-of-fact attitude.
B.   Keep promises made; be honest.
C.   Avoid whispering or acting secretive.
D.   Allow a choice of activities and foods; involve client in treatment plan.

❖   **Goal:** To increase self-esteem by providing successful experiences.
A.   Allow client to set pace in closeness with others.
B.   Avoid involvement in competitive, aggressive activities requiring physical contact (e.g., football, basketball).
C.   Involve client in solitary activities (e.g., drawing, photography, typing) and progress to intellectual activities with others using games (e.g., chess, bridge, Scrabble).
D.   Reward completion of meaningful tasks.
❖   **Goal:** To deal effectively with delusions.
A.   Clarify and focus on reality; use reality testing.
B.   Avoid confirming or approving false beliefs.
C.   Point out that client's beliefs are not shared.
D.   Divert attention from delusions to reality; focus on here and now.

Study Questions: Psychiatric Nursing Concepts and Care

1. The nurse is admitting an older adult client to an extended care facility. The client is confused, very poorly nourished, and has contusions with bruises and welts over the trunk. What would be the most important nursing intervention at this time?
   1 Perform a physical assessment.
   2 Notify the nursing supervisor or PCP regarding client's condition.
   3 Establish communication and rapport with the client.
   4 Notify authorities regarding suspected elderly abuse.

2. The nurse is caring for a client who is confused. What would be a priority of care for this client?
   1 Frequent orientation to person, place, and time.
   2 Offering client frequent meals that are easy to eat.
   3 Assisting the client to select comfortable clothing,
   4 Arranging for a pastor from client's church to visit.

3. A client who does not speak any English is admitted to the unit. What would be the best approach for the nurse to determine the client's immediate needs and collect assessment data?
   1 Contact the nursing office and determine if there is a translator available.
   2 Ask a family member to translate the necessary questions and answers.
   3 Use pictures and pantomime to try to communicate and determine client needs.
   4 Perform the physical assessment and respect the client's privacy.

4. A nurse whose family has a history of drug abuse makes derogatory comments while caring for a substance abuse client. What might be an explanation for the nurse's behavior? The nurse:
   1 Has an issue with denial and repression.
   2 Is unaware of her feelings when working with this type of client.
   3 Is experiencing a need to act out her feelings.
   4 Feels this type of client is insensitive and should be dealt with honestly.

5. A client is suspicious about her surroundings and is paranoid toward the nursing staff. What therapeutic approach should be avoided?
   1 Maintain silence and do not attempt to explain circumstances.
   2 Make sure you have the client's attention and maintain direct eye contact.
   3 Accept the need for the client to be suspicious, and be direct and honest in responses.
   4 Sit with the client and console through touch and being very open and friendly.

6. A client is observed by the nurse opening and closing his fist, and mumbling angrily while walking back and forth in his room. The nurse should:
   1 Attempt to determine source of anxiety.
   2 Give PRN **Ativan** for anxiety.
   3 Call for help to restrain the client.
   4 Leave the client alone.

7. The nurse notes that a client is quite suspicious during an assessment interview and believes that her family is under investigation by the CIA. What would be appropriate nursing intervention with this client? (Select all that apply.)
   1 Use active listening skills to seek information from the client.
   2 Encourage the client to describe the problem as how they see it.
   3 Ask the client to tell you what exactly they think is happening.
   4 Tell the client that they are delusional and you can help them.
   5 Explain to the client that most people are not investigated by the CIA or FBI.
   6 Reassure the client that you are not with the CIA.

8. The nurse is concerned a client is becoming depressed. What nursing observations would support the development of depression?
   1 Insomnia, loss of libido, restlessness.
   2 Anorexia, psychomotor retardation, poor grooming.
   3 Hypervigilance, overeating, poor grooming.
   4 Flight of ideas, weight loss, lack of interest.

9. The nurse on a long-term care unit is planning assignments for the day. What will be important for the nurse to consider in assigning staff to care for a client who is dying?
   1 Change the staff assigned to care for the client daily.
   2 Assign the temporary and part-time staff to this client.
   3 Whenever possible, assign the same staff to care for the client.
   4 To prevent staff depression, rotate staff every other day.

10. What would be important for the nurse to assess for in caring for a client who is schizophrenic?
    1 Delusions and hallucinations.
    2 Depression and delusions.
    3 Self-care deficits and memory loss.
    4 Bradycardia and flat affect.

11. A client is on antipsychotic drug therapy. The client has developed Parkinson-like symptoms. What is the nursing interpretation of this observation?
    1 This is an allergic response to the drug.
    2 The client is demonstrating the therapeutic response to the drug.

3   Observations are classified as extrapyramidal side effects.

4   Symptoms are cholingeric side effects.

12.   A male client is experiencing auditory hallucinations. What would the nurse be most concerned about?
1   Feelings of depression when the voices stop.
2   How the voices are telling him to hurt someone.
3   Feelings of happiness to hear the voices.
4   How the voices sound like a woman's voice.

13.   The family is present as their mother is dying. The family needs assistance as the mother's death becomes imminent. How can the nurse best assist the family to begin preparatory grieving?
1   Assuring them that their mother will suffer no intense pain.
2   Advising the family about ways they can manage after their mother dies.
3   Supporting them while they share feelings about their mother's impending death.
4   Sympathizing with them as they talk about the meaning of their mother's imminent death.

14.   The family of a client with Alzheimer's disease asks the nurse about caring for the client. What advice would the nurse give to the family?

1   Identify ways they can limit the client's behavior.
2   Identify stimuli that may cause recurring episodes.
3   Prioritize client care and family and client needs.
4   Place locks on all rooms to maintain client safety.

15.   Familiar environment and routine for an older adult client fulfills which of Maslow's hierarchy of needs?
1   Self-actualization.
2   Biological integrity.
3   Spirituality.
4   Safety and security.

16.   A child is brought into the emergency department with bruises and raised welts on the child's back. The nurse suspects child abuse. What would be the appropriate action?
1   Demand an explanation from the parents.
2   Observe the child's response to family members.
3   Call the police.
4   Call the emergency room (ER) nursing supervisor for follow-up reporting.

Answers and rationales to these questions are in the section at the end of the book titled Chapter Study Questions: Answers and Rationales.

Appendix 6-1   ALZHEIMER'S MEDICATIONS

GENERAL NURSING IMPLICATIONS

Two types: (1) *cholinesterase inhibitors*, which prevent the breakdown of acetylcholine, thus making it available at the cholinergic synapses and resulting in enhanced transmission of nerve impulses and (2) a new drug—an *NMDA receptor antagonist*—which blocks calcium influx and modulates the effects of glutamate (major excitatory transmitter in CNS).

Drugs do not cure and do not stop disease progression, but they may slow down the progression by a few months.

MEDICATIONS	SIDE EFFECTS	NURSING IMPLICATIONS
Cholinesterase Inhibitors Donepezil (**Aricept**): PO Galantamine (**Razadyne**): PO Rivastigmine (**Exelon**): PO Tacrine (**Cognex**): PO	GI symptoms: nausea, vomiting, dyspepsia, diarrhea Dizziness and headache Tacrine: high risk for liver damage	1. Abrupt withdrawal of medication can lead to a rapid progression of symptoms. 2. Monitor for side effects since drug is typically given in high doses to produce the greatest benefit.
NMDA Receptor Antagonist Memantine (**Namenda**): PO	Dizziness, headache, confusion, constipation	1. Used for moderate to severe cases. 2. Better tolerated than cholinesterase inhibitors.

Appendix 6-2 ANTIANXIETY AGENTS

GENERAL NURSING IMPLICATIONS

- Withhold or omit one or more doses if excessive drowsiness occurs.
- Assess for symptoms associated with a withdrawal syndrome in hospitalized clients: anxiety, insomnia, vomiting, tremors, palpitations, confusion, and hallucinations.
- When discontinuing, the drug dosage should be gradually decreased over a period of days, depending on the dose and length of time the client has been taking the medication.
- Schedule IV drug requires documentation.
- Promote safety with the use of side rails and assistance with ambulation as necessary.
- Teach client and family not to drink alcohol while taking an antianxiety agent and not to stop taking the medication abruptly.

MEDICATIONS	SIDE EFFECTS	NURSING IMPLICATIONS
BENZODIAZEPINES: Reduce anxiety by enhancing the action of the inhibitory neurotransmitter GABA on its receptor; also promote anticonvulsant activity and skeletal muscle relaxation.		
Chlordiazepoxide (**Librium**): PO, IM, IV Diazepam (**Valium**): PO, IM, IV Clonazepam (**Klonopin**): PO Chlorazepate dipotassium (**Tranxene**): PO Midazolam (**Versed**): IM, IV	CNS depression, drowsiness (decreases with use), ataxia, dizziness, headaches, dry mouth. *Adverse effects:* tolerance commonly develops, physical dependency.	1. May cause paradoxical effects and should not be taken by mothers who are breastfeeding. 2. Assess for symptoms of leukopenia, such as sore throat, fever, and weakness. 3. Encourage client to rise slowly from a supine position and to dangle feet before standing. 4. Versed is commonly used for induction of anesthesia and sedation before diagnostic tests and endoscopic exams. 5. Flumazenil (**Romazicon**) is approved for the treatment of benzodiazepine overdose; has an adverse effect of precipitating convulsions, especially in clients with a history of epilepsy. 6. *Uses:* anxiety and tension, muscle spasm, preoperative medication, acute alcohol withdrawal, and to induce sleep.
NONBENZODIAZEPINE AGENTS: Interact with serotonin and dopamine receptors in the brain to decrease anxiety; lack muscle-relaxant and anticonvulsant effects; do not cause sedation or physical or psychologic dependence; do not increase CNS depression caused by alcohol or other drugs.		
Buspirone (**BuSpar**): PO	Dizziness, drowsiness, headache, nausea, fatigue, insomnia.	1. Not a controlled substance. 2. Some improvement can be noted in 7-10 days; however, usually takes 3-4 weeks to achieve effectiveness. 3. *Uses:* short-term relief of anxiety and anxiety disorders.

CNS, Central nervous system; *GABA,* gamma-aminobutyric acid; *IM,* intramuscularly; *IV,* intravenously; *PO,* by mouth (orally).

Appendix 6-3   ANTIMANIC MEDICATIONS

MEDICATIONS	SIDE EFFECTS	NURSING IMPLICATIONS

LITHIUM CARBONATE: Acts to lower concentrations of norepinephrine and serotonin by inhibiting their release; believed to alter sodium transport in both nerve and muscle cells. *Uses:* bipolar affective disorder (manic episode).

Lithium (**Eskalith, Lithane**): PO	*High incidence:* increased thirst, increased urination (polyuria).
	Frequent: 1.5 mEq/L levels or less: Dry mouth, lethargy, fatigue, muscle weakness, headache, GI disturbances, fine hand tremors.
	Adverse effects: 1.5-2.0 mEq/L may produce vomiting, diarrhea, drowsiness, incoordination, coarse hand tremors, muscle twitching.
	2.0-2.5 mEq/L may result in ataxia, slurred speech, confusion, clonic movements, high output of dilute urine, blurred vision, hypotension.
	Acute toxicity: seizures, oliguria, coma, peripheral vascular collapse, death.
		1. Monitor lithium blood levels: blood samples are obtained 12 hours after dose was given.
		2. Teach client the following:
		  a. Symptoms of lithium toxicity.
		  b. Importance of frequent blood tests (every 2-3 days) to check lithium levels at the beginning of treatment (maintenance blood levels done every 1-3 months).
		  c. Importance of dietary intake and taking dose at same time each day, preferably with meals or milk.
		3. Encourage a diet containing normal amounts of salt and a fluid intake of 3 L per day; avoid caffeine because of its diuretic effect.
		4. Report polyuria, prolonged vomiting, diarrhea, or fever to physician (may need to temporarily reduce dosage or discontinue use).
		5. Do not crush, chew, or break the extended-release or film-coated tablets.
		6. Assess clients at high risk for developing toxicity: postoperative, dehydrated, hyperthyroid, those with renal disease, or those taking diuretics.
		7. Blood levels:
		  a. Extremely narrow therapeutic range: 0.5-1.5 mEq/L.
		  b. Toxic serum lithium level is greater than 2 mEq/L.
		8. Management of lithium toxicity: possible hemodialysis.
		9. Long-term use may cause goiter; may be associated with hypothyroidism.

OTHER AGENTS: Both medications listed below were originally developed and used for seizure disorders. Both have mood-stabilizing abilities.

Carbamazepine (**Tegretol**): PO	Drowsiness, dizziness, visual problems (spots before eyes, difficulty focusing, blurred vision), dry mouth. *Toxic reactions:* blood dyscrasias.	1. Used primarily for clients who have not responded to lithium or who cannot tolerate the side effects. 2. Avoid tasks that require alertness and motor skills until response to drug is established. 3. **Tegretol:** monitor CBC frequently during initiation of therapy and at monthly intervals thereafter.
Valproic acid (**Depakene; Depakote**): PO	Nausea, GI upsets, drowsiness, may cause hepatotoxicity.	1. **Depakene; Depakote:** monitor liver function studies.

CBC, Complete blood count; *GI,* gastrointestinal; *PO,* by mouth (orally).

| **Appendix 6-4** | ANTIDEPRESSANT MEDICATIONS | |

GENERAL NURSING IMPLICATIONS

- SSRIs are the drugs of choice for depression.
- Because of the potential interactions with other drugs and certain foods, MAOIs are used as second-line drugs for the treatment of depression.
- Therapeutic effect has a delayed onset of 7-21 days; however, SSRIs may take as long as 6 weeks to become effective.
- Can potentially produce cardiotoxicity, sedation, seizures, and anticholinergic effects and may induce mania in clients with bipolar disorder (SSRIs are less likely to cause these problems).
- Drugs are usually discontinued before surgery (10 days for MAOIs; 2-3 days for TCAs) because of adverse interactions with anesthetic agents.

MEDICATIONS	SIDE EFFECTS	NURSING IMPLICATIONS
TRICYCLIC ANTIDEPRESSANTS: Prevent the reuptake of norepinephrine or serotonin, which results in increased concentrations of these neurotransmitters.		
Imipramine hydrochloride (**Tofranil**): PO, IM Nortriptyline hydrochloride (**Aventyl**): PO Doxepin hydrochloride (**Sinequan**): PO Amitriptyline hydrochloride (**Elavil**): PO, IM	Drowsiness, dry mouth, blurred vision, constipation, weight gain, and orthostatic hypotension. *Adverse reactions:* cardiac dysrhythmias, nystagmus, tremor, hypotension, restlessness.	1. Should not be given at the same time as an MAOI; a time lag of 14 days is necessary when changing from one drug group to the other. 2. Because of marked sedation, client should avoid activities requiring mental alertness (driving or operating machinery). 3. Instruct client to move gradually from lying to sitting and standing positions to prevent postural hypotension. 4. **Sinequan** is tolerated better by older adults; has less effect on cardiac status; dilute the concentrate with orange juice. 5. Contraindicated in clients with epilepsy, glaucoma, and cardiovascular disease. 6. Usually given once daily at bedtime. 7. *Uses:* depression; **Tofranil** is also used to treat enuresis in children.
SELECTIVE SEROTONIN REUPTAKE INHIBITORS (SSRI): Cause selective inhibition of serotonin uptake and produce CNS excitation rather than sedation; have no effect on dopamine or norepinephrine.		
Fluoxetine (**Prozac**): PO Sertraline (**Zoloft**): PO Paroxetine (**Paxil**): PO	Nausea, headache, anxiety, nervousness, insomnia, weight gain, skin rash, sexual dysfunction.	1. Give medication in the morning. 2. *Uses:* depression, obsessive-compulsive disorder, bulimia, appetite suppression in obese clients.
MONOAMINE OXIDASE INHIBITORS (MAOI): Inhibit the enzyme monoamine oxidase, which breaks down norepinephrine and serotonin, increasing the concentration of these neurotransmitters.		
Isocarboxazid (**Marplan**): PO Phenelzine sulfate (**Nardil**): PO Tranylcypromine (**Parnate**): PO	Drowsiness, insomnia, dry mouth, urinary retention, hypotension. *Adverse reactions:* tachycardia, tachypnea, agitation, tremors, seizures, heart block, hypotension.	1. Potentiate many drug actions: narcotics, barbiturates, sedatives, and atropine-like medications. 2. Have a long duration of action; therefore 2-3 weeks must go by before another drug is administered while a client is an taking MAOI. 3. Interact with specific foods and drugs (ones containing tyramine or ympathomimetic drugs). May cause a severe hypertensive crisis characterized by marked elevation of blood pressure, increased temperature, tremors, and tachycardia. Foods and

Continued

drugs to avoid: coffee, tea, cola beverages, aged cheeses, beer and wine, pickled foods, avocados, and figs and many over-the-counter cold preparations, hay fever medications, and nasal decongestants.

4. Monitor for bladder distention by checking urinary output.

5. **Parnate:** most likely to cause hypertensive crisis; onset of action is more rapid.

6. *Uses:* primarily psychotic depression and depressive episode of bipolar affective disorder.

MISCELLANEOUS ANTIDEPRESSANTS

Trazodone (**Desyrel**): PO	Sedation, orthostatic hypotension, nausea, vomiting, can cause priapism (prolonged, painful erection of the penis).	See General Nursing Implications.
Bupropion (**Wellbutrin**): PO	Weight loss, dry mouth, dizziness.	See General Nursing Implications.

CNS, Central nervous system; *IM*, intramuscularly; *MAOIs*, monoamine oxidase inhibitors; *PO*, by mouth (orally); *SSRIs*, selective serotonin reuptake inhibitors; *TCAs*, tricyclic antidepressants.

Appendix 6-5   ANTIPSYCHOTIC (NEUROLEPTIC) MEDICATIONS

GENERAL NURSING IMPLICATIONS
- Use cautiously in older adults.
- Should make the client feel better and experience fewer psychotic episodes.
- Maintain a regular schedule; usually take daily dose 1-2 hours before bedtime.
- Explain to client and family the importance of compliance with medication regimen.
- Medications are not addictive.
- Discuss side effects and importance of notifying PCP if client experiences undesired or side effects.
- When mixing for parenteral use, do not mix with other drugs.
- Inject deep IM; client should stay in reclined position 30 - 60 minutes after dose administration.

MEDICATIONS	SIDE EFFECTS	NURSING IMPLICATIONS
PHENOTHIAZINES: Block dopamine receptors and also thought to depress various portions of the reticular activating system; have peripherally exerting anticholinergic properties (atropine-like symptoms: dryness of mouth, stuffy nose, constipation, blurring of vision).		
Aliphatic types: Chlorpromazine hydrochloride (**Thorazine**): PO, IM, IV suppository Promazine hydrochloride (**Sparine**): PO, IM, IV *Piperazine types:* Prochlorperazine (**Compazine**): PO, IM, IV, suppository Fluphenazine hydrochloride (**Prolixin**): PO, IM Trifluoperazine (**Stelazine**): PO, IM *Piperidine types:* Thioridazine (**Mellaril**): PO Mesoridazine besylate (**Serentil**): PO, IM	**Extrapyramidal effects (movement disorder):** occur early in therapy and are usually managed with other drugs *Acute dystonia*—spasm of muscles of tongue, face, neck, or back; oculogyric crisis (upward deviation of the eyes); opisthotonus. *Parkinsonism*—muscle tremors, rigidity, spasms, shuffling gait, stooped posture, cogwheel rigidity. *Akathisia*—motor restlessness, pacing. **Tardive dyskinesia:** occurs late in therapy; symptoms are often irreversible—earliest symptom is slow, wormlike movements of the tongue; later symptoms include fine twisting, writhing movements of the tongue and face, grimacing; lip smacking; involuntary movements of the limbs, toes, fingers, and trunk. **Neuroleptic malignant syndrome:** rare problem, fever (greater than 41° C, 105° F), "leadpipe" muscle rigidity, agitation, confusion, delirium, respiratory and acute renal failure. *Endocrine*—amenorrhea, increased libido in women, decreased libido in men, delayed ejaculation, increased appetite, weight gain, hypoglycemia, and edema. *Dermatologic*—photosensitivity. *Hypersensitivity reaction*—jaundice, agranulocytosis.	1. Check blood pressure before administration; to avoid postural hypotension, encourage client to rise slowly from sitting or lying position. 2. Be aware of the antiemetic effect of the phenothiazines; may mask other pathology such as drug overdose, brain lesions, or intestinal obstruction. 3. Client teaching: protect skin from sunlight—wear long-sleeved shirts, hats, and sunscreen lotion when out in the sunlight. 4. Explain importance of reporting any signs of sore throat, fever, or symptoms of infection. 5. Encourage periodic liver function studies to be done. 6. Teach that drug may turn urine pink or reddish brown. 7. Extrapyramidal symptoms treated with anticholinergics, (e.g., **Cogentin**). 8. Long-term use of phenothiazines requires assessment of involuntary movement (AIMS testing). 9. *Uses:* severe psychoses, schizophrenia, manic phase of bipolar affective disorder, personality disorders, and severe agitation and anxiety.
OTHER ANTIPSYCHOTIC DRUGS		
Haloperidol (**Haldol**): PO, IM	Significant extrapyramidal effects; low incidence of sedation, orthostatic hypotension; does not elicit photosensitivity reaction.	1. May reduce prothrombin time. 2. Often used as the initial drug for treatment of psychotic disorders.
Risperidone (**Risperdal**): PO	Anxiety, somnolence, extrapyramidal symptoms, dizziness, constipation, GI upset, rhinitis.	1. *Uses:* tics, vocal disturbances, and psychotic schizophrenia. 2. **Risperdal** is the most frequently prescribed antipsychotic because of less serious side effects.
Clozapine (**Clozaril**): PO	Blood dyscrasias (agranulocytosis), sedation, weight gain, orthostatic hypotension, seizures, diabetes.	1. Used with caution in clients with diabetes and those with history of seizures. 2. Treatment is started slowly and gradually increased; it is important that the client not stop taking medication.

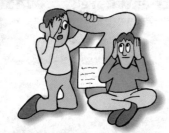

Sensory System

PHYSIOLOGY OF THE EYE

A. Structures of the eye
1. Sclera: tough, protective covering of the outside of the eye; the "white" of the eye.
2. Cornea: transparent tissue that covers the front of the eye over the pupils.
3. Ciliary muscle: muscular body that allows the eye to focus through contraction and relaxation.
4. Iris: controls the amount of light; gives the eye its characteristic color.
5. Retina: thin, innermost lining of the eye that contains millions of nerve cells to coordinate and transmit signals to the optic nerve.
6. Aqueous humor: fluid that fills anterior and posterior chambers; circulates through the pupil and empties into canal of Schlemm.
7. Vitreous humor: fluid that fills the cavity posterior to the lens.
8. Crystalline lens: provides for the convergence and refraction of light rays and images onto the retina; enables vision to be focused.
9. Optic nerve: leaves the eye through the retina at the location of the optic disc.
10. Macula: part of the retina responsible for providing optimal visual focusing.
B. Eyelids: protective coverings of the eye.
1. Conjunctiva: thin, transparent mucous membrane that covers the outer surface of the eye and lines the inner surface of the eyelid.
2. Lacrimal gland: excretes lacrimal fluid (tears) to lubricate, clean, and protect the outer surface of the eye.

Data Collection

A. External data collection.
1. Assess position and alignment of the eyes: Both eyes should fixate on one visual field simultaneously.
2. Evaluate for presence of ptosis (lid lag).
3. Inspect lids and conjunctivae for discharge or inflammation.
4. Assess color of sclera: normally a thin coating; may yellow with aging.
5. Evaluate size and equality of pupils: should be equal in size and shape.
6. Evaluate pupillary reaction to light.
7. Assess extraocular movement: both eyes move together.

B. Evaluate visual health history.
1. Eye pain and headaches.
2. Decreased or blurred vision.
3. Eye infections.
4. Floating or "dots" in field of vision.
5. Chronic illnesses and medications.
6. Surgical procedures.
C. Evaluate visual acuity (see Appendix 7-1).

✔ **OLDER ADULT PRIORITY:** *It is important for older clients to have regular vision checkups and to report any progressive decrease in vision, "floaters" or specks in their visual field or a partial loss of visual field.*

DISORDERS OF THE EYE

 Glaucoma

✳ **Glaucoma is a group of disorders characterized by an increase in intraocular pressure and progressive loss of peripheral vision. It is a chronic condition and a leading cause of blindness.**

Types

A. Primary open-angle glaucoma (POAG): most common form. Flow of aqueous humor is slowed or stopped by obstruction, thus increasing intraocular pressure; characterized by a slow onset; chronic and progressive.
B. Primary angle-closure glaucoma (PACG - acute glaucoma): caused by rapid increase in intraocular pressure. Iris is pushed against drainage system, blocking flow of aqueous humor. Immediate treatment is required.
C. Secondary glaucoma: caused by trauma or optic neoplasm.
D. Treatment can stop progression of condition, but it cannot restore lost peripheral vision.

Data Collection

A. Risk factors.
1. Familial tendency.
2. Aging—occurs most often in clients more than 40 years old.
3. Chronic diseases and eye injury.
B. Diagnostics: increased intraocular pressure (greater than 22 mm Hg) (see Appendix 7-1).

C. Clinical manifestations of primary open-angle glaucoma—develops slowly and frequently without symptoms. (Figure 7-1)
   1. Gradual loss of peripheral vision (i.e., tunnel vision).
   2. Vague headache around lights.
   3. Blindness may eventually occur if untreated.
   4. Central vision is normal, even with loss of peripheral vision.

Treatment

A. Medications (see Appendix 7-2).
   1. Topical drops.
   2. Oral medications to promote diuresis and lower intraocular pressure.
B. Surgical intervention: most often done on outpatient basis with topical anesthetic.
   1. Argon laser trabeculoplasty: microscopic laser to open the fluid channels facilitating outflow of aqueous humor.
   2. Trabeculectomy: creation of an artificial drain to bypass the trabecular meshwork, allowing aqueous humor to flow.

> **TEST ALERT: Assist client to compensate for a sensory impairment (hearing loss or impaired vision).**

Nursing Interventions

❖ **Goal:** To prevent progression of visual impairment.
A. Client must remain on medication in order to control disease.
B. Emphasize the importance of continual follow-up medical care.
C. Stress the importance of wearing a medical alert identification tag.
D. Show client correct administration of eye medication and have client return-demonstrate.
E. Damage to current vision cannot be corrected. Focus of care is to prevent further damage to vision.
❖ **Goal:** To decrease intraocular pressure.
A. Client should avoid straining while defecating, lifting, and stooping.
B. Administer antiemetic, as vomiting causes increased intraocular pressure.
C. Administer medications to decrease intraocular pressure.
❖ **Goal:** To assist client to adapt to visual limitations.
A. Orient clients to objects within visual field.
B. Encourage verbalization regarding fear of blindness and loss of independence.
C. Eliminate potential slip, trip, and fall hazards in the home care environment.

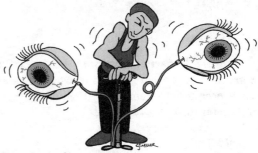

GLAUCOMA
* Increased Intraocular Pressure & Progressive Vision Loss *

Risk Factors - Familial
 - Over Age 40
 - Diabetes, Hypertension
 - History of Ocular Problems

Primary Open-Angle Glaucoma
- Gradual Loss of Peripheral Vision (Tunnel Vision)
- Generally Painless
- Blindness if Untreated
- Decreased Visual Acuity

FIGURE 7-1 Glaucoma (From Zerwekh J, Claborn J, Miller CJ: *Memory Notebook of Nursing,* ed 3, vol 2, Ingram, Texas 2007, Nursing Education Consultants).

❖ **Goal:** To provide preoperative nursing care.
A. Surgery and treatments are frequently done on an outpatient basis and with a local anesthetic. Orient the client to the surroundings and sounds that will occur during the procedure.
B. For outpatient surgery, client should wear comfortable clothes and arrange for someone to provide transportation home.
C. Postoperative instructions should be given to the client or family in writing.
❖ **Goal:** To provide postoperative nursing care (surgery most often done under local anesthesia).
A. Administer medications: miotics, antibiotics, and steroids.
B. Be sure medication is administered in the eye for which it is ordered; the unaffected eye may be treated with a different medication.
C. Client may eat and ambulate as desired after the initial sedative effect is gone.

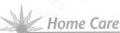 *Home Care*

A. Emphasize the importance of follow-up care.
B. Explain to the client the importance of not rubbing his eyes.
C. Demonstrate how to correctly administer eye medication and have the client return the demonstration.
D. Advise the client to avoid activities that increase intraocular pressure.
E. If pain is not easily relieved by analgesics, the client should call the health care provider.

Cataract

* **A complete or partial opacity of the lens is known as a cataract. It may occur at birth (congenital cataract); however, it occurs most commonly in adults past middle age (senile cataracts).**

Data Collection

A. Clinical manifestations.
   1. Painless with gradual decrease in visual acuity.
   2. Pupil appears gray to milky white.
   3. Decreased perception of colors.
   4. Possible diplopia in affected eye.
B. Diagnostics (see Appendix 7-1).
C. Risk factors.
   1. Age: 70% of adults over age 75 years have cataracts.
   2. Diabetes.
   3. Corticosteroids: long-term systemic use.

Treatment

A. Surgical treatment is the only method of correcting the problem; surgery is usually performed when client begins to experience problems in activities of daily living.
B. Surgical removal of the lens requires lens implant, which usually occurs simultaneously with lens removal.
C. Treatment most often done on outpatient basis.

Nursing Interventions

❖ **Goal:** To provide preoperative nursing care.
A. Orient the client to the surroundings and sounds that will occur during the procedure.
B. Client should wear comfortable clothes and arrange for someone to provide transportation home.
C. Before surgery, the nurse will instill mydriatic eye drops; frequently, cycloplegic drops are also used; client will be photosensitive.
D. Normal for visual acuity to be decreased immediately after surgery.
E. Confirm operative eye according to facility procedure.
F. Client is awake during procedure; frequently a sedative is given preoperatively.

 Home Care (see Box 7-1)

A. Maintain client's orientation to surroundings.
B. Eye patch may be used for about 24 hours or until the client returns to the physician for a follow-up visit.
C. Client should avoid stooping, lifting, or straining in the early postoperative period.
D. Client should avoid sleeping on the affected side.
E. Teach the client to avoid rubbing the eye; there should be minimal discomfort, *report any pain that is not easily relieved by acetaminophen or other analgesic.*
F. Demonstrate to client and/or to family how to administer eye drops (antibiotic and steroid eye drops); have client and/or family demonstrate procedure.
G. *Client should report any signs of increased redness and discharge.*
H. Provide written instructions; make sure the type is large enough for client to read.

Retinal Detachment

* **A separation of the two layers of the retina is called retinal detachment.**

Data Collection

A. Risk factors.
   1. Severe myopia (nearsightedness).
   2. Diabetes.
   3. Trauma.
   4. Degenerative changes in the retina.
   5. Previous cataract surgery.
B. Diagnostics.
   1. Ophthalmoscopic examination.
   2. Evaluation of visual acuity.
C. Clinical manifestations.
   1. Sudden onset.
   2. Flashes of light in visual field.
   3. Sensation of a veil or "cobwebs" over the eye.
   4. Sudden increase in the number of floating spots.
   5. May experience area of blank vision.
   6. Eventually results in loss of vision.

Treatment

There is no medical treatment. The surgical repair may be done on an outpatient basis or may require hospitalization.
A. *Laser photocoagulation:* Laser light beam to create inflammation and sealing of the tear or break.
B. *Cryotherapy:* a "supercooled" probe directed over retinal tear to produce inflammation to seal the tear.
C. *Scleral buckling:* extraocular surgery in which the sclera is depressed from the outside with the application of a silicone "buckle" to weld the retina in contact with the choroid.

BOX 7-1	**OLDER ADULT CARE FOCUS**

Promoting Independent Activities of Daily Living for the Client with Diminished Vision

Medications
- Use containers that have different shapes (square, round, triangular) when client has to take several medications.
- Obtain medication boxes with raised letters or numbers on them representing the days of the week.
- Obtain a "talking clock" that states the time.

Safety
- Remove throw rugs.
- Use unbreakable dishes, cups, and glasses.
- Keep appliance cords short and out of walkways.
- Avoid foot stools, a recliner with a built-in footrest is less of a hazard.
- Cleansers, cleaning fluids, and caustic chemicals should be labeled with large, raised lettering.
- Have hand grips installed in bathrooms.
- Put nonskid stripping on the surface of the tub floor.
- Encourage use of an electric razor.

Communication
- Advise caregivers of client hearing status, encourage everyone who inters the room to always introduce themselves before touching client.
- Teach the client to use telephones that have programmable automatic dialing features. Be sure to include emergency phone numbers.
- Recognize that much communication is nonverbal; therefore frequent clarification of meaning may be required.

Daily Living Considerations
- Provide information on Meals on Wheels for delivery of cooked, ready-to-eat meals.
- Encourage use of a microwave for cooking—it is safer than using a standard stove.
- Encourage the use of large-print books, newspapers, and magazines for reading. Also, many publications are available as audiotapes and CDs at local libraries and vision aid services.
- Avoid rearranging furniture and other belongings.

Nursing Interventions

❖ **Goal:** To prevent further deterioration of vision preoperatively.
A. Restrict activity prior to surgery, especially activities that cause rapid eye movements (e.g., reading, sewing, watching television).
B. Assist client to avoid coughing.
❖ **Goal:** To prevent postoperative complications
A. Local anesthesia may be used; client may be discharged within hours or may remain in hospital—depends on the degree of detachment and the type of repair.
B. Prevent nausea and vomiting.
C. Avoid activities that increase intraocular pressure: bending, lifting, sneezing, coughing, vomiting.
D. Postoperative medications usually include antibiotic eye drops, ophthalmic steroid drops, and dilating agents

 Home Care

A. Orient client to surroundings.
B. Postoperative pain may require narcotic analgesic.
C. Client may experience redness and swelling of the lids.
D. Warm or cool compresses may be used to promote comfort.
E. Have significant other or home health providers identify home environment safety hazards.

Age-Related Macular Degeneration (AMD)

✳ **Most common cause of central vision loss in clients over 40 years old; related to retinal aging.**

Data Collection

A. Risk factors
  1. Familial tendency.
  2. Long-term exposure to UV lights and eye irritants.
B. Clinical manifestations.
  1. Blurred, darkened vision.
  2. Presence of scotomas (blind spots in visual field).
  3. Distortion of vision.
  4. Permanent loss of central vision.
  5. Wet exudative—more severe form.
      a. Development of abnormal vessels in or near macula.
      b. New vessels begin to leak and form scar tissue.
      c. Rapid onset.
  6. Dry nonexudative—less severe, more common form.
C. Diagnostics (see Appendix 7-1).

Treatment

Directed toward stopping progression; affected vision cannot be restored.

Nursing Interventions

❖ **Goal:** To promote prevention and/or early identification of problem and care of client with decreased visual acuity.
A. Encourage regular visual checkups.
B. Encourage diet high in leafy green vegetables and vitamins A and E, beta carotene, and zinc.
C. Promote independence in clients with decreased vision (see Box 7-1).

> **TEST ALERT:** *Identify sensory changes that affect the older client, and encourage regular eye examinations to identify early changes. Identify environmental factors that are a safety hazard to visually impaired client.*

Conjunctivitis

* **Inflammation or infection of the conjunctiva.**

Data Collection

A. Clinical manifestations.
   1. Usually both eyes are affected.
   2. Redness, burning, itching.
   3. Purulent discharge (worse in morning).
   4. Sensitivity to bright light.

Treatment

A. Ophthalmic antibiotic eye ointment for bacterial infection.
B. Drops may be used during day with ointments used at bedtime.

Nursing Interventions

❖ Goal: To prevent transmission.
A. Teach client not to rub eyes, encourage frequent hand washing.
B. Cleanse eyelids with warm saline compresses to remove crusts before administering eye medications.
C. Always clean eye from inner canthus downward and outward to prevent contamination of other eye.
D. Treatment with antibiotic eye drops; instill after eye has been cleaned.
E. Teach client to avoid contamination of tip of medication tube.
F. Client should discard all eye medications after condition is resolved.
G. Highly contagious; spreads easily from one eye to the other and by direct contact from person to person.

Eye Trauma

A. *Chemical injury:* Flush chemicals from the eye. At home use copious amounts of cool tap water; in the hospital use normal saline (see Appendix 7-4).
B. *Corneal abrasion:* May be caused from foreign body or trauma. Fluorescein dye will be used to determine the area of injury.
C. *Intraocular foreign body:* Penetrating foreign bodies must be removed by a physician (ophthalmologist) as soon as possible. Do not attempt to remove foreign objects from eye, but protect from movement while seeking emergency care. If a penetrating foreign body is observed, do not attempt to patch the eye; use a shield if possible, but do not apply pressure to eye.
D. *Subconjuntival hemorrhage:* This eye trauma involves blood between the conjunctiva and the sclera. Most often clears without intervention. Precipitating cause needs to be evaluated.

Nursing Interventions

❖ Goal: To prevent further eye damage.
A. Have client "rest" the eyes: provide dimly lit room; use eye patches if necessary.
B. Irrigate eyes with normal saline solution from inner canthus to outer canthus so solution does not flow into unaffected eye.
C. Eye may remain irritated after foreign body is removed; eye patch may be necessary.
D. If penetrating eye injury is present, decrease activities that cause increased ocular pressure.
E. Keep client immobilized until evaluated by an ophthalmologist.
❖ Goal: To care for a client with an enucleation.
A. Immediate: Determine presence of other injuries; monitor for bleeding.
B. Instillation of topical ointments until prosthesis is fitted.
C. A clear "conformer" may be placed in the eye socket to allow the area to heal so a permanent prosthesis can be fitted.
D. Eye prosthesis.
   1. *Insertion:* notched end of prosthesis should be closest to the client's nose; lift upper eyelid (using non-dominant hand) and insert saline solution-rinsed prosthesis into socket area with top edge slipping under upper lid; gently retract lower lid until bottom edge of prosthesis slips behind it.
   2. *Removal:* retract the lower lid and apply slight pressure just below the eye, this should release the suction holding the eye in place; assess the socket for signs of infection.
   3. The prosthesis is usually cleansed with normal saline.

PHYSIOLOGY OF THE EAR

A. External ear.
   1. Auricle or pinna: the cartilage and connective tissue forming the outside of the ear.
   2. External auditory canal: collects transmitted sound waves to the tympanic membrane; outer half of canal secretes cerumen (wax) that provides a protective function.
   3. Tympanic membrane: a tough membrane separating the external ear and middle ear; transmits vibrations from external ear to the malleus of the middle ear.
B. Middle ear.
   1. Contains three small articulating bones: malleus, incus, stapes.
   2. The eustachian tube in infants and young children is shorter and wider than in adults.
   3. Problems in the external and middle ear cause conductive hearing loss.

C. Inner ear.
1. Assists in maintaining equilibrium.
2. Contains organ of Corti, which is the receptive end organ for hearing.
3. Pathology of the inner ear or nerve pathway can result in sensorineural hearing loss.

Data Collection

A. External assessment of the ear.
1. Assess placement of the ears: Low-set ears may be indicative of congenital anomalies.
2. Movement of the ear lobe should not elicit pain.
3. Note presence of any discharge in the external ear canal.
4. Assess for vertigo: Ask client to close eyes and stand on one foot; have client walk with one foot; client may fall to one side or complain of room spinning.

DISORDERS OF THE EAR

Otitis Media

* **Otitis media is an infection of the middle ear caused by a viral or bacterial agent. Infants and young children are predisposed to the development of acute otitis media because of the physiologic characteristics of the ear—the eustachian tube is shorter, wider, and straighter in children than in adults.**

A. Acute otitis media (AOM) may be purulent (pus-filled) or suppurative (capable of producing pus); repeated or persistent acute infections lead to perforation of the tympanic membrane or more severe complications such as mastoiditis.
B. Otitis media with effusion (OME): a collection of fluid in the middle ear without infection or acute symptoms that results from a blocked eustachian tube; may persist for weeks to months; most common cause of conductive hearing loss.

Data Collection

A. Risk factors.
1. Children: 6 months to 2 years old.
2. History of upper respiratory tract infection.
3. Less common in breast-fed infants.
4. Bottle-feeding in supine position.
5. Respiratory tract allergies.
6. Environment with secondhand smoke.
B. Clinical manifestations.
1. Pain from pressure in the middle ear.
   a. Infants: irritable; pull at their ears; sucking aggravates pain.
   b. Young children verbally complain of severe ear pain.
2. Prevalence of fever varies greatly.
3. Nasal congestion.
4. If tympanic membrane ruptures, purulent drainage may be present in the outer ear; pain will decrease temporarily.
5. Hearing loss with recurrent rupture.

Treatment

A. Medications.
1. Antibiotics: health care provider will determine if infection can be treated with antibiotics.
2. Analgesics, antipyretics, decongestants.
3. Ear drops (antibiotic and steroid combination).
4. OME does not require antibiotics.
B. Surgical: myringotomy drainage of the middle ear with insertion of tubes or grommets (or tympanostomy myringotomy) to relieve pressure and promote healing; used for recurrent cases that do not respond to medication; tubes also known as pressure equalizing tubes (PE tubes).

Nursing Interventions

❖   Goal: To enable parents of clients to describe problem, handle medication schedule, and cope with home care.
A. Recurrent infections cause an increased risk of permanent hearing loss.
B. Antibiotics should be given around the clock, and the prescribed amount should be taken, even after all symptoms are relieved
C. Administer acetaminophen or ibuprofen for pain and fever. Aspirin should not be given.
D. Pain-relieving ear drops (Auralgan, Pramotic) should be used only when there is no tympanostomy tube or rupture of the tympanic membrane.

> ✓ **NURSING PRIORITY:** *Teach the parents to administer the full course of antibiotics regardless of the child's improved status.*

E. Decrease risk of recurrence by preventing fluids from pooling in sinuses and upper airways.
1. Hold or elevate child's head while feeding.
2. Do not prop bottle or allow child to fall asleep while taking a bottle.
3. Encourage juice or water before sleeping.
F. Decongestants may be administered to decrease fluid collection, thereby decreasing prevalence of infection and discomfort.
❖   Goal: Care for child after placement of tympanostomy tubes (myringotomy tubes or grommets).
A. Do not allow soapy or dirty water to get into the child's ears; use of earplugs is currently controversial.
B. Assure parents that if the ear grommet or tube falls out, it is not a significant problem.

Hearing Loss

* **Hearing loss results from an impairment of the transmission of sound waves.**

A. Conductive: results from an impairment in transmission of sound from the outer or middle ear or both. Client will be able to benefit from a hearing aid.
B. Sensorineural (perceptive): results from a problem in the inner ear, or a nerve pathway. Incoming sound cannot be analyzed correctly. Client will not benefit from a hearing aid.
C. Otosclerosis: an immobilization of the small bones in the inner ear; it occurs most often in women.
D. Impacted cerumen can lead to hearing loss; occurs often in the older adult client.

Data Collection

A. Risk factors.
  1. Age-related changes; increased incidence in clients over 65.
  2. Prolonged exposure to high-intensity sound waves.
  3. Repeated, chronic ear infections.
  4. Prenatal problems of rubella and eclampsia.
  5. Female with family history of otosclerosis.
  6. Ototoxic medications - aminoglycosides, diuretics.

> **NURSING PRIORITY:** *Earplugs should be worn when the potential for exposure to loud noise exists.*

B. Diagnostics (see Appendix 7-1).
C. Clinical manifestations.
  1. Speech problems: deterioration of present speech, or delayed speech development.
  2. Fails to respond to oral communication or responds inappropriately.
  3. Social withdrawal.
  4. Decreased self-confidence.
  5. Responds more to facial expressions than to verbal ones.
  6. Inappropriate emotional response.

Treatment

A. Hearing aid, if conductive loss.
B. Speech therapy.
C. Sign language.
D. Stapedectomy for otosclerotic lesions.

> **OLDER ADULT PRIORITY:** *Identify hearing loss; assist client to compensate and to maintain communication.*

Nursing Interventions

❖ **Goal:** To promote communication and socialization of the hearing-impaired client (Box 7-2).
A. Provide information concerning a TDD (telephone device for the deaf) that transmits typed words over the phone line.
B. Suggest light-activated devices rather than sound-activated devices: connect doorbell, smoke, and security alarms to an electrical device that causes lights to flicker on and off.
C. Avoid crowded, noisy environments (such as restaurants) especially if a hearing aid is used, because it amplifies background sound.
D. Teach how to care for hearing aid (Box 7-3).

> **TEST ALERT:** *Provide care for a client using assistive devices: hearing loss and use of hearing aids are common in older adult clients.*

E. Teach client how to remove earwax; if impacted cerumen is a problem, may need ear irrigation (see Appendix 7-3).
❖ **Goal:** To prevent complications for the client who undergoes stapedectomy.
A. Assess client for dizziness, nausea, and vomiting.
B. Teach client to avoid sudden movement to prevent dizziness.
C. Maintain safety measures.
D. Instruct client that hearing may not improve until edema subsides in the operative area.

Home Care

A. Avoid washing hair for about a week; after that keep ear dry.
B. Avoid flying and swimming for about a month or until all edema subsides.

Balance Disorders

* **The vestibular system of the inner ear maintains balance and coordination.**

A. Disorders.
  1. *Ménière's disease:* an inner ear disorder caused by excess endolymph in the vestibular and semicircular canals.
  2. *Labyrinthitis:* an inflammation of the inner ear.

Assessment

A. Diagnostics (see Appendix 7-1).
B. Clinical manifestations.
  1. Vertigo: a sense of moving or spinning that is usually stimulated by sudden movement of the head; may occur when lying down.

2. Sudden, severe paroxysmal episodes of vertigo (Ménière's disease).
   a. Severe nausea, vomiting.
   b. Nystagmus.
   c. Loss of balance.
   d. No pain or loss of consciousness.
3. Fluctuating hearing loss and tinnitus (Ménière's disease).
4. Client may have no symptoms between attacks.
5. Manifestations become less severe with time.

Treatment

A. Medications (Ménière's disease).
   1. Atropine may stop an acute attack.
   2. Sedatives.
   3. Antihistamines, anticholinergics.
   4. Diuretics (to decrease endolymph fluid).
   5. Meclizine hydrochloride (**Antivert**) for prevention and treatment of "motion sickness" symptoms.
   6. Antiemetics.
B. Diet: low-sodium

Nursing Interventions

❖ **Goal:** To provide emotional and physical support during an acute attack.
A. Maintain bed rest in a quiet, dimly lit room; avoid flickering lights and television.
B. Position of comfort.
C. Avoid unnecessary nursing procedures.
D. Minimize stimulation and sudden position changes.
E. If client is severely nauseated, administer medications parenterally.
F. Maintain fall precautions.

> ✔ **NURSING PRIORITY:** *As a safety precaution, instruct the client to lie down immediately if an attack feels imminent.*

BOX 7-2   OLDER ADULT CARE FOCUS
Improving Communication with Hearing Impaired Clients

- Standing in front of client at eye level and speaking with light on your face helps with speech reading (i.e., reading lips).
- Get client's attention by raising your hand or arm.
- Do not walk back and forth in front of client while speaking.
- Speak clearly and in an even tone; do not shout.
- Do not chew gum, cover mouth, or smile excessively while talking.
- Because clients rely on visual cues, watch your facial expressions.
- Encourage professional counseling in speech and sign language.
- If the client is agreeable, assist in obtaining a hearing aid.
- Promote social interaction appropriate for elderly adult.
- Do not avoid conversation with the client; do not depend on family to interpret information.
- Investigate use of TDD (telecommunication device for the deaf).
- Use light-activated devices: door bell, smoke alarms, telephones.
- Client should avoid noisy environments where it is difficult to interpret sound.
- Provide client instruction in a quiet room with minimal distractions.

BOX 7-3   OLDER ADULT CARE FOCUS
Hearing Aid Care

- Keep the hearing aid dry; do not wear it while bathing or swimming or allow it to get wet.
- Clean the ear mold of the hearing aid with soft cloth and recommended cleanser; do not immerse in water.
- Avoid using hair spray, cosmetics, or oils around the ear.
- Always keep extra batteries on hand.
- When not using hearing aid, turn it off and remove the battery before storing it.
- Avoid dropping the hearing aid (has delicate electronics) or exposing it to extremes in temperatures (e.g., leaving it on a window ledge in the sunlight).
- Clean any debris or cerumen from the hole in the middle part that goes in the ear by using a toothpick or pipe cleaner.
- If the hearing aid does not work, change the battery or check the on-off switch, check the connection between the ear mold and receiver, clean it using the steps described above, or take it to an authorized hearing aid service center.

Study Questions: Sensory System

1. The nurse is preparing a client for a cataract removal. Mydriatic eye drops are ordered. What observation by the nurse will indicate the medication is having the desired effect?
   1 The client states his vision is blurred.
   2 The pupil on the client's affected eye is dilated.
   3 The client says his eye feels irritated.
   4. The pupil on the client's unaffected eye is pinpoint size.

2. What is important in the plan of care for a client who has glaucoma?
   1 Prevent secondary infection.
   2 Maintain good visual acuity.
   3 Prevent injury to unaffected eye.
   4 Control intraocular pressure.

3. What is a common finding obtained during data collection on a client experiencing a problem with Meniere disease?
   1 Severe vertigo.
   2 Sloshy feeling in ears.
   3 Watery drainage from ears.
   4 Low-grade temperature.

4. What will the nurse identify as the therapeutic response of a miotic eye medication?
   1 Constriction of the pupil.
   2 Decrease in irritation and pain
   3 Increase in visual acuity
   4 Dilation of the pupil.

5. An infant has a history of frequent otitis media. What would be important teaching information to tell the mother?
   1 Avoid the use of decongestants.
   2 Encourage formula before sleeping.
   3 Stop antibiotics as soon as the fever subsides.
   4 Hold the infant and elevate the head while feeding.

6. The nurse is instructing the client on administration of eye drops. What nursing observation would indicate the client understands how to administer the drops?
   1 Positions himself on his left side to administer drops in the left eye.
   2 Instills the drops into the lower conjunctival sac.
   3 Blows his nose before administering drops.
   4 Cleans the tip of the applicator with a tissue before administering drops.

7. What would be important for the nurse to teach the client about chronic primary open angle glaucoma (POAG)?
   1 The lens of the eye becomes cloudy.
   2 There is an increase in pressure inside the eye.
   3 The cornea becomes stretched, causing blurred vision.
   4 The pupil becomes constricted, allowing minimal vision.

8. Considering the risk factors for hearing loss, what factor would the nurse identify as not being an increased risk for hearing loss?
   1 Prenatal problem of rubella.
   2 Repeated, chronic ear infections.
   3 Taking penicillin and cephalosporin medications.
   4 Exposure to high-intensity sound waves.

9. What would be important for the nurse to teach a client regarding the care of the client's hearing aid?
   1 Always keep extra batteries on hand.
   2 Clean ear mold part by soaking it in alcohol.
   3 Always leave hearing aid turned on when out of the ear.
   4 Continue to wear hearing aid even while sleeping.

10. What medications would the nurse identify as being contraindicated for a client with a diagnosis of glaucoma?
    1 Atropine sulfate (**Atropisol**).
    2 Pilocarpine (**Pilocar**).
    3 Meperidine (**Demerol**).
    4 Fentanyl (**Duragesic**).

11. After a client's eye has been anesthetized, what would the nurse instruct the client to do? He should:
    1 Not watch television for at least 1 day to reduce strain.
    2 Not rub the eye for about 30 minutes.
    3 Irrigate the eye every hour until sensation is felt.
    4 Wear an eye patch for 2 days.

12. A client comes to the clinic with decreased hearing. Examination of the ear canal reveals a large amount of earwax. The nurse prepares for removal of the wax by using:
    1 Forceps.
    2 Normal saline irrigation.
    3 D_5W irrigation.
    4 A cotton swab applicator.

13. The nurse is caring for a client who is hearing-impaired. What nursing action would be least effective in promoting communication?
    1 Provide client with a writing pad.
    2 Increase your voice until client can hear.
    3 Use short sentences or phrases with frequent pauses in the conversation.
    4 Stand directly in front of the client to allow them to see your face.

14. A nurse is teaching a family about the use of a hearing aid. The nurse bases her teaching on the knowledge that the hearing aid does which of the following?
    1 Provides mechanical training for the damaged part of the ear.
    2 Amplifies sound but does not improve the ability to hear.
    3 Amplifies sound and improves the ability to hear.
    4 Assists to heal the damaged part of the ear.

Answers and rationales to these questions are in the section at the end of the book titled Chapter Study Questions: Answers and Rationales.

Appendix 7-1   OPHTHALMIC AND HEARING DIAGNOSTICS

OPHTHALMIC DIAGNOSTICS

Snellen chart is used in screening for visual acuity problems. Client is placed 20 feet from the chart, and visual acuity is expressed as a ratio (what the client *should* see at 20 feet compared with what he or she *can* see at 20 feet). A ratio of 20/50 means that the client can see at 20 feet what he or she should see at 50 feet.

Noncontact tonometer is used to measure intraocular pressure. Normal pressure is 12 to 22 mm Hg. A puff of air is directed toward the cornea, which causes indentation and allows measurement of intraocular pressure, a screen tool for diagnosis of glaucoma.

Direct ophthalmoscopy is examination of the back portion of the interior of the eyeball, which provides for visual evaluation of the retina, vascular patterns, and optic disk.

Biomicroscopy (slit-lamp examination) is used to assess the anterior eye for problems of the cornea, iris, and lens and to evaluate the depth of the anterior chamber.

Refractive error evaluation determines what refractive errors have occurred because light is not correctly focused on the retina. Conditions that occur in refractive errors are:

- Myopia (nearsightedness)—sees near objects clearly; has problem seeing distant objects.
- Hyperopia (farsightedness)—sees distant objects clearly; has problem seeing close objects.
- Presbyopia—a decrease in the elasticity of the lens that causes poor accommodation for near vision (common in older adults)
- Astigmatism—an uneven curvature of the cornea; light rays do not focus on the retina at the same time

HEARING DIAGNOSTICS

Audiometry is used to measure a client's hearing by the use of various tones and intensities of sound produced by an audiometer.

Appendix 7-2   OPHTHALMIC MEDICATIONS

General Nursing Implications

- Instruct client or family in proper administration of eye drops or ointment, (i.e., maintain sterile technique and prevent drop per contamination; clearly mark each container to indicate what eye medication is for).
- Expect some blurriness from ointments; apply at bedtime, if possible, to avoid safety problems from diminished vision.
- Instruct client to report changes in vision, blurring, difficulty breathing, or flushing.
- Teach client to gently close eye and allow medication to distribute evenly.
- Only use ophthalmic preparations of medications.

Medications	Side Effects	Nursing Implications
GLAUCOMA MEDICATIONS: Used to reduce production of aqueous humor and increase outflow, thereby decreasing ocular pressure.		
Alpha$_2$ Adrenergic Agonists Brimonidine (**Alphagan**) topical	Dry mouth, ocular hyperemia, local burning and stinging. Systemic absorption: hypotension.	1. Can be absorbed into contact lens, wait 15 minutes after instilling drops to replace contacts.
Beta Blockers Nonselective Beta$_1$ and Beta$_2$ Blockers Timolol maleate (**Timoptic**) Carteolol (**Ocupress**)	Eye irritation, dry eyes Bradycardia, AV block, bronchospasm	1. Assess for cardiac and respiratory changes with systemic absorption. 2. To decrease systemic absorption of ophthalmic topical medications, teach client to apply gentle pressure to the lacrimal duct (tear duct) during and immediately after instillation of drops.
Selective Beta$_1$ Blockers Betaxolol (**Betoptic**)	Bradycardia, AV block	1. Recommended for use in clients with history of chronic pulmonary disease. Assess for systemic absorption.
Prostaglandin Analogs Latanoprost (**Xalatan**) topical Travoprost (**Travatan**) Bimatoprost (**Lumigan**)	Increases pigmentation of eyelid and growth of eyelashes; conjunctiva hyperemia	1. Minimal systemic effects.
Anticholinergics Pilocarpine hydrochloride (**IsoptoCarpine, Pilocar**): 0.25% to 10% solutions, topical	Conjunctive irritation Provocation of asthma Headache, ciliary spasm	1. Contraindicated in clients with inflammatory eye conditions. 2. Miotic; causes constriction of pupil.
CYCLOPLEGIC AND MYDRIATICS: Block response of sphincter muscle of iris; produce dilation of pupil; may cause paralysis of accommodation. Used in eye examination and diagnosis.		
Atropine sulfate (**Atropisol**): 0.25% to 2% solution, topical Cyclopentolate HCl (**Cyclogyl**): 0.5% to 1% solution, topical Tropicamide (**Mydriacyl**)	Blurred vision, photophobia Headache, hyperemia, Systemic effects: flushing, sweating, dry mouth, dizziness	1. Contraindicated in clients with glaucoma. 2. Dark glasses may be worn to decrease discomfort from photophobia. 3. Use only ophthalmic preparations.
OTHER OPHTHALMIC MEDICATIONS:		
Fluorescein sodium (**Fluorocyte, Fluor-L-Strip**)	Stinging, burning sensation	1. Cornea remains uncolored; abrasions and defects turn green.
Antiinfectives Neomycin-Polymyxin (**Neosporin**) Erythromycin (**Ilotycin**) ointment	Drops and ointment may cause burning or irritation	1. Vision may be blurred. 2. Teach correct application of medication.

CNS, Central nervous system; *GI*, gastrointestinal; *IV*, intravenously; *PO*, by mouth (orally).

Appendix 7-3	NURSING PROCEDURE: EAR AND EYE IRRIGATION

EAR IRRIGATIONS

COMMON SOLUTIONS

- Warm tap water or normal saline solution
- Hydrogen peroxide.

✓ KEY POINTS: Irrigation

- Before irrigation, visually inspect the external ear canal with otoscope to ensure that tympanic membrane is intact and that auditory canal is not obstructed by a foreign body. Do not irrigate an ear with otitis media present.
- Temperature of irrigating solution should be near body temperature (37° C, approximately 98° F). If too cold or hot, dizziness and/or nausea may occur.
- Cerumen may be softened by adding a few drops of warm mineral oil or OTC preparation.
- A rubber bulb syringe or a water pressure device may be used.
- Straighten the ear canal by either pulling the outer ear up for adults or down for children under 3 years.
- Direct water flow toward the top of the ear canal to create a circular motion.
- Do not forcefully push fluid into the ear canal, because this may rupture the eardrum. If severe pain, nausea, vomiting, or dizziness develop, stop the irrigation immediately.
- Position client with irrigated ear dependent to facilitate drainage.

EYE IRRIGATIONS

COMMON SOLUTIONS

- Normal saline or eye irrigation solution

✓ KEY POINTS: Eye Irrigation

- Place client in position in which solution does not run into unaffected eye.
- Small amount of fluid: use a cotton ball moistened in solution.
- Moderate amount of fluid: use a plastic squeeze bottle to direct fluid along conjunctiva and over the eyeball from inner to outer canthus.
- Large amount of fluid: bags of intravenous solutions may be used to provide constant stream and adequate flushing of chemical from the eye.
- Do not allow tip of irrigating equipment to touch the eye.
- Immersion technique: place entire face in basin of lukewarm water and have client open and close eyes repeatedly.
- Avoid use of contact lenses for a period of time after eye irritation.

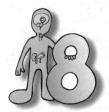

Endocrine System

PHYSIOLOGY OF THE ENDOCRINE SYSTEM

A. Pituitary gland - Often referred to as the "master gland" because it secretes hormones that control hormone secretion of other endocrine glands.

B. Thyroid gland - Primary function of thyroid hormone is to control the level of cellular metabolism by secreting thyroxin (T_4) and triiodothyronine (T_3).

C. Parathyroid gland - Four small parathyroid glands are located near or embedded in the thyroid gland, which secrete parathyroid hormone (PTH) that is primarily involved in the control of serum calcium levels.

D. Pancreas - Produces the enzymes trypsin, amylase, and lipase, which are necessary for the digestion and absorption of nutrients; contains the islets of Langerhans, which contain beta cells that are responsible for the production of insulin. Insulin is necessary for maintaining normal carbohydrate metabolism and glucose utilization.

E. Adrenal glands – Main body is the adrenal cortex that is responsible for the secretion of glucocorticoids, mineralocorticoids, and adrenal sex hormones (androgens and estrogen); adrenal cortical function is essential for life. The adrenal medulla secretes catecholamines, epinephrine, and norepinephrine; under the influence of the sympathetic nervous system.

System Data Collection

A. Pituitary problems.
1. Assess for growth imbalance.
2. Assess for secondary characteristics appropriate for age.
3. Assess for hormonal imbalances throughout the endocrine system organs.

B. Thyroid problems.
1. Assess for changes in weight and appetite: increased or decreased.
2. Assess for intellectual development and mental changes: increased irritability, excitability, nervousness, altered mood and affect, confusion, and coma.
3. Assess for changes in hair and skin, altered general appearance, and sexual dysfunction.

C. Parathyroid problems.
1. History of problems of calcium metabolism and thyroid surgery.

2. Assess for changes in mental or emotional status.
3. Evaluate reflexes and neuromuscular response to stimuli.
4. Evaluate serum calcium levels.

D. Pancreas problems.
1. Evaluate changes in weight, particularly increase in weight in the adult and decrease in weight in the child.
2. Evaluate alterations in fluid balance.
3. Evaluate changes in mental status.
4. Evaluate serum glucose levels.
5. Evaluate pancreatic enzyme studies.
6. Evaluate the abdomen for epigastric pain and abdominal discomfort.

E. Adrenal glands.
1. Adrenal medulla.
   a. Evaluate changes in blood pressure.
   b. Assess for changes in metabolic rate.
2. Adrenal cortex.
   a. Evaluate changes in weight.
   b. Evaluate changes in skin color and texture, and in the presence and distribution of body hair.
   c. Assess cardiovascular system for instability as evidenced by labile blood pressure and cardiac output.
   d. Evaluate GI discomfort.
   e. Assess status of potassium and sodium levels.
   f. Assess for changes in glucose metabolism.
   g. Assess for changes in reproductive system and in sexual activity.
   h. Evaluate changes in muscle mass.

Hyperpituitary: Acromegaly

✳ **Acromegaly is most often the result of a benign slow growing tumor (pituitary adenoma) that secretes growth hormones. It occurs after the closure of epiphyses of the long bones.**

Data Collection

A. Enlargement of the hands and feet and hypertrophy of the skin.

B. Changes in facial features: protruding jaw, slanting forehead, and an increase in the size of the nose.

Treatment

Surgical intervention is primary method of correcting problem; hypophysectomy may be accomplished by the transsphenoidal approach.

Nursing Intervention

❖ **Goal:** To provide supportive preoperative care (see Chapter 3).

❖ **Goal:** To ensure that the client will not experience complications after hypophysectomy.

A. Elevate the head 30 degrees.

B. Discourage coughing, sneezing, or straining at stool to prevent cerebrospinal fluid leak.

C. Assess for symptoms of increasing intracranial pressure (see Chapter 15).

D. Evaluate urine for excessive increase in volume (greater than 200 mL/hr) or specific gravity less than 1.005 (i.e., development of diabetes insipidus).

E. Frequent oral hygiene with nonirritating solutions.

❖ **Goal:** To assist client to reestablish hormone balance after hypophysectomy (adrenal insufficiency and hypothyroidism are most common complications).

A. Administer corticosteroids and ADH-regulating medications (see Appendix 5-7).

 ## Diabetes Insipidus

✳ **Diabetes insipidus (DI) is a problem of the posterior pituitary characterized by a deficiency of ADH (or kidney's inability to respond to ADH). When it occurs, it is most often associated with neurological conditions, surgery, tumors, head injury, or inflammatory problems.**

Data Collection

A. Excretion of excessive amounts urine (greater than 200 mL/hr) (Polyuria).

B. Polydipsia, weakness.

C. Low urine specific gravity (1.001 to 1.005).

D. Severe dehydration (tachycardia, poor skin tugor, dry mucous membranes).

E. Increase in serum sodium level (greater than 147 mEq/L).

Nursing Intervention

❖ **Goal:** To maintain fluid and electrolyte balances (see Chapter 6).

A. Encourage intake of fluids containing electrolytes for clients with DI.

B. Monitor intake and output carefully. Weigh daily.

C. Evaluate urine specific gravity for changes.

D. Assess hydration status.

HYPERTHYROIDISM

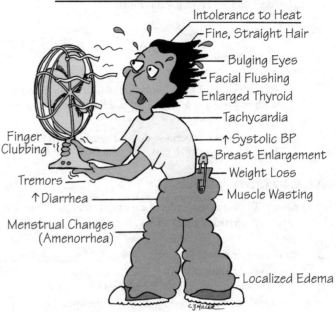

FIGURE 8-1 **Graves' Disease.** (From Zerwekh J, Claborn J, Miller CJ: *Memory notebook of nursing, vol 1,* ed 3, Ingram, 2007, Nursing Education Consultants, Inc.)

 ## Hyperthyroidism

✳ **Hyperthyroidism (also called Graves' disease) or thyrotoxicosis (the signs and symptoms caused by hypermetabolism) is characterized by excessive output of thyroid hormones. (Figure 8-1)**

Data Collection

A. Intolerance to heat.

B. Significant weight loss, despite increased appetite and food intake.

C. Tachycardia, increase in systolic blood pressure.

D. Increased peristalsis, leading to diarrhea.

E. Hand tremors at rest.

F. Visual problems.
   1. Exophthalmos (bulging eyeballs).
   2. Changes in vision, eyelid retraction (lid lag).

G. Changes in menstrual cycle - amenorrhea.

H. Enlarged, palpable thyroid gland.

I. Mood fluctuations.

J. Diagnostics (see Appendix 8-1) - increase in T_3, T_4, and free T_4 serum levels, decrease in TSH, radioactive iodine uptake test (I^{123}) greater than 50%.

Complications

A. Thyroid storm or crisis: may occur after surgery or treatment with radioactive iodine.
   1. Systolic hypertension, tachycardia.
   2. Increased temperature (greater than 102° F).
   3. Increased agitation and anxiety.

B. Calcium deficit may occur as a result of trauma to the parathyroid (see Hypoparathyroid).

Treatment

A. Surgical: thyroidectomy.
B. Medical.
   1. Reduce thyroid tissue: irradiation of thyroid gland with radioactive iodine (I^{131}), eventually resulting in hypothyroid state.
   2. Medications to decrease thyroid synthesis and release (see Appendix 8-2).

Nursing Intervention

❖ Goal: To decrease effects of excess thyroid hormone.
A. Decrease environmental stress (lights, visitors, noise, etc.).
B. Cool environment.
C. Sedatives, if appropriate.
D. Well-balanced meals (high in calories and high in vitamins); small meals served 4 to 6 times per day.

❖ Goal: To protect eyes of client experiencing complications caused by eye changes.
A. Eye drops or ointment.
B. Assess for excess tearing, a sign of dry cornea.
C. Eye patches or mask may be necessary at night.

❖ Goal: To maintain homeostasis in client experiencing thyroid storm (or crisis).
A. Decrease body temperature and heart rate.
   1. Hypothermia blanket.
   2. Acetaminophen to decrease fever.
   3. Propranolol (**Inderal**) and digitalis to treat cardiac issues.
B. Oxygen to meet increased metabolic demands.
C. IV fluids.
D. Antithyroid medications and iodine preparations to decrease T_4 output.

❖ Goal: To provide preoperative nursing measures if surgery is indicated.
A. Demonstrate to client how to provide neck support after surgery.
B. Administer iodine preparations to decrease vascularity of the thyroid gland.

❖ Goal: To maintain homeostasis after thyroidectomy.
A. Maintain semi-Fowler's position to avoid tension on the suture line.
B. Administer analgesics for pain.
C. Administer IV fluids until nausea and swallowing difficulty subside.
D. Check dressings on the side and back of the neck for bleeding and report any bleeding.
E. Apply ice collar to decrease edema.
F. Check calcium levels; parathyroid may have been damaged or accidentally removed.
G. Evaluate temperature elevations; temperature increase may be early indication of thyroid storm.

❖ Goal: To prevent complication of respiratory distress after thyroidectomy.
A. Assess client frequently for noisy breathing and increased restlessness.
B. Evaluate voice changes; increasing hoarseness may be indicative of laryngeal edema. Report any changes immediately.
C. Keep tracheotomy set readily available.

❖ Goal: To decrease radiation exposure in client being treated as an in-patient with radioactive iodine (I^{131}).
A. All body secretions are contaminated because this is a systemic type of radiation.
B. Advise family members to avoid oral contact because saliva is contaminated.
C. For any body fluid spills (urine, vomitus, etc.), contact the radiation safety officer for the facility. Do not clean up the spill.
D. General guideline is to maintain 1 meter (a little more than 3 feet) distance from the client unless direct contact is necessary.
E. Infants and pregnant women should avoid contact with client for approximately 2 days.
F. All health care personnel providing direct care to client should wear a radiation badge.
G. Monitor client for a transient period of several days to weeks when the symptoms of hyperthyroidism may actually worsen after radioactive iodine therapy.

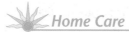 Home Care

A. Thyroid levels checked annually.
B. Lifelong thyroid replacement.
C. If excessive fatigue or tachycardia and tremors become a consistent problem, notify health care provider.

Hypothyroidism

✳ **Hypothyroidism is characterized by a slow deterioration of thyroid function. It occurs primarily in older adults and five times more frequently in women (ages 30 – 60) than in men. Myxedema coma is a life-threatening form of hypothyroidism**

Data Collection

A. Early clinical manifestations.
   1. Extreme fatigue, menstrual disturbances.
   2. Hair loss, brittle nails, and dry skin.
   3. Intolerance to cold, anorexia.
   4. Constipation, apathy.

B. Late clinical manifestations.
1. Subnormal temperature.
2. Cardiac complications (bradycardia, congestive heart failure, hypotension).
3. Weight gain and edema, thickened skin.
4. Change or decrease in level of consciousness.
C. Pediatric implications: cretinism.
1. Identified after birth by mandatory state screening tests.
2. Hypotonia, hyporeflexia, poor feeding.
3. Hypotonic abdominal musculature – constipation, protruding abdomen (umbilical hernia).
D. Diagnostics - decrease in serum T_3 and T_4 levels, increase in TSH level.

Treatment

A. Medical management.
1. Replacement of thyroid hormone.
2. Low-calorie diet to promote weight loss.
3. Decrease in cholesterol intake.
4. Pediatric - If replacement thyroid hormone is accomplished shortly after birth, it is possible that the child will have normal physical growth and intellectual development.

Complications

A. Thyroid hormone replacement will increase the work load of the heart and increase myocardial oxygen requirements.
B. Observe client for development of cardiac failure.

Nursing Intervention

❖ Goal: To assist the client to return to hormone balance.
A. Begin thyroid replacement and evaluate client's response; advise client that it will be about 7 days before he or she begins to feel better.
B. Provide a warm environment.

> ✓ *NURSING PRIORITY: Administer sedatives and hypnotics with caution because of increased susceptibility. These medications tend to precipitate respiratory de-pression in the client with hypothyroidism.*

C. Prevent and/or treat constipation.
D. Assess progress.
1. Decrease in body weight.
2. Intake and output balance.
3. Decrease in visible edema.
4. Energy level and mental alertness should increase in 7 to 14 days and continue to rise until normal.
E. Evaluate cardiovascular response to medication.
❖ Goal: To assist client to understand implications of disease and requirements for health maintenance.
A. Need for lifelong drug therapy.
B. Diabetic client needs to evaluate blood sugar levels

more frequently; thyroid preparations may alter effects of hypoglycemic agents.
C. Continue to reinforce teaching information as client begins to make progress; early in the disease, the client may not comprehend importance of information.

Hyperparathyroidism

✳ **Hyperparathyroidism is characterized by excessive secretion of parathyroid hormone (PTH), resulting in hypercalcemia. Excessive PTH leads to decalcification of the bones, as the calcium moves from the bones into the serum, hypercalcemia results and possible kidney damage.**

Data Collection

A. Bone cysts and pathological fractures.
B. Renal calculi, azotemia.
1. Hypertension caused by renal failure.
2. Repeated urinary tract and renal infections.
C. Central nervous system problems of lethargy, stupor, and psychosis.
D. GI problems.
1. Anorexia, nausea and vomiting.
2. Constipation, development of peptic ulcer.
E. Diagnostics - increased level of serum total calcium; decreased level of serum phosphorous; increased PTH.

Treatment

A. Decrease level of circulating calcium.
B. Parathyroidectomy.

Nursing Intervention

❖ Goal: To decrease the level of serum calcium.
A. High fluid intake to dilute serum calcium and urine calcium levels.
B. Encourage mobility, because immobility increases demineralization of bones.
C. Limit foods high in calcium.
❖ Goal: To assess client's tolerance of and response to increased PTH level.
A. Assess for skeletal involvement – presence of bone pain.
B. Assess for renal involvement.
1. Strain urine for stones.
2. Evaluate for low back pain (renal).
3. Check for hematuria.
4. Assess intake and output carefully.
C. Monitor for cardiac arrhythmias due to increased calcium.
❖ Goal: To provide appropriate preoperative measures if surgery is indicated (see Chapter 3).
❖ Goal: To prevent postoperative complications of parathyroidectomy.
A. Care of client who has undergone parathyroidectomy is same as that for client who has undergone thyroidectomy.

Hypoparathyroidism

* Hypoparathyroidism is characterized by a decrease in the PTH level, resulting in hypocalcemia and elevated serum phosphate levels. Severe hypocalcemia results in tetany.

Data Collection

A. May occur with inadvertent removal of parathyroid gland during thyroidectomy or radical neck dissection.
B. Muscle weakness/spasms.
C. Overt/acute tetany (potentially fatal).
   1. Bronchospasm, laryngospasm.
   2. Seizures, cardiac dysrhythmias.
D. Diagnostics - decreased serum calcium and PTH levels, increased serum phosphate levels.

Treatment

A. Vitamin D to enhance calcium absorption.
B. Increased calcium in the diet.

> 💡 *TEST ALERT: Adjust food and fluid intake to improve fluid and electrolyte balances.*

C. Acute.
   1. Replace calcium through slow IV drip (calcium gluconate, calcium chloride).
   2. Sedatives, anticonvulsants.

Nursing Intervention

❖ **Goal:** To assist client to increase serum calcium levels.
A. Administer calcium preparations.
B. Evaluate increases in serum calcium levels and decreases in serum phosphate levels.
❖ **Goal:** To prevent complications of neuromuscular irritability.
A. Quiet environment.
B. Low lights.
C. Seizure precautions (Appendix 15-5).
❖ **Goal:** To help client avoid complications of respiratory distress.
A. Bronchodilators.
B. Tracheotomy set readily available.
C. Frequent assessment of respiratory status. *Immediately report any significant changes.*

Diabetes Mellitus

* **Diabetes mellitus is a complex, multisystem disease characterized by the absence of or a severe decrease in the secretion or utilization of insulin.**
A. Pathophysiology.
   1. The primary function of insulin is to decrease the blood glucose level.

DIABETES MELLITUS - TYPE 1 SIGNS & SYMPTOMS:

Polyuria
   ↑Urination
Polydipsia
   ↑Thirst
Polyphagia
   ↑Hunger
• Weight Loss
• Fatigue
• ↑Frequency of Infections
• Rapid Onset
• Insulin Dependent
• Familial Tendency
• Peak Incidence From 10 to 15 Years

REST ROOM

FIGURE 8-2 Diabetes, type 1. (From Zerwekh J, Claborn J, Miller CJ: *Memory notebook of nursing, vol 1,* ed 4, Ingram, 2008, Nursing Education Consultants.)

   2. Insulin is secreted by the beta cells in the islets of Langerhans in the pancreas.
   3. Insulin allows the body to use carbohydrates more effectively for conversion of glucose for energy.
   4. If carbohydrates are not available to be used for energy, cells will begin to breakdown the fats and protein stores.
      a. Breakdown of fat results in the production of ketone bodies.
      b. Protein is wasted during insulin deficiency and is broken down.
      c. When fats are used as the primary energy source, the serum lipid level rises and contributes to the accelerated development of atherosclerosis.
   5. When circulating glucose cannot be utilized for energy, the level of serum glucose will increase (hyperglycemia).
B. Classification.
   1. Type 1: absolute deficiency of insulin secretion (Figure 8-2).
      a. Onset is frequently in childhood; most often diagnosed before the age of 18 years. Most common age range is 10 to 15 years.
      b. Previously called juvenile diabetes or insulin-dependent diabetes mellitus.
      c. Client will have Type 1 diabetes for the rest of his or her life.

2. Type 2: combination of insulin resistance and inadequate insulin secretion to compensate (Figure 8-3).
   a. Insulin deficiency caused by defects in insulin production or by excessive demands for insulin; client is not dependent on insulin.
   b. Onset is predominately in adulthood, generally after the age of 40 years, but it may occur at any age.
   c. Previously called adult onset diabetes (AODM) or noninsulin-dependent diabetes mellitus (NIDDM).
   d. Associated with obesity; overweight people require more insulin.
   e. May require insulin for control.
3. Gestational diabetes.
   a. Develops during pregnancy; usually detected at 24-28 weeks gestation by oral glucose tolerance test.
   b. Glucose tolerance usually returns to normal soon after delivery.
   c. Commonly occurs again in future pregnancies; client is at increased risk for development of glucose intolerance and Type 2 diabetes later in life.
   d. Infant may be large for gestational age and may experience hypoglycemia shortly after birth.

Data Collection

A. Clinical manifestations.
   1. Types 1 and 2.
      a. Three P's: polyphagia, polydipsia, polyuria.
      b. Fatigue.
      c. Increased frequency of infections.
   2. Type 1.
      a. Weight loss, excessive thirst.
      b. Bed-wetting, blurred vision
      c. Complaints of abdominal pain.
      d. Onset is rapid, generally over days to weeks.
   3. Type 2. (most clients asymptomatic first 5 to 10 years).

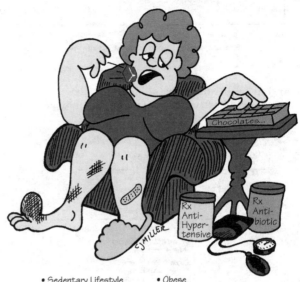

TYPE 2 DIABETES

- Sedentary Lifestyle
- Familial Tendency
- Average Age 50 Years
- Hx of ↑ BP
- Fatigue ↓ Energy
- Obese
- Recurrent Infections
- Polyuria
- Polydipsia
- FBS > 126 mg/dl

FIGURE 8-3 Diabetes, type 2. (From Zerwekh J, Claborn J, Miller CJ: *Memory notebook of nursing, vol 2,* ed 3, Ingram, 2007, Nursing Education Consultants.)

   a. Weight gain (obese), visual disturbances.
   b. Onset is slow; may occur over months.
   c. Onset usually after the age of 40 years; peaks around 45 to 50 years.
   d. Fatigue and malaise.
   e. Recurrent vaginal yeast or monilia infections - frequently initial symptom in women.
   f. Older adult assessment considerations (Box 8-1).
B. Diagnostics (the criteria for diagnosis are two or more abnormal test results with two or more values outside the normal range) (see Appendix 8-1).
   1. Fasting blood glucose level is above 126 mg/dl (normal glucose range 70-100 mg/dl).
   2. Glucose tolerance test: 2-hour glucose values are greater than 200 mg/dl.
   3. Random glucose greater than 200 mg/dl with symptoms (three P's, weight loss).
   4. Prediabetes – intermediate stage between normal and diabetes.
      a. Impaired glucose tolerance (IGT): greater than 140 mg/dl and less than or equal to 200 mg/dl.
      b. Impaired fasting glucose (IFG): fasting blood glucose greater than 100 mg/dl, but less than 126 mg/dl.
   5. Glycosylated hemoglobin (HbA_{1c}) is increased. (Less than 7% is considered good control for diabetic; is not a test to diagnose diabetes).

BOX 8-1	OLDER ADULT CARE FOCUS
	Diabetic Assessment Considerations and Care

- Determine mental status and manual dexterity to handle injections.
- Determine if client can access the injection sites.
- Is client alert and mentally capable of making judgments on medications?
- Determine if the client can pay for supplies.
- What is the client's attitude about needles and injections?
- Assess how many other medications the client is taking; problems with "polypharmacy" (too many medications).
- Determine family's or client's ability to accurately perform serum glucose testing.
- What is the client's support system?

FIGURE 8-4 Profile of Insulins

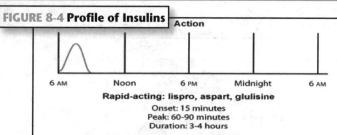

Rapid-acting: lispro, aspart, glulisine
Onset: 15 minutes
Peak: 60-90 minutes
Duration: 3-4 hours

Nursing Implications (rapid acting)
1.   Should be used in combination with longer acting insulin.

✓**NURSING PRIORITY:** *Because of quick onset of action, client must eat immediately.*

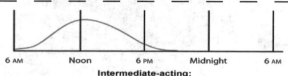

Intermediate-acting: NPH or Lente
Onset: 2-4 hours
Peak: 4-10 hours
Duration: 10-16 hours

Nursing Implications (short acting)
1.   Usually given 20 - 30 minutes before meals.
2.   May be given alone or in combination with longer-acting insulins.
3.   Given for sliding scale coverage.

✓**NURSING PRIORITY:** *When administering injections:*
1. May mix regular insulin with other insulins.
2. Only regular insulin may be given IV.

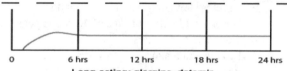

Long-acting: glargine, detemir
Onset: 1-2 hours
Peak: no pronounced peak
Duration: 24+ hours

Nursing Implications (intermediate acting)
1.   Hypoglycemia tends to occur in mid to late afternoon.
2.   Never give IV.
3.   May be mixed with regular insulin.

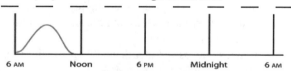

Short-acting: regular
Onset: 1/2-1 hour
Peak: 2-3 hours
Duration: 3-6 hours

Nursing Implications (long acting)
1.   Glargine has low pH (4); **CANNOT** be mixed with other insulins.
2.   Usually given once a day at bedtime, but can be administered during the day.

💡 *TEST ALERT: Intervene to control hypoglycemia/ hyperglycemia. Know various insulins and nursing implications. Specifically, know when to anticipate reaction and what to teach the client about his or her insulin.*

Treatment

A.   Hypoglycemic agents. **High Alert Medications**
1.   Insulin: may be used in both types of diabetes. Primary function of insulin is to transport glucose into muscle and fat cells (Figure 8-4: Profile of Insulins).
     a.   Combination premixed insulin therapy eliminates problem of mixing different types (example: NPH/regular 70/30 – number refers to percentage of each type of insulin).
     b.   Response to insulin mixtures varies with individuals.
2.   Oral hypoglycemic agents for noninsulin-dependent clients (see Appendix 8-2).
B.   Diabetic diet.
1.   Decrease calories for weight loss.
2.   Diet to meet nutritional needs and maintain optimum glucose level. Avoid simple sugars and increase dietary fiber.
3.   Decrease in cholesterol level – reduce saturated and trans fat foods.
4.   Decrease protein for adult due to stress that moderate to high protein places on the kidneys).
C.   Exercise - planned exercise; sporadic exercise is discouraged.

✓*NURSING PRIORITY: Metabolic effects of exercise: 1. Reduces insulin needs by reducing the blood glucose. 2. Contributes to weight loss or maintenance of normal weight. 3. Assists the body to metabolize cholesterol more efficiently. 4. Promotes less extreme fluctuations in blood glucose level. 5. Decreases blood pressure.*

Complications of Insulin Therapy

A.   Hypoglycemia (Table 8-1).
B.   Lipoatrophy (tissue atrophy) and lipohypertrophy (accumulation of extra fat at the site of many subcutaneous injections of insulin).
C.   Somogyi effect.
1.   Rebound hyperglycemia from an unrecognized hypoglycemic state.
2.   Most often occurs at night and treated by decreasing the evening insulin dose or by increasing the calories in the bedtime snack.
D.   Dawn phenomenon
1.   Results from nighttime release of growth hormone and cortisol.
2.   Blood glucose elevates at 5:00 to 6:00 AM (predawn hours).

FIGURE 8-4 Insulin Profiles (Adapted from Lewis S, Heitkemper M, Dirksen S: *Medical-surgical nursing: assessment and management of clinical problems,* "Commercially available insulin preparations showing onset, peak, and duration of action," St Louis, 2007, Mosby).

TABLE 8-1	COMPARISON OF DIABETIC KETOACIDOSIS (DKA) AND HYPOGLYCEMIA	
	DKA	**Hypoglycemia**
Age	All ages, increased incidence in children.	All ages
GI	Abdominal pain, anorexia, nausea, vomiting, diarrhea	Normal; may be hungry
Mental state	Dull, confusion increasing to coma	Difficulty in concentrating, coordinating; eventually coma
Skin temperature	Warm, dry, flushed	Cold, clammy
Pulse	Tachycardia, weak	Tachycardia
Respirations	Initially deep and rapid; lead to Kussmaul respirations	Shallow
Breath odor	Fruity, acetone	Normal
Urine output	Increased	Normal
Lab Values: Serum		
Glucose	Greater than 300 (up to 1500 mg/dL)	Below 70 mg/dL
Ketones	High/large	Normal
pH	Acidotic (less than 7.3)	Normal
Hematocrit	High due to dehydration	Normal
Lab Values: Urine		
Sugar	High	Negative
Ketones	High	Negative
Onset	Rapid (less than 24 hr)	Rapid
Classification of diabetes	Primarily Type 1; Type 2 in severe distress	Type 1 and type 2

DKA, Diabetic ketoacidosis; *GI,* gastrointestinal

3. May be treated by increasing insulin for overnight period.
E.   Insulin requirement increases when:
   1. Serious illnesses, physical trauma, and infections.
   2. Surgical procedures and growth spurts during adolescence.

> ✔ *NURSING PRIORITY: Intensive control of blood glucose levels in clients with type 1 diabetes can prevent or ameliorate the complications. Intervene to control symptoms of hypoglycemia or hyperglycemia.*

Complications Associated with Poorly Controlled Diabetes

A.   Diabetic ketoacidosis.
   1. A severe increase in the hyperglycemic state.
   2. Occurs predominately in type 1 diabetes.
B.   Clinical manifestations of diabetic ketoacidosis (see Table 8-1).
   1. Onset - may be acute or occur over several days.
      a. May result from stress, infection, surgery, or lack of effective insulin control.
      b. Results from poorly controlled diabetes.
   2. Severe hyperglycemia (blood glucose levels of 300-800 mg/dL).
   3. Presence of metabolic acidosis (low pH [6.8-7.3] and serum bicarbonate level less than 15 mEq/L).

4. Hyperkalemia, hypokalemia, or normal potassium level, depending on amount of water loss.
5. Urine ketone and sugar levels are increased.
6. Excessive weakness, increased thirst.
7. Nausea, vomiting, dehydration.
8. Increased temperature caused by dehydration.
9. Fruity (acetone) breath, Kussmaul respirations.
10. Decreased level of consciousness.
C.   Hyperosmolar hyperglycemia syndrome (HHS). Also known as Nonketotic Hyperosmolar Coma and/or Hyperosmolar Hyperglycemic State (see Table 8-1).
   1. Occurs in the adult (older adult) with Type 2 diabetes.
   2. Characterized by extreme hyperglycemia (400-1200 mg/dl) without acidosis.

Complications of Long-Term Diabetes

A.   Angiopathy: premature degenerative changes in the vascular system.
   1. May affect large vessels as in peripheral vascular disease: decreased circulation to lower extremities.
   2. May affect smaller vessels of the kidney, resulting in nephropathy and renal failure.
   3. May affect small vessels of the retina, resulting in blurred vision, retinopathy, cataracts.
   4. Acceleration of atherosclerotic process, resulting in hypertension.

BOX 8-2   IMPLICATIONS IN THE ADMINISTRATION OF INSULIN

1. Do not administer cold insulin; it increases pain and causes irritation at injection site.
2. An open 10-mL vial of unrefrigerated insulin should be discarded after 30 days, regardless of how much was used.
3. Do not allow insulin to freeze and keep it away from heat and sunlight.
4. Insulin pens (NPH and 70/30) should be discarded after 1 week of storage at room temperature. Regular cartridges, which don't contain preservatives, may be left unrefrigerated for up to 1 month.
5. Extreme temperatures (less than 36° F or greater than 86° F) should be avoided.
6. Roll the vial between the palms of the hands to decrease the risk of inconsistent concentration of insulin.
7. The abdomen is the primary site for subcutaneous injections of insulin. Rotate injection sites; injection sites should be 1 inch apart.
8. Abdomen area provides most rapid insulin absorption.
9. Use only insulin syringes to administer insulin.
10. Check expiration date on insulin bottle.
11. When drawing up regular insulin with a long-acting insulin, draw up the regular (clear) insulin before the longer-acting (cloudy) insulin.
12. Regular insulin is used for administration by sliding scale and periods when blood sugar is unstable and difficult to control.
13. Using alcohol to cleanse the skin before injection is not recommended. If used, hold alcohol pad in place for a few seconds but do not massage.
14. Aspirating is not recommended for self-injection.
15. Check dose with another nurse prior to administering.

B. Nerve damage resulting in neuropathy.
1. Peripheral neuropathy: pain and tingling in legs and feet; may progress to painless neuropathy.
2. Very common complication.
C. Infections: Immune system is altered; persistent glycosuria potentiates urinary tract infections.

> ✔ *NURSING PRIORITY: Painless peripheral neuropathy is a very dangerous situation for the diabetic. Severe injury to the lower extremities may occur, and the client will not be aware of it. Clients should be taught to visually inspect their feet and legs.*

Clinical Implications of Diabetes in Pregnancy

A. During the second and third trimester, the *normal* response is for the insulin needs to increase as much as 70% to 100%.
B. Failure of insulin needs to increase may be indicative of placental insufficiency.

C. There is an increased tendency toward the development of metabolic acidosis.
D. There is a tendency to intensify the existing complications of diabetes.
E. Oral hypoglycemic agents are not used to control diabetes in the pregnant client – insulin is used.

Nursing Intervention (All Types)

❖   **Goal:** To return serum glucose to normal level.
A. Initially administer regular insulin on a proportional basis according to need (Box 8-2).
B. Administer insulin 30 minutes before a meal or snack.
C. Maintain adequate fluid intake.
D. Evaluate serum electrolyte levels, especially potassium.
E. Evaluate hydration status.
F. *Evaluate and report clinical manifestations of hypoglycemia and hyperglycemia.*

> *TEST ALERT: Monitor hydration status and electrolyte balance.*

❖   **Goal:** To plan and implement a teaching regimen.
A. Assess current level of knowledge regarding diabetes.
B. Evaluate cultural and socioeconomic parameters.
C. Evaluate client's support system (family, significant others).
D. Instruct regarding sick-day guidelines (Box 8-3).

> *TEST ALERT: Determine ability of family/ support systems to provide care for client. Identify client's and family's strengths.*

E. Administration of insulin (see Box 8-2).
1. Correct injection techniques.
2. Rotate injection site (Figure 8-5).
3. Check expiration date on the insulin.
4. Duration and peak action of prescribed insulin.
5. Allow for ample practice time.
6. Administer at the same time each day.

BOX 8-3   OLDER ADULT CARE FOCUS
Guidelines for Food Selection

- Avoid canned fruits that are in heavy syrup; select fruit packed in water.
- Include fresh fruits and vegetables and whole-grain cereals and breads to provide adequate dietary fiber to prevent constipation.
- Avoid casseroles, fried foods, sauces and gravies, and sweets.
- Fats (oils, margarines) that are liquid at room temperature are better than those that are solid.
- Read food labels: the highest-content ingredient is listed first.
- Select foods in which the majority of calories do not come from a fat source.

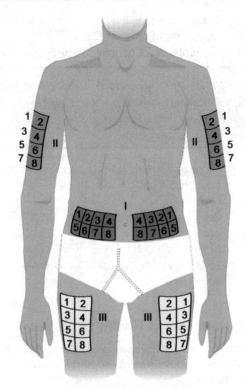

FIGURE 8-5   **Sites Used for Insulin Injection.** The injection site can affect the onset, peak, and duration of action of the insulin. Insulin injected into the abdomen (area I) is absorbed fastest, followed by insulin injected into the arm (area II) and the leg (area III). (From Black J, Hawks, J: *Medical surgical nursing: clinical management for positive outcomes*, ed 8, St Louis, 2009, Mosby.)

7. Clients following an intensive diabetes therapy program may choose to use an insulin pump or to monitor blood glucose levels four to six times a day and take injections at those times.
    a. The insulin pump is battery operated; insertion site is changed every 2 to 3 days; pump is refilled and reprogrammed when site is changed.
    b. Delivers continuous infusion of short-acting insulin over a 24-hour period, allowing for tight glucose control.
    c. Can deliver bolus of insulin based on excessive carbohydrates ingested.
    d. Monitor insertion site for redness and swelling.
8. Insulin pen is a compact portable device that is loaded with insulin; need to change needle with each injection.

F. Oral hypoglycemic agents.
    1. Take medication as scheduled; do not skip or add dose.
    2. Signs and symptoms of hypoglycemia.
    3. Anticipate change in medication with pregnancy.

G. Monitoring blood glucose.
    1. Self-monitoring of blood glucose (SMBG) – not necessary to use alcohol to cleanse site.
    2. Use side of finger pad rather than near the center. If alternative site use (i.e., forearm), may require different equipment.

    3. Need only a large drop of blood.

H. Exercise.
    1. Establish an exercise program.
    2. Avoid sporadic exercise.
    3. Review instructions regarding adjustment of insulin and food intake to meet requirements of increased activity.
    4. Extremities involved in activity should not be used for insulin injection (e.g., arms when playing tennis).

I. Diet (Box 8-4).
    1. Regularly scheduled mealtimes.
    2. Understanding of food groups and balanced nutrition.
    3. Incorporate family tendencies and cultural patterns into prescribed dietary regimen.
    4. Provide client and family with written instructions regarding dietary needs.

J. Infection control.
    1. Report infections promptly.
    2. Insulin requirements may increase with severe infections.
    3. Increased problems with vaginitis, urinary tract infections, and skin irritation.

K. Avoid injury.
    1. Decreased healing capabilities, especially in lower extremities.
    2. Maintain adequate blood supply to extremities; avoid tight-fitting clothing around the legs.
    3. Proper foot care (see Chapter 11).

❖   Goal: To prepare the diabetic client for surgery.
A. Oral hypoglycemic agents should not be given the morning of surgery.
B. For clients with NPO (nothing by mouth) status who require insulin, an IV of 5% dextrose in water (D_5W) is frequently started.
C. Obtain a blood glucose reading about an hour before sending the client to surgery to make sure he or she is not developing hypoglycemia.

> ✓ *NURSING PRIORITY: Evaluate intake; do not give client on NPO status insulin unless IV is in place.*

❖   Goal: To maintain control of diabetic condition in the postoperative client.
A. IV fluids and regular insulin until client is able to take fluids orally.
B. Frequent blood sugar level assessment.
C. Observe for hypoglycemia immediately after surgery.

❖   Goal: To identify diabetic ketoacidosis and assist client to return to homeostasis.
A. Frequent monitoring of vital signs and serum glucose checks (normally hourly).
B. Hourly urine measurements: Do not administer potassium if urine output is low or dropping.

BOX 8-4	DIABETIC "SICK DAY" GUIDELINES

If you do not feel well (not eating regularly, fever, lethargy, nausea and vomiting, etc.):

1. Check your blood glucose every 3 to 4 hours and urine ketones when voiding.
2. Increase your intake of fluids that are high in carbohydrates; every hour, drink fluids that replace electrolytes: fruit drinks, sports drinks, regular soft drinks (not diet beverages).
3. If you cannot eat and you have replaced four to five meals with liquids, notify your health care provider.
4. Get plenty of rest; if possible, have someone stay with you.
5. Do not omit or skip your insulin injections or oral medications unless specifically directed to do so by your health care provider.
6. Follow your health care provider's instructions regarding blood glucose levels and insulin or oral hypoglycemic agents.
7. Stay warm, stay in bed, and do not overexert yourself.
8. Call your health care provider when:
   a. You have been ill for 1 to 2 days without getting any better.
   b. You have been vomiting or had diarrhea for more than 6 hours.
   c. Your urine self-testing shows moderate to large amounts of ketones.
   d. You are taking insulin and your blood glucose level continues to be greater than 240 mg/dl after you have taken two to three supplemental doses of regular insulin (pre-arranged with your provider).
   e. You are taking insulin and your blood glucose level is less than 60 mg/dl.
   f. You have Type 2 diabetes, you are taking oral diabetic medications, and your premeal blood glucose levels are 240 mg/dl or greater for more than 24 hours.
   g. You have signs of severe hyperglycemia (very dry mouth or fruity odor to breath), dehydration, or confusion.
   h. You are sleepier or more tired than normal.
   i. You have stomach or chest pain or any difficulty breathing.
   j. You have any questions or concerns about what you need to do while ill.

Home Care

A. Maintain optimum weight.
B. Continue to receive long-term medical care.
C. Notify all health care providers of diagnosis of diabetes; wear medical alert identification.
D. Recognize problems of the cardiovascular system.
   1. Peripheral vascular disease.
   2. Decreased healing.
   3. Increased risk of stroke.
   4. Increased risk of myocardial infarction.

5. Presence of retinopathy.
6. Increased risk of renal disease.

E. Recognize problems of peripheral neuropathy.

> ✓ *OLDER ADULT PRIORITY: Assess client's ability to take medications correctly and/or client's manual dexterity to handle insulin syringe and visual acuity to measure correct dose.*

❖ **Goal:** To assist the diabetic client to maintain homeostasis throughout pregnancy.

A. Prevent infection.
B. Frequent evaluation of glucose levels and monitoring of changes in insulin requirements.
C. Maintain optimum level of weight gain; labor may be induced or cesarean delivery may be required if complications are evident.

Hypoglycemia (Insulin Reaction)

✳ *Hypoglycemia is a condition characterized by a decreased serum glucose level, which results in decreased cerebral function.*

Data Collection

A. Lability of mood.
B. Emotional changes, confusion.
C. Headache, lightheadedness, seizures, coma.
D. Impaired vision, tachycardia, hypotension.
E. Nervousness, tremors, diaphoresis.
F. Serum glucose below 50 mg/dL.
G. Negative urine acetone test result.

Treatment

A. Carbohydrates by mouth if client is alert and can swallow.
   1. Milk preferred in children with a mild reaction; it provides immediate lactose, as well as protein and fat for prolonged action.
   2. Simple sugars for immediate response: orange juice, honey, candy, glucose tablets.
B. Glucagon can be given intravenously if client is unconscious.

Nursing Intervention

❖ **Goal:** To increase serum glucose level.

A. Administer glucose/carbohydrate preparations as indicated.

> ✓ *NURSING PRIORITY: When in doubt of diagnosis of hypoglycemia versus hyperglycemia, administer carbohydrates; severe hypoglycemia can rapidly result in permanent brain damage.*

B. Thorough assessment of the diabetic client for the development of hypoglycemia.

❖ Goal: To assist client to identify precipitating causes and activities to prevent the development of hypoglycemia.

A. Instruct the diabetic client to carry simple carbohydrates.

B. Administer between-meal snacks at the peak action of insulin.

C. Between-meal snacks should limit simple carbohydrates and increase complex carbohydrates and protein.

D. Client should carry some type of medical alert indentification.

 Pancreatitis

✳ **Pancreatitis is an inflammatory condition of the pancreas that results in autodigestion of the pancreas by its own enzymes.**

Data Collection

A. Severe constant midepigastric pain.
   1. Radiates to the back or flank area.
   2. Exacerbated by eating.
B. Acute.
   1. Persistent vomiting, low-grade fever.
   2. Hypotension and tachycardia.
   3. Jaundice, if common bile duct is obstructed.
   4. Abdominal distention.
C. Chronic.
   1. Decrease in weight, mild jaundice.
   2. Steatorrhea (fatty stools), hyperglycemia.
   3. Abdominal distention and tenderness.
D. Increase in serum amylase and lipase levels.

Treatment

A. Opioid analgesics.
B. Antibiotics, smooth muscle relaxants.
C. Decrease pancreatic stimulus.
   1. NPO status; IV fluids.
   2. Nasogastric suction, bed rest.
   3. Diet: (if not NPO) low-fat, high-carbohydrate.
D. Surgical intervention to eliminate precipitating cause (biliary tract obstruction).

Nursing Intervention

Nursing intervention is the same for the client with acute pancreatitis and for the client with chronic pancreatitis experiencing an acute episode.

❖ Goal: To relieve pain and decrease pancreatic stimulation.

A. Administer analgesics; pain control is essential (restlessness may cause pancreatic stimulation and further secretion of enzymes).

B. Place client on side in knee-chest or in semi-Fowler's position.

C. Evaluate precipitating cause.

D. Maintain NPO status initially.
E. Maintain nasogastric suctioning.
F. Small frequent feedings when food is allowed.

❖ Goal: To prevent complications.

A. Monitor fluid and electrolyte imbalances especially hypocalcemia and hydration.

B. Maintain respiratory status; problems occur because of pain and ascites.

C. Assess for hyperglycemia and development of diabetes.

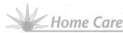 Home Care

A. Avoid all alcohol intake.
B. Know signs of development of diabetes and when to return for evaluation of blood sugar level.
C. Bland diet, low in fat, high in carbohydrates (protein recommendations vary).
D. Replacement of pancreatic enzymes.

 Cancer of the Pancreas

✳ **The majority of tumors occur in the head of the pancreas. As tumors grow, the bile ducts are obstructed, causing jaundice. Tumors in the body of the pancreas frequently do not cause symptoms until growth is advanced. Cancer of the pancreas has a poor prognosis; the 5 year survival rate is low.**

Data Collection

A. Dull, aching abdominal pain.
B. Ascites, nausea, vomiting.
C. Anorexia and progressive weight loss.
D. Jaundice, clay-colored stools.
E. Dark, frothy urine.

Treatment

A. Surgery: Whipple's procedure (radical pancreatic duodenectomy).
B. Radiation therapy.
C. Chemotherapy.

Nursing Intervention

❖ Goal: To maintain homeostasis (see nursing intervention for pancrcatitis).

❖ Goal: To provide preoperative nursing measures if surgery is indicated.

A. Maintain nasogastric suctioning; assess for adequate hydration.

B. Control hyperglycemia.

C. Assess cardiac and respiratory stability.

D. Assess for development of thrombophlebitis.

❖ Goal: To promote comfort, prevent complications, and maintain homeostasis in client who has undergone Whipple's procedure.

A. General postoperative care (see Chapter 3).

B. Evaluate for bleeding tendencies caused by decreased prothrombin activity.

C. Monitor for fluctuation in serum glucose levels.

D. Maintain NPO status and nasogastric suction until peristalsis returns.

E. Encourage adequate nutrition when appropriate.
   1. Decrease fats and increase carbohydrates.
   2. Small, frequent feedings.

Home Care

A. Evaluate for bouts of anxiety and depression caused by severity of illness and prognosis (see Chapter 6).

B. Assist client in setting realistic goals.

C. Encourage ventilation of feelings.

Pheochromocytoma

❋ **Pheochromocytoma is a rare disorder of the adrenal medulla characterized by a tumor that secretes an excess of epinephrine and norepinephrine.**

Data Collection

> ✔ *NURSING PRIORITY: Clients experiencing problems of the adrenal medulla have severe fluctuations in blood pressure related to the levels of catecholamines.*

A. Persistent or paroxysmal hypertension.

B. Palpitations, tachycardia.

C. Hyperglycemia, headache.

Treatment

A. Medications - antihypertensive medications.

B. Surgery: removal of the tumor is the treatment of choice.

Nursing Intervention

❖ **Goal:** To decrease client's hypertension and provide preoperative nursing measures as appropriate (see Chapter 3).

A. Decrease intake of stimulants.

B. Assess vital signs frequently.

❖ **Goal:** To assist client to return to homeostasis after adrenalectomy.

A. Maintain normal blood pressure the first 24 to 48 hours after surgery; client is at increased risk for hemorrhage or severe hypotensive episode.
   1. Assess for blood pressure changes caused by catecholamine imbalance (both hypertension and hypotension).
   2. Administer analgesics judiciously.
   3. Administer corticosteroids as indicated.

❖ **Goal:** To maintain health after adrenalectomy.

A. Continued medical follow-up care.

B. If both adrenals are removed, client will require lifelong replacement of adrenal hormones.

Addison's Disease (Adrenocortical Insufficiency/Adrenal Hypofunction)

❋ **Addison's disease is caused by a decrease in secretion of the adrenal cortex hormones.**

Data Collection

A. Fatigue, weakness.

B. Weight loss, bronze pigmentation of the skin.

C Postural hypotension.

D. Hyponatremia, hyperkalemia.

E. Hypoglycemia.

F. Adrenal crisis (Addisonian crisis) – may be caused by client failing to take medications.
   1. Profound fatigue, dehydration.
   2. Vascular collapse (see cyanosis and signs of shock: pallor, anxiety, weak/rapid pulse, tachypnea, and low blood pressure).

> 💡 *TEST ALERT: Determine if vital signs are abnormal (e.g., hypotension, hypertension); notify others of change in client's condition.*

Treatment

A. Replace adrenal hormones.

B. May require lifelong replacement of adrenal hormones.

Nursing Intervention

❖ **Goal:** To return to homeostasis.

A. Initiate and maintain IV infusion of normal saline solution.

B. Administer large doses of corticosteroids through IV bolus initially, then titrate in a diluted solution.

C. Frequent evaluation of vital signs.

D. Assess sodium and water retention.

E. Evaluate serum potassium levels.

F. Keep client immobilized and quiet.

> ✔ *NURSING PRIORITY: If any client is experiencing difficulty with maintaining adequate blood pressure, do not move him or her unless absolutely necessary. Avoid all unnecessary nursing procedures until the client's condition is stabilized.*

❖ **Goal:** To safely take steroid replacements (see Appendix 5-7).

A. Administer steroid preparations with food or an antacid.

B. Evaluate for edema and fluid retention.

C. Assess serum sodium and potassium levels.

D. Check daily weight.

E. Increase intake of protein and carbohydrates.

F. Evaluate for hypoglycemia.

G. Observe for cushingoid symptoms.

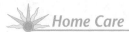Home Care

A.   Lifelong steroid therapy is necessary.
B.   Dosage of steroids may need to be increased in times of additional stress.
C.   Infection, diaphoresis, and injury will necessitate an increase in the need for steroids and may precipitate a crisis state.
D.   Report gastric distress because it may be caused by steroids.
E.   Carry a medical identification card.

Cushing's Syndrome (Adrenal cortex hypersecretion/Hypercortisolism)

*   **Cushing's syndrome occurs as a result of excess levels of adrenal cortex hormones.**

> ✔ *NURSING PRIORITY: The most common cause of Cushing's syndrome is long-term steroid therapy for chronic conditions. Many chronic conditions necessitate the use of long-term steroid therapy. The symptoms of the syndrome are the same regardless of the origin of the problem.*

Data Collection

A.   Marked change in personality (emotional lability), irritability.
B.   Changes in appearance.
  1.   Moon face.
  2.   Deposit of fat on the back.
  3.   Thin skin, purple striae.
  4.   Truncal obesity with thin extremities.
  5.   Bruises and petechiae.
C.   Persistent hyperglycemia.
D.   GI distress from increased acid production.
E.   Osteoporosis.
F.   Increased susceptibility to infection.
G.   Sodium and fluid retention; potassium depletion.
H.   Hypertension.
I.   Changes in secondary sexual characteristics.
  1.   Amenorrhea (females).
  2.   Hirsutism (females).
  3.   Gynecomastia (males).
  4.   Impotence or decreased libido.

Treatment

Treatment depends on the cause of the problem. Cushing's syndrom is most often caused by the intake of steroid medications required to treat a chronic condition (e.g., arthritis, pulmonary inflammation, transplants), and control of the condition requires the client to stay on the medications. At that point, treatment of the condition is supportive.

Nursing Intervention

❖   **Goal:** To assist in return to hormone balance.
A.   Restrict sodium and water intake.
B.   Monitor fluid and electrolyte levels.
C.   Evaluate for hyperglycemia.
D.   Assess for GI disturbances.
E.   Prevent infection.
❖   **Goal:** To prevent complications.
A.   Excessive sodium and water retention: monitor for edema, hypertension, heart failure.
B.   Potassium depletion: monitor for cardiac arrhythmias.
C.   Evaluate client's ability to cope with change in body image.
D.   Predisposed to fractures; promote weight bearing; monitor for joint and bone pain; promote home safety.

Home Care

A.   Stress the need for continuous health care.
B.   Encourage continuation of activities.
C.   Have client demonstrate an understanding of the medication regimen.
D.   Assist client to identify methods of coping with problems of therapy.
E.   Have client demonstrate an understanding of specific problems for which he or she needs to notify the physician.

Study Questions: Endocrine System

1. The nurse is evaluating a client with diabetic ketoacidosis. The nurse would note which respiratory pattern as indicative of complications associated with this condition?
    1   Rapid and deep respirations.
    2   Rapid and shallow respirations.
    3   Normal with sleep apnea.
    4   Cheyne-Stokes respirations.
2. A client in the emergency department has a blood glucose of 40mg/mL. The nurse would anticipate which medication to be ordered?
    1   NPH insulin.
    2   Metformin (**Glucophage**).
    3   Regular insulin.
    4   Glucagon.
3. A client is placed on insulin sliding scale. The nurse would anticipate which medication needing to be administered?
    1   Lente insulin.
    2   Regular insulin.
    3   NPH insulin.
    4   Glargine insulin.
4. While gathering information on a diabetic client, the nurse smells a sweet, fruity odor. What would be important for the nurse to check?
    1   Serum blood glucose level.
    2   Blood urea nitrogen level.
    3   Ketostix of the urine.
    4   Urinary output.
5. A client has an order for a glycosylated hemoglobin test to be done. The nurse understands that the purpose of this test is to:
    1   Determine the glucose levels over the past 120 days.
    2   Evaluate the blood glucose level after a 24-hour fasting.
    3   Determine the level of insulin present in the body.
    4   Evaluate the function of the pancreas.
6. What would be noted on the assessment of a client with hyperthyroidism?
    1   Dry skin, bradycardia, and hypertension.
    2   Difficulty staying awake, increased appetite, and weight gain.
    3   Marked weight gain, hypertension, and tachycardia.
    4   Increased activity, difficulty sleeping, and weight loss.
7. The nurse is caring for a client who is 8-hours post-thyroidectomy. What are important nursing interventions for this client? Select all that apply:
    ____ 1   Have the client speak every 2 hours to determine increasing level of hoarseness.
    ____ 2   Provide a high-calcium diet to replace calcium lost during the procedure.
    ____ 3   Evaluate behind the neck for the presence of blood from the incision.
    ____ 4   Assist client to perform range-of-motion neck exercises to prevent contractures.
    ____ 5   Maintain the client in semi-Fowler's position.
    ____ 6   Check the incision for formation of a hematoma.
8. A client is admitted with a diagnosis of Cushing's syndrome. What is an important consideration for the nurse to make in caring for this client?
    1   The client is going to be intolerant of heat, and pulse rate and blood pressure will be increased.
    2   Due to decreased inflammatory response, the client will be at increased risk for infection.
    3   It is important to maintain strict intake and output due to hypovolemia.
    4   Due to activity intolerance, the client will be kept on bed rest and a high-sodium diet will be prescribed.
9. The nurse is caring for a client who has Addison's disease. How will the nurse evaluate the client for complications associated with this condition?
    1   Evaluate the client for the presence of fluctuating blood pressure readings.
    2   Assess for the development of fever and purulent drainage.
    3   Perform frequent respiratory checks for decreased movement of air.
    4   Maintain strict intake and output records to determine compromised renal function.
10. A diabetic client comes into the emergency department with a diagnosis of diabetic ketoacidosis. The nurse would anticipate what symptoms with this client?
    1   Shallow respirations, bradycardia, confusion.
    2   Pallor, diaphoresis, tachycardia.
    3   Low blood pressure, diaphoresis, nausea and vomiting.
    4   Rapid and deep respirations, tachycardia, confusion.
11. Which client would be most likely to be able to control their diabetes through diet and exercise?
    1   A 10-year-old child.
    2   A 30-year-old woman with onset at age 11 years.
    3   A 1-year-old child.
    4   A 60-year-old woman with onset at age 45 years.
12. When a client returns to his room following a thyroidectomy, what equipment is important for the nurse to have readily available?
    1   Oral airway.
    2   Tracheotomy tray and suction.
    3   Paper and pencil.
    4   A small cassette tape recorder.

Answers and rationales to these questions are in the section at the end of the book titled Chapter Study Questions: Answers and Rationales.

Appendix 8-1	ENDOCRINE DIAGNOSTICS

Diagnostic Test	Normal	Clinical/Nursing Implications
THYROID		
Thyroxine (T$_4$)	5-12 mcg/dl	1. Increased in hyperthyroidism, decreased in hypothyroidism
Triiodothyronine (T$_3$)	70-220 ng/dl	2. When T$_3$ & T$_4$ are low, TSH secretion increases.
Thyroid-stimulating hormone (TSH)	0.2-5.4 mIU/L	3. TSH is increased in hypothyroidism and decreased in hyperthyroidism.
PANCREAS		
Serum glucose	60-110 mg/dl	1. Test is timed to rule out diabetes by determining rate of glucose absorption from serum.
Oral glucose tolerance test	1 hr: less than 200 mg/dl	2. In healthy person, insulin response to large dose of glucose is immediate.
	2 hr: less than 140 mg/dl	3. Insulin and oral hypoglycemic agents should not be administered before test.
Glucose fasting blood sugar (FBS) Also called: fasting blood glucose (FBG) and fasting plasma glucose (FPG)	Same as serum glucose (consistently greater than 126 mg/dl is diagnostic for diabetes)	1. Used as a screening test for problems of metabolism. 2. Maintain client in fasting state for 12 hours until blood is drawn. 3. If client is a known diabetic and experiences dizziness, weakness, or fainting, draw blood for determination of glucose level.
Glycosylated hemoglobin (HbA$_{1c}$)	Nondiabetic usually 4%-6%. 2%-6.4% considered good diabetic control (goal is 7% or less) greater than 8% considered poor diabetic control	1. More accurate test of diabetic control, because it measures glucose attached to hemoglobin (indicates overall control for past 90-120 days, which is the lifespan of the RBC).

> **TEST ALERT:** *Frequently, the level of the FBS is given in a question, and it is necessary to evaluate the level and determine the appropriate nursing intervention.*

2-Hour postprandial blood sugar	65-139 mg/dl	1. Involves measuring the serum glucose 2 hours after a meal; results are significantly increased in diabetic.
Serum amylase	30-200 U/L	1. Used to evaluate pancreatic cell damage. 2. Other intestinal conditions and inflammatory conditions cause increase.
Serum lipase	Normal values vary with method; elevated is abnormal	1. Appears in serum after damage to pancreas.
Urine sugar (**Clinistix, Clinitest, Labstix**)	Negative for glucose	1. Use fresh double-voided specimen. 2. A rough indicator of serum glucose levels. 3. Results may be altered by various medications.
Ketone bodies (acetone)	Negative	1. Ketone bodies occur in the urine before there is significant increase in serum ketones. 2. Use freshly voided urine.
PITUITARY		
Growth hormone (GH)	Less than 5 ng/mL in men Less than 18 ng/mL in women	1. NPO after midnight. 2. Maintain bed rest until serum sample is drawn.
ADRENAL MEDULLA		
Urinary vanillylmandelic acid (VMA)	Less than 8 mg in 24 hr Increased with pheochromocytoma	1. Depending on how test is measured, there may be dietary and medication restrictions. 2. 24-hr urine collection.
ACTH stimulation test	Increase in plasma cortisol levels by more than 7-10 mcg/dl above baseline	1. ACTH is given as IM or IV bolus and samples are drawn at 30 and 60 min to evaluate ability of adrenal glands to secrete steroids.
ADRENAL CORTEX		
ACTH suppression (dexamethasone suppression test)	Normal suppression; 50% decrease in cortisone production (cortisol level less than 3 mcg/dl)	1. An overnight test: A small amount of dexamethasone is administered in the evening, and serum and urine are evaluated in the morning; extensive test may cover 6 days. 2. Cushing's syndrome is ruled out if suppression is normal.
Plasma cortisol levels for diurnal variations	Secretion high in early morning, decreased in evening. 8:00 AM: 5-23 mcg/dl 4:00 PM: 3-13 mcg/dl	1. Elevation in plasma cortisol levels occurs in the morning and significant decrease in evening and night—a diurnal variation.
24-Hour urine for 17-hydroxycorticosteroids and 17-ketosteroids	Male: 3-10 mg/24 hr Female: 2-8 mg/24 hr Child under 15 yr: less than 4.5 mg/24 hr	1. Increase in urine levels indicates hyperadrenal function. 2. Keep specimen refrigerated

ACTH, Adrenocorticotropic hormone; *ADH*, antidiuretic hormone; *NPO*, nothing by mouth; *RBC*, red blood cell.

Appendix 8-2 MEDICATIONS USED IN ENDOCRINE DISORDERS

Medications	Side Effects	Nursing Implications
ADH REPLACEMENT		
Desmopressin (**DDAVP**): nasal spray, PO, IV, SQ	Excessive water retention, headache, nausea, flushing.	1. Monitor daily weight; correlate with intake and output.
Vasopressin (**Pitressin**): IM, SQ Lypressin (**Diapid**): nasal spray		2. Vasopressin more likely to cause adverse cardiovascular and thromboembolic problems.
ANTITHYROID AGENT: Inhibits production of thyroid hormone; does not inactivate thyroid hormone in circulating blood. Medications are not reliable for long-term inhibition of thyroid hormone production.		
Propylthiouracil (**PTU**): PO	Agranulocytosis; abdominal discomfort; nausea, vomiting, diarrhea; crosses placenta.	1. May increase anticoagulation effect of heparin and oral anticoagulants.
Methimazole (**Tapazole**): PO	Same; crosses placenta more rapidly.	2. May be combined with iodine preparations. 3. Monitor CBC. 4. Store Tapazole in light-sensitive container. 5. May be used before surgery or treatment with radioactive iodine.
Lugol's solution: PO Saturated solution of potassium iodide (**SSKI**)	Inhibits synthesis and release	1. Administer in fluid to decrease unpleasant taste. of thyroid hormone. 2. May be used to decrease vascularity of thyroid gland before surgery.
RADIOACTIVE IODINE: Accumulates in the thyroid gland; causes partial or total destruction of thyroid gland through radiation.		
Iodine (I^{123} or I^{131}): PO	Discomfort in thyroid area; bone marrow depression. Desired effect: permanent hypothyroidism.	1. Increase fluids immediately after treatment, because radioactive isotope is excreted in the urine. 2. Therapeutic dose of radioactive iodine is low; no radiation safety precautions are required. 3. Contraindicated in pregnancy.
THYROID REPLACEMENTS: Replacement of thyroid hormone.		
Levothyroxine sodium (**Levothroid, Levoxyl, Levo-T, Novothyrox, Synthroid**): PO, IM, IV	Overdose may result in symptoms of hyperthyroidism: tachycardia, heat intolerance, nervousness.	1. Be careful in reading exact name on label of medications; micrograms and milligrams are used as units of measure. 2. Generally taken once a day before breakfast. 3. Within 3-4 days, begin to see improvement; maximum effect in 4-6 weeks.
Liothyronine (**Cytomel, Triostat**)		
PANCREATIC ENZYMES: Replacement enzyme to aid in digestion of starch, protein, and fat.		
Pancreatin (**Creon**): PO	GI upset and irritation of mucous membranes.	1. Client is usually on a high-protein, high-carbohydrate, low-fat diet.
Pancrelipase (**Pancrease, Pangestyme, Ultrase, Viokase**): PO meals.		2. Enteric-coated tablets should not be crushed or chewed. 3. Pancreatin may be given before, during, or within 1 hr after meals. 4. Pancrelipase is given just before or with each meal or snack.
ANTIHYPOGLYCEMIC AGENT: Increases plasma glucose levels and relaxes smooth muscles.		
Glucagon: IM, IV, SQ	Possible rebound hypoglycemia.	1. Watch for symptoms of hypoglycemia and treat with food first, if conscious. 2. Client usually awakens in 5-20 min after receiving Glucagon. 3. If client does not respond, anticipate IV glucose to be given.

ORAL HYPOGLYCEMIC AGENTS: Stimulate beta cells to secrete more insulin; enhance body utilization of available insulin (see Figure 8-4 for insulin). HIGH ALERT MEDICATIONS

GENERAL NURSING IMPLICATIONS
- Dose should be decreased for elderly.
- Use with caution in clients with renal and hepatic impairment.
- All oral hypoglycemic agents are contraindicated in pregnant clients.
- All clients should be carefully observed for symptoms of hypoglycemia and hyperglycemia.
- Medications should be taken in the morning.
- Long-term therapy may result in decreased effectiveness.

Appendix 8-2	MEDICATIONS USED IN ENDOCRINE DISORDERS—cont'd	

Medications	Side Effects	Nursing Implications
SULFONYLUREAS: Stimulate the pancreas to make more insulin.		
Chlorpropamide (**Diabinase**): PO Glipizide (**Glucotrol**): PO Glyburide (**Micronase, DiaBeta**): PO Glimepiride (**Amaryl**): PO Gliclazide (**Diamicron**): PO Tolbutamide (**Orinase**): PO Tolazamide (**Tolinase**): PO	Hypoglycemia, jaundice, GI disturbance, skin reactions (fewer side effects with 2nd-generation agents).	1. Tolbutamide has shortest duration of action; requires multiple daily doses. 2. Glyburide has a long duration of action. 3. Interact with: calcium channel blockers, oral contraceptives, glucocorticoids, phenothiazines, and thiazide diuretics.
BIGUANIDE: Decrease sugar production in the liver and help the muscles use insulin to break down sugar.		
Metformin (**Glucophage**): PO	Dizziness, nausea, back pain, possible metallic taste.	1. Administered with meals. 2. Has a beneficial effect on lowering lipids. 3. Weight gain may occur.
ALPHA-GLUCOSIDASE INHIBITOR: Slows down how the body absorbs sugar after eating; also known as "starch blockers."		
Acarbose (**Precose**): PO Miglitol (**Glyset**): PO	Diarrhea, flatulence, abdominal pain.	1. Take at beginning of meals; not effective on an empty stomach. 2. Acarbose is contraindicated in clients with inflammatory bowel disease. 3. Frequently given with sulfonylureas to increase effectiveness of both medications.
THIAZOLIDINEDIONES: Enhance insulin utilization at receptor sites (they do NOT increase insulin production); also referred to as "insulin sensitizers."		
Pioglitazone (**Actos**): PO	Weight gain, edema.	1. May affect liver function; monitor LFTs.
MEGLITINIDES: (Non-Sulfonylurea Insulin Secretagogues) Stimulate release of insulin from beta cells.		
Nateglinide (**Starlix**): PO Repaglinide (**Prandin**): PO	Weight gain, hypoglycemia.	1. Rapid onset and short duration. 2. Take 30 min before meals (or right at mealtime). 3. Do not take if meal is missed.
DIPEPTIDYL PEPTIDASE-4 (DDP-4) INHIBITORS: Enhances the incretin system, stimulates release of insulin for beta cells, and decreases hepatic glucose production.		
Sitagliptin (**Januvia**): PO Vildagliptin (**Galvus**): PO	Upper respiratory tract infection, sore throat, headache, diarrhea.	1. Should not be used in Type 1 diabetes or for the treatment of diabetic ketoacidosis.

INJECTABLE DRUGS FOR DIABETES

AMYLIN MIMETICS: Complements the effects of insulin by delaying gastric emptying and suppressing glucagon secretion.		
Pramlintide (**Symlin**): SQ	Hypoglycemia, nausea, injection site reactions.	1. Teach client to take other oral medications at least 1 hour prior to taking or 2 hours after, because of delayed gastric emptying. 2. Injected into thigh or abdomen. 3. Cannot be mixed with insulin.

> ✓   **NURSING PRIORITY:** *Can cause severe hypoglycemia when used with insulin; usually occurs within 3 hours following injection.*

INCRETIN MIMETICS: Stimulates release of insulin, decreases glucagon secretion, decreases gastric emptying, and suppresses appetite.		
Exenatide (**Byetta**): SQ	Hypoglycemia, nausea, vomiting, diarrhea, headache, possible weight loss.	1. Used in conjunction with metformin. 2. Monitor weight. 3. Not indicated for use with insulin.

CBC, Complete blood count; *GI*, gastrointestinal; *IM*, intramuscularly; *IV*, intravenously; *LFTs*, liver function tests; *PO*, by mouth (orally); *SQ*, subcutaneously.

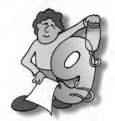

Hematologic System

PHYSIOLOGY OF THE BLOOD

A. Functions of the blood.
1. Transports oxygen from the lungs to the tissues and carbon dioxide from the tissues to the lungs.
2. Transports nutrients from intestines to body cells.
3. Transports waste products to kidneys for excretion.
B. Components.
1. Plasma: 90% water; accounts for about half of the total blood volume.
2. Formed elements (cells): account for about half of the total blood volume.
a. Erythrocytes (red blood cells [RBCs]).
b. Leukocytes (white blood cells [WBCs]).
c. Thrombocytes (platelets).
C. Characteristics of plasma.
1. Plasma is clear and straw colored; it does not contain cellular elements.
2. Globulins: Gamma globulins are protein components; their primary function is prevention of infection.
3. Fibrinogen is a necessary element in normal clot formation; produced in the liver.
4. Prothrombin is a necessary element for normal coagulation.
a. Produced in the liver.
b. Normal production is dependent on availability of adequate vitamin K.
D. Characteristics of erythrocytes (red blood cells).
1. Formed in the red bone marrow; erythropoiesis is the production of red blood cells.
2. Vitamin B_{12} and folic acid are necessary for the production of normal erythrocytes.
3. Hemoglobin is the primary component of the red blood cell and binds with oxygen.
4. Primary function is transportation of oxygen and carbon dioxide.
5. The fraction of the blood occupied by erythrocytes is called the hematocrit.
E. Characteristics of leukocytes (white blood cells).
1. Function is to protect the body against invading microorganisms.
2. Leukocytosis refers to an overall increase in the number of leukocytes; leukopenia refers to an overall decrease in the number of leukocytes.
F. Characteristics of thrombocytes (platelets).
1. Function: primarily involved with hemostasis. When blood vessel wall is damaged, platelets adhere to the area and eventually form a platelet plug to decrease bleeding.
2. Thrombocytosis refers to a marked, abnormal increase in the number of thrombocytes; thrombocytopenia refers to a marked, abnormal decrease in the number of thrombocytes.
G. Blood classification.
1. Major blood groups: A, B, AB, and O.
2. Rh factor may be present (positive) or absent (negative).
a. Rh factor is present on the red blood cell.
b. Rh-positive factor is present in 85% to 95% of the population.

Data Collection

A. Evaluate history.
1. History of disease of bone marrow or organs affecting production of blood.
2. History of treatment that depressed bone marrow activity (especially chemotherapy or radiation therapy).
3. Family history of hematologic problems (inheritance pattern).
B. Bleeding problems occurring during pregnancy, labor and delivery, or immediately after birth in both mother and infant.
C. Presence of disorders, aging, or disease processes other than hematologic disorders (Table 9-1).
D. Evaluate effect hematologic disorder has on client's lifestyle and activities of daily living (ADLs).
1. How long has client experienced symptoms?
2. What are current activities and metabolic requirements of the client?
3. Presence or absence of bleeding episodes.
4. Ability to control pain.
E. Assess client's current nutritional status.
F. Evaluate current blood values.
G. Evaluate status of respiratory and cardiovascular systems in maintaining homeostasis.

Anemias

* **Anemia is characterized by a low RBC count and a decrease to below normal in hemoglobin and hematocrit values. The more rapidly an anemia occurs, the more severe the symptoms will be.**

TABLE 9-1	AGE-RELATED ASSESSMENT FINDINGS FOR THE HEMATOLOGIC SYSTEM	
Assessment Area	**Hematologic System Findings**	**Older Adult Changes and Significance**
Nail beds (check for capillary refill)	Pallor, cyanosis, and decreased capillary refill are often noted in hematologic disorders.	• Nails are typically thickened and discolored. • Need to use another body area, such as the lips, to assess capillary refill.
Hair distribution	Thin or absent hair on trunk and extremities may indicate poor oxygenation and blood supply to area.	• Older adults are losing body hair, but often in an even pattern distribution that has occurred slowly over time. • Lack of hair only on lower legs and toes may indicate poor circulation.
Skin moisture and color	Skin dryness, pallor, and jaundice may occur with anemia, leukemia, etc.	• Dry skin is a normal aspect of aging and thus becomes an unreliable indicator of skin moisture. • Pigment loss and skin changes along with some yellowing occur with aging. • Pallor that is not associated with anemia may be noted in older adults, because they tend not to go outdoors and get exposed to sunlight.

A. Common goal in treatment of all anemias is to identify the origin and correct the problem.
B. Data Collection.
   a. Pale skin, delayed wound healing.
   b. Shortness of breath, dyspnea on exertion, tachypnea.
   c. Tachycardia, palpitations, postural hypotension.
   d. Chronic fatigue, weakness, and apathy.
   e. Anorexia, nausea, weight loss.
   f. Chronic anemia may result in growth retardation in infants and children.

 TEST ALERT: Identify client's ability to maintain activities of daily living.

C. **Iron deficiency anemia:** characterized by inadequate intake of dietary iron or excessive loss of iron.
   1. Common in adolescents; occurs in infants whose primary diet is milk.
   2. May occur in pregnancy or with heavy flow during menses.
   3. Older adults are more prone because of poor dietary iron intake and decreased absorption in the small intestines.
   4. Pallor, glossitis, cheilitis (inflammation of the lips)—three most common findings.
   5. Diagnostics: decreased hemoglobin and hematocrit values (Appendix 9-1).
   6. Treatment: supplemental iron intake (see Appendix 9-2).
      a. Increased dietary iron intake (see Table 2-2).
      b. Supplemental folic acid.

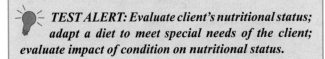 **TEST ALERT: Evaluate client's nutritional status; adapt a diet to meet special needs of the client; evaluate impact of condition on nutritional status.**

D. **Pernicious anemia:** condition characterized by an inability to absorb vitamin B$_{12}$ (cobalamin). It may be associated with loss of intrinsic factor (gastric resection), or it may be an autoimmune problem.
   1. Generally not associated with inadequate dietary intake.
   2. More common in older adult; most common age at diagnosis is 60 years.
   3. May be precipitated by gastric resection, gastritis, or chronic alcoholism.
   4. General symptoms of anemia, confusion.
   5. Paresthesia in the extremities, weakness, reduced vibratory sense.
   6. Smooth, beefy, red tongue (glossitis).
   7. Treatment: injections of vitamin B$_{12}$ may be required indefinitely.
E. **Aplastic anemia:** characterized by depression of the bone marrow in production of all blood cell types—RBCs, WBCs, and platelets.
   1. May be precipitated by chemotherapeutic agents, radiation, and anticonvulsant medications (e.g., **Dilantin**).
   2. Can result from radiation therapy.
   3. General symptoms of anemia.
   4. Fever.
   5. Infections associated with neutropenia.
   6. Bleeding problems associated with thrombocytopenia.

7. Treatment:
   a. Hematopoietic stem cell transplant
      (see Appendix 9-4).
   b. Immunosuppressive medications.
F. Folic acid deficiency anemia: associated with decreased dietary intake of folic acid.
   1. Caused by alcoholism, anorexia, malabsorption syndromes.
   2. Deficiency may occur with increased demands for folic acid: infancy, adolescence, and pregnancy.
   3. May appear ill with malnourishment.
   4. Treatment: folic acid injections may be necessary initially; then oral replacement.

Nursing Interventions

For all clients with anemia.

❖ **Goal:** To assist in establishing a diagnosis.
A. Complete nutritional evaluation.
B. History of possible causes.
❖ **Goal:** To decrease body oxygen needs.
A. Assess client's tolerance to activity.
B. Provide diversional activities but also provide for adequate rest.
C. May need supplemental oxygen.
❖ **Goal:** To prevent infections.
A. Decrease exposure.
B. Evaluate for temperature elevations frequently.
C. Observe for leukocytosis.
D. Maintain adequate hydration.
❖ **Goal:** To assess for complications of chronic anemic state.
A. Evaluate ability of cardiovascular system to maintain adequate cardiac output.
B. Evaluate for symptoms of hypoxia (see Chapter 10).
❖ **Goal:** To help client understand implications of disease and measures to maintain health.
A. Explain medical regimen.
B. Discuss importance of continuing medical follow-up.
C. Explain side effects of medications.
D. Identify foods high in iron and folic acid (see Chapter 2).

Sickle Cell Anemia

* **Sickle cell anemia is a problem characterized by the sickling effect of the erythrocytes, an inherited autosomal recessive disorder.**
A. Sickling problem is not apparent until around 6 months of age; the increased levels of fetal hemoglobin up to that age prevent serious sickling problems.
B. Predominantly a problem of children and adolescents. Child may be asymptomatic between crises. The problems from childhood may cause long-term complications as they become adults.
C. Pathologic changes of sickle cell disease result from:
   1. Increased blood viscosity.
   2. Increased RBC destruction.
   3. Increased viscosity eventually precipitates ischemia

FIGURE 9-1 **Sickle cell anemia crisis.** (From Zerwekh J, Claborn J, Miller CJ: *Memory notebook of nursing,* vol 2, ed 3, Ingram, 2007, Nursing Education Consultants.)

and tissue necrosis caused by capillary stasis and thrombosis.
   4. Cycle of occlusion, ischemia, and infarction to vascular organs.
D. Conditions precipitating sickling effect (Figure 9-1).
   1. Dehydration, acidosis.
   2. Hypoxia, infection with temperature elevation.

Data Collection

A. Splenomegaly, liver failure, hepatomegaly
B. Kidney damage caused by the congestion of glomerular capillaries and tubular arterioles.
C. Vaso-occlusive crisis: blood flow is impaired by sickled cells, causing ischemia and pain.
   1. Extremities - occlusions in the small distal bones of the hands and the feet, characterized by pain, swelling, and decreased function (hand-foot syndrome).
   2. Abdomen – severe abdominal pain.
   3. Pulmonary – symptoms of pneumonia.
   4. Renal – hematuria.
   5. CNS – stroke, visual problems.
   6. Sequestration crisis: pooling of the blood in the liver and spleen with decreased blood volume.

✓ **NURSING PRIORITY:** *Recognize occurrence of a hemorrhage. Bleeding in a client with sickle cell anemia produces different symptoms than bleeding in a client who has undergone surgery; plan and implement nursing care to prevent complications; notify health care provider regarding signs of potential complications.*

D. Diagnostics (see Appendix 9-1): early diagnosis, before 3 months of age, helps to minimize complications.

Treatment

A. Prevention of the sickling problem.
   1. Adequate hydration.
   2. Prevent infections, especially respiratory tract infections; pneumococcal vaccine is recommended.
   3. Clients generally do not require iron because of increased resorption.
   4. Daily folic acid supplement.
   5. Oxygen – assists to prevent a crisis in client with respiratory problems, but it does not reverse a sickling crisis or reduce pain.
B. Treatment of crisis.
   1. Bed rest, hydration, antibiotics.
   2. Analgesics for pain; promote adequate oxygenation.
   3. Blood transfusions and/or exchange transfusions (see Appendix 9-3).
C. Surgery: splenectomy.

Nursing Interventions

❖ **Goal:** To prevent sickle cell disease.
A. Participate in community screening programs and education.
B. Refer persons who are carriers (autosomal recessive trait) for genetic counseling.
❖ **Goal:** To prevent sickling crisis.
A. Maintain adequate hydration; intravenous (IV) fluids may be necessary.
B. Promote respiratory health and tissue oxygenation.
C. Prevent infection.
D. Hydroxyurea (**Droxia**, **Hydrea**): reduces sickling episodes, a long-term complication of leukemia.
❖ **Goal:** To control pain.
A. Assessment of involved area.
B. Administer appropriate analgesics.
C. Allow client to assume a position of comfort; passive range of motion may be beneficial.
D. Maintain rest if movement exacerbates pain.
❖ **Goal:** To maintain adequate hydration and oxygenation.
A. Evaluate adequacy of hydration.
B. Monitor IV fluid administration carefully; maintain accurate intake and output records.
C. Evaluate electrolyte balance.
D. Administer oxygen as indicated.
E. Provide good pulmonary hygiene.

Home Care

A. Increase fluids with physical activity.
B. Seek early intervention for symptoms of infection, especially respiratory tract infection; report temperature elevations, coughing, or pain.
C. Encourage normal growth and developmental activities as tolerated by the child.
D. Client with sickle cell disease should avoid situations

that may precipitate hypoxia.
   1. Traveling to high-altitude areas.
   2. Flying in an unpressurized aircraft.
   3. Participating in overly strenuous exercise.
E. Inform all significant health care personnel that child should wear medical identification.

Polycythemia Vera (Primary)

✳ **Polycythemia vera is a chronic disorder characterized by a proliferation of all red marrow cells due to a chromosomal mutation.**

Data Collection

A. Usually occurs during middle age; median age is 60 years.
B. Early signs: headache, vertigo, tinnitus, pruritus.
C. Ruddy complexion (plethora).
D. Problems of decreased blood flow.
   1. Angina, claudication (pain in muscles during activity).
   2. Thrombophlebitis, hypertension.
E. Complication: stroke secondary to thrombosis.

Treatment

A. Phlebotomy (2-3 times per week initially, then every 2-3 months).
B. Myelosuppressive agents.

Nursing Interventions

❖ **Goal:** To help client understand implications of the disease and long-term health care needs (i.e., prevention of DVT).

Leukemia

✳ **Leukemia is an uncontrolled proliferation of abnormal white blood cells; eventual cellular destruction occurs as a result of the infiltration of the leukemic cells into the body tissue.**

A. Three primary consequences of leukemia.
   1. Anemia from RBC destruction and bleeding.
   2. Infection associated with neutropenia.
   3. Bleeding tendencies caused by decreased platelets.
B. Types of leukemia.
   1. Acute lymphocytic leukemia (blast or stem cell) (ALL).
      a. Peak occurrences: around 4 years of age, then again around 65 years.
      b. Favorable prognosis with chemotherapy.
      c. Leukemic cells will infiltrate the meninges, precipitating increased intracranial pressure.
   2. Acute myelogenous leukemia (AML).
      a. Most common in older adults.
      b. Peak incidence age 60 to 70 years.
   3. Chronic myelogenous leukemia (CML).
      a. Uncommon before the age of 20 years; peak incidence age 45 years.

b. Onset is generally slow.

c. Symptoms are less severe than those in acute stages of disease.

d. Presence of Philadelphia chromosome in 90% of cases.

4. Chronic lymphocytic leukemia (CLL).

a. Common malignancy of older adults; rare before age 30, and more common in men.

b. Frequently asymptomatic; often diagnosed in a chronic fatigue work-up.

Data Collection

A. Clinical manifestations.

1. Anemia, infection, and bleeding tendencies occurring together.

2. Anorexia, weight loss, cough.

3. Central nervous system involvement: headache, confusion, increased irritability.

4. Fatigue, lethargy.

5. Petechiae, bruises easily, epistaxis.

6. Complaints of bone and joint pain.

7. Hepatomegaly and splenomegaly.

B. Diagnostics (see Appendix 9-1): bone marrow aspiration to evaluate cell production.

Treatment

A. Medications.

1. Corticosteroids and antineoplastic agents.

2. Allopurinol (**Zyloprim**) decreases uric acid levels in clients receiving chemotherapy.

B. Hematopoietic stem cell transplantation (see Appendix 9-4).

C. A remission is characterized by absence of leukemic cells and disappearance of all disease symptoms.

Nursing Interventions

❖ **Goal:** To prevent infection.

A. Assess for evidence of infection: fever, inflammation, pain.

B. Monitor temperature elevation closely; notify doctor of increase above 100.5° F (38°C).

C. Meticulous skin care, especially oral hygiene and around perianal area.

D. Protect client from exposure to infection; degree of restriction depends on immunosuppression.

E. Isolate client from persons with communicable childhood diseases, especially those with chicken pox.

F. Polio (IPV), varicella, measles-mumps-rubella, and influenza immunizations are not recommended to be given to children or adults during immunosuppression.

G. Avoid urinary catheterization if possible.

H. Encourage adequate protein and calorie intake, low-bacteria diet.

I. Maintain adequate hydration.

BOX 9-1	BLEEDING PRECAUTIONS

Indications: Clients diagnosed with leukemia, hemophilia, or any condition that causes bleeding; clients receiving anticoagulants or thrombolytic medications.

• Limit number of venipunctures and intramuscular injections.

• Perform guaiac tests on stool as necessary.

• Oral hygiene:

  ✦ Discourage flossing.

  ✦ Use soft toothbrush or no toothbrush; may need to use cotton-tipped swabs while gums are friable.

  ✦ Avoid harsh mouthwashes.

  ✦ Rinse mouth frequently with mild mouthwash.

• Use electric razor for shaving.

• Assess perianal area for fissures and bleeding daily.

• Discourage client from vigorous coughing or nose blowing.

• Avoid aspirin products; evaluate NSAIDs for bleeding properties.

• Avoid catheters (urinary and suctioning) when possible.

• Avoid enemas and suppositories.

• Avoid overinflation of blood pressure cuff or leaving cuff inflated for prolonged period of time.

• Provide safe environment and prevent injury according to age (padded side rails, soft toys, house shoes, etc.).

• Monitor for bleeding episode: nosebleed, hematuria, increased bruising.

NSAIDs, Nonsteroidal antiinflammatory drugs.

✓ **NURSING PRIORITY:** *Identify symptoms of infection and treatment of common infections is a priority in the care of this client.*

❖ **Goal:** To prevent or limit bleeding episodes (Box 9-1).

A. Use local measures to control bleeding (pressure to area; cold packs).

B. Restrict strenuous activity.

C. Involve client in evaluating level of activity; decrease activity when platelet counts are low and anemia is present.

❖ **Goal:** To provide pain relief.

A. Use acetaminophen rather than aspirin.

B. Maintain environment conducive to rest.

C. Position carefully; may coordinate positioning with administration of analgesics.

D. Evaluate effectiveness of pain relief; administer analgesic before pain becomes severe.

E. Do not exercise affected joints.

❖ **Goal:** To decrease adverse effects of chemotherapy (see Table 2-4).

❖ **Goal:** To prevent complications of transfusions (see Appendix 9-3).

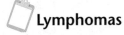
Lymphomas

* **Characterized by malignant neoplasms originating in the bone marrow and lymphocytes. Lymphoma is the fifth most common type of cancer in the U.S.**

A. **Hodgkin's disease:** characterized by painless enlargement of lymph nodes with progression to involve the liver and spleen. Common metastatic sites are the spleen, liver, bone marrow, and lungs. Disease is spread by extension along the lymphatic system. This is the most curable of the lymphomas.
  1. Increased incidence in immunosuppressed clients.
  2. Initially, painless enlargement of cervical, axillary, inguinal, or mediastinal lymph nodes.
  3. Fever, malaise, night sweats.
  4. Weight loss and fatigue are associated with a poor prognosis.
  5. Treatment: chemotherapy and radiation.
B. **Non-Hodgkin's lymphoma:** a neoplastic growth that originates in the lymphoid tissue. It spreads malignant cells unpredictably, infiltrating the lymphoid tissue.
  1. Increased incidence in clients with immunodeficiency or autoimmune conditions who have used immunosuppressant medications.
  2. Symptoms are highly variable, depending on where the disease has spread.
  3. Treatment: chemotherapy and radiation.

Nursing Interventions

❖ **Goal:** To maintain physiologic equilibrium.
A. Maintain hydration and nutrition.
B. Maintain good pulmonary hygiene.
C. Evaluate for shortness of breath; maintain in semi-Fowler's position.
D. Decrease body needs for oxygen.
E. Assess ability of cardiovascular system to maintain cardiac output.
F. Manage pain and effects of therapy.
❖ **Goal:** To prevent infection (see "**Goal:** To prevent infection" in Leukemia section above).
❖ **Goal:** To decrease adverse effects of chemotherapy and radiation therapy (see Table 2-4).

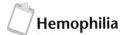
Hemophilia

* **Hemophilia is a defect in the clotting mechanism. The disease is most often recognized during the toddler stage.**

Data Collection

A. Hemophilia is a sex-linked recessive disorders.
  1. Primarily affects males.
  2. Females are carriers.
B. Persistent or prolonged bleeding that occurs from minor trauma/insults.

C. Hemarthrosis: bleeding into joint cavities.
D. Spontaneous hematuria.
E. Hematoma.
F. Intracranial hemorrhage may be fatal.
G. Petechiae are uncommon, because platelet count is normal.

Treatment

A. **Factor VIII concentrate:** must be reconstituted with sterile water immediately before administration; given IV push over 5-10 minutes.
B. **Desmopressin (DDAVP, Stimate):** synthetic vasopressin used to treat mild cases; given IV or intranasal.
C. Treatment may be carried out at home.

Nursing Interventions

❖ **Goal:** To prevent spontaneous bleeding episodes (see Box 9-1).
A. Decrease risk for injury.
  1. Make environment as safe as possible without hampering motor development.
  2. Instruct client to avoid contact sports, but encourage noncontact sports (e.g., swimming).
  3. Regular exercise and physical therapy to promote muscle strength around joints and decrease bleeding episodes.
B. Preventive dental care, and prevent oral infections.
C. Maintain normal weight; increased weight causes increased strain on the joints.
D. Avoid any aspirin compounds.
E. Administer clotting factors before, during, and after invasive medical procedures.
❖ **Goal:** To recognize and treat bleeding episodes.
A. Apply pressure to the area.
B. Immobilize and elevate the joints involved.
C. Do not perform passive range of motion on affected joints.
D. Apply cold pack to promote vasoconstriction.
E. Observe for signs of internal bleeding: tarry stools, slurred speech, headache.
F. Administer clotting factors in a timely manner.
❖ **Goal:** To prepare client and family to administer clotting factors intravenously at home.
A. Correct technique for venipuncture.
B. Indications for use.
C. Encourage child to learn self-administration, generally around age 9 to 12 years.
❖ **Goal:** To prevent permanent joint degeneration.
A. Elevate joint and immobilize during acute bleeding episode.
B. Encourage active range of motion so child will limit movement based on pain tolerance.
C. Physical therapy after the acute phase, no weight bearing until swelling has resolved.
D. Maintain pain relief during physical therapy.

> ✓ **NURSING PRIORITY:** *Apply RICE to the affected joints: rest, ice, compression, elevation.*

Disseminated Intravascular Coagulation

✴ Disseminated intravascular coagulation is a secondary coagulation disorder involving widespread clotting in the small vessels, leading to consumption of clotting factors, thereby precipitating a bleeding disorder. It is not a disease but a result of underlying conditions.

Data Collection

A. Caused by hemolytic processes, extensive tissue damage, shock, sepsis, burns.
B. Petechiae, ecchymosis on skin and mucous membranes are noted.
C. Prolonged bleeding from multiple body areas.
D. Hypotension leading to shock.
E. Multiple organ dysfunction syndrome.

Treatment

A. Correction of the underlying problem.

Nursing Interventions

❖ **Goal:** To identify the problem early and to decrease potential adverse effects.
A. Thorough assessment of bleeding problems in clients severely compromised by other problems (shock and sepsis).
B. Nursing measures to prevent bleeding episodes (see Box 9-1).
C. Assess and support all vital systems.
❖ **Goal:** To help the client's family understand the implications of the disease and demonstrate appropriate coping behaviors.
A. Provide emotional support and encourage visiting as intensive care policies and client's condition allow.
B. Encourage ventilation of feelings regarding critical illness of family member.
C. Be available to family members during visiting time.

Disorders of the Spleen

✴ The spleen is affected by many disorders that can result in splenomegaly (enlarged spleen). The spleen usually contains 20 to 40 mL of blood and does not serve as a reservoir for blood volume or red blood cells.

Data Collection

A. Hypersplenism: splenomegaly with peripheral cytopenias (anemia, leukopenia, thrombocytopenia).
B. Pain due to splenomegaly.
C. Splenic rupture from trauma or inadvertent tearing during other surgical procedures.

Treatment

A. Splenectomy.
B. Analgesics for pain.
C. Platelets, fresh frozen plasma transfusions.

Nursing Interventions

❖ **Goal:** To identify the problem early (splenomegaly, hypersplenism, or splenic rupture) and to decrease potential adverse effects.
A. Thorough assessment of spleen problem and management to address issues of splenomegaly (pain), hypersplenism, or splenic rupture (emergency surgery).
B. Nursing measures to prevent bleeding episodes in hypersplenism (see Box 9-1).
C. Assess and support all vital systems.
D. Monitor for complications following surgery—hemorrhage, shock, fever, abdominal distention, immunologic deficiencies, infection.
❖ **Goal:** To help the client's family to understand the implications of the problem and demonstrate appropriate coping behavior.
A. Provide emotional support and encourage visiting as intensive care policies and client's condition allow.
B. Encourage ventilation of feelings regarding critical illness of family member.
C. Be available to family members during visiting time.
D. Teach about lifelong risk for infection following splenectomy; encourage vaccination for pneumococcus.

Study Questions: Hematologic System

1. The nurse is assessing a client who has been admitted for treatment of his leukemia. What nursing observation should be reported immediately?
   1 Swelling and bleeding into knees.
   2 Increased bruising.
   3 Nausea and vomiting.
   4 Oral temperature of 101° F.

2. What nursing interventions would be important in the care of a client who has severe aplastic anemia? Select all that apply:
   ____ 1 Maintain warm environment.
   ____ 2 Plan all nursing activities early in morning to prevent fatigue.
   ____ 3 Evaluate client for tachycardia.
   ____ 4 Encourage diet that is high in iron and vitamin K.
   ____ 5 Encourage activity, especially ambulating 3 times a day.
   ____ 6 Evaluate respiratory response when ambulating.

3. An older client is being discharged after diagnosis and treatment for leukemia. What will be important to discuss with this client regarding home care?
   1 Maintain a diet that is low in protein and high in carbohydrates.
   2 It is important to regularly check temperature; call physician's office if oral temperature is greater than 101° F.
   3 Always thoroughly wash, cook, or peel fresh vegetables and fruits.
   4 Apply warm packs to joints to prevent further bleeding.

4. A client has developed aplastic anemia. What health problem in the client's past would be associated with this condition?
   1 Hemorrhage and shock after surgery.
   2 Poor dietary intake of iron and folic acid.
   3 Treatment for a pulmonary malignancy.
   4 History of stomach resection and loss of intrinsic factor.

5. A 10-year-old client is admitted in a sickle cell crisis. What would the nurse anticipate to be a priority concern for nursing care?
   1 Pain management.
   2 Swollen, bleeding joints.
   3 Treatment of high temperature.
   4 Decreased bowel sounds.

6. A client is admitted with thrombocytopenia. What will the nurse implement to address this problem?
   1 Contact precautions.
   2 Increase fluid intake.
   3 Cold packs to the joints.
   4 Bleeding precautions.

7. The nurse would expect to find which symptoms in a client who has hemophilia?
   1 Muscle pain and vomiting.
   2 Joint pain and bleeding.
   3 Nausea and fever.
   4 Petechiae and tachycardia.

8. A client is being treated with epoetin alfa (**Epogen**). The nurse would explain to the client that the purpose of the medication is to:
   1 Decrease the availability of prothrombin to decrease bleeding episodes.
   2 Enhance the effectiveness of the chemotherapy medications.
   3 Provide increased availability of iron.
   4 Increase production of red blood cells.

9. The nurse is caring for a client with a hemoglobin level of 8.2 gm/dl. What are important nursing measures?
   1 Increase fluids and ambulate 3 times a day.
   2 Assess for tachycardia; keep warm.
   3 Monitor for bleeding tendencies.
   4 Assess for bradycardia and fever.

10. A child is recovering from a sickle cell crisis. To promote health in this child after discharge, what is important for the nurse to discuss with the parents?
    1 Maintain good hydration status.
    2 Avoid active virus vaccinations.
    3 Avoid contact with peers.
    4 Increase intake of high-calorie foods.

11. Which client would the nurse identify as being at increased risk for development of an iron-deficiency anemia?
    1 An older client receiving radiation therapy weekly.
    2 A client with a history of peptic ulcer disease.
    3 A 2-year-old child with a high milk intake.
    4 A teenager in a sickle cell crisis.

12. A child has a severe laceration on his finger that is bleeding profusely. What is the best nursing action?
    1 Put an ice bag on the finger.
    2 Apply pressure at the site.
    3 Apply pressure at the brachial artery.
    4 Prepare an injection of vitamin K.

13. A client has been placed on bleeding precautions. What is important to include in the nursing care?
    1 Evaluate daily lab values to determine clotting factors.
    2 Discourage flossing and encourage use of a soft toothbrush.
    3 Encourage increased intake of iron-rich foods.
    4 Catheterize the client to determine renal bleeding.

14. The nurse is caring for an older client with leukemia. He is experiencing bleeding into his knees. What is the best nursing care regarding joint mobility and activity?
    1 Encourage walking around the unit every 2 hours.
    2 Gently move each leg through active range-of-motion exercises.
    3 Place warm packs on the joints to promote mobility.
    4 Keep the joints immobilized and maintain bed rest.

15. A client has been diagnosed with pernicious anemia. What will the nurse discuss with the client regarding the vitamin B_{12} he will be prescribed when he is discharged?
    1 He will need to have monthly injections of vitamin B_{12}.
    2 He will need to take the medication with milk.
    3 He should decrease his intake of leafy, green vegetables that are high in vitamin K.
    4 It will be important for him to have weekly lab studies to evaluate the medication.

16. A client is experiencing a problem with epistaxis. What is the first nursing action?
    1 Apply pressure to the nose and have the client lean forward.
    2 Hold the client's head back and put ice on the nose.
    3 Position the client supine and check the blood pressure.
    4 Encourage clear liquids and observe for nausea.

Answers and rationales to these questions are in the section at the end of the book titled Chapter Study Questions: Answers and Rationales.

Appendix 9-1 HEMATOLOGIC DIAGNOSTICS

TEST	NORMAL	CLINICAL AND NURSING IMPLICATIONS

Bone marrow aspiration or biopsy	All formed cell elements within normal range (erythrocytes, leukocytes, and platelets).	1. Evaluates presence, absence, or ratio of cells characteristic of a suspected disease (e.g., hematopoiesis pathology, chromosomal abnormalities).
		2. Preferable site is posterior iliac crest.
		3. Client preparation:
		  a. Local anesthetic is used, as well as analgesics or conscious sedation.
		  b. Feeling of pressure when bone marrow is entered; pain occurs as marrow is being withdrawn.
		4. After test:
		  a. Observe for bleeding at site.
		  b. Apply pressure to site 5 to 10 minutes or longer if client is thrombocytopenic.
		  c. Bed rest for approximately 30 min afterward.
		  d. Analgesics as indicated.
		  e. Monitor for infection.

Sickle cell test **(SICKLEDEX)**	No hemoglobin S present.	1. Routine screening test for sickle cell trait or disorder; does not distinguish between them. 2. False-negative result in infants less than 3 months. 3. False-positive result can occur for up to 4 months after a transfusion of RBCs that are positive for the trait.

COMPLETE BLOOD COUNT

Platelets	150,000-400,000/mm³	1. Decreased platelets (thrombocytopenia) associated with bleeding.
RBC count	4.0-6.0 million/mm³	1. Decreased in clients with bone marrow depression and anemias.
Hemoglobin	Female: 12-16 g/dl Male: 14-18 g/dl Newborn: 14-20 g/dl	1. Components of the RBC responsible for oxygen transport. 2. Decreased in anemias, chronic and acute blood loss, and bone marrow depression.
Hematocrit	Female: 37%-47% Male: 40%-54% Newborn: 52%-62%	1. Values reflect the volume of RBCs found in 100 mL of whole blood. 2. Low levels in anemias, bone marrow depression. 3. An effective indicator of hydration status. An increase in hematocrit may be indicative of a decrease in fluid volume, resulting in hemoconcentration.
WBC count	Adults: 5000-10,000/mm³ Child (2 years): 6000-17,000/mm³	1. White blood cells are an important component in the body's defense against infection. 2. Elevated levels (leukocytosis) are associated with infection. 3. Decreased levels (leukopenia) are associated with diseases of the blood and bone marrow depression.

Appendix 9-2 HEMATOLOGIC MEDICATIONS

MEDICATIONS	SIDE EFFECTS	NURSING IMPLICATIONS

IRON PREPARATIONS REPLACEMENT

MEDICATIONS	SIDE EFFECTS	NURSING IMPLICATIONS

Ferrous fumarate (**Feostat, Span 77, FEM Iron**): IM, PO
 	
Ferrous gluconate (**Fergon, Ferralet**): PO
 	
Ferrous sulfate (**Feosol, Fer-In-Sol**): PO
	GI irritation
	Nausea
	Constipation
	Toxic reactions:
	  Fever
	  Urticaria
		1. Absorbed better on empty stomach; however, may give with meals if GI upset occurs.
		2. Liquid preparations should be diluted and given through a straw to prevent staining of the teeth.
		3. Tell client stool may be black and iron may cause constipation.
		4. Eggs, milk, cheese, and antacids inhibit oral iron absorption.
		5. Iron preparations inhibit oral tetracycline absorption. IM/IV preparations may be used if on oral tetracycline.

Iron dextran injection (**InFeD, Dexferrum**): IV, IM		1. Anaphylactic reaction can occur; test dose should be given. 2. IM should be avoided because of pain and tissue discoloration. 3. If given IM, use Z-track method to prevent tissue staining. 4. IV route recommended if oral route is not acceptable.

VITAMIN K NECESSARY FOR NORMAL PROTHROMBIN ACTIVITY

MEDICATIONS	SIDE EFFECTS	NURSING IMPLICATIONS
Vitamin K: phytonadione (**AquaMEPHYTON**): PO, subQ, IM, IV	GI upset, rash IV not recommended because of hypersensitivity reactions	1. PO and subQ most common routes. 2. Antidote for **Coumadin**. 3. Observe bleeding precautions.

GI, Gastrointestinal; *IM*, intramuscularly; *IV*, intravenously; *PO*, by mouth (orally); *SQ*, subcutaneously.

Appendix 9-3   GUIDELINES FOR MONITORING BLOOD TRANSFUSIONS

General Nursing Implications

- The practical nurse should be familiar with the Nurse Practice Act of the individual state and hospital policies regarding the administration of blood and blood products.
- When blood is brought to the client care unit from the blood bank, it should be started immediately. Blood should never be stored in a unit refrigerator or allowed to sit at room temperature.
- Never add any medication to blood products or to the infusion line of a blood product.
- The usual rate of infusion in an adult is 1 unit of blood over 3 to 4 hours, depending on the condition of the client. *The RN should set the initial rate.*
- Determine if the client has a history of allergy, specifically a previous reaction to transfused blood.
- Baseline vital signs must be obtained immediately before starting the infusion. *Notify the RN if the client's temperature is above 101° F or increases more than 2° F, or if any other vital signs have changed significantly from previous readings.* Check vital signs every hour during and 1 hour after transfusion.
- The client is most likely to experience a reaction during the first 50 mL of blood infused (approximately the first 15 minutes). Monitor for reaction.
- Blood deteriorates rapidly after exposure to room temperature. Blood should not hang longer than 4 hours.

 TEST ALERT: *Monitor the administration of blood or blood products.*

TRANSFUSION REACTIONS

TYPE OF TRANSFUSION REACTION	NURSING MANAGEMENT
Hemolytic Transfusion Reaction 1. Low back pain 2. Hypotension, tachycardia, tachypnea 3. Apprehension, sense of impending doom 4. Fever, chills, flushing 5. Chest pain 6. Dyspnea 7. Onset is immediate	1. *Stop transfusion immediately and notify RN or physician.* 2. Change the IV tubing; do not allow blood in the tubing to infuse into the client; maintain IV access. 3. Obtain first-voided urine specimen to test for blood in the urine. 4. Anticipate blood samples to be drawn by the lab. 5. With suspected renal involvement, treatment with diuretics is initiated to promote diuresis.
Allergic Reaction 1. Urticaria (hives) 2. Pruritus 3. Facial flushing 4. Severe shortness of breath, bronchospasm	1. If client has a history of allergic reactions, antihistamines may be given before starting the transfusion. 2. *Stop transfusion until status of reaction can be determined by the RN or physician; if symptoms are mild and transient, the transfusion may be resumed.*
Febrile Reaction 1. Chills and fever 2. Headache, flushing 3. Muscle stiffness/pain 4. Increased anxiety	1. Keep client covered and warm during transfusion. 2. *Stop the transfusion until status of reaction can be determined by the RN or physician.* 3. Transfusion with leukocyte-poor RBCs or frozen washed packed cells may prevent this reaction in clients susceptible to fever. 4. Most common reaction.

Appendix 9-4 HEMATOPOIETIC STEM CELL TRANSPLANT*

❖ **Goal:** To restore hematologic and immunologic function in clients with immunologic deficiencies, leukemia, congenital or acquired anemias.

PROCEDURE

In the adult client, approximately 400 to 800 mL of bone marrow or harvested stem cells are processed and transfused into the client. (See Appendix 9-1 for care of donor client for bone marrow aspiration.)

COMPLICATIONS

1. Bacterial, viral, or fungal infection from immunosuppressed state.
2. Severe thrombocytopenia resulting in bleeding problems.
3. Rejection of the transplant.

NURSING IMPLICATIONS

1. Preparation of the client for immunosuppression with chemotherapy and radiation therapy.
2. Successful engraftment is indicated by formation of erythrocytes, leukocytes, and platelets, usually 2 to 5 weeks after transplantation.
3. Care of the immunosuppressed client (see Chapter 2).

* *Includes bone marrow transplant and stem cell transplant.*

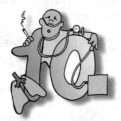

Respiratory System

* The respiratory unit focuses on conditions that interfere with gas exchange. When problems of gas exchange occur, regardless of the precipitating cause, a hypoxic state is frequently the result. A thorough understanding of hypoxia and appropriate nursing interventions for the hypoxic client is necessary for an understanding of the disease processes and ensuing nursing interventions.

PHYSIOLOGY OF THE RESPIRATORY SYSTEM

Organs of the Respiratory System

A. Larynx.
   1. Lies in the middle of the neck.
   2. Controls airflow and prevents foreign objects from entering the airway.
   3. Vocal cords are located in the lower aspect of the larynx.
   4. Glottis: the opening of the vocal cords and the narrowest portion of the laryngeal cavity.
   5. Epiglottis: the area immediately above the glottis.
B. Trachea.
   1. Extends from the larynx downward into the thoracic cavity.
   2. Contains cartilage rings to maintain the patency of the airway to the lungs.
C. Bronchial tree (Figure 10-1).
   1. Trachea divides below the carina into the right and left main stem bronchi, which extend into the lungs.
   2. The right main stem bronchus is shorter, wider, and straighter than the left; therefore foreign objects are more likely to enter the right side.
D. Lungs (organs of respiration).
   1. Divided into lobes.
      a. Right lung: three lobes.
      b. Left lung: two lobes.
   2. Each terminal bronchiole branches into respiratory bronchioles.
   3. The alveolar ducts are located at the end of the respiratory bronchioles.
   4. Alveoli: area of gas exchange; diffusion of O2 and CO_2 between the blood and the lungs occurs across the alveolar membrane.
   5. Surfactant is produced in the alveoli; primary functions are to facilitate alveolar expansion and to decrease tendency of alveoli to collapse.

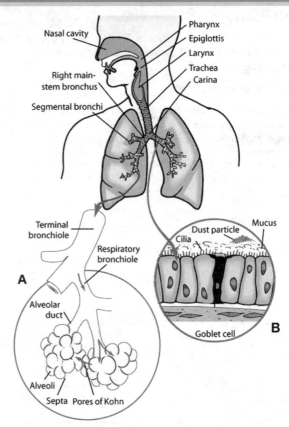

FIGURE 10-1 **Respiratory system.** (From Lewis SL et al: *Medical-surgical nursing: assessment and management of clinical problems,* ed 7, St. Louis, 2007, Mosby.)

   6. Premature infants may have inadequate production of surfactant.
   7. Blood supply to the lungs.
      a. Pulmonary arteries to pulmonary capillaries to alveoli, where exchange of gas occurs.
      b. Bronchial arteries supply the nutrients to the lung tissue and do not participate in gas exchange.

Physiology of Respiration

External respiration is a process by which gas is exchanged between the circulating blood and the inhaled air.

A. Atmospheric pressure: pressure exerted on all body parts by surrounding air.
B. Intrathoracic pressure: pressure within the pleural cavity.

C. Gases flow from an area of high pressure to an area of low pressure; pressure below atmospheric pressure is designated as negative pressure.

D. Inspiration.
1. Stimulus to the diaphragm and the intercostal muscles by way of the central nervous system (CNS).
2. As the diaphragm expands and the chest rises, a negative pressure is created within the lungs.
3. Through the open airways, the lungs are exposed to atmospheric pressure. Air will flow into the lungs to equalize intrathoracic pressure with atmospheric pressure.

E. Expiration.
1. Diaphragm and intercostal muscles relax and return to a resting position; therefore lungs recoil and capacity is decreased.
2. Air will flow out until intrathoracic pressure is again equal to atmospheric pressure.

F. Compliance describes how elastic the lungs are or how easily the lungs can be inflated; when compliance is decreased, the lungs are more difficult to inflate.

G. Control of respiration.
1. Movement of the diaphragm and accessory muscles of respiration is controlled by the respiratory center located in the brainstem (medulla oblongata and pons). The respiratory center will control respirations by way of the spinal cord and phrenic nerve. The diaphragm and intercostal muscles are innervated by the nerves that originate from the spinal cord.
2. The medulla contains the central chemoreceptors responsive to changes in CO_2 blood levels. Increased CO_2 is the normal mechanism stimulating breathing.

> **NURSING PRIORITY:** *In normal clients, when the Paco$_2$ is increased, ventilation is initiated.*

3. Carotid and aortic bodies contain the peripheral chemoreceptors for arterial O_2 levels.
   a. Primary function is to monitor arterial O_2 levels and stimulate the respiratory center when a decrease in Pao$_2$ occurs.
   b. When arterial O_2 concentration decreases to below 60 mm Hg, stimulation to breathe is initiated by the chemoreceptors.
   c. In a person whose primary stimulus to breathe is hypoxia, the receptors in the carotid and aortic bodies that are sensitive to oxygen levels then become the mechanism for control of ventilation.

H. The process of gas exchange.
1. Ventilation: the process of moving air between the atmosphere and alveoli.
2. Diffusion.
   a. The process of moving O_2 and CO_2 across the alveolar capillary membrane.
   b. Gas diffuses across the alveolar capillary membrane from an area of high concentration to an area of low concentration.

> **NURSING PRIORITY:** *Retained mucus that pools in the lung will decrease diffusion as well as provide a reservoir for bacteria and infection.*

3. Perfusion.
   a. The process of linking the venous blood flow to the alveoli.
   b. Dependent on the volume of blood flowing from the right ventricle into and through the pulmonary circulation.

> **TEST ALERT:** *Integrate knowledge of biological sciences in caring for clients.*

Oxygen and Carbon Dioxide Transport

Internal respiration is the exchange of gases between the blood and interstitial fluid. The gases are measured by an analysis of arterial blood.

A. O_2.
1. Transported as a dissolved gas; Pao$_2$ refers to the partial pressure of O_2 in arterial blood.
2. O_2 is bound to hemoglobin; when hemoglobin leaves the pulmonary capillary bed, it is usually 95% to 100% saturated with O_2. It may be referred to as the arterial oxygen saturation (Sao$_2$).
3. Oxygenated hemoglobin moves through the arterial system into the cellular capillary bed, where O_2 is released from the hemoglobin and made available for cellular metabolism.
4. Venous blood contains about 75% O_2 as it returns to the right side of the heart.
5. O_2 delivered to the tissue is dependent on cardiac output.

B. Hemoglobin binds with O_2 in an alkaline condition; hemoglobin releases O_2 more rapidly in an acidotic state.

C. A decrease in the arterial O_2 tension (Pao$_2$) and a decrease in the saturation of the hemoglobin with oxygen (Sao$_2$) results in a state of hypoxemia.

D. Effects of altitude on oxygen transport
1. At high altitudes (above 10,000 feet), there is reduced O_2 in the atmosphere, resulting in a lower inspired O_2 pressure and a lower Pao$_2$. Commercial planes are pressurized to an altitude of 8000 feet.

> **NURSING PRIORITY:** *Clients who require supplemental oxygen should consult with their physician before planning air travel.*

TABLE 10-1	CONSIDERATIONS IN THE RESPIRATORY ASSESSMENT OF THE OLDER ADULT CLIENT
BODY CHANGES	**RESPIRATORY CHANGES**
Kyphosis	Decreased ability to cough and deep breathe effectively
Decreased chest expansion	Decreased O_2 levels, increased risk for atelectasis
Decreased ability to handle secretions	Increased risk for aspiration, atelectasis and pneumonia
Decreased chest expansion	Decreased oxygenation, increased risk for hypoventilation
Altered pulmonary function	Decreased breath sounds, deceased vital capacity, increased residual volume
Decreased/impaired immune response	Increased risk of pulmonary infections

2. The body will increase in the number of red blood cells, thereby increasing the total hemoglobin-carrying and O_2-carrying capacity of the blood.
3. Renal erythropoietic factor (erythropoietin) is released, thereby enhancing the production of red blood cells (secondary polycythemia). It takes approximately 4 to 5 days to actually increase red blood cell production.

 ### System Data Collection

A. History.
   1. Status of immunizations.
      a. Tuberculin (TB) skin test (also known as PPD or Mantoux test).
      b. Determine status of childhood vaccinations.
      c. Adult - tetanus, pneumococcal pneumonia vaccine (Pneumovax).
   3. History of medication use - including OTC, prescriptions, herbs, and vitamins.
   4. Lifestyle and occupational environments.
   5. Tobacco use and alcohol intake.
B. Physical data collection.(Table 10-1)

> ✔ **NURSING PRIORITY:** *Identify progressive changes in respiratory status; primary indicators of respiratory disorders are sputum production, cough, dyspnea, hemoptysis, pleuritic chest pain, fatigue and changes in breath sounds.*

1. Observe client's resting position.
   a. Does client appear comfortable and not in distress?
   b. Determine client's respiratory status in the sitting position if possible.
   c. Is there any dyspnea or respiratory discomfort?

> ✔ **NURSING PRIORITY:** *If there is evidence of respiratory difficulty, keep client at rest in sitting position or in semi-Fowlers position, begin oxygen and request assistance.*

   d. Assess upper airway passages and patency of the airway.
2. Evaluate vital signs.
   a. Are vital signs appropriate for age level?
   b. Establish database and compare with previous data.
   c. Assess client's overall response, pattern of vital signs; normal vital signs vary greatly from one individual to another (see Table 3-1).
3. Inspect the neck for symmetry; determine if the trachea is in midline and observe for presence of jugular vein distention.
4. Assess the lungs.
   a. Visually evaluate the chest/thorax.
      (1) Do both sides move equally?
      (2) Observe characteristics of respirations and note whether retractions are present on the chest wall.
      (3) Note chest wall configuration (barrel chest, kyphoscoliosis, etc.).
      (4) Are retractions present on the chest wall?
   b. Palpate chest for tenderness, masses, and symmetry of motion.
   c. Auscultate breath sounds; begin at lung apices and end at the bases, comparing each area side to side. Breath sounds should be present and equal bilaterally.
   d. Determine presence of adventitious breath sounds (abnormal/extra breath sounds).
      (1) Crackles: usually heard during inspiration and do not clear with cough; occur when airway contains fluid (previously also known as *rales*).
      (2) Wheezes: may be heard during inspiration and/or expiration; are caused by air moving through narrowed passages; sound is music-like and continuous.
5. Assess cough reflex and sputum production.
   a. Is cough associated with pain?
   b. What precipitates coughing episodes?
   c. Is cough productive or nonproductive?
   d. Characteristics of sputum.
      (1) Consistency.
      (2) Amount.

(3) Color (should be clear or white).
   e. Presence of hemoptysis.
6. Assess for abnormal respiratory pattern.
   a. Hyperventilation: increased rate and depth of respirations often associated with loss of CO_2.
   b. Tachypnea: rapid, shallow breathing that may be associated with CO_2 retention.
   c. Bradyphnea: slow, regular breathing; may be induced by anesthetic or narcotics.
   d. Cheyne-Stokes: episodes of apnea alternating with hyperventilation.
   e. Kussmaul's respiration: rapid, deep breathing associated with metabolic acidosis (diabetic acidosis).
7. Assess for and evaluate dyspnea.
   a. Onset of dyspnea and precipitating causes.
   b. Presence of orthopnea.
   c. Presence of adventitious breath sounds.
   d. Noisy expiration.
   e. Level of tolerance of activity.
   f. Correlate with vital signs, pulse oximetry and arterial blood gases.
   g. Cyanosis (a very late and unreliable sign of hypoxia).
      (1) For dark-skinned clients, assess the areas that are less pigmented (oral cavity, nail beds, lips, palms).
      (2) Dark-skinned clients may exhibit cyanosis in the skin as a gray hue, rather than blue.
8. Assess for and evaluate chest pain.
   a. Location of pain.
   b. Character of pain.
   c. Pain associated with cough.
   d. Pain either increased or decreased with breathing.
9. Evaluate fingers for clubbing (characteristic in clients with chronic respiratory disorders).
10. Evaluate pulmonary diagnostics (see Appendix 10-1).
   a. Hemoglobin and hematocrit (presence of polycythemia or anemia).
   b. Electrolyte imbalances.
   c. Arterial blood gases (ABGs, Table 10-2).
   d. Status of pulse oximetry (S_{PO_2}) (Appendix 10-1)

> **TEST ALERT:** *Modify client's care based on the results of diagnostic/lab tests.*

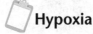

Hypoxia

* **Hypoxia is a condition characterized by an inadequate amount of oxygen available for cellular metabolism.**

> ✓ **NURSING PRIORITY:** *Problems with respiratory status occur in all nursing disciplines. Questions may center around nursing priorities and nursing interventions in maintaining an airway and promoting ventilation in the client with respiratory difficulty. The questions may arise from any client situation (e.g., obstetrics, newborn, surgical, etc.)*

A. Hypoxemia: decreased oxygen saturation of the blood.
B. Hypoxia may be caused by inadequate circulation.
   1. Shock.
   2. Cardiac failure.
C. Anemia precipitates hypoxia caused by a decrease in the O_2-carrying capacity of the blood.
   1. Inadequate red blood cell production.
   2. Deficient or abnormal hemoglobin.

Data Collection

A. Risk factors/etiology.
   1. Chronic hypoxia.
      a. Chronic obstructive pulmonary disease (COPD).
      b. Cystic fibrosis.
      c. Cancer of the respiratory tract.
      d. Heart failure.
      e. Chronic anemia.
   2. Inflammatory problems affecting alveolar surface area and membrane integrity (e.g., pneumonia, bronchitis).
   3. Acute hypoxia.
      a. Acute respiratory failure.
      b. Sudden airway obstruction.
      c. Conditions affecting pulmonary expansion (e.g., respiratory paralysis).

TABLE 10-2	NORMAL ARTERIAL BLOOD GAS VALUES	
Acidity index	pH	7.35-7.45
Partial pressure of dissolved oxygen	PaO_2	80 to 100 mm Hg
Percentage of hemoglobin saturated with oxygen	SaO_2	95% or above
Partial pressure of dissolved carbon dioxide	$PaCO_2$	35 to 45 mm Hg
Bicarbonate	HCO_3-	22 to 28 mEq/L

> ✓ **NURSING PRIORITY:** *An SaO_2 below 95% is indicative of poor ventilation and requires immediate nursing action.*

    d. Conditions causing decreased cardiac output (heart failure, shock, cardiac arrest, etc.).

    e. Hypoventilation (brain attack or stroke, sedation, anesthesia, etc.).

B. Clinical manifestations: underlying respiratory problem, either chronic or acute (Table 10-3).

C. Diagnostics: see Appendix 10-1.
1. Arterial blood gases.
2. Pulse oximetry.
3. Hemoglobin and hematocrit levels.

Nursing Interventions

❖ **Goal:** To maintain good pulmonary hygiene and prevent hypoxic episode.

A. Position client to maintain patent airway.
1. Unconscious client: position on side with the chin extended, and head slightly elevated.
2. Conscious client: elevate the head of the bed and may position on side as well.

B. Encourage effective coughing and deep breathing (Box 10-1).

C. Suction client's secretions as needed and as indicated by amount of sputum and ability to cough.

D. Maintain adequate fluid intake to keep secretions liquefied, 3000 to 4000mL daily (unless contraindicated by cardiac or renal problems).

E. Encourage exercises and ambulation as indicated by condition.

F. Administer expectorants.

G. Administer O_2 if dyspnea is present.

H. Prevent aspiration (Box 10-3).

> **TEST ALERT: Implement measures to manage/ prevent possible complications of a client condition or procedure (aspiration).**

BOX 10-1	EFFECTIVE COUGHING

- Increase activity before coughing: walking or turning from side to side.
- Place client in sitting position, preferably with feet on the floor.
- Client should turn his or her shoulders inward and bend head slightly forward.
- Take a gentle breath in through the nose and breathe out completely.
- Take two deep breaths through the nose and mouth and hold for 5 seconds.
- On the third deep breath, cough to clear secretions.
- Sips of warm liquids (coffee, tea, or water) may stimulate coughing.
- Demonstrate to client how to splint chest or incision during cough to decrease pain.

> ✔ **NURSING PRIORITY:** *Effective coughing is the most effective nursing care to prevent and or treat problems with respiratory acidosis.*

❖ **Goal:** To assess and implement nursing measures appropriate to current level of hypoxia.

A. Assess patency of airway (first/highest priority).
1. Can client speak? If not, initiate emergency procedures (see Appendix 10-3).
2. If speaking is difficult because of level of hypoxia, place in semi-Fowler's position, begin oxygen, obtain assistance, and remain with client.
3. If client is able to speak in sentences and is coherent, continue with assessment of the problem.
4. Evaluate amount of secretions and ability to cough; suction and administer O_2 as indicated.

B. Assess use of accessory muscles, presence of retractions.

TABLE 10-3	SYMPTOMS OF RESPIRATORY DISTRESS AND HYPOXIA

EARLY SYMPTOMS	LATE SYMPTOMS
Restlessness	Extreme restlessness to stupor
Tachycardia	Severe dyspnea
Tachypnea, exertional dyspnea	Slowing of respiratory rate
Orthopnea, tripod positioning	Bradycardia
Anxiety, difficulty speaking	Cyanosis (peripheral or central)
Poor judgment, confusion	
Disorientation	
PEDIATRICS	
Flaring nares (infants)	Mottling, pallor, and cyanosis
Substernal, suprasternal, supraclavicular and intercostal retractions (see Figure 10-2)	Sudden increase or sudden decrease in agitation
	Decrease in breath sounds
Stridor—expiratory and inspiratory	Altered level of consciousness
Increased agitation	Inability to cry or to speak

BOX 10-2 OLDER ADULT CARE FOCUS
RESPIRATORY CARE PRIORITIES

- Provide adequate rest periods between activities, such as bathing, going for treatments, eating, etc.
- Encourage client to eat sitting up to decrease problems with aspiration.
- Increase compliance with medications by scheduling medication administration with routine activities.
- Keep chairs and other supports for client within easy reach when ambulating.
- Encourage annual flu shot for individuals over age 65 and determine whether older adult has received pneumococcal vaccination.
- Evaluate client's response to changes in activity and therapy frequently.
- Maintain adequate hydration but use caution because of increased tendency for fluid volume overload.
- Older adult client may not present with respiratory symptoms, but instead with confusion and disorientation.

C. Maintain calm approach, because increasing anxiety will potentiate hypoxia. Remain with the client who is experiencing severe dyspnea and call for assistance.

> **NURSING PRIORITY:** *Position a dyspneic client in semi-Fowler's or high Fowler's. A pillow placed lengthwise behind the client's back and head may increase comfort; do not flex the client's head backward or forward.*

D. Place adult or older child in a semi-Fowler's position, if not contraindicated.
E. Place infant in an infant seat or elevate the mattress.
   a. Cyanosis that increased with crying is usually of a cardiac origin, cyanosis that decreases with crying is usually a respiratory origin.
   b. Cyanosis may be present in the mucous membranes in the mouth or the inner aspect of the lips and gum.
F. Assess client's color, presence of retractions and presence of diaphoresis.
G. Evaluate vital signs: Are there significant changes from previous readings?
H. Assess for tachycardia.
I. Evaluate chest movements: Are they symmetrical?
J. Evaluate anterior and posterior breath sounds.
K. Assess client for chest pain with dyspnea.
L. Report findings that indicate respiratory compromise.
M. Assess response to O_2 therapy.
N. Monitor levels and changes in pulse oximetry.

> **NURSING PRIORITY:** *Administer fluids very cautiously to a client who is having difficulty breathing. Begin with small sips of water to determine whether the client can swallow effectively—thickened liquids are easier to control. Do not begin with fluids that contain any fat (milk) or caloric value because of the increased risk for aspiration.*

BOX 10-3 PREVENTION OF ASPIRATION

CLIENTS AT HIGH RISK FOR ASPIRATION
- Stroke/brain accident client with facial and tongue weakness.
- Postoperative laryngectomy.
- Tracheotomy.
- Seizures.
- Increased sedation after surgery.
- Older adult clients without their dentures.
- Infants with facial or palate birth defects.
- After a procedure that requires depression of gag reflex: gastroscopy and bronchoscopy.

PREVENTION OF ASPIRATION
- Have suction equipment available.
- Position in semi-Fowler's to high-Fowler's for eating or for tube feedings.
- Put client's dentures in.
- Place food on unaffected side of face (CVA).
- Do not rush client; allow adequate time to chew and swallow.
- Remove drinking straws unless otherwise indicated.
- Encourage thick liquids and soft foods.
- Examine client's mouth for residual food.
- Maintain client in semi-Fowler's to high-Fowler's position for 30 minutes after eating.

Pneumothorax

* **Air in the pleural space results in the collapse or atelectasis of that portion of the lung, which results in a *pneumothorax*.**

* **Tension pneumothorax: the development of a pneumothorax that allows excessive buildup of air and pressure in the pleural space.**

- Causes a shift of the trachea out of the sternal notch to the unaffected side.
- A tension pneumothorax can rapidly become an emergency situation.

Data Collection

A. Risk factors/etiology.
   1. Ruptured bleb (spontaneous).
   2. Thoracentesis.
   3. Infection.
   4. Trauma (penetrating or blunt chest injury).
B. Clinical manifestations.
   1. Dyspnea, hypoxia.
   2. Tachycardia, tachypnea.
   3. Sudden, sharp pleural chest pain, especially on inspiration.
   4. Anxiety with increasing restlessness.
   5. Asymmetrical chest wall expansion.
   6. Diminished or absent breath sounds on the affected side.
   7. Possible development of a tension pneumothorax.
       a. Decreased cardiac filling, leading to decreased cardiac output.
       b. Tracheal shift from midline toward unaffected side.
       c. Increasing problems of hypoxia.
C. Diagnostics: see Appendix 10-1.

> ✓ **NURSING PRIORITY:** *When atmospheric pressure is allowed to disrupt the negative pressure in the pleural space, it will cause the lung to collapse. This requires chest tube placement to reestablish negative pressure and reinflate the lung.*

Treatment

Placement of chest tubes connected to a water-sealed drainage system (see Appendix 10-4 and Figure 10-6).

Nursing Interventions

❖ **Goal:** To recognize the problem and prevent a severe hypoxic episode (see Hypoxia, Nursing Interventions).
A. Report deterioration of client's respiratory status.
B. Maintain client on bed rest in semi–Fowler's position and begin O_2 therapy.
❖ **Goal:** To reinflate lung without complications.
A. Have client cough and deep-breathe every 2 hours.
B. Encourage exercise and ambulation.
C. Establish and maintain water-sealed chest drainage system (see Appendix 10-4).

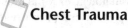 **Chest Trauma**

＊ **An open or "sucking" chest wound is frequently caused by a penetrating injury to the chest.**

> ✓ **NURSING PRIORITY:** *If a chest tube is inadvertently pulled out of the chest, a sucking chest wound may be created.*

Data Collection

A. Clinical manifestations.
   a. Dyspnea and development of hypoxia.
   b. A chest wound with evidence of air moving in and out via the wound.
   c. Flail chest is the loss of stability of the chest wall with respiratory impairment as a result of multiple rib fractures on the same side.
B. Treatment.
   a. Prepare for insertion of chest tubes to water-sealed drainage system.

Data Collection

A. Paradoxical respirations: the movement of the fractured area (flailed segment) inward during inspiration and outward during expiration, or opposite to the other areas of the chest wall.
B. Symptoms of hypoxia.
C. Pneumothorax from fractured ribs.
D. Diagnostics.
   1. Chest x-ray film showing multiple rib fractures.
   2. Crepitus of the ribs.

Treatment

   1. O_2.
   2. Endotracheal intubation with mechanical ventilation for severe respiratory distress (see Appendixes 10-5 and 10-9).
   3. Chest tube placement.

Nursing Interventions

❖ **Goal:** To improve ventilation in client with chest trauma.
A. Open chest wound
   1. Have the client take a deep breath, hold it, and bear down against a closed glottis. Apply a light occlusive, vented dressing (taped/secured on three sides to allow air to escape) over the wound.

> ✓ **NURSING PRIORITY:** *Immediately occlude the chest wound; do not leave the client to go find a dressing. If necessary, place a towel or whatever is at hand over the wound to stop the flow of air.*

   2. After covering the wound with a light occlusive dressing, carefully evaluate the client for development of a tension pneumothorax.
B. Chest trauma
   a. Maintain bed rest in semi-Fowlers position.
   b. Ongoing assessment for level of hypoxia.
   c. Assess for development of tension pneumothorax.
   d. Administer analgesics as necessary for pain control.
   e. Anticipate placement of chest tubes.

Pulmonary Embolism

⁎ An obstruction of a pulmonary artery, most often caused by a blood clot (deep vein thrombosis (DVT) or thrombus that becomes mobile, i.e., embolus). May also be caused by air, fat, amniotic fluid, bone marrow, or sepsis.
A. The severity of the problem depends on the size of the embolus.
B. The majority of pulmonary emboli arise from thrombi in the deep veins of the legs.
C. A pulmonary embolism must originate from the venous circulation, or the right side of the heart.

TEST ALERT: Implement measures to manage/ prevent possible complications of a client condition or procedure (circulatory complication).

Data Collection

A. Common risk factors/etiology.
1. Conditions or immobility predisposing to venous stasis and/or deep vein thrombosis: surgery, stroke, spinal cord injury, and prolonged periods of sitting (e.g. airline flights).
2. DVT: the thrombus spontaneously dislodges secondary to jarring of the area—sudden standing, changes in rate of blood flow (Valsalva maneuver, increased BP).
3. Pregnancy, obesity.
4. Fractures of long bones causing a fat embolus.
B. Clinical manifestations.
1. Classic triad of symptoms: dyspnea, chest pain, and hemoptysis occurs in only 20% if clients.
2. Most common symptoms.
   a. Increased anxiety.
   b. Sudden, unexplained dyspnea.
   c. Tachypnea.
   d. Tachycardia.
   e. Hypoxia.
3. Hypotension and syncope.
4. May result in sudden death if pulmonary embolism is large.
C. Diagnostics: see Appendix 10-1.

Treatment

A. Bed rest, semi-Fowler's position if BP permits.
B. Respiratory support: O₂, possibly assisted ventilation.
C. Anticoagulants (heparin, low-molecular-weight heparin, or warfarin) to prevent further thrombus formation.
D. IV access for fluids and medications to maintain blood pressure.
E. Small doses of morphine sulfate may be used to decrease anxiety, alleviate chest pain, or improve tolerance to endotracheal tube.
F. Thrombolytics.

NURSING PRIORITY: It is far easier to prevent the problem of pulmonary embolism than it is to treat it. Identify clients at increased risk for developing PE and initiate preventive measures.

Nursing Interventions

❖ Goal: To identify clients at increased risk and prevent and/or decrease venous stasis (see Box 11-3).
A. Older adults are at increase risk of DVT.
B. Clients that are at high risk.
1. Orthopedic surgery, knee and hip replacements.
2. Clients with fractures of long bones.
3. Clients requiring bed rest (cardiac, stroke).
C. Prevention of DVT – (see Chapter 11, Box 11-3).
❖ Goal: To identify problem and implement nursing measures to alleviate hypoxia (see Hypoxia, Nursing Interventions).
❖ Goal: To monitor client's respiratory function and response to treatment.

 Croup Syndromes

⁎ The term croup describes a group of conditions characterized by edema and inflammation of the upper respiratory tract.
A. Acute epiglottitis: a severe infection of the epiglottis, characterized by rapid inflammation and edema of the area.
1. Generally occurs in children 2 to 7 years old; may rapidly cause airway obstruction.
2. Cause: most commonly Haemophilus influenza type B.
3. Clinical manifestations: hypoxia (see Table 10-3).
   a. Rapid, abrupt onset.
   b. Sore throat, difficulty in swallowing.
   c. Symptoms of increasing respiratory tract obstruction.
      (1) Characteristic position: sitting with the neck hyperextended (sniffing position) and mouth open (tripod position), drooling.
      (2) Inspiratory stridor (crowing).
      (3) Retractions – intercostal, suprasternal and substernal. (Fig 10-2).
      (4) Increased restlessness and apprehension.
   d. High fever (above 102° F).

NURSING PRIORITY: The presence of drooling with the absence of spontaneous cough are very distinctive symptoms of epiglottitis.

4. Treatment.
   a. Humidified oxygen.
   b. Antibiotics.
   c. Endotracheal intubation for obstruction (see Appendix 10-5).

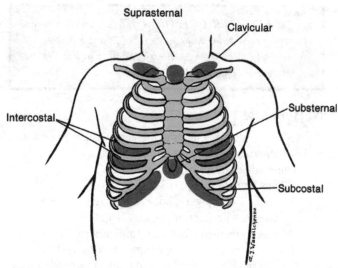

FIGURE 10-2 **Location of retractions.** (From Hockenberry MJ, Wilson D: *Wong's nursing care of infants and children*, 8th ed, St. Louis, 2007, Mosby.)

B. Acute laryngotracheobronchitis (croup): inflammation of the vocal cords, subglottal tissue, trachea, bronchi; most often in children ages 6 mo to 5 years.
1. Onset over several days, frequently preceded by upper respiratory tract infection.
2. Respiratory distress (see Table 10-3).
   a. Inspiratory stridor when disturbed, progressing to continuous stridor.
   b. Flaring of nares, use of accessory muscles of respiration.
   c. "Seal bark" cough is classic sign.
3. Low-grade fever (usually below 102° F).
4. Signs of impending obstruction.
   a. Retractions (intercostals, suprasternal, and substernal) at rest.
   b. Increased anxiety and restlessness.
   c. Tachypnea (rate may be above 60 breaths/min).
   d. Pallor and diaphoresis.
   e. Nasal flaring.

> **TEST ALERT: Implement measures to manage/ prevent possible complication of client condition or procedure, intervene to improve client respiratory status by giving a breathing or respiratory treatment, suctioning, or repositioning; notify health care provider of a change in client's condition.**

5. Treatment.
   a. Cool mist humidification.
   b. Oxygen.
   c. IV fluids if child cannot maintain PO intake.
   d. Maintain patent airway.
   e. Bronchodilators, racemic epinephrine (for moderate to severe croup) by inhalation.

f. No sedatives.
g. Corticosteroids, administered intravenously, intramuscularly, or orally.

Nursing Interventions

❖ **Goal:** To maintain patent airway in hospitalized child.
A. Tracheotomy set or endotracheal intubation equipment easily available.

> ✓ *NURSING PRIORITY: Do not examine the throat of a child with epiglottitis, it may precipitate an airway spasm (laryngospasm).*

B. Endotracheal tube or tracheotomy – suction airway only as necessary.
C. Position for comfort; do not force child to lie down.
D. If child is intubated or in severe distress, do not leave unattended.
E. If transport is required, allow the child to sit upright in parent's lap if possible.

❖ **Goal:** To evaluate and maintain adequate ventilation.
A. Assess for increasing hypoxia.
B. Maintain child in humidified O_2.
C. Conserve energy; promote rest and prevent crying.
D. Monitor pulse oximetry for adequate oxygenation.
E. Report symptoms of increasing respiratory difficulty.

> ✓ *NURSING PRIORITY: Early signs of impending airway obstruction are the same as early signs of hypoxia (Table 10-3).*

❖ **Goal:** To maintain hydration and nutrition.
A. Do not give oral fluids until danger of aspiration is past.

> ✓ *NURSING PRIORITY: In children with severe respiratory distress (rate above 60), do not give anything by mouth due to increased risk for aspiration.*

B. Monitor IV fluids during acute episodes.
C. Provide high-calorie liquids when danger of aspiration is over.
D. Suction nares of infant before feeding.
E. Assess for adequate hydration.

Home Care

A. Teach parents to recognize symptoms of increasing respiratory problems and when to notify physician.
B. Cool mist may assist to decrease edema and/or spasms of airway.
C. Maintain adequate fluid intake.
D. Immunization with *H. influenza* type B vaccine.

Respiratory Syncytial Virus (Bronchiolitis)

A. Respiratory syncytial virus (RSV) is most common cause of bronchitis and lower respiratory tract infections in infants and young children.

B. RSV is transmitted by direct contact with respiratory secretions (Appendix 5-9).

Data Collection

A. Cause: usually begins after an upper respiratory tract infection; incubation period of 5-8 days.

B. Reinfection is common; severity tends to decrease with age and repeated infections.

C. Clinical manifestations.
1. Initial.
   a. Rhinorrhea with copious amounts of secretions.
   b. Low-grade fever, coughing, wheezing
2. Acute phase.
   a. Lethargic.
   b. Tachypnea, air hunger, retractions.
   c. Increased wheezing and coughing.
   d. Periods of apnea, poor air exchange

D. Diagnostics: nasal secretions for RSV antigens.

Treatment

A. Rest, fluids, and high-humidity environment.

B. O_2.

C. Prevention – medication (see Appendix 10-2).

Nursing Interventions

❖ **Goal:** To promote effective breathing patterns.

A. Frequent assessment for development of hypoxia (see Box 10-3); close monitoring of O_2 saturation (oximetry) levels.

B. Increase in respiratory rate and audible crackles in the lungs are indications of cardiac failure and should be reported immediately.

C. Maintain airway via position and removal of secretions.

D. Maintain adequate hydration to facilitate removal of respiratory secretions.

E. Respiratory and nasal secretions make it difficult for an infant to bottle feed or to nurse; instill normal saline drops and suction prior to feeding.

F. Conserve energy; avoid unnecessary procedures, but encourage parents to console and cuddle infant.

❖ **Goal:** To prevent transmission of organisms.

A. If hospitalized, the child should be placed in a private room, with contact/standard precautions in place (Appendix 5-9).

B. Decrease number of health care personnel in client's room.

C. Nurses assigned to care for these children should not be assigned the care of other children who are at high risk for respiratory tract infections.

Home Care

A. Decreased energy level; will tire easily.

B. Small frequent feedings, normal saline nose drops prior to feeding.

C. Teach parents how to assess for respiratory difficulty and to report any signs of respiratory difficulty – paroxysmal cough, dyspnea, increased respiratory secretions.

Tonsillitis

✳ **Tonsillitis is an inflammation and infection of the palatine tonsils.**

Data Colletion

A. Risk factors/etiology.
1. More common in children, increased severity in adults.
2. Generally peaks in winter

B. Clinical manifestations.
1. Edematous, enlarged tonsils; exudate on tonsils.
2. Difficulty swallowing and breathing.
3. Frequently precipitates otitis media.
4. Mouth breathing.
5. Persistent cough, fever.

C. Diagnostics: throat culture for group A *beta-hemolytic streptococci*.

Treatment

A. Antibiotic for identified organism.

B. Surgery: tonsillectomy for severe repeated episodes of tonsillitis.

Nursing Interventions

❖ **Goal:** To assist parents to understand disease process and to promote comfort and healing in home environment.

A. Soft or liquid nonirritating diet.

B. Cool mist vaporizer to maintain moisture in mucous membranes.

C. Throat lozenges, warm gargles to soothe the throat.

D. Explain to parents the importance of giving the child all the medication prescribed in order to prevent reoccurrence.

E. Analgesics, antipyretic (acetaminophen).

❖ **Goal:** To provide preoperative nursing measures if surgery is indicated (see Chapter 3).

❖ **Goal:** To maintain patent airway and evaluate for bleeding after tonsillectomy.

A. No fluids until child is fully awake; then cool, clear liquids initially. Avoid brown- or red-colored fluids and milk products.

B. Position child on side or abdomen to facilitate drainage until fully awake; when awake and alert, child may assume position of comfort but should remain in bed for the day.

C. Evaluate for frequent or continuous swallowing, tachycardia and pallor caused by bleeding; check throat with a flashlight.
D. Have nasopharyngeal suction equipment available.
E. Apply ice collar to decrease edema.
F. Discourage coughing.

> ✔ *NURSING PRIORITY: Before the child is fully awake, position him or her on side or abdomen to prevent aspiration from bloody drainage or vomitus. Always consider the client who has had a tonsillectomy to be nauseated as a result of swallowing blood.*

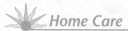Home Care

A. Child will have sore throat for several days; discourage coughing and excessive activity.
B. Bleeding may occur on the 5th to 10th postoperative days, when tissue sloughing may occur as a result of healing and/or infection.
C. Maintain adequate hydration; encourage intake of soft foods and nonirritating fluids.
D. A gray membrane on the sides of the throat is normal; should disappear in 1 to 2 weeks.

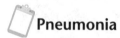 Pneumonia

✱ **Pneumonia is an acute inflammatory process caused by a microbial agent; it involves the lung parenchyma, including the small airways and alveoli. (Figure 10-3)**

Data Collection

A. Predisposing conditions.
 1. Chronic upper respiratory tract infection.
 2. Postoperative
 3. Prolonged immobility.
 4. Smoking.
 5. Decreased immune state (disease and/or age).
 6. Aspiration of foreign material or gastric contents.
 7. Nosocomial pneumonia: caused by tracheal intubation, intestinal/gastric tube feedings.
B. Clinical manifestations.
 1. Fever, chills, tachycardia.
 2. Tachypnea, dyspnea.
 3. Productive cough: thick, blood-streaked, yellow, purulent sputum.
 4. Chest pain.
 5. Malaise, altered mental status.
 6. Respiratory distress (hypoxia) (see Table 10-3).
 7. Diminished breath sounds.
C. Diagnostics: see Appendix 10-1.

> ✔ *OLDER ADULT PRIORITY: An older adult client may initially present with mental confusion and volume depletion rather than respiratory symptoms and fever.*

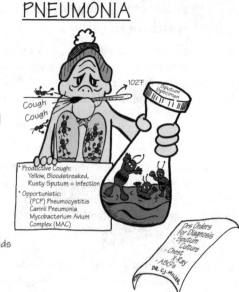

FIGURE 10-3 **Pneumonia.** (From Zerwekh J, Claborn J, Miller CJ: *Memory notebook of nursing,* vol 2, ed 3, Ingram, 2007, Nursing Education Consultants.)

Treatment

A. Antibiotic according to organism identified (see Appendix 5-10).

> ✔ *NURSING PRIORITY: Do not start antibiotics until a good sputum specimen has been collected. An accurate culture and sensitivity test cannot be done if client has already begun receiving antibiotics.*

B. Respiratory precautions: transmitted via airborne droplets (see Appendix 5-9).
C. Inhalation therapy.
 1. Cool O_2 mist.
 2. Postural drainage.
 3. Bronchodilators.
D. Chest physical therapy.

Nursing Interventions

❖ **Goal:** To prevent occurrence.
A. Encourage mobility and ambulation as soon as possible.
B. Good respiratory hygiene; turn, cough, and deep-breathe.
C. Identify high-risk clients.
D. Encourage pneumococcal vaccination.
❖ **Goal:** To decrease infection and remove secretions to facilitate O_2 and CO_2 exchange.
A. Antibiotics.
B. Assist/encourage client to turn, cough, and deep-breathe.
C. Liquefy secretions.

1. Adequate hydration (administer PO fluids cautiously to prevent aspiration).
2. Cool mist inhalation.
D. Evaluate breath sounds and changes in sputum.
E. Position for comfort or semi-Fowler's position.
F. Nursing measures to prevent and evaluate levels of hypoxia (see Hypoxia, Nursing Interventions; also see Table 10-3).
G. Provide adequate pain control measures to facilitate coughing and deep breathing.
H. Droplet/contact with standard precautions, based on identified organism and transmission.
❖ **Goal:** To teach client and family how to provide home care when appropriate.
A. Antibiotics.
B. Cool mist humidification.
C. Maintain high oral fluid intake.
D. Antipyretic: acetaminophen.
E. Encourage activity.
F. Return to primary care provider:
1. Return or increase in fever and chills.
2. Chest pain, hemoptysis.
3. Increase in difficulty breathing.

Tuberculosis

✳ **TB is a reportable communicable disease that is characterized by pulmonary manifestations.**
A. Characteristics.
1. Organism is primarily transmitted through respiratory droplets; it is inhaled and implants on respiratory bronchioles or alveoli; predominately spread by repeated close contact.
2. Characteristic tissue reaction is the formation of a tubercle in the lung, the primary site or tubercle may undergo a process of degeneration or caseation; this area can erode into the bronchial tree, and TB organisms are active and present in the sputum, resulting in further spread of the disease.
3. The tubercle may never erode but may calcify and remain dormant after the primary infection. However, the tubercle may contain living organisms that can be reactivated several years later.
4. The majority of people with a primary infection harbor the TB bacilli in a tubercle in the lungs and will not exhibit any symptoms of an active infection.
5. May occur as an opportunistic infection in clients who are immunocompromised.

Data Collection

A. Predisposing conditions.
1. Frequent close or prolonged contact with infected individual, who frequently has not been diagnosed.
2. Debilitating conditions and diseases.
3. Poor nutrition and crowded living conditions.

B. Cause: *Mycobacterium tuberculosis*, a gram-positive, acid-fast bacillus.
C. Clinical manifestations (up to 20% of clients may be asymptomatic).
1. Fatigue, malaise.
2. Anorexia, weight loss.
3. May have a chronic cough that progresses to more frequent and productive cough.
4. Low-grade fever and night sweats.
5. Hemoptysis is associated only with advanced condition.
6. May present with acute symptoms.
D. Diagnostics (see Appendix 10-1).

✔ **NURSING PRIORITY:** *A positive reaction to a TB skin test means that the person has at some time been infected with the TB bacillus and developed antibodies. It does not mean that the person has an active TB infection.*

---

1. QuantiFERON-TB (QFT) rapid diagnostic: blood test to identify presence of antigens; does not take the place of sputum smears and cultures.
2. Bacteriologic studies to identify acid-fast bacilli in the sputum.
E. Complications.
1. Pleural effusion.
2. Pneumonia.
3. Other organ involvement.

Treatment

A. Chemotherapy (see Appendix 10-2).
1. Medical regimen involves simultaneous administration of two or more medications; this increases the therapeutic effect of medication and decreases development of resistant bacteria.
2. Sputum cultures are evaluated every 2-4 weeks initially; then monthly after sputum is negative. Sputum cultures should be negative within several weeks of beginning therapy, this depends on the medication regimen and the resistance of the bacteria.
3. Direct observed therapy (DOT): health care personnel provide the medications and observe that client swallows medication; preferred strategy for all clients.
4. Prophylaxis chemotherapy
   a. Close contact with a client with a new diagnosis of TB.
   b. Newly infected client with positive skin test reaction.
   c. Client has a positive skin test reaction and is immunocompromised.
   d. Isoniazid (**INH**) most often used for prophylaxis.
B. Most often treated on an outpatient basis.

Nursing Interventions

❖ **Goal:** To understand implications of the disease and measures to protect others and maintain own health.

A. Evaluate client's lifestyle and identify needs regarding compliance with treatment and long-term therapy.

B. Identify community resources available for client.

C. Understand medication schedule and importance of maintaining medication regimen.

   1. Noncompliance is a major contributor to the development of multidrug resistance and treatment failure.

   2. DOT recommended to guarantee compliance; may require client to come to public health clinic for nurse to administer medication.

D. Return for sputum checks every 2 to 4 weeks during therapy.

E. Balanced diet, supplemental vitamins, good hydration.

F. Avoid excessive fatigue; endurance will increase with treatment.

G. Identify family and close contacts who need to report to the public health department for TB screening.

H. Offer client HIV testing.

❖ **Goal:** To prevent transmission of the disease.

A. When sputum is positive for the organism, implement airborne precautions for hospitalized client (see Appendix 5-9).

> 💡 **TEST ALERT: Implement standard precautions; apply infection control measures; use correct equipment to prevent environmental spread of infection.**

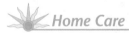 Home Care

A. Teach respiratory precautions.
   1. Cover mouth and nose when sneezing or coughing (Appendix 5-9).
   2. Practice good hand hygiene.
   3. Wear a mask when in contact with other people.
   4. Discard all secretions (nose and mouth) in plastic bags.

B. Re-evaluate periodically for active disease or secondary infection.

Chronic Obstructive Pulmonary Disease

✳ **Chronic obstructive pulmonary disease (COPD) is a group of chronic respiratory disorders characterized by obstruction of airflow.**

Assessment

A. Risk factors/etiology.
   1. Cigarette smoking (including passive smoking)—most common cause.
   2. Chronic infections.
   3. Inhaled irritants (from occupational exposure and air pollution).

B. Clinical manifestations (Figure 10-4).
   1. Distended neck veins, ankle edema.
   2. Orthopnea or tripod positioning, barrel chest.
   3. Prolonged expiratory time, pursed-lip breathing.
   4. Diminished breath sounds.
   5. Thorax is hyperresonant to percussion.
   6. Exertional dyspnea progressing to dyspnea at rest.
   7. Increased respiratory rate.
   8. As a result of a prolonged increase in $Paco_2$ levels, the normal respiratory center in the medulla is affected; when this occurs, hypoxia will become the primary respiratory stimulus.
   9. Emphysema
      a. Cough is not common.
      b. Sensation of air hunger.
      c. Use of accessory muscles of respiration.
      d. Anorexia with weight loss, thin in appearance.
      e. ABGs are often normal until late in disease.
      f. Characteristic tripod position—leaning forward with arms braced on knees.
   10. Chronic bronchitis:
      a. Excessive, chronic sputum production (generally not discolored unless infection is present).
      b. Impaired ventilation, resulting in decreased Pao_2 and symptoms of hypoxia; increased $Paco_2$ (CO_2 narcosis).
      c. Respiratory symptoms: productive cough, exercise intolerance, wheezing, and shortness of breath, progressing to cyanosis.
      d. Dependent edema.
      e. Cardiac enlargement with cor pulmonale.

C. Diagnostics: see Appendix 10-1.

D. Complications.

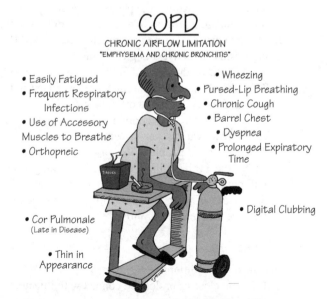

FIGURE 10-4 Chronic obstructive pulmonary disease. (From Zerwekh J, Claborn J, Miller CJ: *Memory notebook of nursing, vol 1*, ed 4, Ingram, 2008, Nursing Education Consultants.)

1. Cor pulmonale (right-side heart failure).
2. Infections (pneumonia).
3. Peptic ulcer and gastroesophageal reflux (GERD; see Chapter 13).
4. Acute respiratory failure.

Treatment

A. Prevention or treatment of respiratory tract infections.
B. Bronchodilators (see Appendix 10-2).
C. Mucolytics and expectorants (see Appendix 10-2).
D. Chest physiotherapy (suctioning, percussion, and postural drainage).
E. Breathing exercises.
F. Exercise to maintain cardiovascular fitness; most common exercise is walking.
G. Low-flow humidified O_2.
H. Corticosteroids (see Appendix 5-7).

> **NURSING PRIORITY:** *The optimum amount of O_2 is the concentration that reverses the hypoxemia without causing adverse side effects. Always notify the RN or health care provider if it is necessary to increase the flow of O_2 for clients with COPD.*

Nursing Interventions

❖ **Goal:** To improve ventilation.
A. Assist client to balance activities and increasing dyspnea.
   1. Teach pursed-lip breathing: inhale through the nose and exhale against pursed lips.
   2. Schedule activities or exercise after respiratory therapy.
   3. Assess for negative responses to activity – increasing dyspnea, tachycardia.
   4. Use portable O_2 tank when walking or exercising.
   5. Avoid respiratory irritants.
B. Humidified O_2 (low flow via nasal cannula at a rate of 1 to 3 L/min) should be used when clients are experiencing exertional or resting dyspnea.
   1. Monitor for increased levels of $PaCO_2$, hypoxia, and respiratory acidosis.
   2. A significant increase in Pao2 may decrease respiratory drive (O_2 toxicity).
   3. Administer O_2 via nasal cannula or Venturi mask (to deliver a more precise Fio_2).
   4. Assess for pressure ulcers on the top of the client's ears where the elastic holds the mask.

> **NURSING PRIORITY:** *Do not withhold O_2 if the COPD client is severely hypoxic, O_2 should be given and the nurse should prepare to provide ventilatory assistance.*

D. Avoid cough suppressants.
E. Position client in high-Fowler's or sitting position.
F. Maintain adequate hydration to facilitate removal of secretions.

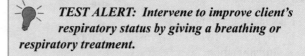

> **TEST ALERT:** *Intervene to improve client's respiratory status by giving a breathing or respiratory treatment.*

❖ **Goal:** To maintain adequate nutrition.
A. Soft, high-protein, high-calorie diet—especially for underweight clients.
B. Postural drainage completed 30 minutes before meals or 3 hours after meals.
C. Good oral hygiene after postural drainage.
D. Small frequent meals; rest before and after meals.
E. Use a bronchodilator before meals.
F. Encourage 3000 mL fluid daily unless contraindicated.
G. Monitor for problems with gastric reflux (GERD).

Home Care

A. Encourage client and family to verbalize feelings about condition and lifelong restriction of activities.
B. Include client in active planning for home care.
C. Discuss with client medication schedule and side effects of prescribed medications.
D. Review with family and client signs and symptoms of upper respiratory tract infection and know when to call physician.
   1. Changes in sputum color –yellow, green, or blood tinged.
   2. Increasing levels of dyspnea.
   3. Fever
E. Encourage activities such as walking—an increase in respiratory rate and shortness of breath will occur, but if respirations return to normal within 5 minutes of stopping activity, it is considered normal.

Asthma

✳ **Asthma is an intermittent, reversible obstructive airway problem. It is characterized by exacerbations and remissions. Between attacks the client is generally asymptomatic. It is a common disorder of childhood but may also cause problems throughout adult life.**

A. Intermittent narrowing of the airway caused by:
   1. Constriction of the smooth muscles of the bronchi and the bronchioles (bronchospasm).
   2. Excessive mucus production.
   3. Mucosal edema of the respiratory tract.
B. Exercise-induced asthma: initially after exercise there is an improvement in the respiratory status, followed by a significant decline; occurs in the majority of clients;

may be worse in cold, dry air and better in warm, moist air.
C. Emotional factors are known to play a role in precipitating childhood asthma attacks.

Data Collection

A. Risk factors/etiology.
1. Hypersensitivity (allergens) and airway inflammation.
2. Air pollutants and occupational factors.
3. Pediatric implications.
   a. *Reactive airway disease* is the term used to describe asthma in children.
   b. General onset before age 3 years.
   c. Children are more likely to have airway obstruction.
4. History of hypersensitivity reactions (history of eczema in children).
B. Diagnostics: see Appendix 10-1.
C. Clinical manifestations:
1. Episodic wheezing, chest tightness, shortness of breath, cough – in absence of infection.
2. Use of accessory muscles in breathing, orthopnea.
3. Symptoms of hypoxia (see Table 10-3); cyanosis occurs late.
4. Increased anxiety, restlessness.
5. Difficulty speaking.
6. Thick tenacious sputum.
7. Diaphoresis.

> ✔ **PEDIATRIC PRIORITY:** *Children who are sweating profusely and refuse to lie down are more ill than children who lie quietly. The child may require immediate medical attention due to hypoxia.*

D. Complications: status asthmaticus is severe asthma unresponsive to initial or conventional treatment; the practical nurse should notify the RN if a client does not respond to initial treatment with bronchodilators.

Treatment

A. Medications (see Appendix 10-2).
1. Bronchodilator.
2. Expectorants.
3. Inhaled steroids and anti-inflammatory drugs to prevent and/or decrease edema.
B. Supplemental humidified O_2 to maintain Sao_2 above 90%.

Nursing Interventions

See Hypoxia, Nursing Interventions.
❖ Goal: To relieve asthma attacks.
A. Position for comfort: usually high-Fowler's position or tripod position.

B. Close monitoring of response to O_2 therapy: maintain Sao_2 levels greater than 95% and monitor for changes in respiratory status.
C. Assess response to bronchodilators and aerosol therapy.
D. Carefully monitor ability to take PO fluids; risk for aspiration is increased.
E. Observe for sudden increase or decrease in restlessness, either may indicate an abrupt decrease in oxygenation.

> ✔ **NURSING PRIORITY:** *Shortness of breath, increase in respiratory rate and decreased breath sounds are highly suggestive of respiratory failure and possibly impending respiratory obstruction – the nurse should seek immediate assistance and anticipate ventilatory support and possible endotracheal intubation.*

Home Care

A. Assess emotional factors precipitating asthma attacks.
B. Discuss with client and family the importance of identifying and avoiding allergens.
C. Implement therapeutic measures (inhalers) before attack becomes severe.
D. Explain purposes of prescribed medications and how to use them correctly (see Appendix 10-2).
E. Administer bronchodilators before performing postural drainage.
F. Use bronchodilators and warm up before exercise to prevent exercise-induced asthma.
G. Encourage participation in activities according to developmental level.

Cystic Fibrosis

* **Cystic fibrosis is a chromosomal abnormality characterized by a generalized dysfunction of the exocrine glands. The disease primarily affects the lungs, pancreas, and sweat glands. The factor responsible for the multiple clinical manifestations of the disease process is the mechanical obstruction caused by thick mucus secretions.**

A. Organs affected by disease process.
1. Pulmonary system: bronchial and bronchiolar obstruction by thick mucus, causing atelectasis and reduced area for gas exchange; the thick mucus provides an excellent medium for bacterial growth and secondary respiratory tract infections.
2. Pancreas: Obstruction of the pancreatic ducts result in a decreased excretion of pancreatic enzymes necessary for normal digestion and absorption of nutrients.
B. Condition is diagnosed in early childhood; with effective treatment, many CF clients are adults and lead active lives.

Data Collection

A. Risk factors/etiology: inherited as an autosomal recessive trait.

B. Clinical manifestations.
1. Wide variation in severity and extent of manifestations, as well as period of onset.
2. Gastrointestinal tract.
    a. Steatorrhea or fatty foul-smelling stools.
    b. Increased bulk in feces from undigested foods; rectal prolapse may occur in infants.
    c. Meconium ileus may occur in newborn.
    d. Abdominal distention.
3. Respiratory tract.
    a. Evidence of respiratory tract involvement generally occurs in early childhood.
    b. Increasing dyspnea, tachypnea.
    c. Paroxysmal, chronic cough.
    d. Pulmonary inflammation: chronic bronchitis.
    e. Increasing problems with hypoxia.
    f. Mucus provides excellent medium for bacteria growth and chronic infections.
4. Excessive salt on the skin: "salty taste when kissed."

C. Diagnostics: see Appendix 10-1.
1. Sweat chloride test: normal chloride concentration range is less than 40 mEq/L, with a mean of 18 mEq/L; chloride concentration 40-60 mEq/L is suggestive of a diagnosis of cystic fibrosis.
2. Pancreatic enzymes: decrease or absence of trypsin and chymotrypsin.
3. Fat absorption in intestines is impaired.

D. Complications.
1. Cor pulmonale and respiratory failure are late complications.
2. Frequent pulmonary infections.
3. Pneumothorax.
4. Glucose intolerance secondary to destruction of pancreatic tissue.

Treatment

Child is usually cared for at home unless complications are present.

A. Nutrition
1. Diet that is high-calorie, high-protein, fats as tolerated; or decrease in fats, increased salt intake.
2. Supplemental fat-soluble vitamins A, D, E, and K in water-soluble forms.
3. Pancreatic enzyme replacement with meals, or with any intake of high fat food. (see Appendix 8-2).

D. Pulmonary therapy.
1. Physical therapy: postural drainage, breathing exercises.
2. Aerosol therapy and chest physical therapy (CPT).
3. Percussion and vibration.
4. Expectorants (see Appendix 10-2).

E. Antibiotics are given prophylactically and when there is evidence of infection.

Nursing Interventions

❖ **Goal:** To prevent or minimize pulmonary complications.

A. Assist child to mobilize secretions.
1. CPT: postural drainage, breathing exercises, nebulization treatments.
2. Encourage active exercises appropriate to child's capacity and developmental level.

B. Prevent respiratory tract infections.

C. Prevent pneumothorax: no power lifting, intensive isometric exercises, scuba diving.

D. Maintain good fluid intake to promote removal of secretions.

❖ **Goal:** To maintain good nutrition.

A. Balanced diet for all food groups with decrease in fat.

B. Perform good oral hygiene before each meal.

C. Administer pancreatic enzymes immediately prior to eating.

D. Perform postural drainage at least 2 hours prior to meals.

❖ **Goal:** Promote optimum home care for child (see Chapter 3 for care of chronically ill child).

A. When appropriate, teach child about heredity aspect of disease.

B. Promote independence in client's ADL's.
1. Encourage children to be responsible for own medications and treatments.
2. Teach children how to avoid respiratory infections at school.
3. Encourage parents to promote child's active involvement in planning and implementing health care routines.

C. Encourage exercises appropriate to child's capacity and developmental level.

Pulmonary Edema

✳ **This condition is caused by an abnormal accumulation of fluid in the lung in both the interstitial and alveolar spaces.**

A. Pressure builds up in the pulmonary circulation secondary to failure of the left ventricle to pump adequately.

B. The severe impairment of the left ventricle to pump effectively and to maintain cardiac output results in an increase in pressure in the pulmonary circulation and movement of fluid into the interstitial spaces and the alveoli of the lung.

Data Collection

A. Risk factors/etiology.
1. Overhydration of IV fluids, especially in older adult clients with cardiac problems.
2. Heart Failure

B. Clinical manifestations: hypoxia (see Table 10-3).
1. Decreasing SaO_2 and PaO_2.

2. Onset of dyspnea may be sudden or gradual.
3. Severe anxiety, restlessness, irritability.
4. Cool, moist skin.
5. Tachycardia (S3, S4 gallop)/ tachypnea.
6. Severe coughing productive of frothy, blood-tinged sputum.
7. Noisy, wet breath sounds that do not clear with coughing.

> ✓ **OLDER ADULT PRIORITY:** *Pulmonary edema can occur very rapidly and become a medical emergency.*

C. Diagnostics: B-type natriuretic peptide (BNP, Appendix 12-1).

Treatment

Condition demands immediate attention; medications are administered intravenously.
A. O_2 in high concentration.
B. Intubation and mechanical ventilation.
C. Rapid acting diuretics, may need to place a urinary retention catheter.
D. Pulmonary therapy - bilevel positive airway pressure (BiPAP).
E. Medications to increase cardiac contractility and cardiac output (see Appendix 10-2).

Nursing Interventions

❖ **Goal:** To assess and decrease hypoxia (see Hypoxia, Nursing Interventions; also Table 10-3).
❖ **Goal:** To improve ventilation
A. Place in high-Fowler's position with legs dependent.
B. Administer high levels of O_2 (Appendix 10-7).
C. Evaluate level of hypoxia and dyspnea; may need endotracheal tube intubation and mechanical ventilation (Appendix 10-5, 10-9).
D. Use caution when suctioning client, prolonged suctioning will decrease the PaO_2.
D. Problem may occur at night, especially in clients who are on bed rest.
E. RN may administer IV sedatives/narcotics.
1. To decrease anxiety and dyspnea and to decrease pressure in pulmonary capillary bed.
2. Closely observe for respiratory depression.
F. Administer bronchodilators and evaluate client's response.
G. Closely monitor vital signs, pulse oximetry, hemodynamic changes, and cardiac dysrhythmias.
❖ **Goal:** To reduce circulating volume (preload) and cardiac workload (afterload).

> ✓ **OLDER ADULT PRIORITY:** *Increased fluid intake in older clients may precipitate a cardiac overload; closely observe clients who are receiving blood and IV fluids.*

A. Administer diuretics to decrease circulating volume (see Appendix 11-5).
B. Medications to decrease cardiac workload and increase cardiac output (see Appendix 12-2).
C. Carefully monitor all IV fluids and continuously evaluate tolerance.
D. Maintain client in semi- to high Fowler's position, but allow legs to remain dependent.
❖ **Goal:** To provide psychological support and decrease anxiety.
A. Approach client in a calm manner.
B. Explain procedures.
C. Remain with client in acute respiratory distress.
❖ **Goal:** To prevent recurrence of problem.
A. Recognize early stages of the problem.
B. Maintain client in semi-Fowler's position.
C. Decrease levels of activity.
D. Use extreme caution in administration of fluids and transfusions.
E. Monitor daily weights and assess weight gain and fluid balance.

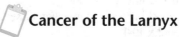

Cancer of the Larnyx

✱ **May involve the vocal cords or other areas of the larynx. If detected early, this type of cancer is curable by surgical resection of the lesion. (see Chapter 2).**

Data Collection

A. Risk factors/etiology.
1. More common in older adult men.
2. History of tobacco use.
B. Clinical manifestations (may be asymptomatic)
1. Early changes.
   a. Voice changes, hoarseness.
   b. Persistent unilateral sore throat, difficulty swallowing.
   c. Feeling of foreign body in throat.
   d. Oral leukoplakia whitish or red patch on oral mucosa or tongue (premalignant lesion)
2. Late changes.
   a. Pain.
   b. Dysphagia and decreased tongue mobility.
   c. Airway compromise.
C. Diagnostics: direct laryngoscopic examination with biopsy.

Treatment

Based on the extent of the malignancy, and the client choice of therapy.
A. Radiation: brachytherapy—placing a radioactive source into or near the area of the tumor; may also be used with external radiation treatments (see Chapter 2).
B. Surgical intervention.
1. Partial laryngectomy: preserves the normal airway and normal speech mechanism; if a trache-

otomy is performed, it is removed after the risk for swelling and airway obstruction has subsided.

2. Radical neck dissection or total laryngectomy, involves resection of the trachea, a permanent tracheotomy for breathing, and an alternative method of speaking (Appendix 10-5).

Complications

A. Airway obstruction.
B. Hemorrhage.
C. Fistula formation.

Nursing Interventions

❖ **Goal:** To prevent oral and laryngeal cancer.
A. Avoid chemical, physical, or thermal trauma to the mouth.
B. Maintain good oral hygiene: regular brushing and flossing.
C. Prevent constant irritation in the mouth; repair dentures or other dental problems.
D. See a doctor for any oral lesion that does not heal in 2 to 3 weeks.

❖ **Goal:** To prepare client for surgery.
A. General preoperative preparation (see Chapter 3).
B. The surgeon should discuss with the client the method of postoperative airway management – permanent or temporary tracheotomy.
C. Plan follow up discussion with client regarding type of tracheotomy anticipated.
D. Encourage ventilation of feelings regarding a temporary or permanent loss of voice after surgery, as well as alteration in physical appearance.
E. If total laryngectomy is anticipated, a visit from a speech pathologist to discuss postoperative speech may be helpful in reducing anxiety.
F. Establish a method of communication for immediate postoperative period.
G. With a permanent tracheotomy, there will be a loss or significant reduction in the ability to smell.

❖ **Goal:** To prevent aspiration and maintain a patent airway.
A. If tracheotomy is not performed, evaluate for hematoma and increasing edema of the incisional area that can precipitate airway occlusion respiratory distress.
B. Place in semi-Fowler's position.
C. Administer humidified O_2 therapy.
D. Observe for signs and symptoms of hypoxia.
E. Avoid analgesics that depress respiration.
F. Promote good pulmonary hygiene.
G. If tracheotomy is present, suction as indicated (see Appendix 10-6).

> 💡 **TEST ALERT: Maintain client tube patency (tracheostomy tube)**

❖ **Goal:** To maintain airway; to prevent complications after tracheotomy (see Appendix 10-5).
❖ **Goal:** To promote nutrition postoperatively.
A. Method of nutritional intake depends on the extent of the surgical procedure (see Appendix 13-6 for tube feedings).
B. IV fluids initially.
C. Gastrostomy, nasogastric, or nasointestinal tubes may be placed during surgery and used until edema has subsided and incisional area begins to heal.
D. Provide good oral hygiene; may need to suction oral cavity if client cannot swallow.
E. Evaluate tolerance of tube feedings; treat nausea quickly to prevent vomiting (see Appendix 13-6).
F. Closely observe for swallowing difficulty with initial oral feedings.
   1. Bland, nonirritating foods.
   2. Thicker foods allow more control over swallowing, thin watery fluids should be avoided.
G. For a partial laryngectomy, the possibility of aspiration is a primary concern during the first few days after surgery.
H. Maintain client in semi-Fowler's or high Fowler's position during eating or during tube feeding and maintain position after eating or tube feeding.

❖ **Goal:** To promote wound healing
A. Assess pressure dressings and presence of edema formation.
B. Monitor wound suction devices (Hemovac, Jackson-Pratt) drainage should be serosanguineous.
C. Monitor patency of drainage tubes every 3-4 hours, fluid should gradually decrease.
D. If skin flaps were used, the wound is often left uncovered for better visualization of flap and to prevent pressure on area.
E. When drainage tubes are removed, carefully observe area for increased swelling.

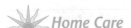 *Home Care*

> 💡 **TEST ALERT: Identify significant body image change that may affect recovery; monitor client progress toward achieving improved body image (see Chapter 6).**

Total Laryngectomy with Permanent Tracheotomy

A. Encourage client to begin own suctioning and caring for the tracheostomy before he or she leaves the hospital.
B. Assist the family in obtaining equipment for home use.
   1. System for humidification of air in home environment.
   2. Suction and equipment necessary for tracheostomy care.
C. Care of stoma.
   1. No swimming.

2. Wear plastic collar over stoma while showering.
3. Maintain high humidification at night to increase moisture in airway.
4. Avoid use of aerosol sprays.

D. Nutritional considerations: client cannot smell; taste will also be affected.

E. Client should carry medical identification.

F. Encourage client to put arm and shoulder on affected side through range of motion exercises to prevent functional disabilities of the shoulder and neck.

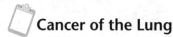 Cancer of the Lung

* **Cancer of the lung is a tumor arising from within the lung. It may represent the primary site or may be a metastatic site from a primary lesion elsewhere (see Chapter 2).**

Data Collection

A. Risk factors.
1. Smoking, including passive smoking.
2. Occupational exposure to and/or inhalation of carcinogens.

B. Clinical manifestations: nonspecific; appear late in disease.
1. Persistent chronic cough.
2. Change in respiratory pattern – wheezing or dyspnea.
3. Hemoptysis or blood streaked sputum.
4. Common sites of metastasis.
   a. Liver, bones, brain.
   b. Lymph nodes: mediastinum.
5. Pain is a late manifestation.

C. Diagnostics: bronchoscopy with biopsy.

Treatment

Varies with the extent of the malignancy (see Chapter 2).

A. Radiation: may be used preoperatively to reduce tumor mass.

B. Surgery: treatment of choice early in condition.
1. Lobectomy: removal of one lobe of the lung.
2. Pneumonectomy: removal of the entire lung.
3. Lung conserving resection: removal of a small area (wedge) or a segment of the lung.

C. Chemotherapy.

D. Treatment may involve all three therapies.

E. Palliative – may include radiation to decrease size of tumor, pain management, and comfort.

Nursing Interventions

❖ Goal: To prepare client for surgery.

A. General preoperative preparations (see Chapter 3).

B. Improve quality of ventilation before surgery.
1. No smoking.
2. Bronchodilators.
3. Good pulmonary hygiene.

C. Discuss anticipated activities in the immediate postoperative period.
1. Chest tubes and thoracic incision.
2. Pain control.
3. Shoulder exercises to promote mobility

D. Encourage ventilation of feelings regarding diagnosis and impending surgery.

E. Establish baseline data for comparison after surgery.

F. Orient client to the intensive care unit, if indicated.

❖ Goal: To maintain patent airway and promote ventilation after thoracotomy.

A. Removal of secretions from airway, either by coughing or suctioning.

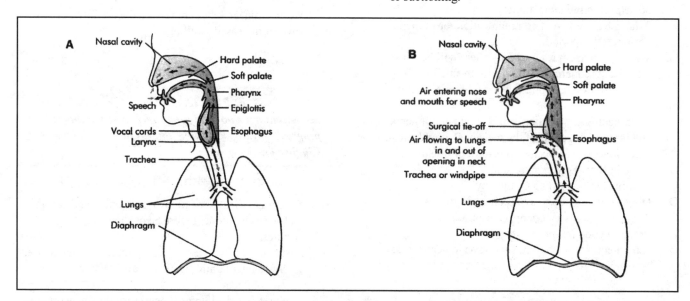

FIGURE 10-5 **A, Normal airflow in and out of lungs. B, Airflow in and out of the lungs after total laryngectomy.** Clients using esophageal speech trap air in the esophagus and release it to create sound. (From Lewis S. Heitkemper M, Dirksen S: *Medical-surgical nursing: assessment and management of clinical problems*, ed 6, St. Louis, 2004, Mosby.)

B. Have client cough frequently, deep-breathe, and use incentive spirometer.

C. Assess vital signs; closely evaluate changes in vital signs and breath sounds.

D. Closely observe pulse oximetry – *report levels that are constantly changing or decreasing*; provide supplemental O_2 as indicated.

E. Control pain so that client can take deep breaths and cough.

F. Do not position the client who has undergone a wedge resection or lobe resection on the affected side for extended periods of time; this will hinder the expansion of the lung remaining on that side. If client is in stable condition, place in semi-Fowler's position to promote optimum ventilation.

✔ **NURSING PRIORITY:** *Postoperative positioning of the client who has had thoracic surgery is important to remember, especially the client who has undergone pneumonectomy.*

G. If the client who has undergone pneumonectomy experiences increased dyspnea, place him or her in semi-Fowler's position. If tolerated, positioning on the operative side is recommended to facilitate full expansion of lung on unaffected side.

H. Encourage ambulation as soon as possible.

I. Assess presence if or level of dyspnea at rest and with activity.

J. Maintain water-sealed drainage system (see Appendix 10-4). The client who has undergone pneumonectomy will not have chest tubes for lung reexpansion because there is no lung left in the pleural cavity. Occasionally a chest tube will be placed to remove excessive fluid that collects in the pleural cavity, but not establish negative pressure.

❖ **Goal:** To assess and support cardiac function after thoracotomy.

A. Monitor for dysrhythmias – especially tachycardia.

B. Evaluate urine output.

C. Administer IV fluids and transfusions with extreme caution; client's condition is very conducive to development of fluid overload.

D. Evaluate hydration and electrolyte status.

E. *Report any significant changes in vital signs, activity tolerance, or respiratory status.*

F. Encourage shoulder and arm exercises to maintain mobility.

 Home Care

A. No more smoking; avoid respiratory irritants.

B. Discuss positions that enhance deep breathing and coughing.

C. Decreased strength is common.

D. Continue exercises and activity: stop any activity that causes shortness of breath, chest pain, or undue fatigue.

E. Avoid lifting heavy objects until complete healing has occurred.

F. Return for follow-up care as indicated.

Study Questions: Respiratory System

1. A client is to have a pulse oximetry to measure arterial oxygen levels. How will the nurse explain this procedure to the client?
   1. It will involve deep breathing and blowing into a spirometer.
   2. A probe with a light is placed on the finger to determine oxygen levels.
   3. Arterial blood is drawn to determine the levels of absorbed oxygen.
   4. Medication is inhaled and a pulmonary scan is performed.

2. Clients with pulmonary obstructive disease are usually on low levels of oxygen via nasal cannula. What problem would occur if these clients received too high an oxygen concentration?
   1. Increased sputum production with decreased oxygen exchange.
   2. Respiratory rate greater than 30 breaths per minute.
   3. Decrease in rate and depth of respirations.
   4. Increased wheezing and irritability.

3. A thoracentesis procedure is to be done in the client's room. The nurse would place the client in which position for this procedure?
   1. Prone position with feet elevated.
   2. Sitting with upper torso over bedside table.
   3. Lying on left side with right knee bent.
   4. Semi-Fowler's with lower torso flat.

4. What findings would the nurse expect to find in a client who is developing pneumonia as a complication of immobility?
   1. Diminished breath sounds.
   2. Use of accessory respiratory muscles.
   3. Dry hacking cough at night.
   4. Bradypnea and lethargy.

5. An expectorant has been ordered for a client. How will the nurse evaluate the client to determine the effectiveness of the medication?
   1. Decrease in the thickness of the sputum, making it easier to cough up sputum.
   2. Decrease in the amount of mucus by drying the mucous membrane.
   3. Decrease in respiratory rate with a decrease in dyspnea.
   4. Increased depth and quality of respirations.

6. Why should a client with a history of increased blood pressure be cautious about using a decongestant?
   1. May cause a problem with urinary frequency.
   2. Bradycardia is a common untoward effect.
   3. Increases vascular vasoconstriction.
   4. Frequently causes a headache.

7. What assessment findings would indicate a positive response in the client who is being treated for an acute asthmatic problem?
   1. Respiratory rate of 18 breaths per minute.
   2. Pulse oximetry of 90%.
   3. Pulse rate of 110 beats per minute.
   4. Nonproductive cough.

8. Which of the following clients would be at an increased risk for development of a deep vein thrombosis and potential for pulmonary emboli?
   1. Client in chronic renal failure on hemodialysis.
   2. Client with history of hypertension and current pressure of 180/110.
   3. Older adult client with kyphosis from osteoporosis and respiratory difficulty.
   4. Older adult client who is postoperative after repair of a fractured femur.

9. A client is experiencing progression of his chronic pulmonary condition. What characteristic data would be found on assessment of this client?
   1. Increased temperature and headache.
   2. Hyperventilation and bradycardia.
   3. Increasing dyspnea with cough and fatigue.
   4. Production of sputum and frequent cough.

10. A client's condition is described as progressing to hypoxemia. How would the nurse interpret this information?
    1. There is an abnormally low level of oxygen in the blood.
    2. Infection has been identified in the blood.
    3. The client's respirations are greater than 24 breaths per minute.
    4. The client is retaining excessive amounts of carbon dioxide.

11. What is important for the nurse to anticipate in providing care for a client who is 2-days postoperative for a total laryngectomy?
    1. He will have a hoarse voice and difficulty speaking.
    2. The tracheotomy stoma will require cleansing and protection.
    3. He will experience respiratory fatigue with activity.
    4. Hourly suctioning will be required to reduce secretions.

12. A client is 3-days postoperative from a thoracotomy. What would be a normal finding on the nursing evaluation of the chest tube?
    1. Dark drainage with no fluctuation of the fluid in the tubing.
    2. Bubbling in the collection chamber on expiration.
    3. 300 mL daily of serosanguineous drainage.
    4. Moderate amount of bright red drainage in tubing.

13. The nurse auscultates the upper lung fields of a client with asthma and hears wheezing bilaterally. What causes the wheezing sounds?
    1. Tachypnea and bradycardia.
    2. Increased thickness of mucus.
    3. Movement of air through narrowed airways.
    4. The sound of oxygen delivered via nasal cannula.

14. What statement is correct regarding the procedure for suctioning a client with a tracheotomy and increased respiratory secretions?
   1 The catheter is inserted into the tracheotomy tube; intermittent suction is applied until there are no further secretions present.
   2 Suction is applied to the nose and upper airways; then the tracheotomy is suctioned.
   3 With suction applied, the catheter is inserted into the tracheotomy tube until resistance is met; then the catheter is withdrawn.
   4 The catheter is inserted into the tracheotomy until slight resistance is met; suction is applied as the catheter is withdrawn.

15. When transporting a client to the radiology department, how should the nurse provide for the water-sealed chest drainage system?
   1 Hang the drainage apparatus on the head of the bed.
   2 Clamp the chest tube until the client reaches the radiology department.
   3 Keep the collection system below the level of the client's chest.
   4 Disconnect chest tube from drainage collections chamber.

16. What would create an increased risk of pulmonary infection in the client with chronic pulmonary disease?
   1 Fluid imbalance with pitting edema.
   2 Pooling of respiratory secretions.
   3 Increase in anterior-posterior chest diameter.
   4 Decreased activity and dehydration.

17. The nurse is assigned to work with a client with active tuberculosis. What assessment findings would the nurse anticipate to be present?
   1 Cough, low-grade fever, night sweats.
   2 Tachycardia, oliguria, night sweats.
   3 Upper body rash, night sweats, coughing.
   4 Dyspnea, pleural edema, lack of appetite.

18. A client had a Mantoux skin test; 72 hours later the client's forearm has a raised red area about 16 mm in diameter. What is the correct interpretation of this Mantoux skin test?
   1 A negative skin reaction.
   2 An allergy to the serum.
   3 Active tuberculosis is present.
   4 Positive for exposure to the tubercle bacillus.

19. A client is 1-day postoperative thoracotomy. What nursing observations would indicate the chest tubes are working correctly?
   1 Good bilateral breath sounds; fluctuation of fluid level in drainage tube.
   2 Bubbling in the water-sealed chamber with each expiration.
   3 Bloody drainage in the drainage chamber of the collection device.
   4 No drainage or fluctuation of fluid level in tubing coming from the client.

20. What nursing observation indicates the cuff on an endotracheal tube is leaking?
   1 An increase in peak pressure on the ventilator
   2 Client is able to speak
   3 Increased swallowing efforts by client
   4 Increased crackles (rales) over left lung field

Answers and rationales to these questions are in the section at the end of the book titled Chapter Study Questions: Answers and Rationales.

Appendix 10-1   PULMONARY DIAGNOSTICS

X-RAY STUDIES

Chest X-Ray Film: An x-ray film of the lungs and chest wall; no specific care is required before or after x-ray study.

SPUTUM STUDIES (Appendix 10-8)

Culture and Sensitivity (C&S) Test: Sputum is obtained to determine the presence of bacteria (culture); also identifies antibiotic that bacteria will be sensitive to. Sputum should be collected prior to beginning antibiotics.

Acid-Fast Bacilli: Sputum collection and analysis when tuberculosis (TB) is suspected; morning sputum may contain a higher concentration of organisms.

Cytologic Exam: Tumors in pulmonary system may slough cells into the sputum.

BRONCHOSCOPY

Provides for direct visualization of larynx, trachea, and bronchi; client is generally NPO for 6 hours before the exam; premedication is given for sedative and or amnesia. The client's upper airway is anesthetized topically.

Nursing Implications: Before the test determine if dentures need to be removed. If biopsy is done, assess for bleeding and possible pneumothorax, do not give anything by mouth until the gag reflex returns. After the exam, monitor for the return of gag and cough reflex; maintain client's NPO status until return of gag reflex.

PULMONARY FUNCTION STUDIES

Purpose: (1) to evaluate pulmonary function; (2) to evaluate response to bronchodilator therapy; (3) to differentiate diagnosis of pulmonary disease; and (4) to determine the cause of dyspnea.

Nursing Implications: The test requires client participation, client must be alert and cooperative; client should not be sedated. Study is done in the pulmonary function laboratory; client will be directed to breathe into a cylinder from which a computer interprets and re cords data in specific values. Client should not smoke (for 12 hours), nurse should determine if bronchodilating medications are to be given or not.

COMPUTERIZED AXIAL TOMOGRAPHY (CAT SCAN) (See Appendix 15-1)

LUNG SCAN

(V/Q Scan): A procedure to determine the integrity of the pulmonary vessels. Particularly useful in the client suspected of having a pulmonary embolus or a ventilation/perfusion problem A radioactive dye is injected or is inhaled and the specific uptake is recorded. Client is not sedated or on dietary restrictions.

PULSE OXIMETRY

Measurement is made by placing a sensor on the finger or earlobe; a beam of light passes through the tissue and measures the amount of oxygen-saturated hemoglobin. If probe is placed on the finger, any nail polish should be removed. Provides a method for continuously evaluating the oxygen saturation levels (SaO_2) It is noninvasive, and there are no pre- or postoximetry preparations. Normal range is 95% or higher. SaO_2 levels below 90% are critical and require immediate attention. Oximetry is not valid in clients who are experiencing shock and vasoconstriction.

PULMONARY ANGIOGRAM

Contrast material is injected into the pulmonary arteries to visualize pulmonary vasculature. It is a definitive diagnosis for pulmonary emboli. The client should be well hydrated prior to the procedure.

Contraindications: (1) dye or shellfish allergies, (2) unstable condition, (3) uncooperative client, (4) pregnancy.

MAGNETIC RESONANCE IMAGING (MRI) (See Appendix 15-1)

THORACENTESIS

A needle is inserted into the pleural cavity, fluid and air are removed. May be used for diagnosis as well as for therapeutic purposes.

Nursing Implications

1. Explain procedure to client – it is important for the client to remain very still during the procedure.
2. Position client.
   a. Preferably, client should sit on the side of the bed with the arms and head over the bedside table.
   b. If client is unable to assume sitting position, place on affected side with the head of the bed slightly elevated. Area containing fluid collection should be dependent.
3. Closely monitor client's respiratory status and general appearance during the procedure.
4. Support and reassure the client during the procedure.
5. After the procedure, position the client on his or her side with puncture side up (or in semi-Fowler's position) and monitor respiratory status and breath sounds for possible development of a pneumothorax.
6. Anticipate a chest x-ray after completion to check for possible pneumothorax.

Continued

Appendix 10-1	PULMONARY DIAGNOSTICS—cont'd.

ARTERIAL BLOOD GAS STUDIES (Table 10-2)

Measurement of the pH and partial pressures of dissolved gases (oxygen, carbon dioxide) of the arterial blood; requires approximately 3 mL of arterial blood, obtained through an arterial puncture. Arterial puncture most commonly performed on the radial artery.

Nursing Implications:
1. If client's oxygen concentration or ventilatory settings have been changed, or if a client has been suctioned, blood should not be drawn for at least 30 minutes.
2. An Allen's test should be done prior to the arterial puncture to assess adequacy of collateral circulation.

   Allen's Test: Hold client's hand, palm up. While occluding both the radial and ulnar arteries, have the client clench and unclench his or her hand several times; the hand will become pale. While continuing to apply pressure to the radial artery, release pressure on ulnar artery. Brisk color return (5-7 seconds) to the hand should occur with the radial artery still occluded. If color does not return, then ulnar artery does not provide adequate blood flow, and cannulation or puncture of radial artery should not be done.
3. Pressure should be maintained at the puncture site for a minimum of 5 minutes, hand should be warm and of good color.

 TEST ALERT: Monitor lab values that are deviations from normal arterial blood gases.

MANTOUX SKIN TEST

Mantoux test, or purified protein derivative (PPD) test, is a method of tuberculin skin testing. PPD is injected intradermally in the forearm. Results are read in 48 to 72 hours. A positive reaction means the individual has been exposed to M. tuberculosis recently or in the past and has developed antibodies (sensitized). It does not determine if client has an active TB infection.

Nursing Implications
1. Intradermal injection: A small (25-gauge) needle is used to inject 0.1 mL of PPD under the skin. The needle is inserted bevel up; a raised area or "wheal" (6-10 mm) will form under the skin.
2. The most common area for injection is the inside surface of the forearm.
3. Do not aspirate; do not massage area.
4. The client should be given specific directions to return, or plans should be made to read the test in 48 to 72 hours.
5. Interpretation: The area of induration (only the part of the reaction that can be felt; induration may not be visible) is measured, it is not the area of erythema or inflammation.
   a. An induration of 5 mm or more is a positive reaction in immunosuppressed clients, IV drug users, and persons who have been recently exposed to active TB.
   b. An induration of 10 mm is a positive reaction for persons who are at increased risk for infection. This includes IV drug users, clients with chronic medical conditions, children under 4 years of age, institutionalized clients, clients in long-term care facilities, and health care workers.
   c. An induration of 15 mm is a positive reaction for members of the general population who do not meet any of the other criteria.
6. A chest x-ray film, prophylactic medication, and medical follow-up are used to determine whether TB is dormant or active or whether the person was exposed and has an adequate immune response. It is also important to determine when and where the person came in contact with the TB bacillus.

Appendix 10-2   RESPIRATORY MEDICATIONS

BRONCHODILATORS - Relax smooth muscle of the bronchi, promoting bronchodilation and reducing airway resistance; also inhibit the release of histamine.

General Nursing Implications

- Metered-dose inhalers (MDIs): Hand-held pressurized devices that deliver a measured dose of drug with each "puff." When two "puffs" are needed, 1 minute should elapse between the two "puffs." A spacer may be used to increase the delivery of the medication.
- Dry powder inhalers (DPIs) deliver more medication to lungs and do not require coordination as with an MDI; medication is delivered as a dry powder directly to the lungs; 1 minute should elapse between "puffs."
- Bronchodilators: Beta2 agonists and theophylline are given with caution to the client with cardiac disease, because tachydysrhythmias and chest pain may occur.
- Aerosol delivery systems have fewer side effects and are more effective.

Medications	Side Effects	Nursing Implications
Epinephrine (**Adrenaline**): subQ, IV Racemic (nebulized) epinephrine	Headache Dizziness Hypertension Tremors Dysrhythmias	1. Do not administer to clients with hypertension or tachydysrhythmias. 2. Primarily used to treat acute asthma attacks and anaphylactic reactions. 3. With racemic epinephrine, results should be observed in less than 2 hours. 4. High alert medication.
Theophylline (**Theodur**): PO, rectal, IV Aminophylline: IV	Tachycardia Hypotension Nausea/vomiting Seizures	1. Theophylline blood levels should be determined for long-term use; therapeutic levels are between 10 and 20 mcg/mL; levels above 20 mcg/mL are toxic. 2. Monitor client with IV administration, it may cause rapid changes in vital signs. 3. Considered to be a third-line drug for use with asthma.

RAPID-ACTING CONTROL

Beta₂ Agonists		
Albuterol (**Proventil, Ventolin**): MDI, DPI, PO, aerosol Terbutaline (**Brethine**): aerosol, PO Pirbuterol (**Maxair**): MDI Levalbuterol (**Xopenex**): nebulizer Metaproterenol (**Alupent**): nebulizer, MDI	Tachycardia, tremors, and angina can occur but are rare with inhaled preparations.	1. Used for short-term relief of acute reversible airway problems. 2. Not used on continuous basis in absence of symptoms. 3. Client teaching regarding proper use of MDI and/or DPI.

ANTICHOLINERGICS

Ipratropium bromide (**Atrovent**): aerosol, MDI	Nasal drying and irritation. Minimal systemic effects.	1. Nasal spray may be used for clients with allergic rhinitis and asthma. 2. MDI used to decrease bronchospasm associated with COPD. 3. Therapeutic effects begin within 30 seconds.

LONG-ACTING CONTROL

Beta₂ Agonists		
Salmeterol (**Serevent**): DPI	Headache, cough, tremors, dizziness.	1. Administered two times daily (q 12 hours). 2. Not used for short-term relief; effects begin slowly and last for up to 12 hours.
Corticosteroids Beclomethasone (**Beclovent, Vanceril**): MDI Triamcinolone acetonide (**Azmacort**): MDI Fluticasone (**Flovent**): MDI	Oropharyngeal candidiasis, hoarseness, throat irritation, bad taste, cough, minimal side effects.	1. Works well with seasonal and exercise-induced asthma. 2. Prophylactic use decreases number and severity of attacks. 3. May be used with beta2 agonist. 4. Gargle after each dose and use a spacer to decrease candidiasis.
Nonsteroidal Antiinflammatory Drugs Cromolyn sodium (**Intal**): MDI	Inhalation: cough, dry mouth, throat irritation, and bad taste.	1. Prophylactic use decreases number and severity of attacks. 2. Prevents bronchoconstriction before exposure to known precipitant (e.g., exercise). 3. Not for an acute attack.
Nedocromil sodium (**Tilade**): MDI	Unpleasant taste.	1. Given to children over 6 years old. 2. Maximal effects develop within 24 hours. 3. Does not treat an acute asthmatic attaack.

Continued

Appendix 10-2 RESPIRATORY MEDICATIONS—cont'd.

Leukotriene Modifiers

Montelukast (**Singular**): PO   Headache,   1. Once daily dose in the evening.
Zafirlukast (**Accolate**): PO   GI disturbance   2. Administer within 1 hour before or 2 hours after eating.

ANTITUBERCULAR - Broad-spectrum antibiotic specific to TB bacilli.

General Nursing Implications

- Client is not contagious when sputum culture is negative for three consecutive cultures.
- Use airborne respiratory precautions when sputum is positive for bacilli.
- Treatment includes combination of medications for about 6 to 8 months.
- Monitor liver function studies for clients receiving combination therapy.
- After initial therapy, medications may be administered once daily or on a twice-weekly schedule.
- Teach clients they should not stop taking the medications when they begin to feel better.
- Advise clients to return to the doctor if they notice any yellowing of the skin or eyes or begin to experience pain or swelling in joints, especially the big toe.
- Medication regimens always contain at least 2 medications to which the infection is sensitive; inadequate treatment is primary cause of increased incidence.

Medications	Side Effects	Nursing Implications
Isoniazid (**INH**): PO, IM	Peripheral neuritis Hypersensitivity Hepatotoxicity Gastric irritation	1. Administer with (pyridoxine) vitamin B6 to prevent peripheral neuritis. 2. Primary medication used in prophylactic treatment of TB.
Rifampin (**Rifadin**): PO Rifapentine (**Priftin**): PO (a derivative of rifampin)	Hepatotoxicity—Hepatitis Hypersensitivity Gastric upset	1. May negate the effectiveness of birth control pills and warfarin. 2. May turn body secretions orange: urine, perspiration, tears—can stain soft contacts.
Ethambutol (**Myambutol**): PO	Optic neuritis Allergic reactions—dermatitis, pruritus. Gastric upset	1. Give with food if GI problems occur. 2. Observe for vision changes.
Pyrazinamide (**PZA Pyrazinamide, Tebrazid**): PO	Hepatotoxicity Increased uric acid levels	1. May take with food to reduce GI upset.
Rifabutin (**Mycobutin**) PO	Rash, GI disturbances, Hepatotoxicity	1. May turn body secretions orange: urine, perspiration, tears—can stain soft contacts. 2. Use with caution in pregnancy.

NASAL DECONGESTANTS -Produce decongestion by acting on sympathetic nerve endings to produce constriction of dilated arterioles.

Phenylephrine hydrochloride (**Neosynephrine**): intranasal
Oxymetazoline (**Afrin**): nasal spray
Pseudoephedrine (**Sudafed**): PO, nasal aerosol spray

Large dose will cause CNS stimulation, anxiety, insomnia, increased blood pressure, and tachycardia.

1. With intranasal preparations, rebound congestion may occur.
2. Not recommended for children under 6 years old.

 TEST ALERT: Monitor client's use of medications – over the counter and home remedies.

3. Medications are frequently found in OTC combination decongestants.
4. Caution clients with high blood pressure to check with their health care provider before using.

ANTIHISTAMINE - Blocks histamine release at H1 receptors (see Appendix 5-13).

EXPECTORANT - Stimulates removal of respiratory secretions; reduces the viscosity of the mucus.

Guaifenesin (**Robitussin, Mucinex**): PO   Nausea GI upset   1. Increase fluid intake for effectiveness.

CNS, Central nervous system; *GI*, gastrointestinal; *IM*, intramuscularly; *IV*, intravenously; *OTC*, over-the-counter; *PO*, by mouth (orally); *subQ*, subcutane-

Appendix 10-3   SUDDEN AIRWAY OBSTRUCTION

 NURSING PRIORITY: *The procedure to remove airway obstruction is not effective in the child with epiglottitis or sudden airway obstruction caused by inflammation of the upper airways.*

❖ Goal: To identify foreign body airway obstruction.

 NURSING PRIORITY: *If the adult client is coughing forcefully, do not interfere with attempts to cough and expel the foreign body. Do not administer any forceful blows to the back.*

1. If the victim can speak or cry, there is probably adequate air exchange.
2. If the victim cannot speak or cry but is conscious, proceed to implement abdominal thrusts to clear the obstructed airway.
3. If the victim is unconscious:
   a. Call for help: dial 911/announce code blue, etc.
   b. Place client supine.
   c. Open airway using head-tilt/chin-lift method.
   d. Observe for presence of foreign body; perform finger sweep and remove if visible.
   e. Maintain open airway; if there is no evidence of breathing, deliver two effective breaths (breaths that cause visible chest rise) either mouth-to-mouth or mouth-to-nose and mouth resuscitation.
   f. If effective breaths cannot be delivered, reposition head, reopen airway, and attempt to ventilate victim again.
   g. If still unable to ventilate, initiate procedure for relieving obstructed airway.

💡 **TEST ALERT: Identify and intervene in life-threatening situations; evaluate and document client's response to emergency procedures.**

❖ Goal: To clear obstructed airway—adult and child (conscious and unconscious).
1. Conscious: Perform Heimlich (abdominal thrusts) maneuver (chest thrusts if pregnant or obese) until obstruction is removed or client becomes unconscious.
   a. Stand behind client and wrap arms around waist.
   b. Make a fist and place thumb side against client's abdomen; place fist midline, just above the umbilicus, and below the xiphoid.
   c. Place other hand over fist and press into client's abdomen using quick upward thrusts.
   d. Repeat upward thrusts until foreign body is dislodged or client becomes unconscious.
   e. When client becomes unconscious, evaluate for presence of foreign body in the airway, remove if identified and attempt to ventilate.
2. Unconscious: Evaluate airway. Open airway and attempt to ventilate; if unable to ventilate, then proceed with steps for removal of foreign body.
   a. Position client supine, kneel astride the client's thighs; with the heel of the hand, apply forceful upward thrust to the abdomen well below the xiphoid and above the umbilicus.
   b. Administer five abdominal thrusts, return to the client's head, open the airway, and assess for breathing; if absent, provide two effective breaths.
❖ Goal: To clear obstructed airway—infant (conscious and unconscious).
1. Straddle the infant over the forearm with the head dependent.
2. Deliver up to five forceful back blows between the shoulder blades.
3. Supporting the head, turn the infant back over and administer up to five chest compressions (lower one-third of the sternum, approximately one finger breadth below the nipple line).
4. Attempt to remove foreign body only if it can be visualized.
5. If infant becomes unconscious, check the mouth before giving breaths to see if foreign body can be identified.

 PEDIATRIC PRIORITY: *Do not do a blind sweep of the infant or child's mouth; the foreign body should be visualized before you attempt to sweep the mouth.*

Appendix 10-4   WATER-SEALED CHEST DRAINAGE

PURPOSES

1. To remove air and/or fluid from the pleural cavity.
2. To restore negative pressure in the pleural cavity and promote reexpansion of the lung.
3. Placement of chest tubes. (Figure 10-6).

PRINCIPLE OF WATER-SEALED CHEST DRAINAGE

The water seal (or dry seal on some equipment) serves as a one-way valve; it prevents air, under atmospheric pressure, from reentering the pleural cavity. On inspiration, air and fluid leave the pleural cavity via the chest tube; the water or dry seal keeps the air and fluid from reentering.

> ✓ *NURSING PRIORITY: There must be a seal (either water or dry seal) between the client and the atmospheric pressure.*

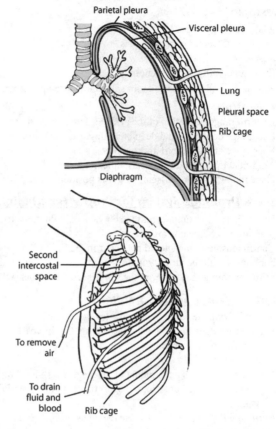

FIGURE 10-6 Placement of chest tubes.
(From: Lewis SL et al: *Medical-surgical nursing: assessment and management of clinical problems*, ed 7, St. Louis, 2007, Mosby.)

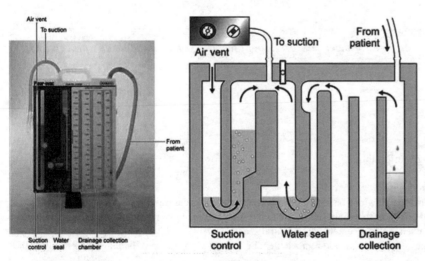

FIGURE 10-7 Water-sealed chest drainage. (From Ignatavicius, D., Workman, L. (2010). *Medical-Surgical Nursing: Patient-Centered Collaborative Care*, ed 6, Elsevier.

EQUIPMENT

Three-chamber disposable chest drainage system: A molded plastic system that provides a collection chamber, a water-sealed chamber, and a suction-control chamber. When "wet" suction is applied, there should be a continuous, gentle bubbling in the water in the suction-control chamber (see Figure 10-7).

Two-chamber disposable chest drainage system: A molded plastic system that provides a water-sealed chamber where atmospheric pressure is prevented from going into client's pleural cavity via a one-way valve. The second chamber serves as a collection chamber.

Continued

Appendix 10-4   WATER-SEALED CHEST DRAINAGE—cont'd.

Nursing Implications

Assessment
1. Evaluate for hypoxia.
2. Evaluate character of respirations.
3. Assess for symmetrical chest wall expansion.
4. Evaluate breath sounds bilaterally.
5. Palpate around insertion site for subcutaneous emphysema.

Intervention
1. Perform range of motion of the affected arm and shoulder.
2. Encourage coughing and deep breathing every 2 hours.
3. Encourage ambulation if appropriate.
4. Administer pain medications as indicated.
5. Place in low Fowler's or semi-Fowler's position.

Observe Drainage System for Proper Functioning
1. Drainage level in tubing from the client should fluctuate (tidal): rise on inspiration and fall on expiration. The opposite occurs with positive-pressure mechanical ventilation.
2. Continuous bubbling should not occur in the fluid where water seal is maintained; continuous bubbling indicates an air leak; continuous bubbling should occur only in the system that maintains a third chamber for suction control.
3. Initial bubbling may occur in the water-sealed chamber with coughing or with deep respiration as air is moved out of the pleural cavity.

Maintain Water-Sealed System
1. Keep all drainage equipment below level of client's chest.
2. Evaluate for dependent loops in the tubing; this increases resistance to drainage. All extra tubing should be coiled in the bed and flow in a straight line to the system.
3. Tape all connections.
4. Note characteristics and amount of drainage. Mark level on the drainage system as needed and every 8 hours.
5. Vigorous "milking" or stripping chest tubes is controversial. Stripping should not be done routinely on clients because it increases pleural pressures.
6. *Notify the RN when the collection chamber is approximately half full.* The increased volume in the collection chamber increases the resistance to the flow of drainage.
7. Do not clamp chest tubes during transport.

 TEST ALERT: Maintain client tube patency (chest tubes); reinforce client teaching on treatments and procedures.

Chest Tube Removal
1. Criteria for removal of the tube:
   a. Minimum or no drainage.
   b. Fluctuations stop in the water-seal chamber.
   c. Chest x-ray film reveals expanded lung.
   d. Client has good breath sounds and is breathing comfortably.
2. Procedure.
   a. Provide pain relief about 30 minutes before procedure.
   b. Generally, the physician will want the client in a low Fowler's or semi-Fowler's position, unless contraindicated.
   c. The physician will ask the client to exhale and hold it or to exhale and bear down (a Valsalva maneuver). Either of these procedures will increase the intrathoracic pressure and prevent air from entering the pleural space.
   d. With the client holding his or her breath, the physician will quickly remove the tube and place an occlusive bandage over the area; the client can then breathe normally.
   e. Assess the client's tolerance of the procedure; a chest x-ray film should be obtained to determine that the lungs remain fully expanded.

Appendix 10-5 ARTIFICIAL AIRWAYS

Endotracheal Intubation - Placement of an endotracheal (ET) tube through the mouth or nose into the trachea (Figure 10-8).

Purpose

To provide an immediate airway in an emergency situation; to maintain a patent airway; to facilitate removal of secretions and provide airway for controlled ventilation.

Nursing Interventions

1. Provide warm, humidified oxygen.
2. Establish method of communication because the client cannot speak; child is unable to cry.
3. Maintain safety measures.
   a. Prevent client from accidentally removing tube: soft hand restraints, mittens, etc.
   b. Secure ET tube to the face.
   c. Child with an ET tube requires constant attendance.
4. As soon as tube is inserted, assess symmetry of chest expansion and bilateral breath sounds. Assess for presence of bilateral breath sounds every 2 hours. If tube slips farther into the trachea, it may pass into the right main stem bronchus, obliterating the left main stem bronchus. Determine placement by checking breath sounds.
5. Cuff must remain inflated if client is on a volume ventilator. If the client has adequate spontaneous respiration and is not on a ventilator, the cuff may be left deflated.
6. Minimal occluding volume (MOV) should be used when inflating the cuff to prevent aspiration or to maintain mechanical ventilation. This is accomplished by placing a stethoscope over the trachea or by listening to the client's breath sounds to determine when air stops moving past the cuff. A safe pressure on the cuff is 20 to 25 mm Hg.
7. Provide frequent oral hygiene; assess for pressure areas on the nose or the mouth.
8. Client's nothing-by-mouth (NPO) status is maintained as long as tube is in place.
9. Suction as indicated (see Appendix 10-6).

Tracheostomy - A surgical opening in the trachea (Figure 10-8).

Purpose

To maintain airway over an extended period of time; to facilitate removal of secretions.

Nursing Interventions

Initially After Tracheostomy
1. Provide warm, humidified oxygen.
2. Small amount of bleeding around the tube is expected.
3. Observe for pulsations of the tube; it may be resting on the innominate artery; notify RN or physician of observation.
4. Maintain frequent contact and communication with client and provide reassurance.

Maintenance of Tracheostomy
1. Provide warm, humidified oxygen.
2. Establish method of communication because client cannot speak; child is unable to cry.
3. Maintain safety measures.

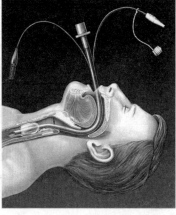

FIGURE 10-8 Artificial airways. Position of endotracheal tube. (From Potter PA, Perry AG: *Fundamentals of nursing*, ed 7, 2009 Mosby.)

Continued

Appendix 10-5 ARTIFICIAL AIRWAYS—cont'd.

 TEST ALERT: *Maintain tube patency – tracheostomy tube; provide care for a client with a tracheostomy.*

    a.   Secure tracheal tube to the client's neck.
    b.   Use safety measures to prevent client from dislodging tube: soft restraints, trach ties, etc.
    c.   Prevent clothing or bed covers from occluding area of tracheal opening.
    d.   Child with a tracheostomy requires continuous attendance.
4.   Assess for symmetrical expansion of chest wall and bilateral breath sounds.
5.   Assess levels of pulse oximetry.
6.   Provide frequent oral hygiene; turn every 2 hours.
7.   Inflate tracheostomy cuff during tube feedings or feedings by mouth (minimal occluding pressure).
8.   Cuff must remain inflated if client is on a ventilator. If the client has adequate spontaneous respiration, the cuff may be left deflated.
9.   Suction as indicated (see Appendix 10-6).
10. If the tracheal tube has an obturator, it should be taped to the head of the bed. If the tracheostomy tube is accidentally removed, the obturator will be necessary for replacing the tube.
11. A fenestrated tracheostomy tube can be adapted so that air will flow throughout normal passages; frequently used when client is beginning to be weaned from the ventilator. If client has respiratory difficulty when the inner cannula is removed, immediately reinsert the cannula to provide a tracheal airway. The tube can also be plugged so that client can speak or cough through normal airway. Make sure the cuff is deflated before plugging the tracheostomy.
12. Establish means of communication; keep call light within easy reach of client.
13. If the client accidentally removes the tube, use the obturator to attempt to replace the tube in the tracheal opening. If unable to replace tracheotomy tube, hold the opening open with a hemostat until physician is available to replace the tube.

    ✔ **NURSING PRIORITY:** *The purpose of the cuff on a tracheostomy tube or on an ET tube is to facilitate the delivery of air to the lungs, not to secure the tube position.*

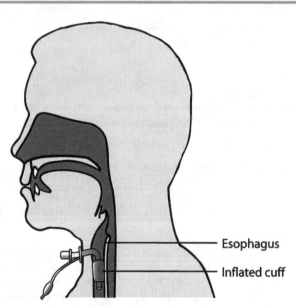

Esophagus

Inflated cuff

FIGURE 10-9 Artificial airways. Position of tracheostomy tube. (From: Lewis SL et al: *Medical-surgical nursing: assessment and management of clinical problems*, ed 6, St. Louis, 2004, Mosby.)

Appendix 10-6   SUCTIONING THROUGH ARTIFICIAL AIRWAYS

> *NURSING PRIORITY: Suctioning the endotracheal tube or the tracheostomy is done to remove excess secretions and to maintain patent airway. Suctioning should always be done before a cuff is deflated.*

1. Determine that the client needs to be suctioned.
   a. Auscultate lungs to detect presence of secretions.
   b. Observe to see whether client is experiencing immediate difficulty with removal of secretions.
2. Explain procedure if client is not familiar with it, or simply indicate you are going to assist with the removal of the secretions.
3. All equipment introduced into the trachea or the ET tube must be sterile.
4. Prepare equipment by attaching the suction catheter to the suction source while maintaining sterile technique.
5. If client is not in immediate danger of airway occlusion, hyperoxygenate with 100% O_2 for three to four hyperinflations.
6. Gently insert sterile catheter into the opening without applying suction. Insert catheter to the point of slight resistance; then pull catheter back 1 to 2 cm.
7. Apply intermittent suction as the catheter is gently rotated and withdrawn.
8. Each suctioning pass should not exceed 10 to 15 seconds in duration.
9. Reconnect client to oxygen source and evaluate whether one suctioning episode was sufficient to remove secretions.
10. Hyperoxygenate client for 1 to 5 minutes after suctioning; assess vital signs and pulse oximetry—SaO_2 levels should return to normal or to the previous levels before suctioning.
11. Avoid suctioning client before drawing blood for determination of arterial blood gas values. Client should be allowed to stabilize for approximately 30 minutes before blood is drawn.
12. Monitor pulse oximetry while suctioning; if oximetry does not come back to normal level immediately after suctioning, do not attempt to suction client again; replace oxygen and or ventilatory connection and call for assistance.

COMPLICATIONS OF SUCTIONING

1. *Hypoxia:* If possible, preoxygenate with high percentage of O_2 before and after suctioning.
2. *Dysrhythmias:* Limit suctioning to 10 to 15 seconds; monitor rhythm during suctioning; if bradycardia or tachycardia develops, discontinue suctioning immediately.
3. *Bronchospasm:* Try to time the suctioning with client's own cycle; insert tube during inspiration.
4. *Airway trauma:* Maintain suction level below 120 mm Hg.
5. *Infection:* Use sterile technique; assess the color and quantity of sputum suctioned.
6. *Atelectasis:* Use suction catheters that are approximately one-third or less of the diameter of tube.

> *TEST ALERT: Intervene to improve client respiratory status by suctioning.*

Appendix 10-7 OXYGEN

❖ **Goal:** The goal of oxygen therapy is to maintain an optimum level of oxygenation at the lowest effective level of fraction of inspired oxygen (Fio_2).

Methods of Administration

1. *Low-flow systems:* nasal cannula, standard mask, nonrebreather mask. Oxygen is measured in liters per minute flow (LPM): a range of 2 to 8 LPM is the most common order.
2. *High-flow systems:* Venturi mask, nebulizer mask, and ventilators. Oxygen is measured as Fio_2 in concentrations from 24% to 100%: 10 LPM oxygen flow is required to obtain accurate percentage flow.

Humidification

1. Adds water vapor to inspired gas.
2. Prevents drying and irritation of respiratory membranes.
3. Loosens thick secretions, allowing them to be more easily removed.

Indications for Oxygen Administration

1. A decrease in oxygen in the arterial blood (hypoxemia).
2. An increase in the work of breathing.
3. To decrease the cardiac workload.

 TEST ALERT: *Intervene to improve client's respiratory status by giving a breathing or respiratory treatment.*

Oxygen Safety in Administration

1. Properly ground all electrical equipment.
2. Do not permit any smoking by anyone in the area.
3. Use water-based, not oil-based, lubricants.
4. Use oxygen with caution in clients with chronic airway disease; most often administered via mask or nasal cannula at 2 to 4 LPM, unless client is in severe distress.
5. Oxygen supports combustion but is not explosive.

OXYGEN TOXICITY: A medically induced condition produced by inhalation of high concentrations of oxygen over a prolonged period of time. Toxicity is directly related to concentration of oxygen, duration of therapy, and degree of lung disease present.
1. Tracheal irritation and cough.
2. Dyspnea and increasing cough.
3. Decrease in vital capacity.
4. The Pao_2 continues to decrease, even with an increasing Fio_2.
5. Atelectasis.

 TEST ALERT: *Assure safe functioning of client care equipment, follow facility protocols for safe use of equipment.*

Appendix 10-8   NURSING PROCEDURE: SPUTUM SPECIMEN COLLECTION

Nursing Implications

1. Sputum for culture and sensitivity should be collected as soon as possible to facilitate identification of bacteria and treatment.
2. Specimens for cytology and for acid-fast bacilli for TB diagnostics should be collected in the morning when bacteria and cells are most concentrated.
3. No mouthwash should be used before collection of specimen; have client rinse his mouth with water or brush his teeth with water, but do not use toothpaste.
4. Aerosol mist will assist in decreasing thickness of sputum and increasing effectiveness of coughing.
5. Maintain strict asepsis and standard precautions in collecting and transporting specimen; use sterile specimen collection container.
7. Acid-fast bacillus: Sputum collection should be done on three consecutive days.
8. Culture and sensitivity: Initial specimen should be obtained before antibiotics are administered.

 TEST ALERT: *Collect specimens for diagnostic testing; reinforce client teaching on purpose of laboratory tests; monitor diagnostic or laboratory test results.*

Clinical Tips for Problem Solving

If client experiences pain while coughing:
Support painful area with roll pillows to minimize pain and discomfort.
Encourage client to take several deep breaths before beginning. This assists in triggering the cough reflex and aerates the lungs (see Box 10-2).
If client is unable to produce sputum specimen:
Attempt procedure early in the morning, when mucus production is greatest.
Notify physician to obtain orders for a bronchodilator or nebulization therapy.

Appendix 10-9   MECHANICAL VENTILATORS

 TEST ALERT: *Monitor and maintain clients on a ventilator.*

Mechanical ventilators regulate the rate and depth of respirations. Settings are frequently evaluated and adjusted based on ABG results to maintain optimum ventilation and gas exchange. An endotracheal tube or a tracheostomy are used to maintain airway.

PATTERNS OF VENTILATION

1. *Assist control (AC):* The client may initiate the cycle with inspiration.
2. *Continuous mandatory ventilation (CMV):* The machine controls rate and volume of the client's ventilatory cycle.
3. *Intermittent mandatory ventilation (IMV)/synchronized intermittent mandatory ventilation (SIMV):* Delivers ventilation at inspiratory phase of client's spontaneous ventilation; may be used for weaning from ventilator.
4. *Positive end-expiratory pressure (PEEP):* Maintains positive pressure at alveolar level at end of expiration to facilitate the diffusion of oxygen. PEEP will increase the intrathoracic pressure, thus further decreasing the venous return and causing a decrease in blood pressure. *Indications for use:* Acute respiratory distress syndrome (ARDS); clients unable to maintain patent airway; neuromuscular diseases causing respiratory failure.
5. *Continuous positive airway pressure (CPAP):* Used to augment the functional residual capacity (FRC) during spontaneous breathing. Used to wean clients from ventilators and may be administered by face mask. Client or infant must have spontaneous respirations.

 TEST ALERT: *Provide care to a client on a ventilator; implement measures to manage/prevent possible complication of client condition or procedure.*

NURSING IMPLICATIONS

1. All alarms should be set and checked each shift, especially low pressure and low exhaled volume.
2. A bag-valve mask resuscitator is placed in the client's room in case of mechanical failure of equipment.
3. Ventilator setting for fraction of inspired oxygen (Fio_2), tidal volume, respiratory rate, pattern of control (AC/IMV, etc.), and PEEP should be checked and charted.
4. Assess client's tolerance of the ventilator; intravenous medications are frequently used. If changes, weaning, or removal of the ventilator are anticipated, do not sedate the client.
5. The client frequently experiences a high level of anxiety and fear. Explain equipment and alarms to the client and to the family. Maintain a calm, reassuring approach to the client.
6. When ventilator changes are made, carefully assess the client's response (pulse oximetry, vital signs, ABGs).
7. Never allow the condensation in the tubing to flow back into fluid reservoir.

COMMON VENTILATOR ALARMS

1. High pressure alarm: Sounds when tidal volume cannot be delivered at set pressure limit.
   Nursing Care: Increased secretions—suction; client biting tube—place oral airway; coughing and increased anxiety—administer sedative.
2. Low pressure alarm: Sounds when the machine cannot deliver the tidal volume because of a leak or break in the system.
   Nursing Care: Disconnection—check all connections for break in system; tracheostomy or endotracheal (ET) tube cuff is leaking—check for air escaping around cuff, may need to replace tracheostomy tube if cuff is ruptured.

WEANING FROM VENTILATORS

May be done via SIMV, or T-piece on ET or tracheotomy with heated mist and oxygen, or by pressure support ventilation from the ventilator. During weaning it is imperative for the nurse to maintain close observation for increasing dyspnea and hypoxia. If client experiences dyspnea, he or she should be returned to the ventilator at whatever parameters were being used, and the doctor should be notified; anticipate drawing blood for determination of arterial blood gas values.

> ✓ **NURSING PRIORITY:** *Focus on the client not on the ventilator. In case of problems with the ventilator, assess the client; if adequate ventilation is not being achieved, take client off the ventilator, maintain respirations via a bag-valve mask resuscitator, and call for assistance.*

Vascular System

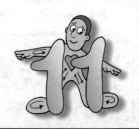

PHYSIOLOGY OF THE VASCULAR SYSTEM

Vessels

A. Arteries.
1. Primary function is to transport nutrients and oxygen to the cellular level.
2. Arterial vascular system is a high-pressure system with a rapid blood flow.
B. Capillaries.
1. Microscopic vessels at the cellular level.
2. Capillary bed is the area of circulation where the arterioles branch into capillaries and exchange between the circulating blood volume and the interstitial fluid occurs.
C. Veins.
1. Primary function of the veins is to return blood to the heart.
2. Veins contain valves to maintain direction of blood flow and to prevent the backflow of blood.
3. Venous system is a low-pressure system.
D. Circulatory systems.
1. Systemic circulation: the flow of blood from the left ventricle into the aorta and through the arteries to the capillary beds, where cellular nutrition and oxygenation occur; then blood returns to the right atrium of the heart via the veins.
2. Pulmonary circulation: the flow of blood from the right ventricle into the pulmonary artery and then into the lungs; in the capillary beds of the lungs, the blood picks up oxygen and releases carbon dioxide and then returns to the left atrium through the pulmonary veins.
3. Hepatic-portal circulation: the flow of blood from the venous system of the stomach, intestines, spleen, and pancreas into the portal vein and through the liver for absorption of nutrients and removal of toxins. Venous blood leaves the liver through the hepatic vein and flows into the inferior vena cava for return to the right atrium.
E. Lymphatic system: primary function is to return fluid and protein to the blood from the interstitial fluid.

Mechanics of Blood Flow

A. Blood flow is controlled by:
1. The diameter of the vessel.
2. The length of the vessel.
3. The pressure at either end of the vessel.
4. The viscosity of the blood.

B. Physiological control.
1. Autoregulation: the ability of tissue to control its own blood flow. Autoregulatory system enables blood supply to vital organs (brain, kidney, heart) to remain relatively constant, even though blood pressure may fluctuate within normal ranges.
2. Nervous system control.
a. Parasympathetic nervous system: influence on blood flow is the regulation of the heart rate by the vagus nerve.
b. Sympathetic nervous system.
(1) Primary influence of sympathetic system is on arterioles for dilation and constriction of the vessels in order to maintain peripheral resistance and vasomotor tone.
(2) Peripheral resistance is resistance of arterioles to flow of blood.
(3) Dilation decreases peripheral resistance, thereby decreasing blood pressure; vasoconstriction increases peripheral resistance, thereby increasing blood pressure.

Blood Pressure

A. Systolic blood pressure is the arterial pressure at the peak of ventricular contraction. The systolic pressure is determined primarily by the amount of blood ejected.
B. Diastolic pressure represents the pressure exerted in the arteries at the end of systole; it is the resting ventricular pressure. Diastolic pressure depends on the ability of the arteries to stretch and handle the blood flow.
C. Pulse pressure is the difference between the systolic and diastolic pressures.

DISORDERS OF THE VASCULAR SYSTEM

Atherosclerosis

✳ **Atherosclerosis is the most common disease of the *arteries*. The word means "hardening of the arteries."**
A. Atherosclerosis: most common classification of arteriosclerosis; characterized by stenosis and obstruction in the lumen of the vessel (Figure 11-1).
1. Process is slow; generally no evidence of problems until a major artery is affected and there is severe decrease in blood supply to tissue supplied by artery involved.

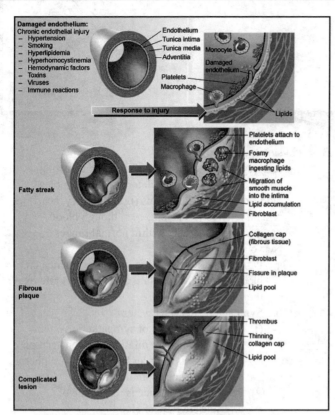

FIGURE 11-1 Pathophysiology of Atherosclerosis - (From Ignatavicius, DD, Workman, ML: *Medical Surgical Nursing Patient-Centered Collaborative Care, ed 6*, St Louis, 2010, Saunders.)

2. Arteries commonly affected by atherosclerosis:
   a. Coronary arteries.
   b. Cerebrovascular arteries.
   c. Aorta: may lead to aortic aneurysm.
   d. Peripheral arteries.

Data Collection

A. Modifiable risk factors.
   1. Diet high in saturated fats (cholesterol).
   2. Smoking.
   3. Obesity.
   4. Decreased activity.
   5. Stress.
B. Nonmodifiable risk factors.
   1. Familial tendencies.
   2. Age.
C. Conditions accelerating atherosclerotic development.
   1. Diabetes mellitus.
   2. Hypertension.
   3. High cholesterol/triglyceride levels.
D. Clinical manifestations: depend on artery involved.
E. Diagnostics.
   1. Clinical manifestation of specific area involved.
   2. Increased levels of serum triglycerides, lipids, and cholesterol.

Treatment

A. Low-cholesterol diet.
B. Decrease risk factors.
C. Antihyperlipidemic medications (see Appendix 11-2).
D. Peripheral vasodilating medications.
E. Vascular surgery.

Nursing Interventions

See Nursing Intervention for specific areas involved.

Hypertension

✳ **Hypertension is a consistent increase in blood pressure.**
A. Classification.
   1. Essential (primary, benign, idiopathic): etiology unknown; accounts for approximately 85% to 95% of hypertensive clients.
   2. Secondary: accounts for approximately 10% to 15% of hypertension cases; the sustained elevation is due to an identifiable cause.
      a. Increased intracranial pressure.
      b. Renal disease.
      c. Pregnancy-induced hypertension (eclampsia).
      d. Cushing's syndrome.
      e. Thyrotoxicosis.
   3. Malignant hypertension: a sustained increase in the diastolic pressure that is unresponsive to treatment.
   4. Hypertensive crisis: when the degree of hypertension is a life-threatening situation.

Data Collection

A. Risk factors in essential hypertension (Table 11-1).
B. Clinical manifestations of essential hypertension.

> ✔ *NURSING PRIORITY – Encourage blood pressure monitoring in clients with increased risk, hypertension is most often asymptomatic.*

   1. Increase in blood pressure.
   2. Headache.
   3. Dizziness.
   4. Palpitations.
   5. Increase in the rate of atherosclerosis.
   6. Heart failure.
   7. Left ventricular hypertrophy.
   8. Visual disturbances.
C. Diagnostics.
   1. Increase in blood pressure, especially diastolic pressure on two separate occasions at least 2 weeks apart (Box 11-1).
      a. Diastolic pressure of 80 mm Hg or higher.
      b. Systolic pressure of 125 mm Hg or higher.

TABLE 11-1	RISK FACTORS IN ESSENTIAL HYPERTENSION

Nonmodifiable Factors	Modifiable Factors
Age: B/P progressively increases with age, commonly increases between ages 30-50 years. Gender: more prevalent in men until age 55, and then more prevalent in women. Ethnic group: higher in African Americans than in whites. Family history: especially if close relative has hypertension.	Obesity: central abdominal obesity. Stress: repeated, prolonged stress; prevalent in woman. Excess sodium intake: causes fluid retention and contributes to increased blood pressure. Elevated lipid levels: hyperlipidemia is common in clients with high B/P. Substance abuse: excessive alcohol intake, tobacco use. Sedentary life style: regular physical activity helps to decrease risk.

 TEST ALERT: *Review with client understanding of health promotion behaviors.*

BOX 11-1   OLDER ADULT CARE FOCUS
Evaluation of Blood Pressure

- If a client has been hypertensive for a long period of time, the client's "normal" systolic blood pressure may need to be greater than 120 mm Hg to maintain adequate blood flow and allow client to perform ADLs.
- Teach client how to avoid increased problems with orthostatic hypotension.
- Obtain blood pressure readings with client standing, lying, and sitting and in both arms.
- Make sure client has not had any nicotine or coffee for about an hour before taking blood pressure measurements.
- Do not allow client to cross legs during blood pressure measurement.
- Compliance problems occur when the client has to take several medications for BP as well as cope with other chronic health problems.

2. Diagnostics to rule out problem of secondary hypertension.
D. Complications.
   1. Coronary artery disease.
   2. Cerebral vascular disease (see Chapter 15).
      a. Reversible ischemic neurologic deficit (RIND).
      b. Stroke (brain attack).
   3. Nephrosclerosis: ischemia of the intrarenal vessels.
   4. Retinal damage: ischemia of the arterioles in the retina.
   5. Hypertensive crisis.
   6. Peripheral vascular disease.

TEST ALERT: *Compare current data to client baseline data (e.g., vital signs). Determine if vital signs are abnormal.*

Treatment
A. Diet.
   1. Low sodium.
   2. Weight reduction.
   3. Decreased cholesterol and saturated fats.
B. Regular exercise.
C. Antihypertensive medications (see Appendix 11-4).
D. Diuretics to decrease circulating volume (see Appendix 11-5).
E. Limit alcohol intake to 1 to 2 ounces per day.
F. Stress management.
G. Stop smoking.

Nursing Interventions
❖   **Goal:** To identify and educate high-risk individuals.
A. Encourage client to participate in community blood pressure screening programs.
B. Educate public regarding risk factors.
C. Identify health-promoting behavior for high-risk individuals (Box 11-2).
❖   **Goal:** To reduce blood pressure and assist client to maintain control. (Figure 11-2).
A. Assess response to medication.
   1. Antihypertensives (see Appendix 11-4).
   2. Diuretics (see Appendix 11-5).
B. Evaluate blood pressure measurement (Box 11-1)

✓ **OLDER ADULT PRIORITY:** *Older adults are more sensitive to blood pressure changes. A drop in blood pressure to less than 120 mm Hg systolic may cause orthostatic hypotension.*

C. Maintain low-sodium diet.
D. Assess changes in weight with regard to low-sodium intake and use of diuretics.
E. When blood pressure (BP) is initially decreased, evaluate client's tolerance to drop in BP.

BOX 11-2 LIFESTYLE MODIFICATIONS FOR HYPERTENSION PREVENTION AND CONTROL

- Lose weight if indicated.
- Limit alcohol and caffeine intake.
- Follow a regular program of aerobic exercise (30 to 45-minutes; 3 to 4 days a week).
- Limit sodium intake.
- Maintain adequate potassium intake.
- Maintain adequate intake of dietary calcium, magnesium, and fiber.
- Stop smoking.
- Reduce intake of dietary saturated fat and cholesterol.

 TEST ALERT: Review client/family understanding of health promotion behaviors.

1. Presence of postural hypotension.
2. Change in urinary output.
3. Change in energy level.
4. Changes in level of consciousness.

F. *Report significant changes in BP to the charge nurse.*

✔ ***NURSING PRIORITY:** Obtain hemodynamic measurements: the BP of a hypertensive person should be measured lying down, sitting and standing; measure the BP in both arms.*

HYPERTENSION NURSING CARE

Diuretic — **D**aily weight
I & **O**
Urine Output
Response of B/P
Electrolytes
Take Pulses
Ischemic Episodes (TIA)
Complications: 4 C's
CAD
CRF
CHF
CVA

FIGURE 11-2 **Hypertensive Nursing Care** - (From: Zerwekh, JA, Claborn, JC, Miller, CJ, *Memory Notebook of Nursing, Vol 1, ed 4*, Ingram, Texas, 2008, Nursing Education Consultants.)

 Home Care

A. Continue low-cholesterol, low-sodium diet.
B. Decrease weight if appropriate.
C. Assist to identify an appropriate, consistent, regular exercise program.
  1. A gradually increasing exercise program.
  2. Episodic strenuous activity should be avoided.
  3. Walking, swimming, slow jogging.
  4. Avoid weight lifting and heavy isometric exercises.
D. Take medications as prescribed.
  1. Take medication at regular times.
  2. Know the names and common side effects of the medications.
  3. Inform health care provider (HCP) if unable to afford medications.
  4. Do not stop taking medications unless advised to by HCP.

TEST ALERT: Identify side effects and adverse reactions of medications.

E. Avoid hot baths, steam rooms, spas (increase vasodilating effect of medications).
F. Side effects of medication are frequently temporary.
G. Avoid drugs that interact with BP medications (e.g., antacids, cold/sinus medications).
H. If sexual problems or impotence develops, contact HCP; do not stop taking medication.
I. Take measures to control effects of orthostatic hypotension.
  1. Get up slowly, sit at the bedside to regain equilibrium, and then stand slowly.
  2. Wear elastic support hose.
  3. Lie or sit down when dizziness occurs.
  4. Do not stand or sit for prolonged periods of time.
J. Lifestyle modifications (Box 11-2)

Peripheral Arterial Disease (Peripheral Vascular Disease)

✳ **Also known as peripheral vascular disease (PVD), this disorder primarily involves narrowing and obstruction of the extremities, especially the lower extremities. The atherosclerotic lesions cause chronic arterial obstruction that progressively leads to decreased oxygen delivery to the tissues.**

A. Lesions are predominantly found in the lower aorta, from below the renal arteries extending through the popliteal area.
B. By the time symptoms occur, the artery is approximately 85% to 95% occluded.
C. The renal, femoral, popliteal, and aortic iliac arteries are the most commonly affected sites.

Data Collection

A. Risk factors (same as for hypertension – Table 11-1).
B. Clinical manifestations.

> 💡 **TEST ALERT: Recognize the client with conditions resulting in inadequate circulation of lower extremities.**

1. Intermittent claudication (pain with activity, relieved by rest).
2. Ischemic pain at rest, or pain at night indicates advanced stages of PVD.
3. Paresthesia of the feet.
4. Decreased or absent peripheral pulses (Figure 11-3).
   a. Dorsalas pedis, posterior tibial.
   b. Popliteal.
   c. Femoral.
5. Arterial ulcers.
   a. Commonly found on metatarsal heads and tips of toes.
   b. Painful, sharp edges, pale color base, frequently occurs on the large toe.
   c. Poor healing of injuries on the extremities due to lack of circulation.
6. Changes in the skin.
   a. Cool to touch.
   b. Shiny, fragile, poor turgor.
   c. Dry, scaly.
   d. Loss of hair on the lower leg.
7. Brittle, thick toenails.
8. Dependent rubor (dusky redness) when legs are in a dependent position, pallor with elevation of the legs.
C. Diagnostics - see Appendix 11-1.

Treatment

A. Medical.
1. Vasodilating medications.
2. Decrease progression of atherosclerosis.
   a. Decrease dietary cholesterol intake.
   b. Initiate an exercise program as tolerated.
   c. Stop all tobacco use.
   d. Decrease weight if appropriate.
3. Prevent and control infections.
4. Treatment of diabetes.
B. Surgical: Procedures are performed when intermittent claudication interferes with the client's activities of daily living or when the circulation must be restored in order to salvage the limb.
1. Peripheral atherectomy: removal of plaque within the artery.
2. Bypass graft: bypass of an obstruction by suturing a graft proximally and distally to the obstruction.
3. Patch graft angioplasty: artery is opened, plaque is removed, and a patch is sutured in the opening to widen the lumen.

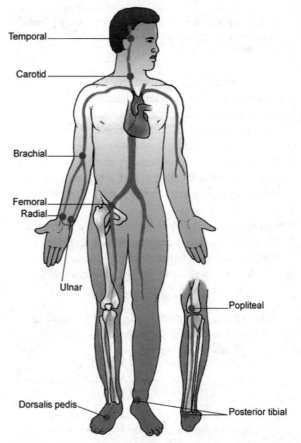

FIGURE 11-3 **Pulse Points for assessment of arterial pulse,** (From: Ignatavicius, DD, Workman, ML: *Medical Surgical Nursing Patient-Centered Collaborative Care, ed 6*, St Louis, 2010, Saunders.)

4. Amputation: used as a last resort when other therapies have failed and gangrene or infection is extensive.
C. Nonsurgical.
1. Percutaneous transluminal angioplasty: use of a balloon catheter to compress the plaque against the arterial wall.
2. Laser-assisted angioplasty: a probe is advanced through a cannula to the area of occlusion; a laser is used to vaporize the atherosclerotic plaque.
3. Intravascular stent: placement of a stent within a narrowed vessel to maintain patency.

Nursing Interventions

❖ **Goal:** To evaluate level of involvement of the extremity.
A. Assess peripheral pulses; compare quality of pulses in the lower extremities.
B. Evaluate skin on the affected extremity.
1. Color, skin temperature.
2. Capillary refill.
3. Condition of the skin and nail beds.
4. Presence of ulcers or lesions, stages of healing.
5. Assess tolerance to activity; at what point does pain occur.

TEST ALERT: *Review assessment of peripheral pulses, report signs of potential complications.*

❖ Goal: To prevent injury and infection.
A. Avoid vigorous rubbing of the extremity.
B. Prevent pressure to heels, ankles, toes.
C. Use heel covers and bed cradle to prevent pressure on the toes and heels.
D. Maintain good skin hygiene and proper care of toenails.
   1. Do not trim the toenails, report problems to RN or encourage client to see podiatrist.
   2. Do not trim calluses or corns.
   3. *Advise RN or HCP if client has ingrown toenails.*
   4. Keep feet clean and dry, do not soak feet, use lubricating lotion to prevent skin cracks.
   5. Teach client to always wear shoes; avoid shoes or socks that are too tight.

 TEST ALERT: *Identify methods for preventing complications associated with illness. Identify factors that affect wound healing.*

❖ Goal: To increase arterial supply and decrease venous congestion to the extremity.
A. Encourage moderate exercise (e.g., walking).
B. Perform active postural exercises (Buerger-Allen exercises).
C. Maintain constant warm temperature; do not use hot water bottles or heating pads on lower extremities.
D. Avoid pressure in the posterior popliteal area.
   1. Do not raise knee gatch of the bed without raising the foot of the bed to eliminate pressure behind the knee.
   2. When the client is sitting in a chair, make sure the feet are flat on the floor to decrease the pressure from the edge of the chair behind the knee.
   3. Teach client to avoid clothing that is tight and restricts circulation to the lower extremities (e.g., knee high hose, girdles).
E. Elevate extremities while at rest.
F. Promote blood flow to legs.
   1. Avoid standing in one position for prolonged periods.
   2. Avoid crossing legs at the knees or ankles while in bed.
F. Prevent vasoconstriction.
   1. Decrease caffeine intake.
   2. Stop all tobacco use.
   3. Avoid becoming chilled, keep lower extremities warm.
G. Control diseases precipitating arterial problems.
   1. Diabetes.
   2. Hypertension.

✓ **NURSING PRIORITY:** *In planning and caring for the diabetic client, problems of peripheral vascular disease must be considered. Poor peripheral circulation is a common complication.*

❖ Goal: To provide appropriate preoperative care.
A. See Chapter 3.
❖ Goal: To evaluate and promote circulation in the affected extremity following vascular surgery.
A. Perform extremity circulation checks: initially every 15 minutes, then hourly, then every 4 hours. Report immediately any changes in quality of pulses.
B. Encourage movement of the extremity as soon as client is awake. Avoid flexion in the area of the graft (femoral or popliteal areas).
C. Encourage client to be out of bed and ambulate as soon as indicated; perform pulse checks when client returns to bed.
D. Do not allow the raised knee gatch of the bed to put pressure on the popliteal area.
E. Assess client's response to anticoagulants; maintain bleeding precautions (see Chapter 14).
F. Continue measures to protect the feet.
G. Assess for development of dependent edema; may require compression dressings or use of diuretics.
H. Monitor for potential complications of bleeding (e.g., clot formation, compartment syndrome).
I. Assess type of pain – pain from increased perfusion is different than pain of ischemia prior to surgery.
J. Notify surgeon or HCP immediately of any symptoms suggestive of a further decrease in circulation or of occlusion of graft.
❖ Goal: To provide general postoperative care as indicated (see Chapter 3).

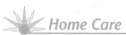 Home Care

A. Lose weight if appropriate through a low-fat, low-cholesterol, high-fiber diet.
B. Avoid:
   1. Standing or sitting for prolonged periods of time.
   2. Avoid tight socks, constrictive clothing, stockings.
   3. Smoking.
C. Avoid trauma to the extremities.
D. Care of extremities:
   1. Visually inspect feet daily
   2. Avoid bath water that is too hot.
   3. Dry well between toes.
   4. Prevent drying of skin; no lotion between toes.
   5. Clip nails straight across.
   6. Seek care promptly for ulcerations or blisters.
   7. Always wear well-fitting/protective shoes; do not go barefoot.
   8. Elevate feet if they are swelling.
   9. Evaluate bruises and discolored areas.
   10. Assess for any breaks in the skin.

E. Do not apply direct heat to the legs.
F. Exercise as tolerated; stop if pain occurs.
G. Maintain good nutrition.
H. Teach client methods to increase circulation during normal work day (do not cross legs; use a good chair; get up and walk every hour if working at a desk).

> **TEST ALERT:** *Review client adaptations to illness and/or disease. Assist client in identifying behaviors that could impact health.*

Thromboangiitis Obliterans (Buerger's Disease)

* **Thromboangiitis obliterans is a condition that causes vasculitis of the small and medium-size arteries and veins of the extremities.**

Data Collection

A. Intermittent claudication.
B. Pain is predominant symptom.
C. Cyanosis and redness of the extremity.
D. Increased sensitivity to cold in the extremity.
E. Ischemic ulcerations may develop in fingers, toes, and then may progress upward.
F. Decreased sensation.
G. Peripheral pulses may be diminished or absent (see Figure 11-3).
H. Closely associated with tobacco use, especially young men who smoke.

Treatment

No cure; treatment is based on symptoms; cessation of all tobacco use frequently stops disease progress.

Nursing Interventions

❖ **Goal:** To evaluate level of involvement of the extremity and increase circulation to the extremity.
A. Encourage client to decrease or stop all tobacco use.
B. Evaluate tolerance to activity.
C. Inspect feet for vascular changes.
D. Have client perform postural exercises to decrease venous congestion.
E. Perform circulatory checks of the affected extremity.
F. Protect extremities from exposure to cold.
❖ **Goal:** To assist client to understand implications of the disease and measures to maintain health.
A. See PVD goals about assisting client to understand implications of the disease.

> ✔ *NURSING PRIORITY: The vascular problem has a direct relationship to cigarette smoking. The client should understand that in order for the condition to be controlled, he must quit smoking.*

Raynaud's Disease

* **A disease characterized by episodic spasms of the small cutaneous arteries. It occurs primarily in the fingers.**

Raynaud's Phenomena

A. Intermittent episodic spasms of the arterioles of the fingers, toes, nose, and ears. Spasms are not necessarily correlated with other peripheral vascular problems.
B. Condition usually occurs in the hands and is bilateral and symmetrical.

Data Collection

A. Increased incidence in females 20 to 49 years old.
B. Symptoms are precipitated by:
   1. Exposure to cold.
   2. Emotional stress.
   3. Smoking.
   4. Caffeine consumption.
C. Associated with connective tissue diseases such as systemic lupus erythematosus, scleroderma, and rheumatoid arthritis.
D. Initially there is pallor or cyanosis due to the vaso spasm, causing numbness and tingling. As digits warm, there is redness, warmth, and throbbing as hyperemia occurs.
E. Involvement generally is bilateral.
F. Pulses may remain adequate.
G. Attacks are usually intermittent and only last a few minutes.

Treatment

A. No cure; diagnosis and treatment are based on symptoms.
B. Vasodilating medications.

Nursing Interventions

❖ **Goal:** To assist client to understand disease implications and measures to increase arterial circulation.
A. Stop all tobacco use, especially smoking.
B. Evaluate client's response to activities.
C. Perform circulatory checks of the affected extremity.
D. Perform visual inspection of the skin of the affected extremity.
E. Protect extremities from exposure to cold.
F. Limit caffeine intake.
G. Avoid vasoconstrictive drugs.

Aneurysm

* **An aneurysm is a dilation or sac formed within the wall of an arterial vessel. The aneurysm may involve one layer or all layers of the arterial wall.**

A. Types of aneurysms.
   1. Berry aneurysm (see Chapter 15).
   2. Abdominal aortic aneurysm: occurs primarily in the abdominal aorta below the renal arteries.
   3. Thoracic aortic aneurysm: located in the aorta in the thoracic area.
   4. Dissecting aneurysm: bleeding occurs between the layers of the vessel wall.
B. Common locations.
   1. Abdominal aortic aneurysm (AAA): occurs most often in the abdominal aorta below the renal arteries.
   2. Thoracic aortic aneurysm: located on the aorta in the thoracic area.
   3. Femoral aneurysm.
   4. Popliteal aneurysm.

Data Collection

A. Abdominal aortic aneurysm (AAA).
   1. May be asymptomatic.
   2. Epigastric, back, flank or abdominal pain.
   3. Pulsating abdominal mass may be palpable.
   4. Signs of rupture.
      a. Severe back pain.
      b. Rapid hypotension and shock.
      c. Abdominal distention and tenderness.
      d. Hematoma formation in the flank region.
B. Thoracic aortic aneurysm.
   1. Frequently asymptomatic.
   2. Compression of structures in the adjacent area.
      a. Dysphagia due to pressure on the esophagus.
      b. Hoarseness due to pressure on the laryngeal nerve.
      c. Pressure on the vena cava may cause edema of head and arms.
   3. Signs of dissection and rupture.
      a. Sudden constant, excruciating back and/or chest pain.
      b. Rapid hypotension progressing to shock.
C. Diagnostics (see Appendix 11-1).
   1. Chest x-ray.
   2. Aortography.
   3. Abdominal ultrasound.

Treatment

Directed toward prevention of rupture (e.g., surgical resection of the aneurysm).

Nursing Interventions

❖   **Goal:** To prepare client and family for anticipated surgery.
A. Provide appropriate preoperative care (see Chapter 3).
B. Identify other chronic health problems that will have implications postoperatively (hypertension, diabetes, PVD).

C. Evaluate characteristics of pulses in the lower extremities; mark locations and document status for evaluation postoperatively.
❖   **Goal:** To monitor, prevent, and recognize complications before surgical intervention.
A. Control hypertension.
   1. Administer antihypertensives.
   2. Decrease risk factors.
B. Observe closely for signs of rupture/dissection.
C. Do not vigorously palpate abdomen.

 TEST ALERT: *Determine if client is prepared for surgery. Monitor client after surgery.*

❖   **Goal:** To promote graft patency and optimal circulation postoperative aneurysm resection.
A. Follow general postoperative care as indicated (see Chapter 3).
B. Maintain adequate blood pressure to facilitate tissue perfusion and filling of the graft.
C. Monitor client response to (IV) fluids and blood components.
D. Initially perform hourly checks of peripheral circulation; monitor characteristics of pulses in lower extremities (see Figure 11-3). Symptoms of graft occlusion include:
   1. Changes or decrease in quality of pulse.
   2. Extremity cool below level of graft.
   3. Change in color of extremity.
   4. Increase in abdominal distention and increased severity of pain in extremities.
E. Evaluate urine output hourly.
F. Evaluate blood urea nitrogen (BUN) and serum creatinine levels to assess renal function.
G. Maintain adequate body warmth to prevent temperature-induced vasoconstriction.
H. Immediately report any changes in the status of circulation of a client's extremity.

TEST ALERT: *Recognize client conditions that result in insufficient vascular perfusion; review assessment of peripheral pulses of client. Pulse checks are critical in vascular surgery client. The nurse should compare the peripheral pulses in the lower extremities and initiate protective and preventative actions.*

❖   **Goal:** To maintain homeostasis and prevent postoperative complications.
A. Maintain adequate body warmth.
B. Assess and maintain adequate hydration.
C. Assess for elevation of temperature.
D. Evaluate for return of GI function.
   1. Bowel sounds.
   2. Distention.
   3. Passage of flatus.
   4. Diarrhea.

E. Nasogastric suction is frequently used in the immediate postoperative period to prevent gastric distention from causing increased pressure around area of the graft.

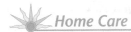 *Home Care*

A. Activity restrictions.
   1. No heavy lifting for 6-12 weeks.
   2. Avoid activities that involve pushing, pulling, or straining.
B. Report any signs of infection, redness, swelling, drainage, or fever.

 Shock (Severe Hypotension)

✳ **Shock is characterized by inadequate blood flow and tissue perfusion.**

A. For adequate circulation to occur, all parts of the circulatory system must function effectively together.
   1. Adequate vascular tone to maintain normal resistance of the vessels.
   2. Ability of the heart to maintain cardiac output.
   3. Adequate amount of total blood volume.
B. The initial problems precipitating shock and the specific treatment for the problems are very different. However, regardless of the precipitating cause of shock, the underlying problem is inadequate tissue perfusion.
C. Classifications of shock.
   1. Hypovolemic shock: size of vascular compartment remains the same while the volume of blood or plasma decreases; may be relative or absolute.
      a. Hemorrhage.
      b. Burns.
      c. Severe fluid loss.
   2. Cardiogenic shock: heart is unable to effectively circulate the intravascular volume.
      a. Dysrhythmias.
      b. Myocardial infarction (MI).
      c. Heart failure.
   3. Distributive shock: an increase in the blood volume on the venous side with a decrease in the venous return to the heart.
      a. Neurogenic: spinal cord shock; loss of nerve supply to blood vessels.
      b. Septic: vasodilation from severe infection.
      c. Anaphylactic: vasodilation secondary to histamine release (allergic reactions).
   4. Obstructive shock: physical impediment to blood flow.
      a. Pulmonary embolism.
      b. Vena cava compression.
      c. Tension pneumothorax.

Data Collection

Signs and symptoms of shock are essentially the same regardless of the precipitating cause.

> 💡 *TEST ALERT: Implement interventions to manage potential client circulatory complications. Be able to recognize clients at increased risk; know the early symptoms of shock and initiate protective and preventive actions.*

A. Risk factors.
   1. Increased incidence in the very young and in the very old.
   2. Increased incidence in clients with chronic progressive disease states.
   3. Trauma.
   4. Postoperative hemorrhage.
B. Clinical manifestations.
   1. Compensatory stage (early).
      a. Client is oriented to time, place, and date but may be restless or apprehensive with increased anxiety.
      b. BP—low normal; pulse—increased or normal; respirations—increased; temperature—normal or subnormal.
      c. Urine output may be slightly decreased, but within normal range.
      d. Complaints of thirst and feeling cool; skin pale and cool.
      e. Nausea/vomiting common as BP decreases.
   2. Progressive stage (intermediate).
      a. Decreasing sensory perception; decreased responsiveness to stimuli.
      b. Vital signs.
         (1) BP continues to decrease.
         (2) Pulse rate increased with weak or thready peripheral pulses.
         (3) Respirations—rate is increased with dyspnea.
      c. Cold, moist skin; pallor.
      d. Decrease in urine to oliguric levels.
      e. Development of acidosis
   3. Refractory (irreversible, late).
      a. Progressively decreasing level of consciousness to unresponsiveness.
      b. BP—not measurable (unable to perfuse vital organs); pulse—slow and irregular; respirations—irregular, shallow, labored.
      c. Anuria.
      d. Client becomes hypoxic with skin pallor, cyanosis and mottling.
   4. Diagnostics: based on the clinical manifestations and history of underlying problems.

Treatment

Depends on the underlying problem.

Nursing Interventions

❖ Goal: To identify and monitor progress.

A. Maintain bed rest.
B. Position supine to increase venous return but not compromise pulmonary status.
C. Maintain airway; provide supplemental oxygen.
D. Keep warm; no chilling.
E. Protect from falls and injury.
F. Evaluate for progression of shock—compensating to noncompensating.

❖ Goal: To maintain ventilation and prevent hypoxia (see Chapter 10).

A. Monitor levels of pulse oximetry, ABGs.
B. Determine quality and changes in breath sounds, characteristics of respirations.
C. Monitor changes in orientation and presence of confusion.
D. Maintain airway patency.

❖ Goal: To correct acid-base imbalance (see Chapter 5).

❖ Goal: To assess and support the cardiovascular and respiratory systems.

A. Monitor blood pressure closely in individuals at increased risk.
B. Evaluate tissue perfusion in response to dysrhythmias.
C. Protect integrity of venous access lines.
D. Hypovolemic shock requires an increase in the circulating volume; monitor client response to fluid resuscitation.

❖ Goal: To evaluate renal response to decrease in cardiac output.

> 💡 **TEST ALERT: Identify client factors that could interfere with elimination. Decreased urinary output is often an early observable sign of decreased renal perfusion secondary to decrease in cardiac output.**

A. Evaluate urine output hourly.
B. Carefully assess renal response to increase in IV fluids.
C. Monitor BUN and creatinine for evidence of renal complications.

❖ Goal: To maintain homeostasis and decrease effects of shock.

A. Monitor client response to medications to counteract effects of shock (see Appendix 11-6).
B. Continue to orient client.
C. Decrease unnecessary sensory stimuli.
D. Maintain NPO; provide oral hygiene.
E. Evaluate for bowel sounds and distention due to intestinal ischemia.
F. Keep client comfortably warm; do not allow chilling.
F. Do not administer medications PO, IM, or subcutaneously because of decreased tissue perfusion. (RN or HCP will administer medications IV push.)
G. Provide emotional support; continue to talk with client and describe procedures before they are done.
H. Avoid unnecessary nursing procedures.

📋 Chronic Venous Insufficiency and Venous Stasis Ulcers

✳ **Chronic venous insufficiency (CVI) results from damage to the valves of the veins in the legs.**

A. The primary cause of chronic venous insufficiency is incompetent valves of the deep veins, primarily in the lower extremities.
B. Compression and relief of venous congestion are the key factors to treatment and prevention of CVI.
C. This valvular incompetence leads to regurgitation of blood, venous pooling, and edema in the lower extremities; eventually resulting in development of venous stasis ulcers.

Data Collection

A. Risk factors.
 1. Valve incompetence.
 2. Chronic disease (diabetes).
 3. Previous episode of DVT.
B. Clinical manifestations.
 1. Brown or "brawny" skin on lower legs.
 2. Edema.
 3. Stasis dermatitis or stasis eczema is often the first indication.
 4. Ulcers occur above the outer ankle.
 5. Ulcers typically have irregularly shaped margins and red in color.
 6. Copious serosanguineous drainage from ulcers.
 7. Ulcerations are very painful.
C. Diagnostics: history and clinical manifestations.
D. Complications.
 1. Infection and cellulitis are common.
 2. Delayed or poor healing.

Treatment

A. Medical therapy.
 1. Compression therapy.
  a. Elastic compression stockings.
  b. Sequential compression devices.
  c. Unna boot (a paste bandage).
 2. Moist dressings for open wound care.
 3. Good nutritional status.
 4. Treatment of varicose veins.
B. Surgical therapy: excision of ulcer with skin grafting.

Nursing Interventions

❖ Goal: To prevent/relieve venous congestion; this is the key to ulcer management (Box 11-3).

BOX 11-3 NURSING MEASURES TO DECREASE VENOUS STASIS

- Encourage mobility; even standing at the bedside promotes venous tone.
- Elastic support stockings:
  1. Hospitalized clients should wear them all the time.
  2. Home clients generally wear them during the day; they should put stockings on before getting out of bed and remove them when going to bed.
  3. Make sure the stockings are not causing increased pressure behind the knee, and do not allow stockings to bunch up and cause constriction behind the knee.
  4. Toe hole should be under the toes and heel patch over the heel.
  5. Do not hang feet dependent when putting stockings on; elevate or place them parallel on the bed.
- Pneumatic sequential compression devices (SCDs) may be used in the hospital on clients at increased risk for complications secondary to venous stasis.
  1. Remove every 8 hours to inspect skin.
  2. If client is at high risk for development of thrombophlebitis, measure area to determine if there is an increase in size of calf or thigh.
  3. Assess legs for areas of warmth, tenderness, or inflammation.
- Teach client to elevate legs for about 20 minutes every 4 to 5 hours.
- Avoid prolonged sitting; get up an walk for 5 minutes every 1 to 2 hours.
- Do not cross legs when sitting or lying in bed.
- Do not wear clothing that restricts circulation to lower extremities.
- Maintain good fluid intake; avoid dehydration.

> **TEST ALERT:** *Implement interventions to promote venous return. Plan interventions to prevent complications of cardiovascular system.*

A. Compression devices: prevention of venous stasis is the key to healing.
  1. Compression boots/stockings: extremity may be covered with continuous compression bandage, boot, or stocking.
  2. Intermittent or sequential pneumatic compression devices: always check arterial circulation with any type of compression device.
  3. Assess adequacy of arterial circulation prior to initiating compression therapy.
B. Keep feet clean and dry; assess for development of venous ulcers.
C. Keep feet/legs elevated.
D. Avoid prolonged sitting/standing.
E. Institute a daily walking program once ulcers have healed.
❖ **Goal:** Promote healing of venous stasis ulcers.
A. Apply moist oxygen permeable dressings (e.g., hydrocolloids, foams).

B. Change dressings as necessary due to excessive wound drainage.
C. Dressing may be used in combination with compression devices.
D. Encourage increase in protein and vitamins to promote healing.
❖ **Goal:** To teach clients about self-care as recurrence of CVI is high.
A. Avoid trauma to limbs.
B. Use moisturizing lotions to prevent skin from cracking; do not use fragrant products.
C. Seek medical care at first sign of wound infection
  1. Pain
  2. Purulent drainage
  3. Offensive odor.

> **TEST ALERT:** *Implement measures to promote venous return, to manage potential circulatory complications, and to monitor wounds for signs and symptoms of infection.*

Varicose Veins

✳ **Varicose veins occur when veins in the lower trunk and extremities become congested and dilated because of incompetent valves in the vessels, as well as loss of elasticity of the vessel wall. As venous pressure increases, the-muscle around the vein fails to constrict effectively, and there is increased congestion and decreased venous return.**

Data Collection

A. Risk factors.
  1. Congenital weakness of the vein walls.
  2. Obesity.
  3. Pregnancy.
  4. Work settings requiring prolonged sitting or standing.
B. Clinical manifestations.
  1. Dilated, tortuous subcutaneous veins.
  2. Objectionable cosmetic appearance.
  3. Aching or pain after prolonged standing.
  4. Pain generally relieved by elevating the extremity.
  5. Nocturnal leg cramps.

Treatment

A. Medical.
  1. Rest with feet elevated.
  2. Elastic support hose.
B. Surgical.
  1. Scleropathy: injection of sclerosing agents into affected vein.
  2. Surgical ligation of the veins; may be combined with vein stripping as well.

Nursing Interventions

❖ **Goal:** To identify client at high risk and prevent development of varicosities.

A. Encourage client to avoid sitting or standing for prolonged periods of time.

B. Prevent injuries to extremities.

C. Encourage client to avoid constrictive clothing.

D. Teach client to avoid rubbing extremities.

❖ **Goal:** To assist client to understand implications of the disease and measures to maintain health.

A. Elastic stockings should be put on before getting out of bed in the morning.

B. Maintain good skin care of lower extremities.

C. Decrease weight if appropriate.

D. Avoid prolonged standing or sitting in the work environment.

E. Avoid constrictive clothing.

Thrombophlebitis

✳ **Problem begins with an inflammation of the *vein*. The inflammatory process may initiate a clot formation and the development of deep vein thrombosis (DVT). Thrombi occurring in the deep veins of the pelvis, legs, and abdomen are of particular concern because there is increased incidence of embolus formation.**

> **TEST ALERT:** *Identify complications of immobility. Monitor client responses to interventions for preventing complications from immobility. With any condition that causes an increase in venous stasis or inflammation to a vein, there is a significant increased risk for the development of thrombophlebitis and DVT.*

Data Collection

A. Risk factors (Virchow's Triad).

1. Venous stasis.
    a. Surgery (hip, pelvic and orthopedic surgery are associated with high risk).
    b. Pregnancy, obesity.
    c. Prolonged immobility (bed rest, long trips, prolonged sitting).
    d. Heart disease (atrial fibrillation, congestive heart failure).

2. Hypercoagulability.
    a. Malignancies, dehydration.
    b. Blood dyscrasias.
    c. Oral contraceptives, hormone replacement therapy.
    d. Pregnancy and postpartum.

3. Endothelial damage.
    a. IV fluids and drugs (IV catheterization, drug abuse, caustic solutions or drugs)
    b. Abdominal and pelvic surgery.

c. Fractures and dislocations (especially of the pelvis, hip, or leg).

d. History of DVT.

B. Clinical manifestations.

1. Redness, warmth, and tenderness along vein.
2. Cramping calf pain.
3. Swollen extremity.
4. Warm, cyanotic skin.
5. Increased temperature.
6. Homans' sign: this is no longer considered an accurate indicator of thrombophlebitis.

> ✔ **NURSING PRIORITY:** *Do not attempt to check Homans' sign on a client with a diagnosis of thrombophlebitis. This can cause embolization of a thrombus that is present.*

C. Diagnostics (Appendix 11-1).

D. Complications.

1. DVT associated with high risk for pulmonary emboli.
2. Chronic venous insufficiency and venous stasis ulcers.

> **TEST ALERT:** *Implement measures to manage potential circulatory complications. Due to the multiple types of conditions that precipitate circulatory complications, questions may be incorporated into the care of the surgical client, the obstetric client, or any client with problems of circulation or immobility.*

Treatment

A. Medical (primary method of treatment).

1. Bed rest with elevation of affected extremity.
2. Warm, moist heat.
3. Anticoagulants, anti-inflammatory and fibrinolytic medications (see Appendix 11-3, and 5-7).
4. Elastic stockings if edema is present after client is ambulatory.
5. Elastic stocking on *unaffected leg* during period of bed rest.
6. Range-of-motion exercises on *unaffected leg* during bed rest.

B. Surgical intervention: done to prevent pulmonary emboli.

1. Venous thrombectomy.
2. Vena cava ligation.
3. Umbrella filter device in the vena cava.

Nursing Interventions

> ✔ **NURSING PRIORITY:** *The best way to prevent the development of a pulmonary emboli is to prevent the development of DVT or thrombophlebitis. It is much easier to prevent the problem than it is to treat it.*

❖ **Goal:** To prevent problem of thrombophlebitis in clients at high risk.

A. Use prophylactic measures for the surgical client (see Chapter 3).

B. Prevent complications of immobility (see Chapter 3).

C. Provide prophylactic anticoagulation medications for the high-risk client (e.g., hip and prostate surgery clients).

D. Implement nursing measures to decrease venous stasis (see Box 11-3).

   1. Do not cross legs in the bed or while sitting.

   2. Do not place a pillow under the knees.

   3. Do not stand or sit in one position for a prolonged period of time.

   4. Perform isometric exercises of the calf and thigh muscles.

   5. Intermittent pneumatic compression devices may be used to facilitate venous return.

❖ **Goal:** To decrease inflammatory response and prevent emboli formation.

A. Maintain bed rest with the feet elevated.

B. Warm, moist soaks may be used to dilate arteries and veins and to decrease lymphatic congestion and promote healing.

C. Observe client for adverse reactions to anticoagulants (see Appendix 11-3).

D. Elastic stockings may be used if client's legs become edematous after ambulating.

E. Do not use pillow under the knees or elevate the knee gatch of the bed.

F. Measure circumference of client's calf daily to determine changes.

☀ Home Care

A. Avoid oral contraceptives.

B. Decrease/stop smoking.

C. Avoid constrictive clothing on lower extremities.

D. Stand and walk every hour if working at a desk or sedentary activity.

E. Lose weight if indicated.

F. Decrease sodium in diet if edema is present.

G. Follow instructions regarding anticoagulation therapy at home.

H. Follow measures to prevent venous stasis and promote venous return (see Box 11-3).

I. Report increased pain, swelling, redness, or skin changes.

Study Questions: Vascular System

1. A client had an aortic femoral bypass graft. The nurse assists the client back to bed after he has ambulated. What will be a priority nursing assessment?

   1 Determine fluctuations in client's blood pressure.

   2 Assess pulse rate to determine tolerance of activity.

   3 Evaluate the temperature of the client's affected extremity.

   4 Determine quality of pulse in the client's affected extremity.

2. The nurse is teaching a client about home care and treatment of the venous stasis ulcers on his leg. What would be included in the nurse's instructions? Select all that apply.

   ____ 1 Dressings do not need to be changed frequently because there is minimal drainage.

   ____ 2 Healing will be facilitated by wearing leg compression devices.

   ____ 3 When in the sitting position, legs should be kept elevated.

   ____ 4 Claudication pain may be relieved by stopping all activity.

   ____ 5 Cool packs can be applied to the ulcers to decrease inflammation.

3. The nurse is told in report that a hypertensive client has been started on medications and has been experiencing orthostatic hypotension. What considerations will the nurse make in caring for this client?

   1 Assist the client to a sitting position and allow him to sit on the side of the bed before standing.

   2 When ambulating the client, observe for the presence of tachycardia and decreased blood pressure.

   3 Assess the client's blood pressure with him in a sitting and in a lying position.

   4 Obtain assistance when ambulating the client due to his tendency toward syncope.

4. The nurse is administering heparin. What is the correct procedure for administration of this medication?

   1 Check the prothrombin time and administer the medication if it is below 30 seconds.

   2 Use a 22-gauge, ½-inch needle and inject the medication subcutaneously.

   3 Inject the medication into the deltoid and rub carefully to disperse medication.

   4 With a 25-gauge, ⅝-inch needle, inject the medication into the abdomen.

5. What would the nurse identify as modifiable risk factors to prevent the development of essential hypertension?
    1   Obesity, drug abuse, smoking.
    2   Obesity, smoking, history of cancer in the family.
    3   Sedentary lifestyle, obesity, vegetarian diet.
    4   Sedentary lifestyle, obesity, smoking.

6. A hypertensive client is concerned about her medications. She asks the nurse how long she will have to take medication. What is the best nursing response?
    1   When the client returns to see her doctor in 2 months, the medications may be discontinued at that time.
    2   When the client's blood pressure returns to normal for a period of 6 months, her medication will be discontinued.
    3   To maintain stable control of her blood pressure, the client will remain on the medication indefinitely.
    4   The medication may be adjusted every month; the client needs to talk with the doctor.

7. The nurse is caring for a client with venous blood pooling in the lower extremities secondary to chronic venous insufficiency. The nurse would identify what assessment data that would correlate with this diagnosis? Select all that apply.
    _____ 1   Stasis dermatitis.
    _____ 2   Diminished peripheral pulses.
    _____ 3   Peripheral edema.
    _____ 4   Gangrenous wounds.
    _____ 5   Venous stasis ulcers.
    _____ 6   Skin hyperpigmentation.

8. A client has peripheral vascular disease with compromised circulation in the lower extremities. What would the nursing assessment reveal?
    1   Diminished pedal pulses.
    2   3+ edema bilaterally.
    3   Dusky gray color of the feet.
    4   Muscle spasms in the feet.

9. The nurse is assessing a client who is 4 hours postoperative for a repair of his aortic aneurysm. The nurse would immediately report which findings?
    1   Total urinary output of 80 mL since surgery.
    2   No bowel sounds in any of the four quadrants.
    3   Legs and feet cool to touch bilaterally.
    4   Pulses weak and equal in both extremities.

10. What is included in the nursing management of a client with deep vein thrombosis?
    1   Ambulate the client in the room to decrease venous stasis.
    2   Assist the client with active range of motion to affected extremity.
    3   Maintain the client on bed rest and elevate the foot of the bed.
    4   Elevate the legs when the client is out of bed.

11. A client has been diagnosed with left leg thrombophlebitis. Which findings would *not* be typical of this condition?

1   Pain and tenderness in the left leg.
2   Warmth over infected area.
3   Redness over infected area.
4   Decreased quality of pulse in left leg.

12. An older adult client has peripheral vascular disease and the nurse is advised that the client also experiences intermittent claudication. What are the characteristics of intermittent claudication?
    1   Pain in the client's hands being aggravated by smoking and cold temperatures.
    2   Pain occurring in the lower part of the extremity when the client is sitting down.
    3   The need for analgesics prior to walking due to increased pain.
    4   Presence of pain on ambulation, pain is relieved by sitting down.

13. What client profile indicates a high risk for the development of peripheral vascular disease?
    1   A 76-year-old client with hypertension and diabetes mellitus.
    2   A 65-year-old client with a history of hypertension and alcohol abuse.
    3   A 35-year-old athlete with a family history of diabetes.
    4   A 35-year-old client with a family history of cardiovascular disease.

14. A client has a diagnosis of deep vein thrombosis. What would be typical assessment findings?
    1   Extremity is cool to touch and edematous.
    2   Bilateral, swollen, red extremities.
    3   Thready pulse and slow capillary return.
    4   Pain with swelling in affected part of leg.

15. A client is to be discharged and the physician has changed the anticoagulant from heparin to warfarin sodium (**Coumadin**). Why is the medication being changed from heparin to **Coumadin** when the client is discharged?
    1   The client cannot safely take heparin when he gets home.
    2   **Coumadin** may be taken by mouth and heparin cannot.
    3   **Coumadin** does not require monitoring of coagulation studies.
    4   As the client becomes more mobile, the **Coumadin** is more effective.

16. The nurse is caring for a client following a thoracotomy. What assessment finding would be present if the client is experiencing hypovolemic shock from excessive bleeding?
    1   Urine output below 30 mL per hour.
    2   Jugular vein distention with head elevated.
    3   Chest tube drainage of 50 mL per hour for 4 hours.
    4   Blood pressure 110/70 mm Hg, pulse rate 120 beats per minute.

17. Which of the following would cause the most problems for a client with hypertension?
    1   Caffeine, sugar, milk products.
    2   Chocolate, tea, nicotine.

3 Caffeine, amphetamines, nicotine.
4 Fruits, sugar, amphetamines.

18. A client is taking a diuretic for treatment of his hypertension. What foods would the nurse encourage the client to eat?
1 Orange juice and apricots.
2 Cranberry juice and dairy products.
3 Leafy, green vegetables and apple juice.
4 Grains, legumes, and fish.

19. What would the nurse expect to find on the assessment of a client with a diagnosis of arterial insufficiency?
1 Thin, fragile toenails.
2 Dependent rubor.

3 Bounding arterial pulses.
4 Warm, erythematous legs.

20. The nurse is caring for a client with Buerger's disease. What would be the most important information to discuss with this client regarding his condition?
1 Elevate extremities several times a day.
2 Protect the extremities from cold.
3 Stop smoking.
4 Stop activity when pain occurs.

Answers and rationales to these questions are in the section at the end of the book titled Chapter Study Questions: Answers and Rationales.

Appendix 11-1 VASCULAR DIAGNOSTICS

	Normal Value	Therapeutic Value	Nursing Implications
SERUM STUDIES			
Activated coagulation time (ACT)	70-120 sec	150-210 sec	1. Used to evaluate heparin level changes. 2. Correlate results with APTT.
Fragment D-dimer (D-dimer test)	less than 250 ng/mL	less than 250 ng/mL	1. Confirms thrombin and plasmin generation have occurred. 2. Used in diagnosis of disseminated intravascular coagulation (DIC) and to screen for thrombosis and acute MI.
Prothrombin time (PT)	10-13-sec range	1½ to 2½ times control level	1. Used to evaluate liver function and monitor warfarin (Coumadin) medications.
Activated prothrombin time (APTT)	Activated: 30-45 sec	1½ to 2½ times normal	1. Indicator of adequacy of anticoagulation with heparin. 2. Do not draw sample from extremity with a heparin lock or infusion.
International normalized ratio (INR)	Mathematically calculated to maintain consistency	1.5-2.0 (anticoagulation) (0.7-1.8)	1. Calculated level based on PT; method of standardizing values.
INVASIVE STUDIES			
Peripheral arteriography (angiography) Venogram	Involves injection of a radiopaque dye into either the artery or the vein; x-rays are taken to identify atherosclerotic plaques, presence of aneurysms		1. Explain procedures to client; mild sedative may be indicated. 2. After procedure: a. Circulatory checks distal to the puncture site. b. Observe client for allergic reactions to the dye. c. Pressure dressings to arterial puncture sites.

NONINVASIVE STUDIES

Doppler ultrasonography: Hand-held Doppler device used to detect flow of blood in peripheral arterial disease. Is not sensitive to early disease changes.
Venous /arterial duplex scan: Uses ultrasound to assess veins for flow and pressure. Has become the primary diagnostic tool for DVT because it permits visualization of the vein.
Ankle-brachial index (ABI): Calculated index using a handheld Doppler; divide the ankle systolic blood pressure (SBP) by the highest brachial SBP; normal = 0.91 to 1.30; moderate PAD = 0.41 to 0.70.
Computerized tomography (CT): Allows for visualization of the arterial wall and adjacent structures. Used for diagnosis of abdominal aortic aneurysm or graft occlusions.
Trendelenburg's test: Client lies supine with leg elevated to drain the veins. A tourniquet is then applied at mid thigh and the client is asked to stand. Veins normally fill from below (or distally); a varicose vein will fill from above (or proximally) because of the incompetent valves. Do not leave tourniquet in place longer than 1 minute.

Appendix 11-2 ANTIHYPERLIPIDEMIC MEDICATIONS

Medications	Side Effects	Nursing Implications
Antihyperlipidemics: Decrease LDL cholesterol, but preferably do not decrease the HDL cholesterol. Used in combination with dietary restrictions, exercise, and smoking cessation to reduce blood lipid levels.		

General Nursing Implications

- Advise client that serum liver enzymes should be monitored throughout therapy.
- Medications should be taken with the evening meal or at bedtime.
- Medications should be used in conjunction with other lipid-lowering therapies (exercise, low-cholesterol diet, smoking cessation).
- Serum cholesterol and triglyceride levels should be monitored periodically throughout therapy.

Medications	Side Effects	Nursing Implications
Cholestyramine (**Questran**): PO Colestipol (**Colestid**): PO	GI disturbances Constipation	1. Supplemental fat-soluble vitamins in long-term therapy. 2. Mix powder or granules with several ounces of fluid for administration, do not take the medication dry. 3. Use with caution in presence of constipation; increase fiber and fluid intake to prevent constipation.
Colesevelam (**Welchol**): PO		1. Take all tablets with food and water 2. Does not have side effects of **Questran** or **Colestid**.
Nicotinic acid (**Niacin, Nicolar**): PO	Intense flushing GI disturbances Hyperglycemia	1. Immediately report signs of hepatotoxicity (darkening of urine, light colored stools, anorexia). 2. Flushing occurs in almost all clients; will diminish over several weeks.
Gemfibrozil (**Lopid**): PO	Diarrhea GI disturbances Abdominal pain	1. Assess for increase in muscle pain. 2. Will potentiate warfarin-derivative anticoagulants (**Coumadin**). 3. Do not confuse with hyoscyamine (**Levbid**).
Lovastatin (**Mevacor**): PO Simvastatin (**Zocor**): PO Fluvastatin (**Lescol**): PO Atorvastatin (**Lipitor**): PO Pravastatin (**Pravachol**): PO Crestor (**Rosuvastatin**) PO	Muscle breakdown Hepatotoxic GI disturbances	1. Should not be given to clients with pre-existing liver disease. 2. Advise client to report any increase in muscle pain. 3. Do not confuse pravastatin (**Pravachol**) with lansoprazole (**Prevacid**).

GI, Gastrointestinal; *HDL*, high-density lipoprotein; *LDL*, low-density lipoprotein; *PO*, by mouth (orally).

Appendix 11-3   ANTICOAGULANTS/ANTIPLATELETS

Medications	Side Effects	Nursing Implications

General Nursing Implications

- Increased risk for bleeding when used concurrently with other drugs, herbal remedies, or foods affecting coagulation.
- Initiate bleeding precautions (Box 9-1).
- Do not automatically discontinue according to automatic stop policies (procedures, surgery) without verifying the order; reevaluate all clients whose anticoagulants are being held for procedures and assess the need to reorder the anticoagulant therapy.

> ✔ **NURSING PRIORITY:** *If heparin is discontinued, within hours the client is not adequately anticoagulated and is at increased risk for complications.*

Medications	Side Effects	Nursing Implications
Heparin: IV, subQ May not be given PO. Short-term anticoagulation	Bleeding tendencies: hematuria, bleeding gums, or frank hemorrhage Heparin-induced thrombocytopenia: associated with increase in thrombosis	1. Check the APTT for therapeutic levels. 2. Protamine sulfate is the antidote. 3. Will not dissolve established clots. 4. Evaluate client for decreased platelets. 5. Effective immediately after administration; anticoagulation effect has a half life of 1.5 hours. 6. Do not store in same area as insulin; both are given by units. 7. Prophylactic use does not require daily APTT levels. 8. Determine if heparin is being used to treat thromboembolic problem or as prophylaxis for thromboembolic problems.
Low-Molecular Weight-Heparin Enoxaparin (**Lovenox**): subQ Dalteparin sodium (**Fragmin**): subQ		1. Use: prophylaxis for thromboembolic problems in high-risk clients (immobility, hip or knee replacement). 2. Dosage is not interchangeable with heparin. 3. Leave the air lock in the prefilled syringe to prevent leakage. 4. Lovenox should be injected into the "love handles" of the abdomen.

Warfarin sodium
(**Coumadin**): PO
Long-term anticoagulation
		1. Check the PT and INR to evaluate level of anticoagulation.
		2. Vitamin K is the antidote.
		3. Half-life is 3-5 days; discontinue 3 days before any invasive procedure.
		4. Client teaching:
		  • Bleeding precautions (Box 9-1).
		  • Advise all health care providers of medication – drug interactions are common.
		  • Maintain routine checks on coagulation studies.
		  • Do not stop taking medication unless told to do so by health care provider.

> **TEST ALERT:** *Observe for effects of medications. Review the nursing implications associated with administration of anticoagulants.*

Antiplatelet Medications		
Aspirin: PO	GI bleeding, hemorrhagic stroke	1. Given in small doses (e.g., 81 mg daily). 2. Prophylactic therapy for prevention of MI and thrombotic stroke in clients with TIAs.
Clopidogrel (**Plavix**): PO	Abdominal pain, dyspepsia, diarrhea Blood dyscrasias	1. Prophylactic treatment for prevention of MI, strokes in clients with established peripheral artery disease. 2. Expensive and slightly more effective than aspirin. 3. Monitor for bleeding tendencies.
Cilostazol (**Pletal**): PO	Headache, dizziness, GI bleeding	1. Monitor for relief of intermittent claudication. 2. Grapefruit juice inhibits metabolism. 3. Administer on an empty stomach.
Ticlopidine (**Ticlid**): PO	Diarrhea, bleeding, aplastic anemia	1. Monitor coagulation studies throughout therapy. 2. Monitor cholesterol/triglyceride levels.

GI, Gastrointestinal; *MI*, myocardial infarction; *PO*, by mouth (orally); *TIA*, transient ischemic attack

Appendix 11-4   ANTIHYPERTENSIVE MEDICATIONS

Medications	Side Effects	Nursing Implications

General Nursing Implications

- Advise client that postural (orthostatic) hypotension may occur and how to decrease effects:
    Sit on side of bed before standing, make sure client is stable before standing.
    Do not stand for prolonged periods of time.
    Older client is at increased risk
    May occur with first dose or subsequent doses.
    Problem is most often temporary.
- Hypotension may be increased by hot weather, hot showers, hot tubs, and alcohol ingestion.
- Client should not abruptly discontinue medication or change dosage without consulting health care provider. Abrupt withdrawal can cause rebound hypertension.
- Encourage a low-sodium diet and weight maintenance or reduction.
- Discourage use of all tobacco products.
- Have client report unpleasant side effects related to sexual dysfunction.
- Advise client not to take over-the-counter cough medications or decongestants that contain pseudoephedrine; these medications cause an increase in BP.

 TEST ALERT: *Observe for effects of medications. Evaluate client's use of medications.*

Medications	Side Effects	Nursing Implications
Vasodilator: Acts directly on vascular smooth muscle to produce vasodilation.		
Hydralazine HCl (**Apresoline**): PO, IM, IV	Tachycardia, headache, sodium retention, drug-induced lupus syndrome	1. Advise client that postural hypotension may occur. 2. May be used in combination with other antihypertensive medications.
Minoxidil (**Loniten**): PO	Tachycardia, sodium and water retention	1. Used in clients with severe hypertension that is not responding to other medications. 2. Requires very close monitoring of blood pressure.
Centrally Acting Inhibitors (antiadrenergics): Decrease sympathetic effect (norepinephrine), resulting in decreased BP and peripheral resistance, decrease in heart rate, and no change in cardiac output.		
Methyldopa: PO Methyldopate: IV	Hepatotoxicity, hemolytic anemia, sexual dysfunction, orthostatic hypotension	1. If withdrawn abruptly, may precipitate a hypertensive crisis. 2. Do not confuse methyldopa with levodopa or L-dopa 3. Monitor for depression or altered mental status in older adults.
ACE Inhibitors: Reduce peripheral vasculature resistance without increasing cardiac output, rate, or contractility; angiotension antagonists.		
Captopril (**Capoten**): PO Enalapril (**Vasotec**): PO Lisinopril (**Zestril**): PO Ramipril (**Altace**): PO Moexipril (**Univase**): PO Benazepril (**Lotensin**): PO	Postural hypotension, hyperkalemia, insomnia, nonproductive cough, loss of taste	1. Monitor closely on first dose; hypotension and first-dose syncope frequently occurs. 2. Conserve potassium; may not need a potassium supplement when given with a diuretic. 3. Skipping doses or stopping drug may result in rebound hypertension.
Beta-Adrenergic Blockers and ***Calcium Channel Blockers*** See Appendix 12-2.		

ACE, Angiotensin-converting enzyme; *BP*, blood pressure; *ECG*, electrocardiogram; *GI*, gastrointestinal; *IM*, intramuscularly; *IV*, intravenously; *PO*, by mouth (orally).

Appendix 11-5   DIURETICS

®

General Nursing Implications

- In hospitalized clients, evaluate daily weights for fluid loss or gain.

- Evaluate intake and output records and compare to weight gain or loss.

a Monitor for hypokalemia, anorexia, muscle weakness, numbness, tingling, paresthesia, confusion, and excessive thirst.

- Advise client of foods that are rich in potassium (Table 2-2).

- Administer medications in the morning to allow diuresis to occur during the day.

- Teach client how to decrease effects of postural hypotension.

- Monitor BP response to medication.

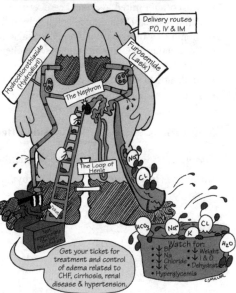

FIGURE 11-4 Diuretic Water Slide - (From: Zerwekh, JA, Claborn, JC, Miller, CJ, *Memory Notebook of Nursing: Pharmacology and Diagnostics, ed 2,* Ingram, Texas, 2009, Nursing Education Consultants.)

Medications	Side Effects	Nursing Implications
Loop Diuretics: Block sodium and chloride reabsorption. Prevent reabsorption of water back into the circulation causing an increase in excretion of the water, and produces diuresis.		
Furosemide (**Lasix**): PO, IM, IV Bumetanide (**Bumex**): PO, IM, IV Torsemide (**Demadex**): PO, IV	Dehydration, hypotension; excessive loss of potassium, sodium, chloride; hyperglycemia, hyperuricemia; muscle weakness	1. Strong diuretic that provides rapid diuresis. 2. Use with caution in older adults; CNS problems of confusion, headache. 3. Monitor closely for tinnitus/hearing loss. 4. Do not confuse Bumex with buprenorphine (**Buprenex**).
Thiazide Diuretics: Inhibit NaCl reabsorption, which causes an increase in the excretion of water, sodium, and chloride.		
Chlorothiazide (**Diuril**): IV, PO Chlorthalidone (**Hygroton**): PO Hydrochlorothiazide (**HydroDIURIL, Esidrix**): PO Metolazone (**Zaroxolyn**): PO (a thiazide-like diuretic)	Dehydration, hypotension; excessive loss of potassium, hyperglycemia, hyperuricemia; muscle weakness	1. Frequently used as first-line drug to control essential hypertension. 2. Increased risk for digitalis toxicity if taking digoxin products.
Potassium-Sparing Diuretics: Block the effect of aldosterone on renal tubules		
Spironolactone (**Aldactone**): PO Triamterene (**Dyrenium**): PO	Hyperkalemia, hyponatremia, impotence, hypotension	1. May be used in combination with other diuretics to reduce potassium loss. 2. Potassium-sparing effects may result in hyperkalemia. 3. Client should not take potassium supplements. 4. Avoid salt substitutes and foods containing large amounts of sodium or potassium.
Osmotic Diuretic: Increases osmotic pressure of the fluid in the renal tubules, preventing reabsorption of sodium and water.		
Mannitol (**Osmitrol**): IV	Pulmonary edema, CHF, tissue dehydration, nausea, vomiting	1. Stop infusion if client begins to show symptoms of respiratory complications. 2. Monitor infusion site closely for infiltration and/or extravasation. 3. May be used to decrease intracranial pressure.

BP, Blood pressure; *CHF,* congestive heart failure; *CNS,* central nervous system; *IM,* intramuscularly; *IV,* intravenously; *PO,* by mouth (orally).

| Appendix 11-6 | MEDICATIONS USED FOR TREATMENT OF SHOCK | |

General Nursing Implications

- Most often limited to critical care settings; constant monitoring is required.
- Administered IV in diluted solution by infusion pump.
- Monitor IV infusion site closely; leakage into tissue may cause tissue sloughing.
- Continuous ECG monitoring; observe client closely for cardiac dysrhythmias.
- Monitor urinary output every hour.
- Medications should not be administered to clients receiving MAOIs or tricyclic antidepressants.
- Primary responsibility of PN is to monitor client and keep RN and HCP closely advised of client's response.

Medications	Side Effects	Nursing Implications
Adrenergics: Increases myocardial contractility, thereby improving cardiac output, BP, and urine output.		
Dopamine (**Intropin**): IV	Dysrhythmias (tachycardia), angina, hypertension, headaches	1. Should not be given to clients with tachydysrhythmias or ventricular fibrillation 2. **High Alert Medication** – consequences of a medication error can be fatal, always check with RN and HCP. 3. *If extravasation occurs, stop infusion immediately and notify RN or HCP.* 4. Closely monitor VS, cardiac rhythm, and urinary output during administration.
Dobutamine (**Dobutrex**): IV	Tachycardia, dysrhythmias, hypertension	1. *Closely observe client for development of angina, notify RN or HCP.* 2. *If extravasation occurs, stop infusion and notify RN or HCP.*
Epinephrine hydrochloride (**Adrenalin**): IV	Nervousness, restlessness, tremors, angina, dysrhythmias, tachycardia, hypertension.	1. Be sure to read label correctly and use correct strength / concentration. 2. **High-Alert Medication** - dosages are easily confused and mistakes are made. 3. Use in treatment of anaphylactic shock and cardiac arrest.

ECG, Electrocardiogram; *IV,* intravenous; *MAOIs,* monoamine oxidase inhibitors; *VS,* vital signs.

Cardiac System

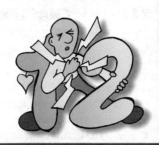

PHYSIOLOGY OF THE CARDIAC SYSTEM

A. The heart is located in the mediastinal space of the thoracic cavity.

B. The apex of the heart points downward and to the left; the apex contacts the chest wall at about the fifth to sixth intercostal space; in the normal individual, the point of maximum impulse (PMI) may be palpated here; this is also the area to auscultate and evaluate the apical heart rate.

C. Myocardial wall.
   1. Epicardium: the outer surface.
   2. Myocardium: the middle layer of cardiac muscle.
   3. Endocardium: the lining of the inner surface of the cardiac chambers.

D. Cardiac chambers (Figure 12-1).
   1. Four chambers are located within the heart; these chambers represent two pumps.
      a. Right-side pump: the right atrium and right ventricle, separated by the tricuspid valve.
      b. Primary function of the right side of the heart is to receive venous blood return from the vascular system and to pump blood through the lungs.
      c. Left-side pump: left atrium and left ventricle, separated by the mitral valve.

d. Primary function of the left side of the heart is to receive oxygenated blood from the lungs and to pump the blood through the aorta into the systemic circulation.
   2. Both atria are the receiving chambers; both ventricles are the ejecting chambers.
   3. The atrioventricular septum separates the respective chambers.
   4. The right side of the heart has a thinner myocardium than the left side and is a lower pressure system.
   5. The left ventricle is composed of thicker muscle, is a high-pressure system, and is capable of generating enough force to eject blood through the aortic valve and through the systemic circulation.
   6. Pericardium: a fibroserous sac that surrounds the heart.

E. Cardiac valves: maintain the directional flow of blood through the heart chambers.

F. Direction of blood flow through the heart structure (see Figure 12-1).
   1. From the venous system, the blood enters the right atrium via the superior vena cava and inferior vena cava; it then flows through the tricuspid valve into the right ventricle; blood is ejected from the right ventricle through the pulmonary valve into the pulmonary artery; then it goes to the lungs for oxygenation.
   2. Oxygenated blood returns to the left atrium via the pulmonary veins; it flows through the mitral valve into the left ventricle; blood from the left ventricle is ejected through the aortic valve into the aortic arch, where it enters the systemic circulation.
   3. The pulmonary artery is the only artery in the circulatory system to carry unoxygenated blood; the pulmonary vein is the only vein in the circulatory system to carry oxygenated blood.

G. Cardiac function.
   1. One complete cardiac cycle consists of contraction of the myocardium (systole) and subsequent relaxation of the myocardium (diastole).
   2. The amount of blood ejected from the ventricles is the stroke volume.
   3. The heart pumps approximately 5 L of blood every minute.
   4. The heart rate increases with exercise; therefore cardiac output increases.

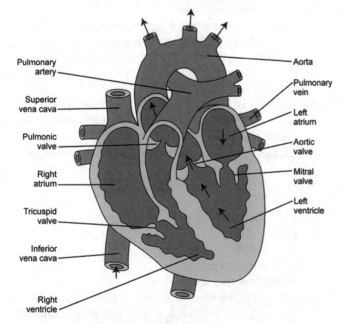

FIGURE 12-1 **Heart structures and path of oxygenated blood through the heart.** (From deWit, S: *Medical-surgical nursing: Concepts and practices,* ed 7, St Louis, 2009, Saunders.)

5. The cardiac output will vary according to the amount of venous return (preload).
H. Myocardial blood flow.
   1. Coronary arteries supply the heart muscle with oxygenated blood.
   2. Collateral circulation.
      a. There are 3 main coronary arteries that branch from the aorta and supply oxygenated blood to the cardiac muscle.
      b. With a gradual occlusion of the large coronary arteries by atherosclerotic heart disease (ASHD), the smaller vessels increase in size and branch out to provide alternative sources of blood flow (collateral circulation).
      c. Because of the development of the collateral circulation, coronary artery disease (CAD) may be well-advanced before the client experiences symptoms.
I. Conduction System (Appendix 12-4)

System Data Collection

A. Health history.
   1. Identify presence of risk factors for the development of arteriosclerotic disease (Box 12-1).
   2. Respiratory system.
      a. History of difficulty breathing.
      b. Medications taken for respiratory problems.
      c. Determine normal activity level.
   3. Circulatory system.
      a. History of chest discomfort.
      b. History of edema, weight gain.
      c. History of syncope.
      d. Medications taken for the heart or for high blood pressure.

> **TEST ALERT: Teach health promotion information. Know the risk factors for ASHD and be able to teach the client how to effectively reduce risk factors.**

B. Physical assessment.
   1. What is the overall general appearance of the client? Is there any evidence of distress? What is the level of orientation and ability to think clearly?
   2. Evaluate blood pressure.
      a. Pulse pressure: the difference between the systolic and diastolic pressures.
      b. Assess for postural (orthostatic) hypotension: decrease in blood pressure when the client stands.
   3. Evaluate character of pulse.
      a. Rate, base rhythm.
      b. Regularity, presence of irregular or ectopic beats.

BOX 12-1 RISK FACTORS IN ARTERIOSCLEROTIC HEART DISEASE

Modifiable Risk Factors
- Elevated serum cholesterol levels
- High blood pressure
- Cigarette smoking
- Sedentary lifestyle
- Obesity
- Type A personality (high-pressure lifestyle, driving, competitive)
- Poorly controlled diabetes mellitus

Nonmodifiable Risk Factors
- Genetic predisposition
- Positive family history of heart disease
- Increasing age
- Gender: occurs more often in men; increase in women after menopause

      c. Pulse deficit: the difference in the rate of the pulse at the radius and at the apex (or apical rate). If there is a pulse difference, the radial pulse rate will be less than the apical pulse rate.
      d. Pulse quality: the amplitude or quality of the pulse; pulses should be evaluated bilaterally.
         (1) +1: thready, weak, rapid pulse.
         (2) +2: diminished pulse; cannot be obliterated.
         (3) +3: easy to palpate, full; cannot be obliterated.
         (4) +4: strong bounding pulse; may be abnormal.
      e. Palpitations: client describes a feeling or sensation of rapid, bounding, or irregular heartbeat.
   4. Assess quality and pattern of respirations and evidence of respiratory difficulty.
   5. Apical heart rate: listen for the apical pulse and count the apical rate at the fifth intercostal space, mid-clavicular line.
   6. Evaluate peripheral pulses and observe for presence of peripheral edema.
   7. Weight gain: 3 or more pounds in 24 hours represents fluid gain.
   8. Evaluate for presence of chest discomfort (Box 12-2).
      a. Location.
      b. Intensity of pain.
      c. Precipitating causes.
   9. Determine client's activity level; increasing fatigue with mild exercise occurs with clients with cardiac disease.

BOX 12-2   ASSESSING CHEST PAIN-PQRST

P: Precipitating Factors

- May occur without obvious cause
- Physical exertion
- Emotional stress
- Eating a large meal
- Sexual activity

Q: Quality

- Pressure
- Squeezing
- Heaviness
- Smothering
- Burning
- Severe pain
- Increases with movement

R: Region and Radiation

- Substernal or retrosternal
- Spreads across the chest
- Radiates to the inside of either or both arms, the neck, jaw, back, upper abdomen

S: Symptoms and Signs (Associated with)

- Diaphoresis; cold, clammy skin
- Nausea, vomiting
- Dyspnea
- Orthopnea
- Syncope
- Apprehension
- Dysrhythmias
- Palpitations
- Weakness
- Feeling of impending doom

T: Timing and Response to Treatment

- Sudden onset
- Constant
- Duration
- Response to rest or nitroglycerin
- Relief with narcotics

Angina Pectoris (Chronic Angina)

*   **Coronary artery disease (CAD) occurs as a result of the atherosclerotic process (see Chapter 11) in the coronary arteries.** *Angina pectoris* **is caused by myocardial ischemia due to narrowed or blocked coronary arteries. The buildup of plaque or fatty material in the coronary artery causes a narrowing of the lumen of the artery and precipitates myocardial ischemia that causes chest pain.**

A.   Pain (angina) occurs when the oxygen demands of the heart muscle exceed the ability of the coronary arteries to deliver it.

B.   Temporary ischemia does not cause permanent damage to the myocardium. Pain frequently subsides when the precipitating factor is removed.

C.   Types of angina.
1.   Chronic stable angina
2.   Unstable angina (acute coronary syndrome).
3.   New onset angina – first symptoms of angina that most frequently occur after exertion.

Data Collection

A.   Risk factors/etiology.
1.   Arteriosclerotic heart disease (see Chapter 11).
2.   Cardiac ischemia.
3.   Increased cardiac demands.
a.   Exercise.
b.   Emotional stress.
c.   Heavy meals.
B.   Clinical manifestations—chronic stable angina.
1.   Pain in varying levels of severity (see Box 12-2).
a.   Predictable with level of stress or exertion; consistently responds well to nitroglycerin.
b.   Pain rarely occurs at rest.
2.   Pain most often is located behind or just to the left of the sternum.
3.   Pain may radiate to neck, jaw, and shoulders.
4.   Client may describe pain as squeezing, choking, or constricting or as a vague feeling of pressure and indigestion.
5.   Client will frequently deny seriousness of the pain.
6.   Most clients correlate pain with activity and increased cardiac demands.
7.   Pain is of short duration, generally lasting about 5 minutes.
8.   Accompanying symptoms may include diaphoresis, increased anxiety, pallor, and dyspnea.
C.   No permanent damage to myocardium.
D.   Diagnostics—chronic stable angina (see Appendix 12-1).

Treatment—Chronic Stable Angina

A.   Primary goal of treatment is to relieve pain and prevent future attacks.
B.   Medication – vasodilators, beta-adrenergic blockers (Appendix 12-2).
C.   Procedures/surgical intervention.
1.   Percutaneous transluminal angioplasty (PTA), percutaneous coronary intervention (PCI): A balloon is passed through an artery in the groin into the affected coronary artery to the area of obstruction. The balloon is inflated in an attempt to compress the plaque in the affected area and re-establish blood flow to the cardiac muscle.
2.   Atherectomy: a catheter is threaded into the coronary arteries, there is a rotating shaver on the tip that cuts away the plaque.

3. An intracoronary stent is an expandable wire mesh that can be inserted during any of the above procedures. A stent serves as a scaffold to support the coronary artery and increase the blood flow to the cardiac muscle.

4. Cardiac revascularization: coronary artery bypass graft (CABG) surgery, open heart surgery.

D. Restricted activity.

E. Supplemental oxygen.

F. Control of the modifiable risk factors (see Box 12-1).

Complications

A. Dysrhythmias.

B. Myocardial infarction.

> ✓ **OLDER ADULT PRIORITY:** *In the older adult client, dyspnea, not angina, may be the presenting symptom of myocardial ischemia.*

Nursing Interventions—*see acute angina (coronary artery syndrome)*

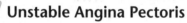

Unstable Angina Pectoris

✳ **Unstable Angina Pectoris (acute coronary syndrome [ACS]) according to the American Heart Association, includes degrees of coronary artery occlusion that can develop with coronary atherosclerosis. This includes unstable angina that occurs when a thrombus partially occludes a coronary artery causing prolonged symptoms of ischemia which can occur at rest.**

Assessment

A. Risk factors/etiology.
   1. Family history of coronary artery disease.
   2. Hypertension, hypercholesterolemia.
   3. Diabetes, smoking.
   4. Average age for first MI - men over 64.5 years, women over 70.5 years.
   5. Women are at increased risk after menopause.

B. Clinical manifestations.
   1. Two or more episodes of angina within 24 hours, pain occurs when client is at rest.
   2. Chest pain lasting longer than 20 minutes and unrelieved by nitroglycerin.
   3. Presenting symptoms in women: indigestion, pain between the shoulders, shortness of breath, and anxiety.
   4. Hypotension, dysrhythmias.

C. Diagnostics (Appendix 12-1).

D. Treatment (initial).
   1. Bed rest.
   2. Monitor vital signs, including oxygen saturation level.

3. Supplemental oxygen to maintain O_2 sat at or above 90%.

4. Reduce coronary reocclusion with antiplatelet medications. (Appendix 12-2)

5. Reduce and control ischemic pain: vasodilators (nitroglycerin, morphine sulfate IV if pain not relieved by the nitroglycerin).

Complications

A. Dysrhythmias (see Appendix 12-4).

B. Myocardial infarction (MI).

Nursing Interventions for Angina and Acute Coronary Syndrome

❖ **Goal:** To decrease pain and increase myocardial oxygenation.

A. Maintain bed rest; position client in reclining position with head elevated.

B. Begin supplemental O_2.

C. Assess characteristics of pain.

D. Administer medications.
   1. Nitroglycerin sublingual, IV, or translingual spray (Box 12-3; Appendix 12-2), evaluate client's response; pain from chronic angina is usually relieved; pain from acute angina may not be relieved.

> **BOX 12-3   CLIENT EDUCATION FOR NITROGLYCERIN ADMINISTRATION**
>
> 1. Keep in a tightly closed, dark glass container.
> 2. Carry supply at all times—either sublingual (SL) tablets or translingual spray; do not swallow sublingual tablets.
> 3. Fresh tablets (sublingual) should cause a slight burning/tingling under the tongue.
> 4. Date all opened containers and discard all medication that is 24 months old.
> 5. Take nitroglycerin prophylactically to avoid pain—before sexual intercourse, exercise, walking, etc.
> 6. Take nitroglycerin when pain begins; stop all activity.
> 7. If pain is not relieved in 5 minutes, call 911 and activate EMS.
> 8. While waiting for EMS response, if chest pain continues, take another SL pill or 1 metered sublingual spray.
> 9. Remain lying down; orthostatic hypotension can be a problem.
> 10. Long-acting preparations should not be abruptly discontinued; this may precipitate vasospasm.
> 11. To decrease development of tolerance in long-acting preparations, schedule an 8-hour nitro-free period each day, preferably at night.
> 12. Do not take erectile dysfunction drugs with nitroglycerin.
>
> **TEST ALERT: Instruct clients about self-administration of medications.**

2. Narcotic analgesics (morphine), monitor response to small increments of IV morphine.
E. *Immediately report presence of chest pain and or any changes in characteristics of chest pain to the RN.*
F. Protect venous access.
G. Maintain calm, reassuring atmosphere.
H. Evaluate vital signs.
I. *Do not leave a client alone if they are experiencing chest pain.*

> 💡 **TEST ALERT: Check client's discomfort and pain levels. Evaluate client's response to interventions.**

❖ **Goal:** To evaluate characteristics of anginal pain and client's overall response (see Box 12-2).
A. Does pain increase with breathing? (Anginal pain is generally not affected by breathing or changes in position.)
B. Assess activity tolerance or precipitating factor.
C. Assess characteristics of pain (Box 12-2).
D. Evaluate response of pain to treatment and or progression to more severe level.
E. Assess respiratory status and response to pain; presence of dyspnea, or wet breath sounds.
F. Assess for presence of irregular heartbeat and tolerance of dysrhythmias.
G. Assess adequacy of cardiac output – peripheral pulses, urinary output, level of consciousness.
H. Continuous ECG monitoring - assess for presence of dysrhythmia and impact on cardiac output.
I. Assess client's psychosocial response – denial is common; anger, fear and depression occur in both client and family.
❖ **Goal:** To provide care after cardiac interventional therapies (e.g., angioplasty, stent placement).
A. Monitor for chest pain and hypotension.
B. Frequent reassessment of status of circulation distal to area of catheter insertion.
C. A sheath may be left in place; monitor area for bleeding. If bleeding occurs, put manual pressure on the area and *notify the RN.*
D. Prevent flexion of affected extremity and maintain bed rest for 6 to 8 hours.
E. Immediately report any *bleeding at site and occurrence of chest pain or syncope.*

> 💡 **TEST ALERT: Intervene in response to client's unexpected response to therapy; document response, promote recovery.**

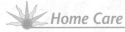 *Home Care*

A. Education regarding ASHD.
1. Assist client to identify personal risk factors and appropriate health practices to decrease risk factors.

2. Assist client to identify factors precipitating pain.
B. Avoid activities that precipitate pain (e.g., large meals, smoking, exercise, extremes in weather).
C. Understand medication (see Box 12-3 and Appendix 12-2), activity, and diet regimen.
D. If chest pain persists and is not relieved by medication, client should call primary care provider (PCP) or physician and/or go to closest emergency department.
E. Advise client to not take erectile dysfunction drugs (Appendix 17-1) if on nitrates for chest pain.

> 💡 **TEST ALERT: Review client/family understanding of health promotion behaviors/activities.**

 ## Myocardial Infarction

✳ **A myocardial infarction (MI, coronary occlusion, heart attack) is a total occlusion of a portion of a coronary artery. Immediately following the occlusion, there is myocardial ischemia. In the hours following an MI, the tissue becomes necrotic.**
A. Most common site of infarction is the left ventricle.
B. The severity of the event depends on the area of the heart involved, as well as the size of the artery occluded.
C. The presence of preestablished collateral circulation will assist in decreasing the size of the necrotic area.

Data Collection

A. Risk factors/etiology – see unstable angina.
B. Clinical manifestations.
1. Typical pain is severe, substernal, crushing, and unrelieved by nitroglycerin (see Box 12-2).
2. Frequently client will deny seriousness of the pain.
3. Pain may radiate down the arm or up to the jaw.
4. Dyspnea, nausea, vomiting and indigestion.
5. Pale, dusky skin, syncope.
6. Onset is usually sudden.
7. Diaphoresis; extreme weakness.
8. Decrease in blood pressure, tachycardia, syncope.
9. Dysrhythmias: tachycardia, irregular rhythm.
C. Diagnostics (Appendix 12-1).

> ✔ **NURSING PRIORITY:** *Danger of death from an MI is greatest during the first 2 hours.*

D. Complications
1. Dysrhythmias (see Appendix 12-4).
2. Cardiogenic shock.
3. Heart failure.

Treatment

A. Reperfusion (fibrinolytic) therapy: most effective if administered immediately or within the first 3 to 6 hours after the MI.

B. Supplemental oxygen 4 L/min via nasal cannula (maintain O_2 sat above 95%).

C. Bedrest.

D. Maintain intravenous (IV) line for medications.

E. Pain control: most often morphine; pain increases cardiac workload.

F. Medications (see Appendix 12-2).

G. Dietary restrictions.
1. Progress to diet as tolerated: low sodium and low cholesterol.
2. Decrease intake of stimulants (e.g., coffee, tea).

H. Percutaneous coronary intervention (PCI).

I. Open heart surgery for myocardial revascularization.

Nursing Interventions

❖ **Goal:** To decrease pain and increase myocardial oxygenation (see previous related goal for angina pectoris).

> ✓ *NURSING PRIORITY: As long as a client is experiencing chest pain myocardial ischemia is present. If client experiences tachycardia, decrease activity whether client has chest pain or not.*

❖ **Goal:** To evaluate characteristics of cardiac pain and client's overall response (see previous related goal for angina pectoris).

❖ **Goal:** To maintain homeostasis and decrease effects of MI.

A. Maintain IV access; report infiltration or phlebitis at site.

B. Maintain bed rest initially.

C. Evaluate urinary output and renal response to changes in circulation.

D. Continuous cardiac monitoring, assess cardiac rate and rhythm; dysrhythmias are major cause of death after an MI.

E. Assess respiratory system for increasing dyspnea and pulmonary congestion.

F. Evaluate peripheral circulation; assess for presence of dependent edema.

G. Frequent assessment of vital signs; evaluate urinary output in response to changes in vital signs.

H. Frequent assessment for presence of chest pain.

> 💡 *TEST ALERT: Meet client's pain management needs; provide medication for pain relief; monitor for effects of pain medication.*

I. Maintain NPO initially; then allow clear liquids and progress to light meals that are low in sodium and cholesterol.

J. Promote normal bowel pattern.
1. Stool softeners.
2. Bedside commode.
3. Caution against straining while defecating (Valsalva maneuver).
4. Increase fiber in diet.

K. Decrease anxiety.
1. Administer pain medication promptly.
2. Keep client informed regarding progress and immediate plan of care.
3. Decrease sensory overload.
4. Encourage verbalization of concerns and fears.
5. *Immediately report presence of chest pain.*

L. Monitor for changes in neurological status (e.g., confusion, disorientation).

M. Monitor progressive activity.
1. Early activities should not increase heart rate greater than 25% of resting rate
   a. Walking in hallway 3-4 times a day with gradual increasing increments.
   b. Decrease in 20mm Hg in systolic B/P, changes in heart rate greater than 20 bpm, shortness of breath and or chest pain indicate poor tolerance to activity.
2. Assess heart rhythm, fatigue, blood pressure (BP) after each activity.
3. Resting tachycardia is a contraindication to activity.

 Home Care

A. Participate in organized cardiac rehabilitation program.
1. Monitored exercise.
2. Dietary modifications.
3. Continued education regarding ASHD and methods to decrease personal risk factors.

B. Understand medication regimen (see Box 12-3 and Appendix 12-2).

C. Teach client how to check radial pulse for rate and regularity.

D. Teach client how to evaluate response to increased exercise, such as chest pain, shortness of breath and tachycardia.
1. When beginning walking program, remain close to home.
2. Always carry nitroglycerin when walking or exercising.
3. Check pulse rate before, halfway through and at the end of activity.
4. Stop activity for pulse increase of more than 20bpm, shortness of breath, chest pain, or dizziness.

E. Exercise in climate-controlled areas.
F. Call the physician for pain not controlled by nitroglycerin, significant changes in pulse rate, decrease in activity tolerance, syncope, or increase in dyspnea.
G. Sexual intercourse generally is resumed 4 to 6 weeks following an MI, or when client can climb two flights of stairs, or walk one block without experiencing chest pain.
   1. Do not drink alcohol or eat a large meal before sexual activity.
   2. Take nitroglycerin before sexual activity.
   3. Do not take erectile dysfunction medications (Appendix 17-1) if taking nitrates.
H. Return to physician for regular checkups.

Heart Failure

* **Heart failure (cardiac insufficiency, ventricular failure) is the inability of the heart to pump adequate amounts of blood into the systemic circulation to meet tissue metabolic demands.**

Physiology of Heart Failure

A. Left-sided failure (congestive heart failure [CHF]) (Figure 12-2).
   1. Results from failure of the left ventricle to maintain adequate output.
   2. Blood backs up into the left atrium and into the pulmonary veins.
   3. Increasing pressure in the pulmonary capillary bed causes lungs to become congested, resulting in respiratory distress.
   4. Increasing pulmonary pressure results in increased pressure on right side of heart.
B. Right-sided failure (cor pulmonale).
   1. Results from failure of the right ventricle to maintain adequate output.
   2. Blood backs up into the systemic circulation and causes peripheral edema.
   3. Most common cause is secondary to left-sided failure and chronic pulmonary disease.
C. Each side of the heart is dependent on the other for adequate function.
   1. Left-sided failure results in pulmonary congestion; this causes an increase in pulmonary pressure, which puts increased workload on the right side of the heart and precipitates right-sided failure.
   2. Although the origin of the problem may begin solely on one side, the majority of clinical situations involve failure on both sides.

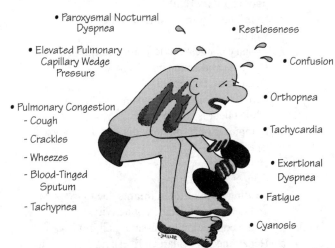

LEFT SIDED ♥ FAILURE

- Paroxysmal Nocturnal Dyspnea
- Elevated Pulmonary Capillary Wedge Pressure
- Pulmonary Congestion
  - Cough
  - Crackles
  - Wheezes
  - Blood-Tinged Sputum
  - Tachypnea
- Restlessness
- Confusion
- Orthopnea
- Tachycardia
- Exertional Dyspnea
- Fatigue
- Cyanosis

FIGURE 12-2 Left-Sided heart failure. (From Zerwekh J, Claborn J, Miller CJ: *Memory notebook of nursing, vol 1*, ed 4, Ingram, 2008, Nursing Education Consultants.)

   3. Left-sided failure rapidly causes right-sided failure. However, right-sided failure may occur alone for an extended period of time. Frequently associated with chronic lung problems.
D. The heart will attempt to maintain the body requirements for cardiac output (increasing cardiac rate, vasoconstriction) when these mechanisms become ineffective, cardiac decompensation or failure will occur.
E. *In children,* HF occurs most often as the result of a congenital defect of the heart.
F. Edema development in heart failure.
   1. Decreased cardiac output leads to decrease in renal perfusion, the kidneys respond by increasing the retention of sodium and water.
   2. Dependent pitting edema occurs with an increase in circulating volume (venous pressure).

TEST ALERT: *If a test question states that a client is in heart failure, assume that both sides are in failure unless indicated otherwise.*

Data Collection

A. Risk factors/etiology.
   1. Disease of cardiac valves, most often involves the mitral valve.
   2. History of myocardial disease.
   3. History of congenital heart disease.
   4. Fluid overload; excessive IV fluids.
   5. Chronic pulmonary disease.
B. Clinical manifestations.
   1. Impaired cardiac function.
      a. Tachycardia evaluated according to age group (see Table 3-1).
      b. Enlarged heart from dilatation and hypertrophy.

c. Poor perfusion: cool extremities, weak pulses, poor capillary refill.

d. In infants, failure to thrive and gain adequate weight.

2. Pulmonary congestion (left-sided failure).
   a. Dyspnea and cough on exertion.
   b. Orthopnea, tachypnea.
   c. Paroxysmal nocturnal dyspnea (PND) occurs while client is asleep.
   d. Symptoms of respiratory distress and hypoxia (see Table 10-3).
   e. Hemoptysis.
   f. Congested breath sounds.
   g. Feeding difficulties in infants due to dyspnea and decreased tolerance of activity.

3. Systemic congestion (right-sided failure).
   a. Hepatomegaly (enlarged liver): may be an early sign in children.
   b. Peripheral edema and weight gain.
   c. Dependent edema or generalized edema in infants; evaluate by weight gain.
   d. Ascites.
   e. Increase in central venous pressure (CVP).
   f. Jugular vein distention (JVD) with head elevated 30 degrees.

C. Diagnostics – Appendix 12-1

> **TEST ALERT: Determine changes in client's cardiovascular status as related to the client's CHF; interpret what data need to be reported immediately.**

Treatment

A. Treatment of the underlying problem.
B. Prevention.
   1. Early treatment of hypertension.
   2. Early treatment of dysrhythmias.
C. Oxygen.
D. Bed rest: semi-Fowler's or high-Fowler's position.
E. Medications (see Appendix 12-2).
   1. Angiotensin-converting enzyme (ACE) inhibitors will decrease systemic vascular resistance; this will decrease cardiac workload (see Appendix 11-4).
   2. Cardiac glycoside (digitalis) will increase contractility of cardiac muscle and increase cardiac output.
   3. Medications to decrease platelet aggregation or clumping.
F. Decrease sodium in diet.
G. Fluid restriction: adults and older children. Infants seldom need fluid restrictions due to feeding difficulty.

Nursing Interventions

❖ **Goal:** To decrease cardiac demands and improve cardiac function.
A. Early identification and treatment of dysrhythmias.
B. Limit physical activity.

C. Maintain normal body temperature; avoid chilling because it will increase oxygen consumption.
D. Provide supplemental oxygen, especially when needed with increased activity.
E. Provide uninterrupted sleep when possible.
F. Monitor urinary output: assess for any correlation of decreased urine output with decreased cardiac output.
G. Minimize crying in children and infants.
H. Decrease stress and anxiety; encourage parents to remain with child.
I. Carefully assess vital signs and compare with other physical assessment data.

> ✓ **NURSING PRIORITY:** The goals for care of a client with CHF are to:
> - Improve cardiac output: digitalis and oxygen.
> - Decrease cardiac workload (afterload): decrease activity, administer vasodilator.
> - Decrease venous return (preload): diuretics; decrease sodium and fluid intake; place client in semi-Fowler's position.

❖ **Goal:** To decrease circulating volume.
A. Diuretics (see Appendix 11-5).
B. Decreased sodium diet and fluid restriction in adults.
C. Calculate fluids carefully; client frequently on fluid restriction.
D. Evaluate fluid retention by obtaining accurate daily weights; teach client to weigh daily (1 kg or 2.2 lb weight gain = 1 L of fluid retention).
E. Accurate intake and output records; assess response to diuretics; *notify RN if client gains 2 to 4 pounds over 24-hours.*

❖ **Goal:** To reduce respiratory distress and promote gas exchange.
A. Position client carefully.
   1. Position adult client in semi-Fowler's or in an arm chair; do not elevate client's legs because this increases venous return.
   2. Infants and small children may breathe better side-lying with the knees drawn up to the chest.
   3. Infants may be placed in an infant seat.
   4. Make sure diapers are loosely pinned and safety restraints do not hinder maximum expansion of the chest.
   5. Hold infant upright over the shoulder with knees flexed (knee-chest position).
B. Administer humidified oxygen *to keep saturation levels at or above 90%*
C. Decrease exposure to upper respiratory tract infections.
D. Evaluate breath sounds; check for distended neck veins and peripheral edema.
E. Promote gradual activity. Determine client's respiratory response to increased activity.
F. Do not allow infants to cry for extend periods.

❖   **Goal:** To monitor for development of hypoxia (see Chapter 10).

❖   **Goal:** To maintain nutrition.

A.   Due to dyspnea, eating is sometimes difficult.

B.   Provide small, frequent feedings; allow client adequate time to eat.

C.   Infants may need to be gavaged, due to increased caloric need and increased work of sucking.

D.   Infants generally not on fluid restriction, due to decreased intake from dyspnea.

E.   Do not prop the bottle, but do burp the infant frequently.

Home Care

A.   Client should begin walking short distances, 250 to 300 feet, at least three to four times per week; distance can be increased as tolerated (no shortness of breath, dizziness, chest pain, or tachycardia).

B.   Teach client how to count his or her pulse.

C.   Client should weigh daily, before breakfast and with similar clothes on (nightgown, pajamas, etc.).

D.   Discuss use of and safety factors for home oxygen.

E.   Contact health care provider for:
   1.   Weight gain of 3-5 pounds over a week, or 1-2 pounds overnight.
   2.   Increase in dyspnea or angina, especially with decreased activity or at rest.
   3.   Decrease in activity tolerance that exceeds 3 or 4 days.
   4.   Increased urination at night, presence or increase in peripheral edema.
   5.   Cough or respiratory congestion that lasts longer than 3 or 4 days.

F.   Provide written instructions for medications.

Rheumatic Heart Disease

✱   **Rheumatic heart disease occurs in about 40% of clients with rheumatic fever; it primarily affects the cardiac valves. Myocardial involvement is characterized by an inflammatory response, causing scarring of the cardiac valves. The mitral valve is the most common area affected.**

A.   Usually preceded by a group A beta-hemolytic streptococcal infection.

B.   Rheumatic carditis is the only symptom that produces permanent damage, most often involves damage to the mitral valve.

C.   Rheumatic fever usually occurs during childhood, but manifestations of cardiac damage may not be evident for years.

Data Collection

A.   Clinical manifestations of rheumatic fever symptoms vary; no specific symptom or lab test is diagnostic of rheumatic fever. Criteria for the diagnosis require a combination of symptoms to be present.
   1.   Polyarthritis.
   2.   Carditis and fever.
   3.   Chorea: CNS involvement characterized by involuntary purposeless movement; no residual damage occurs.
   4.   Possible rash.
   5.   Subcutaneous nodules.

B.   Clinical manifestations of rheumatic carditis.
   1.   Heart murmur, tachycardia.
   2.   Pericarditis, pericardial friction rub, and chest pain.

> ✔ **NURSING PRIORITY:** *Prevention and adequate treatment of streptococcal infections prevent the development of rheumatic heart disease.*

Treatment

A.   Prevention: adequate treatment of streptococcal infections.

B.   Rest and decreased activity to decrease cardiac workload.

C.   Salicylates to control inflammatory response and arthritic pain.

D.   Prophylactic treatment.
   1.   Initiated after acute therapy.
   2.   Administration of penicillin over extended period of time. Duration depends on presence and level of cardiac involvement.
   3.   Before invasive medical procedures, client will need additional antibiotics due to increased risk of bacterial endocarditis.

Complications

Severe valve damage secondary to infective endocarditis may precipitate the development of congestive heart failure which may require open heart surgery for replacement of diseased valve.

Nursing Interventions

Child is generally cared for in the home environment.

❖   **Goal:** To assist parents and family to provide home environment conducive to healing and recovery.

A.   Decrease activity; maintain bed rest if pulse rate is increased or if febrile.

B.   Encourage routine activities within the home.

C.   Friends may visit for short periods; child is not contagious.

D.   Arrange for school work to be continued at home as appropriate.

E.   Maintain adequate nutrition and hydration.

F.   Administer analgesics for joint pain.

❖   **Goal:** To assist parents and client to understand need for long-term prophylactic antibiotic therapy.

A. Discuss the importance of preventing recurring infections.
B. Importance of prophylactic therapy before invasive medical procedures.
C. Continued medical follow-up care for the development of valve problems as child grows.
D. Follow-up required with females; cardiac problems may not be manifested until woman is pregnant.

Infective Endocarditis (Bacterial)

✳ **Endocarditis is an infection of the valves and inner lining of the heart.**
A. Organism may enter from any site of localized infection.
B. Organism grows on the endocardium and produces a characteristic lesion consisting of vegetation, fibrin deposits, and collagen; the lesion then progresses to damaged adjacent valves.
C. Lesion is fragile and particles may break off and form emboli.

Risk Factors

A. Congenital heart disease.
B. Prosthetic valve replacement.
C. IV drug abuse.
D. History of rheumatic fever with carditis.

Data Collection

A. Onset is gradual with nonspecific symptoms.
    1. Intermittent fever, high or low grade.
    2. Anorexia, weight loss.
    3. Joint pain.
    4. Petechiae (common) in conjunctiva, lips, buccal mucosa, on the ankle, and in the antecubital and popliteal areas.
    5. Splinter hemorrhages in nail beds.
B. Cardiac murmur, symptoms associated with heart failure.
C. Symptoms secondary to emboli.
    1. Spleen: splenomegaly, upper left quadrant pain.
    2. Kidney: flank pain, hematuria.
    3. Brain: hemiplegia, decreased level of consciousness.
    4. Pulmonary: dyspnea, chest pain, hemoptysis.

Treatment

A. Identification of infectious organism and appropriate antibiotic therapy for 4-6 weeks (see Appendix 5-10).
B. Bed rest if high fever or if evidence of heart failure is present.
C. Prophylactic antibiotics for 3 to 5 years, especially in children with history of rheumatic carditis or congenital abnormalities.

D. Prophylactic antibiotics before dental work, invasive diagnostic procedures, or surgery.

Nursing Interventions

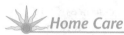

❖ **Goal:** To assist parents/client to understand need for long-term prophylactic therapy in high-risk candidates (see related goal for rheumatic heart disease).
❖ **Goal:** To maintain homeostasis and prevent complications over long-term hospitalization.
A. Maintain pattern of decreased activity; assess activity tolerance.
B. Evaluate for complications of emboli and congestive heart failure.

Home Care

A. Explain the purpose of long-term antibiotic therapy.
B. Good oral hygiene
    1. Daily care and regular dental visits.
    2. Inform dentists and PCPs before any invasive procedure (e.g., tooth extraction, cystoscopy). Antibiotics will be ordered prophylactically.
C. Monitor temperature; report fever, chills, malaise, increasing fatigue, weight loss to the PCP.
D. Follow a progressive activity schedule until back to previous level of activity; avoid excessive fatigue; plan rest periods and activity.
E. Advise all health care providers of history of endocarditis.

Pericarditis

✳ **Pericarditis is an inflammation of the pericardium. The pericardial space is a cavity between the inner and the outer layers of the pericardium.**

Data Collection

A. Acute form may occur 2 to 3 days after a myocardial infarction.
B. Chronic pericarditis (Dressler's syndrome) may occur 1 to 4 weeks after an MI.
C. Chest pain aggravated by breathing, swallowing, lying supine.
D. Pain increases with deep inspiration and lying supine; sitting may relieve pain; pain may radiate, making it difficult to differentiate from angina.
E. Pericardial friction rub caused by myocardium rubbing against inflamed pericardium.
F. Fever, dyspnea, tachypnea.
G. Restlessness, irritability, anxiousness.

Treatment

A. Acute.
    1. Treat underlying problem.
    2. Restricted activity.
    3. Antiinflammatory medications.

Nursing Interventions

❖ **Goal:** To maintain homeostasis and promote comfort.
A. Assess characteristics of pain; administer appropriate analgesics.
B. Position client upright; client leaning forward frequently relieves pain.
C. Decrease anxiety as client often associates problem with an MI; assist client to distinguish the difference.
   1. Pain does not increase with activity.
   2. Pain is not relieved by rest.
   3. Pain is relieved by sitting up and leaning forward.
D. In a client with chronic pericarditis, evaluate for symptoms of CHF and initiate appropriate nursing intervention.

Cardiovascular Disease in Pregnancy

* **Rheumatic heart disease and congenital heart defects account for the greatest incidence of cardiac disease in pregnancy. Of these, mitral valve stenosis is by far the most common problem.**

A. Normal physiological alterations of pregnancy that increase cardiovascular stress.
   1. Increase in oxygen requirements.
   2. Increase in cardiac output.
   3. Weight gain.
   4. Hemodynamic changes during delivery.
B. As normal pregnancy advances, cardiovascular system is unable to maintain adequate output to meet increasing demands.

Data Collection

Clinical manifestations indicative of cardiac decompensation are those of impending cardiac failure.
A. Frequent cough.
B. Progressive general edema (face, feet, hands); excessive weight gain.
C. Progressive dyspnea.
D. Excessive fatigue for level of activity.
E. Dysrhythmias: tachycardia greater than 100 beats/min.
F. Congested breath sounds.
G. Cardiac decompensation increases with length of gestation; increased incidence of heart failure at 28- to 32-weeks gestation.

Treatment

A. Management of the pregnant client.
   1. Balanced nutritional intake; adequate calories to maintain weight (avoid attempts to lose weight).
   2. Restricted activity, frequent rest periods.
   3. If severe, may be hospitalized and placed on bed rest at 28 to 32 weeks, due to impending cardiac failure.
   4. Prophylactic penicillin to prevent infection: especially important in women with mitral valve disease from rheumatic fever.

B. Management of the client during labor and delivery.
   1. Continuous monitoring of fetus and mother.
   2. Supplemental oxygen.
C. Management of the client during postpartum.
   1. Because of dramatic changes in the hemodynamic system of the mother, the first 24 hours postpartum is a period of increased risk.
   2. Client is treated symptomatically according to status of cardiovascular system; the first 24-48 hours postpartum is period of highest risk for HF in the mother.

Nursing Interventions

❖ **Goal:** To assist client to maintain homeostasis during pregnancy.
A. Provide written information regarding nutritional needs.
B. Assess for early symptoms of cardiac failure.
C. Encourage frequent rest periods; stop any activity that increases shortness of breath.
❖ **Goal:** To maintain homeostasis in postpartum period.
A. Assess pulmonary and cardiac adaptation to changes in hemodynamics.
B. Increased blood flow due to decreased abdominal pressure may cause a reflex bradycardia.
C. Maintain semi-Fowler's position or left lateral position with the head elevated.
D. Promote gradual progression of activities depending on cardiac status as indicated by:
   1. Normal pulse rate.
   2. Good respiratory status.
   3. Activity tolerance.
E. Encourage progressive ambulation as soon as possible to prevent venous stasis and development of DVT.
F. Assist mother and family to prepare for discharge.

 TEST ALERT: *Provide care for client experiencing complications of pregnancy.*

Congenital Heart Disease

A. Clinical manifestations depend on the severity of the defect and the adequacy of pulmonary blood flow.
B. Normal pressure in the right side of the heart is lower than pressure in the left side; there is an increased blood flow from an area of high pressure to an area of low pressure.
   1. When there is an opening between the right and left side of the heart, oxygenated blood will shunt from the left side of the heart to the right side (right-to-left shunt).
   2. When the pressures on the right side of the heart exceed the pressure on the left side of the heart, unoxygenated blood from the right side will flow into the left side and unoxygenated blood will flow into the systemic circulation (left-to-right shunt).
C. Physical consequences of congenital heart defects.

1. Delayed physical development.
   a. Failure to gain weight, caused by inability to maintain adequate caloric intake to meet increased metabolic demands.
   b. Tachycardia and tachypnea precipitate increase in caloric requirements.
2. Excessive fatigue, especially during feedings.
3. Frequent upper respiratory tract infections.
4. Dyspnea, tachycardia, tachypnea.
5. Hypercyanotic spells (called "blue" spells or "tet" spells): infant suddenly becomes acutely cyanotic and hyperpneic; occur most often in children 2 months to 1 year of age.
D. Diagnostics (see Appendix 12-1).

Nursing Interventions

❖ **Goal:** To evaluate infant's response to cardiac defect.
A. Determine infant's Apgar score at birth.
B. Evaluate adequacy of weight gain.
C. Assess for feeding problems.
   1. Poor sucking reflex.
   2. Poor coordination of sucking, swallowing, breathing.
   3. Fatigues easily during feeding; may result in inadequate intake.
D. Frequency of upper respiratory tract infections.

E. Determine if cyanosis occurs at rest or is precipitated by activity.
F. Presence and quality of pulses in extremities.
G. All fevers should be reported, bacterial endocarditis is a primary concern before and after correction of congenital defect.

> ✔ *PEDIATRIC PRIORITY: Cyanosis that decreases with crying is associated with respiratory function; cyanosis that increases with crying is associated with cardiac function.*

❖ **Goal:** To assist parents in adjusting to diagnosis.
A. Allow family to grieve over loss of perfect infant.
B. Evaluate parents' level of understanding of the infant's problem.
C. Foster early parent-infant attachment; encourage touching, holding, and general physical contact.
D. Assist the family to develop a relationship which fosters optimal growth and development of all family members. (See Chapter 2 for psychosocial aspect of chronically ill children.)
❖ **Goal:** To detect, prevent, and treat HF – see earlier discussion of heart failure.
❖ **Goal:** To provide appropriate nursing interventions for the client undergoing open heart surgery for repair of a defect.

Study Questions: Cardiac System

1. The nurse is preparing a client for a cardiac catheterization. What is important for the nurse to explain to the client regarding his care after the test?
   1 It will be important for you to lie flat for several hours.
   2 It will be necessary for you to ambulate soon after the test.
   3 You will be very sleepy; let the nurse know if you are hurting.
   4 There will be a catheter in your bladder because you cannot get up.
2. A cardiac catheterization is scheduled for a client. In considering allergic reactions to the dye used in the procedure, an allergic reaction to what food would cause the nurse the most concern?
   1 Eggs.
   2 Milk products.
   3 Shellfish.
   4 Penicillin.
3. Cardiac isoenzymes are ordered for a client who is admitted with a diagnosis of "rule out myocardial infarction." What information will this test provide?
   1 Identifies myocardial tissue damage.
   2 Determines the area of myocardial involvement.
   3 Evaluates the ability of heart muscle to contract.
   4 Identifies presence of endocarditis.
4. The nurse is assessing the apical heart rate on a client.

Where on the chest wall should the nurse place the stethoscope?
   1 Midline and to the left of the mediastinum.
   2 Mid-clavicular line, fifth intercostal space on the left.
   3 Fifth intercostal space, left mid-axillary line.
   4 Right of mediastinum, anterior to the axillary area.
5. A client with bacterial endocarditis is being discharged. What will be important for the nurse to review with the client?
   1 Begin exercise regimen in about 2 weeks.
   2 Increase your fluid intake of fruit juices.
   3 Keep taking your antibiotic.
   4 Return weekly for an electrocardiogram.
6. What is the rationale for a low-sodium diet in the client with congestive heart failure?
   1 Fluid retention will decrease, and this will improve cardiac output.
   2 Fluids will be retained to maintain cardiac output.
   3 A decrease in sodium level will cause a decrease in potassium levels.
   4 Myocardial contractility depends on normal serum sodium levels.
7. The nurse is administering nitroglycerin to a client who says he is experiencing midsternum chest pain. What would the nurse identify as a common side effect of this medication?

1   Pulse rate of 120 beats per minute.
2   Increase in systolic blood pressure.
3   Onset of nausea and vomiting.
4   Client says his head is hurting.

8.   A client has a diagnosis of left-sided heart failure, and he is tells the nurse he is having difficulty breathing. The nurse determines the client's pulse rate to be 120 beats per minute; respirations are 32 breaths per minute. What is the immediate nursing action?
1   Determine when he last had his medications.
2   Evaluate the adequacy of urinary output.
3   Put him in supine position with feet elevated.
4   Place him in high-Fowler's position with feet dependent.

9.   A client with a diagnosis of chronic angina is being discharged. What is important for the nurse to teach the client regarding how to take the sublingual nitroglycerin tablets?
1   Take the medication with a full glass of water.
2   Keep the medication in a clear container.
3   The medication has a rapid onset of action of 2 to 5 minutes.
4   Take the medication at the first onset of chest pain.

10.   Digitalis has been ordered for a client in congestive heart failure. What would the nurse expect to find when evaluating the client for the therapeutic effectiveness of the drug?
1   Improved respiratory status and increased urinary output.
2   Increased heart rate and blood pressure.
3   Diaphoresis with decreased urinary output.
4   Increased heart rate with increased respirations.

11.   When should the nurse determine the client's pulse rate by checking the apical heart rate? Select all that apply:
_____ 1   Determining pulse rate before the administration of digitalis.
_____ 2   Checking the vital signs on a hypertensive client.
_____ 3   Determining the heart rate in a client with an irregular pulse.
_____ 4   Evaluating vital signs within the first 24 hours after a myocardial infarction.
_____ 5   Evaluating a client with orthostatic hypotension.
_____ 6   Determining vital signs on an infant.

12.   As edema decreases in a client with heart failure, what physiological response would the nurse expect to find?
1   Increase in body weight.
2   Rales across all lung fields.
3   Respiratory rate greater than 24 breaths per minute.
4   Increase in the urinary output.

13.   The nurse is caring for a client with a chronic pulmonary condition who has developed a complication of right-sided heart failure. Which nursing observation is associated with this complication?
1   Decreasing urinary output.
2   An irregular pulse rate.
3   Jugular vein distention.
4   Increasing pulmonary congestion.

14.   The nurse is assessing a client 2 days after he was diagnosed with a myocardial infarction. What finding would cause the most immediate concern?
1   Urinary output of 40 mL per hour.
2   Jugular vein distention in the supine position.
3   Shooting pain in the left upper thigh.
4   Irregular pulse rate of 120 beats per minute.

15.   An older adult client is admitted in congestive heart failure. What observation by the nurse indicates that the client's condition is getting worse?
1   1+ edema in lower extremities.
2   Blood pressure of 160/98 mm Hg.
3   Urinary output of 60 mL/hr.
4   Increasing irritability and confusion.

16.   A client with a history of cardiac problems tells the nurse he is beginning to have chest pain while he is sitting in a bedside chair. What would be the first nursing action?
1   Assess the characteristics of the chest pain.
2   Return the client to bed and begin oxygen.
3   Advise the physician regarding the client's status.
4   Determine when the client last ate any food.

17.   What is considered a modifiable risk factor for coronary artery disease?
1   Age.
2   Race.
3   Diet.
4   Heredity.

18.   A client is admitted to the hospital due to malfunction of his permanent pacemaker. What would be important to include in the nursing care of this client?
1   Encourage increased fluid intake.
2   Maintain fall precautions.
3   Encourage daily ambulation in the hall.
4   Assess for development of hypoxia.

19.   A client returns to the room after placement of a permanent pacemaker via the right subclavian vein. What is an important nursing action to prevent complications?
1   Ambulate the client and encourage deep breathing.
2   Check the radial pulse rate to evaluate the pacemaker function.
3   Limit movement and abduction of the right arm.
4   Assess the status of incision and external pacemaker wire.

20.   Why is the client placed on a firm surface when CPR is performed?
1   The heart is compressed between the sternum and the spine.
2   It is easier to establish and maintain an open airway.
3   It promotes venous return back to the heart.
4   It decreases the potential for damage to the xiphoid process.

Answers and rationales to these questions are in the section at the end of the book titled Chapter Study Questions: Answers and Rationales.

Appendix 12-1   CARDIAC DIAGNOSTICS

SERUM LABORATORY STUDIES

Cardiac Enzymes

Enzymes are drawn to evaluate myocardial muscle and determine if there has been damage to the muscle.

1. **Creatine kinase (CK-MB).** Increases greater than 4%-6% of total CK are highly indicative of an MI. Increases greater than 5% of total creatine kinase are strongly supportive of an highly indicative of MI.
2. **Cardiac troponin T and cardiac troponin I:** normal levels are less than 0.2 ng/mL (for T) and less than 0.03 ng/dl (for I); levels are elevated within 3 to 6 hours after an MI and peak within 10 to 24 hours. Any elevation is significant because it is not found in healthy clients.

Nursing Implications

1. Enzymes must be drawn on admission and obtained at regular intervals. There is a characteristic pattern to the increases and decreases of enzyme levels in a client with an MI.
2. The larger the infarction, the larger the enzyme response.
3. Increased levels of troponin are the most significant and diagnostic of myocardial damage.
4. Cardiac-specific troponin helps discriminate from other tissue injury.

C-Reactive Protein (CRP), Highly Sensitive C-Reactive Protein (hs-CRP)

Highly sensitive CRP (hs-CRP) may be used to identify risk for developing an MI. The response to the test assists in evaluating the severity and course of inflammatory conditions.

Normal: Less than 1 mg/L or 8 mg/dL; increasing level is significant and may indicate some degree of inflammatory response caused by plaque formation.

B-Type Natriuretic Peptide (BNP)

First whole blood marker for identifying and treating heart failure. Serial BNP values may be used to evaluate left ventricular function; assists to identify heart failure versus respiratory failure as cause of dyspnea. Normal is less than 100 pg/mL.

NONINVASIVE

Electrocardiogram (ECG)

A graphic representation of the electrical activity of the heart, generally conducted using a 12-lead format. Test to identify conduction in rhythm disorders as well as specific electrical changes that correlate with cardiac ischemia and injury.

Holter Monitor

Client is connected to a small portable ECG unit with a recorder that records the client's heart activity for approximately 24 hours. The client is directed to keep a log of activity, pain, or palpitations. The client should not shower or bathe while the monitor is in place. The recording is then analyzed, comparing the heart rate and rhythm to the client's activity log.

Event Monitor

Client is connected to an ECG portable unit with a recorder. The client can activate the recorder at any time he feels any dizziness or palpitations. Monitor may be worn for extended periods of time. Monitor leads and battery unit may be removed for showering, but should be reconnected immediately after bathing. Recordings are transmitted over the phone.

Exercise Stress Test

This test involves the client exercising. This may be done on a treadmill or a stationary bicycle that increases in speed and degree of incline to increase the heart rate and blood pressure. ECG leads are attached to the client, and the response of the heart to exercise is evaluated.

Nursing Implications

1. Appropriate pretest client education; establish baseline vital signs and cardiac rhythm.
2. Client should:
   a. Avoid smoking, or drinking alcohol immediately before test, a light meal may be give 2 hours prior to the test.
   b. Avoid stimulants (caffeine), and extreme temperature changes immediately after test.
3. Cardiac rhythm and vital signs are monitored constantly during test.
4. Reasons for terminating an exercise stress test: predetermined heart rate is reached, chest pain, excessive fatigue, dyspnea, vertigo, hypotension or ventricular dysrhythmias occur; ECG changes of significant ST segment depression or T-wave inversion occurs.
5. If any of the above changes occur and the test is terminated, it is said to be a positive stress test.

Thallium 201 Test

A small dose of thallium is administered, and a camera records the uptake of thallium through the heart. Normal tissue has a rapid uptake of thallium; areas of scarring or damage have slower or no uptake of thallium. Clients should not ingest caffeine or smoke before this test.

Echocardiogram

An ultrasound procedure to evaluate valvular function, cardiac chamber size, ventricular muscle, and septal motion. The ultrasound waves are displayed on a graph and interpreted. Provides more specific information that an ECG. Nurse should determine if any medication needs to be given and/or withheld prior to the test. Sedation is not used.

Continued

Appendix 12-1	CARDIAC DIAGNOSTICS—cont'd.

Transesophageal Echocardiography

This test is an endoscopy ultrasound and provides a higher quality picture and additional diagnostic data than a regular echocardiogram. The throat is anesthetized, and a flexible endoscope is passed into the esophagus to the level of the heart and an echocardiogram is conducted from the esophageal view.

Sedation is used during the procedure.

Nursing Implications

1. NPO for 4 to 6 hours before test.
2. After the test, check for gag reflex before resuming PO fluids.

Magnetic Resonance Imaging

This is a noninvasive diagnostic scan. A magnetic field and radio waves are used to detect and define the differences between healthy tissue and diseased tissue. Provides images in three dimensions.

Nursing Implications

1. The client cannot have any metal on his/her body; remove all jewelry, hair clips, etc.
2. Clients with permanent metal implanted in the body (pacemakers, implanted clips and wires, insulin pumps) are not candidates for MRI.
3. Client must be cooperative and remain very still during the procedure.
4. No specific care required after the procedure.

Positron Emission Tomography (PET)

Very sensitive in identifying viable and nonviable cardiac tissue. The procedure takes about 2 to 3 hours, and a radioactive dye is injected intravenously, followed by glucose. A client's glucose must be between 60-140 mg/dL prior to the test.

INVASIVE DIAGNOSTICS

Cardiac Catheterization

An invasive procedure in which a catheter is passed through an artery or vein into the heart. Cardiac catheterization will provide data regarding status of the coronary arteries, as well as cardiac muscle function, valvular function, and left ventricular function (ejection fraction).

Right-side catheterization: Provides information regarding the function and structure of the right atrium, right ventricle, pulmonic valve, and tricuspid valve.

Left-side catheterization: Provides information regarding the function and structure of the left atrium, left ventricle, aortic valve, and mitral valve. The catheter is manipulated through the aorta and dye is injected into the coronary arteries (coronary angiogram).

Nursing Implications

1. Pretest preparation.
   a. NPO 4 to 8 hours before test.
   b. Record quality of distal pulses for comparison post-test.
   c. Check for dye allergy, especially iodine and contrast media.
   d. Determine whether any medications need to be withheld.
   e. Client education: report any chest pain or discomfort or difficulty breathing. Client will need to lie still on hard table; a flushed feeling may occur when dye is injected.
   f. Client is awake during procedure; sedative may be given.

2. Post-test.
   a. Evaluate catheterization entry site (most often femoral) for hematoma formation. *Notify the RN or the physician immediately for excessive bleeding at the site, and for significant changes in blood pressure.*
   b. Evaluate pulses distal to catheterization site, color, sensation of the extremity. *Notify the RN or the physician immediately for a decrease in peripheral circulation or neurovascular changes in affected extremity.*
   c. Assess for dysrhythmias, if identified, *notify RN immediately.*
   d. Maintain bed rest for 4 to 8 hours; avoid flexion, keep the extremity straight.
   e. Keep head of bed elevated at 30 degrees or less.
   f. Fluids will be encouraged to flush the dye out of the body.

 TEST ALERT: *Monitor peripheral pulses; identify and intervene to prevent circulatory complications.*

Appendix 12-2 CARDIAC MEDICATIONS

NITRATES: Increase blood supply to the heart by dilating the coronary arteries; cardiac workload is reduced due to decrease in venous return because of peripheral vasodilation.

Medications	Side Effects	Nursing Implications
Nitroglycerin (**NTG, Nitrostat**): sublingual Nitroglycerin (**Nitro-BID, Nitrol**): topical (patch) Nitroglycerin ointment (**Nitropaste**): topical, by the inch Nitroglycerin translingual spray	Headaches (will diminish with therapy), postural hypotension, syncope, blurred vision, dry mouth, reflex tachycardia	1. Advise client that alcohol will potentiate postural hypotension. 2. Educate client regarding self-medication (see Box 12-3). 3. Do not take with erectile dysfunction drugs. 4. Topical or transdermal application is used for sustained protection against anginal attacks. 5. Avoid skin contact with topical form; remove all previous applications on client's skin. 6. Sublingual tablets and translingual spray given for an immediate response.

Calcium Channel Blockers: Blockade of calcium channel receptors in the heart causes decreased contractility and dliation of arteries for treatment of hypertension and angina; some medications have cardiac specific properties.

Medications	Side Effects	Nursing Implications
Diltiazem (**Cardizem**): PO, IV Nifedipine (**Procardia**): PO Verapamil (**Calan, Isoptin**): IV, PO	Constipation, exacerbation of CHF, hypotension, bradycardia, peripheral edema	1. Nifedipine is less likely to exacerbate preexisting cardiac conditions; is not effective in treating dysrhythmias. 2. Intensifies cardiosuppressant effects of beta-blocker medications. 3. Assess for bradycardia.

Beta-Adrenergic Blocking Agents (adrenergic antagonists): Blockade of beta receptors in the heart causes decreased heart rate, and decreased rate of AV conduction. Used to treat hypertension as well as angina. Beta blockers should be administered to all clients experiencing unstable angina or having an MI unless contraindicated.

Medications	Side Effects	Nursing Implications
Labetalol (**Trandate**): PO, IV Metoprolol (**Lopressor, Toprol XL**): PO, IV Propranolol (**Inderal**): PO, IV Atenolol (**Tenormin**): PO, IV Carvedilol (**Coreg**): PO Note: Carvedilol, bisoprolol, and metoprolol sustained release are used to treat HF.	Bradycardia, hypotension, depression, lethargy and fatigue	1. Closely monitor cardiac client—may precipitate heart failure, but is also used to treat heart failure. 2. Teach client how to decrease effects of postural hypotension. 3. Teach client to continue medication regardless of feeling better. 4. Check pulse for bradycardia before administering. 5. If client has diabetes, blood glucose control may be impaired. 6. Give with caution to clients with history of bronchospasm.

Antidysrhythmic Medications: Decrease cardiac excitability; delay cardiac conduction in either the atrium or ventricle. Atropine is cardiac stimulant for bradycardia.

General Nursing Implications

- Assess client for changes in cardiac rhythm and impact on cardiac output.
- Evaluate effect of medication on dysrhythmia and resulting effects on cardiac output.
- Have atropine available for cardiac depression resulting in symptomatic bradycardia.
- All cardiac depressant medications are contraindicated in clients with sinus node or AV node blocks.
- Digitalis will enhance cardiac depressant effects.
- Closely monitor for dysrhythmias that are precipitated by the treatment.
- All of these medications can make existing dysrhythmias worse and also create new ones.
- RN or physician will administer IV medications; LPN may assist in monitoring the client.

Continued

Appendix 12-2	CARDIAC MEDICATIONS—cont'd.	

Medications	Side Effects	Nursing Implications
Quinidine sulfate (**Quinidine Sulfate, Quinidex**): PO	Hypotension Diarrhea, nausea, vomiting	1. Administer with food. 2. Monitor for ECG changes for toxicity—widened QRS and prolonged QT. 3. *Uses:* supraventricular tachycardia and ventricular dysrhythmias.
Atropine: subQ, IV	Tachycardia Dry mouth, blurred vision, dilated pupils	1. *Use:* symptomatic bradycardia. 2. Assess client's cardiac output in response to the bradycardic episode.
Amiodarone hydrochloride (**Cordarone**): PO, IV	AV heart block, hypotension Toxicity—lung and visual problems	1. *Use:* life-threatening ventricular arrhythmias, atrial fibrillation. 2. Monitor for severe bradycardia. 3. Monitor for indications of pulmonary toxicity – dyspnea and cough. 4. **High Alert Medication** - caution with administration and maintain close client observation.
Lidocaine hydrochloride (**Xylocaine**): IV	Drowsiness, confusion, seizures, severe depression of cardiac conduction	1. *Use:* ventricular dysrhythmias. 2. Must use IV preparatioin of Lidocaine for IV infusion. 3. Monitor for seizures and bradycardia. 4. **High Alert Medication** - use only cardiac preparation for IV.
Procainamide (**Pronestyl**): PO, IV	Abdominal pain, cramping, hypotension, prolonged QT interval Blood dyscrasias	1. *Use:* short- and long-term control of ventricular and supraventricular dysrhythmias. 2. Closely monitor for bradycardia and hypotension. 3. Do not take OTC cold preparations. 4. May develop autoimmune problems – systemic lupus erythematosus.
Propranolol hydrochloride (**Inderal**): PO, IV	See previous discussion of beta-adrenergic blockers	1. *Use:* long- and short-term treatment and prevention of tachycardia. 2. **High Alert Medication** - give with caution and closely monitor client response.

Fibrinolytic (thrombolytic) medications: Initiate fibrinolysis of a clot. Medications will break up a clot anywhere in the body – in a surgical incision as well as in the heart.

General Nursing Implications
- Therapy should begin as soon as the MI is diagnosed or when there is a history of prolonged angina—for best results, from admission in the ED (emergency department) until medication is administered is 30 min (door-to-needle), or within 60 min of onset of symptoms.
- Used to treat: acute coronary thrombosis (MI), deep vein thrombosis (DVT), and massive pulmonary emboli.
- Medication should be administered by an RN or physician; LPN may monitor client after infusion.
- Bleeding precautions (see Table 9-1).

Medications	Side Effects	Nursing Implications
Alteplase (**tPA, Activase**): IV Reteplase (**Retavase**): IV Streptokinase (**Streptase, Kabikinase**): IV	Bleeding and hypotension	1. Obtain base vital signs, monitor for hypotension. 2. Monitor for allergic reactions with streptokinase. 3. Monitor for bleeding. 4. Avoid venipunctures during and after infusion. 5. **High Alert Medication** - monitor client closely. 6. *Use:* MI, PE, DVT; brain accident, contraindicated in clients with active bleeding.

Continued

| Appendix 12-2 | CARDIAC MEDICATIONS—cont'd. | |

ANTIPLATELETS (PLATELET AGGREGATION INHIBITORS): Inhibit the aggregation and clumping of platelets which reduces the risk of stroke, or MI or peripheral vascular occlusion in clients with peripheral vascular.

Medications	Side Effects	Nursing Implications
Aspirin: PO Clopidogrel (**Plavix**) PO Ticlopidine (**Ticlid**): PO	GI bleeding, dyspepsia, hemorrhagic stroke GI disturbances, skin reactions, blood dyscrasias. **Plavix and Ticlid**: Thrombotic thrombocytopenic purpura (TTP) is a rare, but serious side effect.	1. Aspirin is given in small doses (e.g., 81 mg daily). 2. Take aspirin and Ticlid with food to decrease gastric irritation. 3. Prophylactic therapy for prevention of MI and ischemic stroke (thrombotic) in clients with TIAs. 4. Monitor coagulation studies throughout therapy.
Cilostazol (**Pletal**): PO	Headache, dizziness,	1. Primary use is for relief of intermittent claudication in PVD. 2. Grapefruit juice inhibits metabolism. 3. Administer on an empty stomach.

Blood Viscosity Reducing Agent:

Pentoxifylline (**Trental**): PO	Nausea, vomiting, dizziness, headache, diarrhea,	1. Primary use is for relief of intermittent claudication from PVD. 2. Therapeutic effect may not be noted for 2-4 weeks. 3. Do not chew, crush or break tablets.

GI, Gastrointestinal; *MI*, myocardial infarction; *PO*, by mouth (orally); *TIA*, transient ischemic attack; *PVD*, peripheral vascular disease.

Cardiac Glycosides: Increase myocardial contractility and cardiac output. Decrease heart rate by slowing conduction of impulses through the AV node.

General Nursing Implications
- Take the apical pulse for a full minute; if the rate is below 60 beats/min in an adult or below 90-110 beats/min in infants and young children, or below 70 in a child, hold the medication and *notify the RN or the physician.*
- Evaluate for tachycardia, bradycardia, and irregular pulse. *If there is significant change in rate and rhythm, hold the medication and notify the RN or primary care provider.*
- Evaluate serum potassium levels and response to diuretics; *hypokalemia potentiates action of digitalis.*
- Gastrointestinal symptoms are frequently the first indication of digitalis toxicity.
- Teach client not to increase or double a dose in the case of a missed dose; if client vomits, do not give an additional dose.
- To achieve maximum results rapidly, an initial loading dose is administered; then dose is reduced to a maintenance dose.

Medications	Side Effects	Nursing Implications
Digoxin (**Lanoxin**): PO, IV	Most common: anorexia, nausea, vomiting. Most serious: drug-induced dysrhythmias Visual disturbances, fatigue Children/infants: frequent vomiting, poor feeding, or slow heart rate may indicate toxicity	1. Therapeutic plasma levels of digoxin are 0.5-2.0 ng/mL. 2. First sign of toxicity is usually GI symptoms. 3. Uses: supraventricular tachycardia, CHF. 4. Monitor serum potassium levels – low potassium potentiates action of digitalis. 5. **High Alert Medication** - monitor client closely for side effects and toxicity.

✔ ***OLDER ADULT PRIORITY:*** *Older adults are more sensitive to digitalis and are more likely to experience toxicity.*

GI, Gastrointestinal; *MI*, myocardial infarction; *PO*, by mouth (orally); *TIA*, transient ischemic attack; *PVD*, peripheral vascular disease.

Appendix 12-3	CARDIOPULMONARY RESUSCITATION (CPR) FOR HEALTH CARE PROVIDERS

The American Heart Association (AHA) has established standards for cardiopulmonary resuscitation for the health care provider. For further delineation of the procedure, consult the American Heart Association Cardiopulmonary Resuscitation Guidelines. For health care providers, the American Heart Association uses the term infant to refer to individuals between birth and 1 year of age; child is used to refer to those who are between 1 year of age and the onset of puberty.

1. AIRWAY.

1. Identify that the victim is unconscious.
2. Activate the emergency medical services (EMS) system.
3. Repeat and/or obtain an automated external defibrillator (AED). Use AED as soon as it is available for all adults and children for sudden, witnessed collapse and for in-hospital clients.
4. Place client in position to open airway.
5. Open the airway: head-tilt/chin-lift maneuver.
6. Check for adequate breathing (look, listen, and feel for breaths).
7. If victim is breathing, place in recovery position.
8. If victim is not breathing, give 2 rescue breaths using mouth-to-mouth, or a pocket mask or bag mask.

2. Breathing.

1. Maintain the open airway.
2. Pinch nostrils closed.
3. Give two breaths that make the chest rise, at 1 sec per breath, using mouth-to-mouth technique (mouth–to–nose and mouth technique may be used for small children and infants).
4. Do not give "extra" breaths; do not give large, forceful breaths.
5. When an advanced airway is present, ventilate at the rate of 8-10/min; do not pause for cardiac compressions.

3. Check the pulse for no more than 10 sec.

1. Adult and child: Check the carotid pulse.
2. Infant: Check the brachial or femoral pulse.
3. If the pulse is absent, begin chest compressions—cycles of 30 compressions and 2 breaths until ACLS or PALS standards are initiated.
4. If the pulse is present, continue rescue breathing, and recheck pulse every 2 min. If despite adequate ventilation, the heart rate of an infant or child remains under 60 bpm, chest compressions should be started.
5. Adult: 1 breath every 5-6 sec, 10-12 per min.
6. Child and infant: 1 breath every 3-5 sec, 12-20 breaths per min.
7. Advanced airway present (laryngeal mask airway, endotracheal tube): 1 breath every 6-8 sec without trying to synchronize breaths with compressions.

> ✔ **PEDIATRIC PRIORITY:** *Be careful not to hyperextend the infant's head; this may block the airway. Don't pinch the infant's nose shut—cover the nose with your mouth instead. Breathe slowly, just enough to make the chest rise.*

4. External cardiac compression.

1. Place the victim on a firm surface. If the client is in a bed, put a cardiac board behind him or her. DO NOT attempt to remove the client from the bed.
2. Locate the lower half of the sternum in the adult. For the adult, place one hand over the lower sternum; place the other hand on top of the previous hand. For a child (age 1 year to puberty), use the heel of one hand, or two hands based on the size of the child, and press on the center of the chest at the nipple line. For an infant, locate the nipple line; the area for compression is one finger's width below the line.
3. Depress the sternum 1½ to 2 inches in the adult; in children and infants depress approximately one-third to one-half of depth of chest.
4. Push hard and fast; allow the chest to recoil completely between compressions and as few interruptions as possible.

Adult and child:
One rescuer and two rescuers: 30 compressions (rate of 100 per min) to 2 ventilations.
Infant:
One rescuer: 30 compressions (rate of 100 per min) to 2 ventilations.
Two rescuers: 15 compressions to 2 ventilations.

Continued

| **Appendix 12-3** | CARDIOPULMONARY RESUSCITATION (CPR) FOR HEALTH CARE PROVIDERS—cont'd. |

Defibrillation: Use automatic electronic defibrillator (AED) as soon as available for sudden collapse and for in-hospital clients.

Steps for using an automated external defibrillator (AED):

1. Provide CPR until the AED arrives.
2. On arrival, open the case and turn the power on.
3. Select the correct pads for the size and age of the victim (only use the child pads/system for children less than 8 years old).
4. Attach the adhesive electrodes—one on the upper-right side of the chest directly below the clavicle, the other below the left nipple below the left armpit.
5. Attach the connecting cable to the AED.
6. Compressions will need to be discontinued while the rhythm is analyzed.
7. If shock is indicated, loudly state "Clear!" and visually check to ensure that no one is touching the client.
8. Press the SHOCK button.
9. Resume CPR immediately with cycles of 30 compressions to 2 breaths.
10. After 2 min, the AED will prompt you to repeat steps 6 through 9.

5. Termination of CPR. A rescuer who is not a physician should continue resuscitation efforts until one of the following occurs:

1. Spontaneous circulation and ventilation have been restored.
2. Resuscitation efforts are transferred to another equally responsible person who continues the resuscitation procedure.
3. A physician or physician-directed person assumes responsibility for resuscitation procedure.
4. The victim is transferred to an emergency medical service (e.g., paramedics and ambulance).
5. The rescuer is exhausted and unable to continue resuscitation.

 TEST ALERT: *Identify and intervene in life-threatening client situations. Notify primary health care provider about unexpected response/emergency situation of client.*

Appendix 12-4 CARDIAC CONDUCTION AND DYSRHYTHMIAS

CHARACTERISTICS OF NORMAL SINUS RHYTHM

Pulse Characteristics:

Rate: 60 to 100 beats/min
Rhythm: regular

Electrocardiograph Characteristics (Figure 12-3):

1. P wave: indicative of the impulse generated from the sinoatrial node. A P-wave is present and precedes each QRS complex.
2. PR interval: delay of the impulse at the atrioventricular node to promote ventricular filling, normal interval is 0.12 to 0.20 second.
3. QRS complex: passage of the impulse through the bundle of His, down the bundle branches, through the Purkinje fibers; depolarization of the ventricle occurs. A QRS is present for each P-wave, QRS interval is less than 0.10 second.
4. T wave: ventricular repolarization and return to the resting state.
5. S-T segment: above the baseline in cardiac injury and below the baseline with ischemia.

Dysrhythmias:

Dysrhythmias may be classified according to:
Rate—either bradycardia or tachycardia.
Origin—atrial or ventricular. Ventricular dysrhythmias are more life-threatening than atrial dysrhythmias.

Nursing Implications

1. Evaluate client's tolerance of the dysrhythmia.
   - Level of consciousness, increased lethargy
   - Hypotension or postural hypotension
   - Pulse rate: tachycardic/bradycardic
   - Urinary output
2. Maintain adequate cardiac output: keep client on bed rest until client's response to the dysrhythmia is determined.
3. Provide supplemental oxygen immediately with any client who complains of chest pain or shortness of breath.

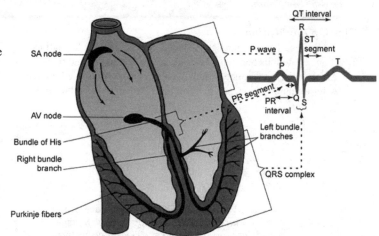

FIGURE 12-3 The Cardiac Conduction system. (From deWit, S: *Medical-surgical nursing: Concepts and practices,* ed 7, St Louis, 20009, Saunders.)

Life Threatening Dysrhythmias

Ventricular tachycardia		
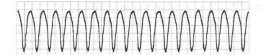	Wide, bizarre, erratic or regular ORS complexes occurring at a very rapid rate of 125 to 200 beats/min	Severe decrease in cardiac output; potentially life-threatening situation. May have a pulse or be pulseless. If unconscious and pulseless initiate CPR. *Treatment:* lidocaine, amiodarone, procainamide, cardioversion.
Ventricular fibrillation		
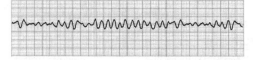	Very rapid, erratic conduction with undetermined rate; cannot identify QRS complexes;	Client is unresponsive, with no pulse; initiate a code and begin CPR. *Treatment:* defibrillation, lidocaine.

FIGURE 12-4 Life threatening dysrhythmias (From deWit, S: *Medical-surgical nursing: Concepts and practices,* St Louis, 2009, Saunders).

Appendix 12-5   PACEMAKERS

PERMANENT

An internal generator is inserted into soft tissue of upper chest or abdomen, and electrodes are positioned in the heart according to the pacing mode; procedure planned and conducted under highly controlled environment. Most often done in same-day surgery (Figure 12-5).

Demand Pacing Mode

The heart is stimulated to beat when the client's pulse rate falls below a set value or rate. The majority of pacemakers have a set rate between 60 and 72 beats per minute; if client's pulse rate falls below the set value, the pacemaker will be initiated. The pacemaker "senses" the initiation of a beat and the following conduction. If a normal cardiac impulse or beat is initiated and conducted, the pacemaker does not initiate an impulse.

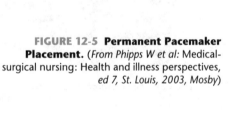 **NURSING PRIORITY:** *Pacemaker failure - An ECG must be available to validate pacemaker failure. If a client with a pacemaker experiences syncope or a bradycardia below the rate set on the pacemaker, it needs to be investigated immediately.*

Nursing Implications

1. Assess insertion site for signs of bleeding or hematoma formation.
2. If pulse rate falls below preset level, keep client in bed and report it immediately.
3. Assess client's tolerance of activity: syncope or orthostatic hypotension should not occur.
4. After initial insertion, avoid moving affected arm above the head.

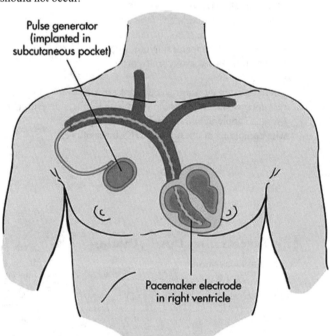

Pulse generator (implanted in subcutaneous pocket)

Pacemaker electrode in right ventricle

FIGURE 12-5 Permanent Pacemaker Placement. (*From Phipps W et al:* Medical-surgical nursing: Health and illness perspectives, *ed 7, St. Louis, 2003, Mosby*)

Client Education

1. Wear a medical alert identification, and advise all health care professionals regarding the pacemaker.
2. Avoid irritating or tight clothing that puts pressure on or irritates the site; report any signs of infection over site.
3. Safe environment: avoid close contact with areas of high voltage, magnetic force fields, large running motors; microwaves are not a problem.
4. Avoid activity that requires vigorous movement of arms and shoulders or any direct blows to PM site.
5. Advise the client of the set rate of pacemaker; teach client how to count their radial pulse. Notify the cardiac center or primary care provider immediately if the pulse rate is lower than the set rate.
6. Advise client to immediately report episodes of syncope.
7. Follow-up care and monitoring of the pacemaker are very important. Follow-up is usually done on a monthly basis via a trans-telephonic device; it does not require client to come into office.
8. Client may travel without restrictions.

 TEST ALERT: *Determine pacemaker malfunction.*

Gastrointestinal System

PHYSIOLOGY OF THE GASTROINTESTINAL (GI) SYSTEM

Organs of the Gastrointestinal System

(Figure 13-1)

A. Mouth, pharynx, esophagus.
B. Stomach.
   1. Lies in the upper left portion of the abdominal cavity.
   2. Gastroesophageal sphincter (cardiac sphincter): opening of the esophagus into the upper portion of the stomach.
   3. Length of time food remains in stomach depends on type of food, gastric motility, and psychologic factors; average time is 3 to 4 hours.
   4. Chyme (food mixed with gastric secretions) moves through the pylorus into the small intestine.
C. Small intestine.
   1. Digestion and absorption of food occurs in the small intestine, where villi provide absorptive surface area; minimal amount of nutrients are absorbed in the stomach.
   2. Carbohydrates are broken down and are absorbed through the villi of the small intestine.
   3. Intrinsic factor is secreted in the stomach and promotes absorption of vitamin B_{12} (cobalamin) in the small intestine.
   4. Movement of food (chyme) through the small intestine stimulates release of bile for digestion of fats.
D. Large intestine.
   1. Reabsorption of water; peristalsis moves the residue toward the descending colon and rectum.
   2. Large intestine absorbs water and electrolytes and forms feces.
E. Rectum and anus.
   1. Serves as a reservoir for fecal mass until defecation occurs.
   2. During defecation the rectum and colon contract; the individual takes a deep breath and initiates a voluntary contraction of the diaphragm and the abdominal wall with the glottis closed; this action results in increased pressure in the rectum.
      a. Valsalva maneuver is the voluntary pressure exerted against a closed glottis during defecation or straining at stool.
      b. This activity increases intrathoracic pressure and impedes venous return to the heart.

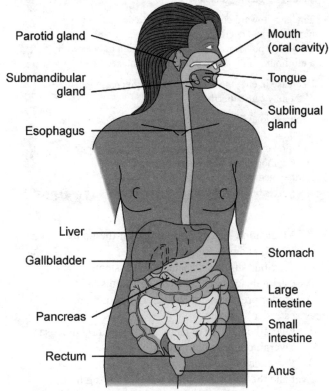

FIGURE 13-1 Organs of the digestive system (From deWit, S, *Medical surgical nursing: concepts and practices*, St Louis, 2009, Saunders).

   c. When the strain is released, there is an increase in venous return to the heart. This may precipitate problems in the client with cardiac disease.
F. Changes in the gastrointestinal system related to aging (Box 13-1).

System Data Collection

A. Evaluate client's history.
   1. Changes in bowel habits.
   2. Evaluate dietary pattern and fluid intake, note recent changes in dietary habits.
   3. Weight loss or gain, intentional on non-intentional.
   4. Pain; location of pain.
   5. Nausea and vomiting.
      a. Associated with pain.
      b. Precipitating factors.
   6. Presence or problems with flatulence.

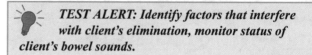

BOX 13-1   OLDER ADULT CARE FOCUS

Changes in Gastrointestinal System Related to Aging

- Decrease in production of hydrochloric acid and a decrease absorption of vitamins; encourage frequent, small well balanced meals.

- Tendency toward constipation due to a decrease in peristalsis and decrease in sensation to defecate; encourage physical activity and a diet high in fiber with a minimum of 2000 mL of daily fluid intake.

- Decrease in enzymes for fat digestion; increase intake of fat may cause diarrhea.

- Decrease in ability of liver to produce enzymes to metabolize drugs, therefore a tendency, toward accumulation of medications; instruct clients not to double up or withhold any of their medications, especially cardiac medications.

    7. Medication history, including over-the-counter (OTC) and prescription drugs.

    8. Previous surgeries related to GI system.

B. Assess vital signs in client's overall status.

C. Assess for presence and characteristics of pain.

D. Assess client's mouth.

    1. Overall condition of teeth, gums, and oral mucosa.

    2. Overall condition of tongue.

    3. Presence of gag reflex.

E. Evaluate the abdomen (client should be lying flat); sequence of assessment: inspection, auscultation, percussion, palpation.

    1. Divide the abdomen into four quadrants (Figure 13-2) and visually inspect contour and presence of scars, masses, and movement (aortic pulsation may be visible).

    2. Assess for presence of and characteristics of bowel sounds; should be audible within 1 minute.

      a. Intensity and frequency.

      b. Sounds are usually loudest just to the right and below the umbilicus.

      c. Bowel sounds are considered absent if no sound is heard for 2-5 minutes in any one of the 4 quadrants.

      d. Normally soft gurgles should be heard every 5 to 30 seconds.

    3. Percuss the abdomen for areas of distention and air.

    4. Palpate the abdomen. Begin with nontender areas first.

      a. Soft to palpation.

      b. Presence of distention.

      c. Presence of masses.

F. Assess rectal area for lesions, hemorrhoids, or ulcerations.

G. Assess stool specimen.

    1. Color, consistency, and odor.

    2. Presence of blood or mucus.

H. Evaluate elimination patterns and effects of aging on GI tract (Box 13-1).

 TEST ALERT: *Identify factors that interfere with client's elimination, monitor status of client's bowel sounds.*

Nausea and Vomiting

✳ **Nausea is an unpleasant feeling that vomiting is imminent. Vomiting is an involuntary act in which the stomach contracts and forcefully expels gastric contents.**

A. Loss of fluid and electrolytes is the primary consequence of repeated vomiting; the very young and the elderly are more susceptible to complications of fluid imbalances.

B. Prolonged vomiting will precipitate a metabolic problem with acid-base balance.

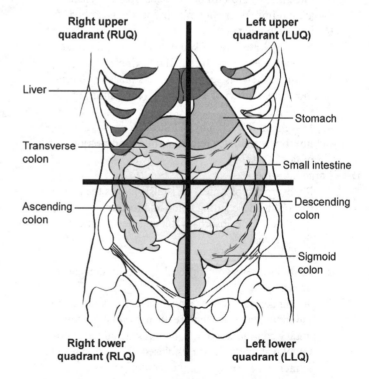

FIGURE 13-2 Abdominal quadrants. (From deWit, S, *Medical surgical nursing: concepts and practices*, St Louis, 2009, Saunders.)

Data Collection

A.   Clinical manifestations.
1.   Identify precipitating cause.

> 💡 **TEST ALERT:** *Recognize and intervene to prevent complications of surgery; recognize signs and symptoms of dehydration; monitor client's response to restore fluid and electrolyte balance.*

   a.   Postoperative clients may experience abdominal distention and vomiting.
   b.   May be associated with medications.
   c.   If problem is a result of food intolerance, client generally feels better after vomiting.
   d.   May be associated with virus, upper respiratory tract infections, and postnasal drainage.
   e.   Gastritis associated with food poisoning.
   f.   Vomiting may be associated with chemotherapy and radiation.
   g.   Vomiting may occur in first trimester of pregnancy.
2.   Assess frequency of vomiting, amount of vomiting, and contents of vomitus.
3.   Hematemesis: presence of blood in vomitus.
   a.   Bright red blood is indicative of bleeding in the stomach or the esophagus.
   b.   Coffee-ground material is indicative of blood retained in the stomach. The digestive process has broken down the hemoglobin.
4.   Projectile vomiting: vomiting not preceded by nausea; expelled with excessive force.
5.   Presence of fecal odor in vomitus indicates a back flow of intestinal contents into stomach.
B.   Diagnostics: clinical manifestations.

Treatment

A.   Eliminate the precipitating cause.
B.   Antiemetics (see Appendix 13-2).
C.   Parenteral replacement of fluid if loss is excessive.

Nursing Interventions

❖   **Goal:** To prevent recurrence of nausea and vomiting, and ensuing complications.
A.   Administer prophylactic antiemetics for clients with a tendency toward vomiting (e.g., chemotherapy clients, postoperative clients).
B.   Provide prompt removal of unpleasant odors, including the used emesis basin, used equipment, and soiled linens.
C.   Encourage good oral hygiene.
D.   Position conscious client on his side or in semi-Fowler's position; position unconscious client on side with head of bed slightly elevated.
E.   Withhold PO food and fluid initially after vomiting; begin oral intake slowly with clear liquids; begin with weak tea or an oral hydrating solution (ORS) at room temperature; for infants and children begin ORS.
F.   Support abdominal incisions during prolonged vomiting.
❖   **Goal:** To relieve nausea and vomiting.
A.   Administer antiemetics as indicated.

> ✔ **NURSING PRIORITY:** *Determine causes of nausea and vomiting; do not treat symptomatically until cause is investigated.*

B.   Evaluate precipitating causes; relieve if possible.
C.   Gastric decompression with a nasogastric tube may be indicated.
❖   **Goal:** To assess client's response to prolonged vomiting.
A.   Correlate changes in vital signs with fluid loss.
B.   Evaluate electrolyte loss and monitor urine specific gravity; assess for adequacy of hydration.
C.   Observe for continued presence of gastric distention.
D.   Record intake and output, correlate with weight loss or gain.

Constipation

✳   **Constipation exists when the interval between bowel movements is longer than normal for the individual and the stool is dry and hard.**

Data Collection

A.   Precipitating causes.
1.   Inadequate bulk in the diet.
2.   Inadequate fluid intake.
3.   Immobilization.
4.   Ignoring the urge to defecate.
5.   Diseases of the colon and rectum.
6.   Side effects of medications.
B.   Clinical manifestations.
1.   Abdominal distention.
2.   Decrease in the amount of stool.
3.   Dry, hard stool, straining to pass stool.
4.   Impaction – client is unable to pass dry hard stool, liquid stool may be passed around impaction.
C.   Diagnostics: clinical manifestations.

Treatment

See Appendix 13-2 and Box 13-2.

Nursing Interventions

❖   **Goal:** To identify client at risk of developing problems and institute preventive measures.
❖   **Goal:** To implement treatment measures.

BOX 13-2   OLDER ADULT CARE FOCUS

Preventing Fecal Impaction

- Increase intake of high-fiber foods to increase bulk of stool: raw vegetables, whole-grain breads and cereals, fresh fruits.

- Increase fluid intake, minimum intake should be at least 2000mL daily.

- Encourage daily physical activity: walking, swimming, or biking. If confined to wheelchair, change position frequently, perform leg raises and abdominal muscle contractions.

- Discourage use of laxatives and enemas: client can easily become dependent on them. If absolutely necessary, warm mineral oil enemas may soften and lubricate stool.

- Encourage use of bulk-forming products to provide increased fiber (methylcellulose, psyllium).

- Encourage bowel movement at same time each day.

- Try to position client on bedside commode rather than on a bedpan.

- If client is experiencing diarrhea, check to see if stool is oozing around an impaction.

Diarrhea

✳   **Diarrhea occurs when there is a significant increase in the number of stools and stools are more liquid.**

A.   Infants and older adults are most susceptible to complications of dehydration and hypovolemia.

B.   Acute diarrhea is most often caused by an infection and is self-limiting when all causative agents or irritants have been evacuated.

Data Collection

A.   Precipitating causes.
1.   Bacteria, parasites and viruses of the intestinal tract.
2.   Food and drug intolerance, food poisoning.
3.   Bowel disorders, malabsorption problems.
B.   Clinical manifestations.
1.   Frequent, liquid bowel movements.
2.   Stools may contain undigested food, mucus, pus, or blood.
3.   Frequently foul-smelling.
4.   Abdominal cramping, distention, and vomiting frequently occur with diarrhea.
5.   Weight loss.
6.   Hyperactive bowel sounds.
7.   May precipitate dehydration, hypovolemia, electrolyte imbalance; can progress to hypovolemia and shock.

8.   Infants and older adults are most susceptible to complications of diarrhea.
9.   Rotavirus is the most common pathogen in young children hospitalized for diarrhea.
   a.   Affects all age groups; children 6 months to 24 months are most susceptible; is most common in cool weather.
   b.   Incubation period is 1 to 3 days.
   c.   Important source of hospital acquired infections.
   d.   Is frequently associated with an upper respiratory tract infection.
C.   Diagnostics.
1.   Clinical manifestations.
2.   Stool culture.
D.   Complications of severe diarrhea.
1.   Dehydration resulting in hypovolemia.
2.   Acid-base imbalances.

Treatment

A.   Treat the underlying problem.
B.   Decrease activity and irritation of the GI tract by decreasing intake.
C.   Increase clear liquids (ORS) as tolerated.
D.   Parenteral replacement of fluids and electrolytes if diarrhea is severe.
E.   Antidiarrheal medications (see Appendix 13-2).
F.   Antidiarrheal medications may not be administered if causative agent is bacterial or parasitic. Antidiarrheals prevent client from purging the bacteria or parasite and traps the causative organism(s) in the intestines and prolongs the problem.
G.   Viral infections may be treated with medication or left to run their course, depending on the severity and type of virus.

Nursing Interventions

❖   **Goal:** To decrease diarrhea and prevent complications.
A.   Identify precipitating causes and eliminate if possible.
B.   Decrease food intake; offer soft, nonirritating food, clear liquids or ORS.
C.   Maintain good hygiene in the rectal area to prevent skin excoriation.
D.   Decrease activity.

> ✓ *NURSING PRIORITY: With nausea, vomiting and diarrhea, do not offer high carbohydrate or carbonated fluids initially; offer small amounts of clear liquids (ORS) at room temperature.*

❖   **Goal:** To evaluate client's response to diarrhea.
A.   Evaluate changes in vital signs correlating with fluid loss.
B.   Evaluate electrolyte changes, urine specific gravity and overall hydration status (Chapter 5).

C. Monitor intake and output as well as daily weight if diarrhea is progressive.
D. Assess changes in abdominal distention and cramping.
E. Provide ongoing evaluation of characteristics of diarrhea.
❖ Goal: To prevent spread of diarrhea.
A. Promote good hand hygiene: teach family importance of hand hygiene.
B. Institute contact precautions if diarrhea is of infectious origin (Appendix 5-9).
C. Maintain clean and dirty areas in the client's room - dispose of diapers and soiled linens; keep soiled objects away from clean area in room.

> 💡 **TEST ALERT: Identify client risk factors for infection, apply principles of infection control – standard plus contact precautions for client with diarrhea.**

📋 Oral Cancer

A. May occur in any area of the mouth; frequently curable if discovered early.
B. Sites of oral cancer.
   1. Lips.
   2. Tongue.
   3. Salivary glands.
   4. Floor of the mouth.

Data Collection

A. Risk factors/etiology.
   1. Smoking.
   2. Continuous oral irritation due to poor dental hygiene.
   3. Chewing tobacco.
B. Clinical manifestations.
   1. Leukoplakia: whitish patch on oral mucosa or tongue.
   2. Painless oral lesions that are fixed and hard with raised edges.
   3. Advanced symptoms include dysphagia, difficulty chewing or speaking, and enlarged lymph nodes.
C. Diagnostics: biopsy of suspected lesion.

Treatment

A. Surgery.
   1. Surgical resection.
   2. Reconstructive surgery.
B. Radiation.
C. Chemotherapy.

Nursing Interventions

❖ Goal: To prepare client for surgery.
A. Follow general preoperative care guidelines (see Chapter 3).

B. *Discuss with RN/surgeon the anticipated extent of surgery; reiterate and reinforce information with client.*
C. Emphasize good oral hygiene.

> 💡 **TEST ALERT: Monitor and provide support to client with unexpected changes in body image; identify family and client's coping mechanism.**

❖ Goal: To maintain patent airway postoperatively.
A. In the immediate postoperative period, elevate head of bed slightly to promote venous and lymphatic drainage, and to promote airway maintenance.
B. *Immediately report any swelling at incision site.*
C. Evaluate ability of client to handle oral secretions; prevention of aspiration is a priority.
D. Frequent respiratory assessment to identify problems of airway compromise.
E. The client may have a tracheostomy; depends on the extent of surgery (see Appendix 10-5).
F. Encourage good pulmonary hygiene.
G. In clients without a tracheotomy, aspiration is a primary concern.

> ✔ **NURSING PRIORITY: Airway maintenance and respiratory distress are potential problems with any operative procedure that involves the face and neck.**

❖ Goal: To maintain oral hygiene and prevent injury and infection postoperatively.
A. Type of oral hygiene is indicated by the extent of the procedure.
   1. Soothing mouth rinses of normal saline or a weak bicarbonate solutions.
   2. Avoid antiseptic or commercial mouthwashes.
   3. If dentures are present, clean mouth well before replacing.
   4. Oral hygiene before and after PO intake.
❖ Goal: To maintain nutrition postoperatively.
B. Tube feedings may be indicated initially.
C. May be necessary to maintain nutrition by total parenteral nutrition or by tube feedings (see Appendix 13-9).
D. Monitor oral intake; assess client's ability to swallow and control fluids.
   1. Liquid, soft, nonirritating foods.
   2. No extremes in temperature of food.
   3. Small, frequent feedings.
   4. Provide privacy and do not rush during meals.

 Home Care

A. Assist client to identify community resources for individual problems in rehabilitation - speech therapist, dietitian, counseling.
B. Avoid upper respiratory tract infections.
C. Instruct client regarding oral hygiene, dressing care, and medications.

D. Teach client symptoms of complications and to notify health care provider (HCP) if any of the following occur: infection, suture line bleeding or disruption, airway problems, swallowing problems, increased pain.

> **TEST ALERT: Monitor a client's ability to eat, determine impact of disease on nutritional status.**

Gastroesophageal Reflux Disease (GERD)

* **Gastroesophageal reflux disease is caused by a reflux of gastric contents into the esophagus (esophageal reflux). When reflux occurs, the esophagus is exposed to gastric acid.**

A. Prolonged GERD is an increased risk for development of cancer.

B. Gastric acid breaks down the esophageal mucosa and initiates an inflammatory response.

C. Hiatal hernia is the herniation of a portion of the stomach into the esophagus; it presents with same symptoms as GERD and the management is the same.

D. Not uncommon in clients with chronic respiratory problems.

Data Collection

A. Clinical manifestations
   1. Reflux esophagitis (heartburn, dyspepsia).
   2. May be associated with nicotine, or intake of high-fat foods, and caffeine.
   3. Pain after meals; may be relieved with antacids.
   4. Regurgitation (effortless return of stomach contents into the mouth), not associated with belching or nausea.
   5. Discomfort occurs with increase in abdominal pressure (e.g., lifting, straining).

B. Diagnostics: esophagoscopy, 24-hour monitoring of esophageal pH.

Treatment

A. Medications (see Appendix 13-3).

B. Surgical correction if hiatal hernia is present.

Nursing Interventions

❖ **Goal:** To decrease symptoms of esophageal reflux.

A. Administer antacids.

B. Modify diet.
   1. Decrease intake of highly seasoned foods and tomato products.
   2. Eat frequent, small meals (4 to 6 daily) to prevent gastric dilation.
   3. Avoid carbonated beverages and alcohol.
   4. Avoid any food that precipitates discomfort (e.g., fats, caffeine, chocolate; nicotine will decrease esophageal sphincter tone).

   5. Do not lie down after eating; avoid eating 2 to 3 hours before bedtime.

C. Decrease or stop smoking.

D. Elevate head of bed on 6- to 8-inch blocks.

E. Lose weight to decrease abdominal pressure.

F. Avoid activities that increase intraabdominal pressure (e.g., bending, weight-lifting, working in bent-over position).

G. Avoid NSAIDs and salicylates.

> ✓ **OLDER ADULT PRIORITY: GERD is often underreported in the older client; clients who awaken from coughing should be evaluated for GERD; clients are also at increased risk for aspiration.**

Obesity

An imbalance between energy expenditure and caloric intake that results in an abnormal increase in fat cells.

A. According to the CDC, 65% of people in the United States over age 20 are obese.

B. Children are considered overweight if their weight is in the 95th percentile or higher for their age, gender, and height on the growth chart.

Assessment

A. Risk factors.
   1. Genetic predisposition.
   2. Sedentary lifestyle: energy intake (food) exceeds energy expenditure.
   3. Obesity puts client at increased risk for cardiovascular, respiratory, and musculoskeletal problems, as well as increased risk for development of diabetes.

B. Clinical manifestations.
   1. A recommended body mass index is 18.5 to 24.9, a BMI of 25 to 29.9 is considered over weight, and a BMI of over 30 is considered obese.
   2. A BMI is calculated by multiplying the weight in pounds by 705 and dividing this figure by the square of the height in inches.

Treatment

A. Lifestyle changes and modification of dietary intake.

B. Bariatric surgery.
   1. Laproscopic adjustable-banded gastroplasty (LABG) involves placing an adjustable band around the fundus of the stomach.
   2. Malabsorptive: Roux-en-Y bypass (REG) or gastric bypass involves bypassing segments of small intestine so less food is absorbed.

Nursing Interventions

❖ **Goal:** To prepare client for surgery (Chapter 3).

A. Discuss the importance of early ambulation to reduce complications.

B. Length of time in hospital depends on procedure.

C. Dietary changes.

❖ **Goal:** To maintain homeostasis postoperatively (Chapter 3).

A. Immediately postoperative airway may be a problem; maintain good pulmonary hygiene; positive end expiratory pressure (PEEP) and or ventilator support may be necessary.

B. Increased risks for thromboembolic problems: sequential compression stockings, encourage early ambulation and thromboprophylaxis with low-molecular-weight heparin.

C. Do not adjust an NG tube, and do not insert NG tube even if there is protocol to do so for nausea and vomiting; *notify RN or surgeon.*

D. Observe client for development of anastomotic leaks: increasing back, shoulder and or abdominal pain, unexplained tachycardia or decrease urine output; *notify RN or surgeon of these findings.*

E. May use abdominal binder to protect incision.

F. Prevent skin excoriation – monitor areas in skin folds; keep area dry, may require use of padding.

F. In client with diabetes, assess for fluctuations in serum blood glucose; may require less antihypoglycemics.

G. Client with malabsorption surgery may experience dumping syndrome (Box 13-3).

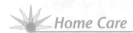 *Home Care*

A. Diet.
1. Eat at least 3 small meals a day; chew food completely.
2. Drink fluids throughout the day, but do not drink fluids with meals.
3. Avoid high-calorie, high-sugar, and high-fat foods.
4. Stop eating when you feel full.
5. Try to get 50 to 60 g of protein daily; may need to take a protein supplement.
6. Learn how to avoid dumping syndrome (see Box 13-3).

B. Take a chewable or liquid multivitamin with iron.

C. Can expect to lose 50% to 70% of excess body weight over 5 years.

D. For women, do not try to get pregnant for about 18 months after surgery.

Peptic Ulcer Disease (PUD)

❋ **PUD is the ulceration or erosion of the gastric mucosa as a result of the digestive action of hydrochloric acid and pepsin. The condition may be classified as acute or chronic. Duodenal ulcer is the most common type.**

BOX 13-3 DUMPING SYNDROME

Condition occurs when a large bolus of food that has mixed with gastric fluids (chyme) and hypertonic fluid enter the intestine. May occur in clients after a gastric resection for treatment of a perforated peptic ulcer, cancer or bariatric surgery.

ASSESSMENT

• Symptoms often occur within 15 to 30 minutes after eating.
• Initial symptoms frequently include: weakness, dizziness, tachycardia, and diaphoresis frequently occur.
• Epigastric fullness, abdominal cramping, hyperactive bowel sounds may also occur.
• Usually self-limiting and resolves in about 6 to 12 months.

PREVENTING DUMPING SYNDROME.

• Eat 5-6 small meals daily; decrease amount of food eaten at one meal.
• Decrease intake of simple carbohydrate and salt.
• Increase proteins and high-fiber foods as tolerated.
• Do not drink fluids with meals or for 1 hour following or before a meal. Drink fluids between meals only.
• Position client in semi-recumbent position during meals; client may lie down on the left side for 20 to 30 minutes after meals to delay stomach emptying.
• Hypoglycemia may occur 2 to 3 hours after eating, caused by rapid entry of carbohydrates into jejunum.

TEST ALERT: Assist with teaching client about dietary modifications.

Data Collection

A. Characteristics
1. Factors contributing to the development.
   a. Presence of *Helicobacter pylori* bacteria in the stomach.
   b. Frequently associated with increased acid production.
   c. Increased stress in lifestyle.
   d. Smoking and alcohol.
   e. Increase in physical stress (e.g., surgery, trauma).
   f. Associated with medications (e.g., NSAIDs and steroids).
2. Clinical manifestations.
   a. Burning, cramping, midepigastric pain.
   b. Duodenal ulcers: pain may occur 1 to 3 hours after eating; may be relieved by eating.
   c. Dyspepsia syndrome occurs with both duodenal and gastric ulcers: fullness, epigastric discomfort, distention, anorexia, and weight loss.

B. Diagnostics
1. Clinical manifestations.
2. Gastric analysis with possible biopsy.
3. Endoscopy: gastroscopy with test for *H. pylori*.

Treatment

A. Medical (see Appendix 13-3).
1. Antacids.
2. Histamine receptor antagonists and antisecretory agents to decrease acid production.
3. Medication regimen to treat *H. pylori*.
4. Dietary modifications: highly individual; foods precipitating pain are to be avoided.
5. Avoid use of NSAID's and other anti-inflammatory medications.
B. Surgical interventions: gastric resection.

> ✓ **NURSING PRIORITY:** *Carefully evaluate the client's blood pressure, observe for orthostatic hypotension – decrease in blood pressure when standing may be an early sign of hypovolemia.*

Complications

A. Hemorrhage when ulcer erodes through a vessel in the gastric musosa.
1. Pain, nausea and vomiting.
2. Hematemesis or melena, or both.
3. Hypovolemic shock (see Chapter 11).
B. Perforation of ulcer into the peritoneal cavity.
1. Sudden, severe, diffuse, upper abdominal pain.
2. Abdominal muscles contract as abdomen becomes rigid.
3. Hyperactive bowel sounds progressing to absent.
4. Respirations become shallow and rapid.
5. Severity of the peritonitis is proportional to size of perforation and amount of gastric spillage.

Nursing Interventions

❖ **Goal:** To promote health in clients with PUD.
A. Assist client to understand disease process.
B. Assist client to identify factors that precipitate pain and discomfort.
C. Provide information regarding dietary implications.
D. Use acetaminophen instead of aspirin products.
❖ **Goal:** To relieve pain and promote healing.
A. Modify diet.
1. Encourage small, frequent meals.
2. Nonstimulating bland foods are generally tolerated better during healing of acute episodes.
3. Assist client to identify specific dietary habits that accelerate or precipitate pain.
4. Promote good nutritional habits.
B. Decrease and/or change activity as indicated by discomfort.

❖ **Goal:** To assess for complications of hemorrhage, perforation, and peritonitis, and to initiate nursing actions accordingly.

> 💡 **TEST ALERT:** *Implement interventions to manage potential client circulatory complications; monitor client for bleeding.*

A. Assess stools and nasogastric drainage for presence of blood.
B. Assess for distention, increase in pain, and tenderness.
C. Monitor vital signs and evaluate changes.
D. Maintain client NPO.
E. Elevate head of bed unless vital signs are unstable.
1. Decrease risk of aspiration if vomiting.
2. Prevent chemical irritation of the diaphragm.
F. Prepare client for immediate surgery.
❖ **Goal:** To assist client to return to homeostasis postoperative gastric resection.
A. Follow general postoperative care as indicated (see Chapter 3).
B. Assess for the bowel sounds that indicate return of peristalsis.
C. Maintain nasogastric suction until peristalsis returns: assess color and consistency of drainage, do not adjust nasogastric tube.
D. After removal of nasogastric tube, assess for:
1. Increasing abdominal distention.
2. Nausea, vomiting.
3. Changes in bowel sounds.
E. Keep client NPO until removal of nasogastric tube.
F. Begin PO fluids slowly: clear liquids; then progress to bland soft diet.
G. Encourage ambulation to promote peristalsis.

> ✓ **NURSING PRIORITY:** *Carefully monitor drainage from the nasogastric tube, distention and vomiting will occur if tube is not draining properly.*

❖ **Goal:** To identify complication of dumping syndrome and initiate preventive nursing measures postoperative gastric resection.
A. Assess for symptoms of this condition.
B. Prevent dumping syndrome (Box 13-3).
❖ **Goal:** To initiate measures to prevent the development of pernicious anemia postoperative total gastric resection (see Chapter 9).
❖ **Goal:** To assist client to understand implications of the disease and measures necessary to maintain health postoperative total gastric resection.
A. Encourage modification of dietary habits.
B. Stop smoking.
C. Client should understand importance of monthly vitamin B_{12} injections.
D. Continue medical follow-up.

E. Identify factors in lifestyle that precipitate stress and if necessary obtain counseling to decrease stress in lifestyle.

> ✔ *NURSING PRIORITY: Clients with PUD should check with their health care provider prior to taking any over-the-counter medications – especially aspirin or NSAIDs.*

Pyloric Stenosis

✱ **The obstruction of the pyloric sphincter by hypertrophy and hyperplasia of the circular muscle of the pylorus. Most often occurs in infants between 3 and 6 weeks old.**

Data Collection

A. Onset of vomiting may be gradual, or may develop forceful, projectile vomiting.
B. Vomiting occurs shortly after feeding.
C. Vomitus does not contain bile.
D. Infant is hungry and nurses well.
E. Infant does not appear to be in pain or acute distress.
F. Failure to gain weight.
G. Stools decrease in number and in size.
H. Evidence of dehydration as condition progresses.
I. Upper abdomen is distended and an "olive-shaped" mass may be palpated in the right epigastric area.

Treatment

Surgical release of the pyloric muscle (pyloromyotomy).

> 💡 *TEST ALERT: Monitor infant's ability to eat and maintain fluid and nutritional status; position infant to prevent complications.*

Nursing Interventions

❖   **Goal:** To restore and maintain hydration and electrolyte balance; to initiate appropriate preoperative nursing activities.
A. Monitor vital signs and correlate with problems of dehydration.
B. Monitor electrolyte balance.
C. If infant is dehydrated, may be placed NPO with continuous IV infusion.
D. Maintain accurate intake and output records: complete description of all vomitus and stools.
E. Gastric decompression and suction may be used preoperatively; maintain patency of tube and accurate record of drainage.
F. Provide preoperative teaching for parents.
G. Infant should have optimal hydration and electrolyte balance preoperatively.
❖   **Goal:** To maintain adequate hydration and promote healing postoperative pyloromyotomy.

A. Postoperative vomiting in the first 24 to 48 hours is not uncommon.
B. Assess infant's response to surgery.
C. Continue to monitor infant's hydration status in the same manner as in the preoperative period.
D. Feedings are initiated early, beginning with clear liquids including oral rehydrating solutions and glucose.
   1. Offer small feedings at frequent intervals.
   2. Feed infant slowly in upright position and "bubble" frequently.
   3. Decrease activity with minimal handling after feeding.
E. Monitor infant's response to feedings.
❖   **Goal:** To assist parents to provide appropriate home care postoperative pyloromyotomy.
A. Generally, there are no residual problems after surgery.
B. Modifications of feedings should be continued at home.

Appendicitis

✱ **Appendicitis is characterized by an inflammation of the appendix and is the most common reason for abdominal surgery during childhood.**
A. Obstruction of the blind sac of the appendix precipitates inflammation, ulceration, and necrosis.
B. Problems arise when the necrotic area ruptures, spilling intestinal contents into the peritoneal cavity, causing peritonitis.

Data Collection (Figure 13-3)

A. More common in older children between 10 and 12 years old.
B. Child may complain of severe abdominal pain and may not be able to stand upright; pain may increase with coughing.
C. Pain becomes more persistent and consistent; more intense at McBurney's point (right lower quadrant).
D. Pain may be characterized as rebound pain or tenderness; may have referred pain around the perimeter of the abdomen near umbilicus.
E. Anorexia, nausea and vomiting, diarrhea.
F. Low-grade fever.
G. Client assumes a characteristic position of side-lying with the knees flexed.
H. Sudden relief from pain may be indicative of ruptured appendix.
I. Elevated WBC count.
J. No specific, definitive diagnostics.
K. Complications: peritonitis.

Treatment

A. Appendectomy to remove appendix if inflammatory condition is localized.
B. More extensive abdominal surgery must be done if appendix has ruptured (abdominal laparotomy).

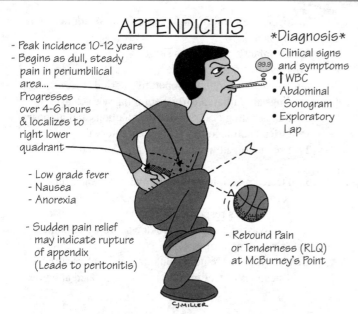

APPENDICITIS

- Peak incidence 10-12 years
- Begins as dull, steady pain in periumbilical area... Progresses over 4-6 hours & localizes to right lower quadrant

- Low grade fever
- Nausea
- Anorexia

- Sudden pain relief may indicate rupture of appendix (Leads to peritonitis)

Diagnosis
- Clinical signs and symptoms
- ↑ WBC
- Abdominal Sonogram
- Exploratory Lap

– Rebound Pain or Tenderness (RLQ) at McBurney's Point

FIGURE 13-3 Appendicitis. (From Zerwekh J, Claborn J, Miller CJ: *Memory notebook of nursing,* vol 2, ed 3, Ingram, 2007, Nursing Education Consultants.)

Nursing Interventions

❖ **Goal:** To assist in evaluating child for clinical manifestations and to prepare the child for surgery as indicated.

A. Perform a careful nursing assessment for clinical manifestations.
B. Maintain child NPO until otherwise indicated.
C. Maintain bed rest in position of comfort.
D. Do not apply heat to the abdomen; cold applications may provide some relief or comfort.
E. Do not administer enemas.
F. Avoid unnecessary palpation of abdomen.
G. *Immediately report changes in pain or sudden decrease in pain.*
H. Diagnosis cannot be confirmed until surgery; protocol for undiagnosed abdominal pain should be followed (Box 13-4).

> ✔ *NURSING PRIORITY: Pain medication should not be used indiscriminately in the client with abdominal pain. It may mask the symptoms of complications.*

❖ **Goal:** To maintain homeostasis and healing postoperative appendectomy (see Chapter 3).

❖ **Goal:** To prevent abdominal distention and promote bowel function postoperative abdominal laparotomy (ruptured appendix).

A. Maintain NPO.
B. Provide gastric decompression by nasogastric tube; maintain patency and suction.
C. Monitor abdomen for distention and increased pain.
D. Assess for return of peristaltic activity.

BOX 13-4   UNDIAGNOSED ABDOMINAL PAIN

DO NOT
- Give anything by mouth.
- Put any heat on the abdomen.
- Give an enema.
- Give strong narcotics.
- Give a laxative.

DO
- Maintain bed rest.
- Place in a position of comfort.
- Assess hydration.
- Assess abdominal status: distention, bowel sounds, passage of stool or flatus, generalized or local pain.
- Maintain client NPO until notified otherwise.

E. Evaluate and record character of bowel movements.
F. Encourage ambulation as soon as indicated.

❖ **Goal:** To decrease infection and promote healing postoperative abdominal laparotomy.

A. Position client in semi-Fowler's to localize infection and to prevent spread of infection and development of abdominal abscess.
B. Antibiotics are usually administered via IV infusion, then as oral preparations; monitor response to antibiotics as well as status of IV infusion site.
C. Provide wound care; evaluate drainage from abdominal Penrose drains and incisional area.
D. Assess abdomen for increase in distention and/or tenderness, and for presence of bowel sounds.
E. Monitor vital signs frequently and assess for presence of infection.

❖ **Goal:** To maintain adequate hydration and nutrition and to promote comfort postoperative abdominal laparotomy.

A. Maintain adequate hydration via IV infusion.
B. Evaluate tolerance to PO liquids when nasogastric tube is removed.
C. Begin clear liquids PO when peristalsis returns.
D. Progress diet as tolerated.
E. Administer analgesics as indicated.

Acute Abdomen

❉ **An acute abdomen covers a broad spectrum of urgent conditions that require immediate surgical intervention. May also be referred to as peritonitis which is characterized by a generalized inflammation of the peritoneal cavity.**

> 💡 *TEST ALERT: Identify the client at risk for infection and signs and symptoms of infection.*

A. Intestinal motility is decreased and fluid accumulates as a result of the inability of the intestine to reabsorb fluid.

B. Fluid will leak into the peritoneal cavity, precipitating fluid, electrolyte, and protein loss as well as fluid depletion.

Data Collection

A. Risk factors/etiology: primary source of problem is rupture of an area of the gastrointestinal tract.

> ✔ *NURSING PRIORITY: Monitor the status of the postoperative client. Peritonitis is a potential complication whenever the abdomen is entered – either from trauma or from surgery.*

B. Clinical manifestations (Figure 13-4)
1. Presence of precipitating cause (ulcer perforation, ruptured appendix, trauma, ruptured diverticuli).
2. Pain over involved area; rebound tenderness.
3. Abdominal distention.
4. Abdominal muscle rigidity ("board-like" abdomen) and "guarding."
5. Fever.
6. Anorexia, nausea, vomiting.
7. Increased pulse rate, decreased blood pressure, shallow respirations.
8. Decreased or absent bowel sounds.
9. Dehydration leading to hypovolemia.
C. Diagnostics.
1. Increased white cell count.
2. X-ray of abdomen.
3. Peritoneal lavage (aspiration) to evaluate presence and characteristics of intra-abdominal fluid.
4. Clinical manifestations.

Treatment

A. Identify and treat precipitating cause (may require surgical intervention).
B. Antibiotics.
C. IV fluids.
D. Decrease abdominal distention with nasogastric tube and suction.

Nursing Interventions

❖ Goal: To provide adequate pain control and wound care.
❖ Goal: To maintain fluid and electrolyte balance and reduce gastric distention (Chapter 3).
A. Maintain nasogastric suction.
B. Monitor IV fluid replacement and hydration status.
C. Evaluate peristalsis and return of bowel function.
D. Maintain intake and output records.
E. Assess for problems of dehydration.
F. Encourage ambulation as soon as possible to facilitate return of bowel function.
❖ Goal: To reduce infectious process.

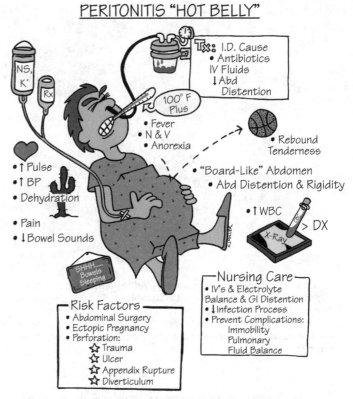

FIGURE 13-4 **Peritonitis.** (From Zerwekh J, Claborn J, Miller CJ: *Memory notebook of nursing,* vol 2, ed 3, Ingram, 2007, Nursing Education Consultants.)

A. Assess client's tolerance of antibiotics and status of infusion site.
B. Evaluate vital signs and correlate with progress of infectious process.
C. Maintain semi-Fowler's position to enhance respirations as well as to decrease irritation of diaphragm.
❖ Goal: To prevent complications associated with immobility (see Chapter 3).
❖ Goal: To provide postoperative care as indicated (see Chapter 3).

> 💡 *TEST ALERT: Identify factors that may interfere with wound healing. Monitor the client for infections and provide emergency care of wound disruption.*

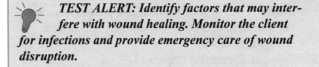 **Intestinal Obstruction**

❋ **Interference with normal peristalsis and impairment of forward flow of intestinal contents is known as an intestinal obstruction.**
A. Regardless of the precipitating cause, the ensuing problems are a result of the obstructive process.
B. The higher the obstruction in the intestine, the more severe the symptoms.

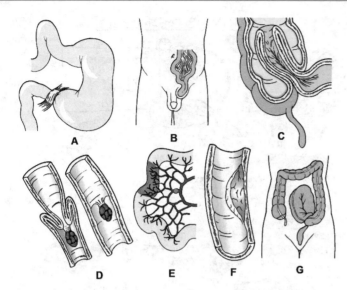

FIGURE 13-5 **Bowel obstructions. A,** Adhesions. **B,** Strangulated inguinal hernia. **C,** Ileocecal intussusception. **D,** Intussusception from polyps. **E,** Mesenteric occlusion. **F,** Neoplasm. **G,** Volvulus of the sigmoid colon. (From Lewis SI, et al: *Medical-surgical nursing: assessment and management of clinical problems*, ed 7, St. Louis, 2007, Mosby.)

C. The location of the obstruction determines the extent of fluid and electrolyte imbalance and acid-base imbalance.
   1. Dehydration and electrolyte imbalance do not occur rapidly if obstruction is in the large intestine.
   2. If obstruction is located high in the intestine, dehydration occurs rapidly due to the inability of the intestine to reabsorb fluids.

D. Fluid, gas, and intestinal contents accumulate proximal to the obstruction. This causes distention proximal to the obstruction and bowel collapse distal to the obstruction.

E. As fluid accumulation increases, so does pressure against the bowel. This precipitates extravasation of fluids and electrolytes into the peritoneal cavity. Increased pressure may cause the bowel to rupture.

F. Increased pressure causes an increase in capillary permeability and leakage of fluids and electrolytes into peritoneal fluid; this leads to a severe reduction in circulating volume.

G. Types of obstruction (Figure 13-5).
   1. Mechanical obstruction.
     a. Strangulated hernia.
     b. Intussusception: the telescoping of one portion of the intestine into another (occurs most often in infants and small children).
     c. Volvulus: twisting of the bowel.
     d. Tumors: cancer (most frequent cause of obstruction in older adults).
     e. Adhesions.
   2. Neurogenic: interference with nerve supply in the intestine.
     a. Paralytic ileus or adynamic ileus occurring as a result of abdominal surgery or inflammatory process.
     b. Potential complication from spinal cord injury.
   3. Vascular obstruction: interference with the blood supply to the bowel.
     a. Infarction of superior mesenteric artery.
     b. Bowel obstructions related to intestinal ischemia may occur very rapidly and may be life-threatening.

Data Collection

A. Clinical manifestations.
   1. Vomiting occurs early and is severe if obstruction is high.
   2. Vomiting may be caused by lower obstructions occurs more slowly and may be foul smelling due to presence of bacteria.
   3. Abdominal distention.
   4. Bowel sounds initially may be hyperactive proximal to the obstruction and decreased or absent distal to the obstruction; eventually all bowel sounds will be absent.

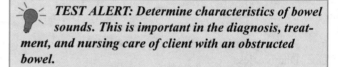

     TEST ALERT: Determine characteristics of bowel sounds. This is important in the diagnosis, treatment, and nursing care of client with an obstructed bowel.

   5. Colicky-type abdominal pain.
   6. Intussusception
     a. Sudden occurrence of acute abdominal pain.
     b. Child may pass bloody mucous stool described as "currant jelly".
     c. A "sausage shaped" mass may be palpated in the abdomen.

B. Diagnostics.
   1. X-ray of the abdomen to assist in differentiating obstruction from perforation.
   2. Evaluation of history of abdominal problems.

Treatment

A. Mechanical and vascular intestinal obstructions are generally treated surgically; ileostomy or colostomy may be necessary.

B. Treatment of neurogenic obstruction (paralytic ileus) may consist of intestinal intubation and decompression.

C. Maintain fluid and electrolyte replacement.

Complications

A. Infection/septicemia.
B. Gangrene of the bowel.
C. Perforation of the bowel.
D. Fluid and electrolyte imbalance.

Nursing Interventions

❖ **Goal:** To prepare client for diagnostic evaluation and to maintain ongoing nursing assessment for pertinent data (see Appendix 13-1).

A. Monitor all stools, passage of normal stool may indicate the obstruction is resolved.

B. Classic symptoms of intussusception may not be present - observe child for diarrhea, anorexia, vomiting and acute episodic abdominal pain.

❖ **Goal:** To decrease gastric distention and to maintain hydration and electrolyte balance.

A. Maintain NPO.

B. Maintain nasogastric suction (Appendix 13-5).

C. Monitor IV fluid replacement.

D. Evaluate peristalsis and return of bowel function.

E. Maintain accurate intake and output records.

F. Assess for problems of dehydration and hypovolemia.

G. Measure abdominal girth to determine if distention is increasing.

H. Encourage activities to facilitate return of bowel function.

1. Encourage activity, ambulate client as often as possible.

2. May attempt to decrease pain medication to facilitate return of bowel function.

3. Maintain good hydration.

❖ **Goal:** To provide appropriate preoperative preparation when surgery is indicated (see Chapter 3).

❖ **Goal:** To maintain homeostasis and promote healing postoperative abdominal laparotomy (see Chapter 3).

❖ **Goal:** To maintain fluid and electrolyte balance and prevent gastric distention postoperative abdominal laparotomy (see preoperative goal).

❖ **Goal:** To decrease infection and promote healing postoperative abdominal laparotomy.

A. Antibiotics are usually administered via IV infusion. Monitor client's response to antibiotics as well as status of IV infusion site.

B. Monitor vital signs frequently and evaluate for presence of infectious process.

C. Provide wound care; evaluate drainage from abdominal Penrose drains as well as from abdominal incisional area (Appendix 3-2).

> 💡 **TEST ALERT:** *Empty and reestablish negative pressure of portable wound suction devices (Hemovac, Jackson-Pratt drains).*

❖ **Goal:** To reestablish normal nutrition and to promote comfort postoperative abdominal laparotomy.

A. Evaluate tolerance of liquids when nasogastric tube is removed.

B. Begin clear liquids initially and evaluate presence of peristalsis.

C. Progress diet as tolerated.

D. Administer analgesics as indicated.

Diverticular Disease

✳ **The condition in which an individual has multiple diverticula is known as diverticulosis.**

A. Diverticulum: dilatation or outpouching of a weakened area in the intestinal wall.

B. Diverticulitis: circulation to the diverticulum is compromised, allowing for bacterial invasion and an inflammatory reaction.

C. Meckel's diverticulum is a diverticula in the ileum in children; most common congenital anomaly of the GI tract in children.

Data Collection

A. Risk factors/etiology.

1. Increased incidence in clients over 45 years of age.

2. Low-fiber diet and chronic constipation.

3. Most frequently occurs in the sigmoid colon.

4. Indigestible fibers (seeds, corn, etc) may precipitate diverticulitis, but do not contribute to the development of the diverticula.

B. Clinical manifestations.

1. Diverticulum is usually asymptomatic; symptoms vary with degree of inflammation.

2. Intermittent left quadrant tenderness, abdominal cramping.

3. Constipation or alternating constipation and diarrhea.

4. Occult blood and/or mucus in the stool.

5. Inflammatory changes may precipitate perforation or abscess formation.

6. Diverticulitis occurs when undigested food and bacteria are trapped in the diverticula.

a. Fever.

b. Left lower quadrant pain, usually accompanied by nausea and vomiting.

c. Abdominal distention.

d. Frequently constipated.

e. May progress to intestinal obstruction, abscess, or perforation.

C. Diagnostics.

1. Stool examination.

2. Barium enema.

3. Colonoscopy.

Treatment

A. Medical management of uncomplicated diverticulum.

1. High-fiber diet (restrict indigestible fiber such as corn, popcorn, and sesame seeds).

2. Decrease intake of fat and red meat.

3. Prevent chronic constipation: use bulk laxatives and stool softeners.

4. Increase physical activity.

B. Treatment for acute diverticulitis.

1. Antibiotics.

2. May be NPO or on a low-residue diet.
3. IV fluids if dehydrated.
4. Possible surgery and colon resection if abscess, obstruction, bleeding, or perforation occurs.

Nursing Interventions

❖   **Goal:** To assist client to understand dietary implications and maintain prescribed therapy to prevent exacerbations.
A. Understand high-fiber diet.
B. Avoid indigestible roughage such as nuts, popcorn, small fruit seeds.
C. Maintain high-fluid intake.
D. Avoid large meals.
E. Avoid alcohol.
F. Weight reduction if indicated.
G. Avoid activities that increase intra-abdominal pressure (straining while defecating, bending, lifting, wearing tight restrictive clothing).

> 💡 **TEST ALERT: Use measures to improve client's nutrition – clients with diverticulitis need specific dietary instructions.**

 ## Hernias

✳   **A hernia is a protrusion of the intestine through an abnormal opening or weakened area of the abdominal wall.**
A. Types.
1. Inguinal: a weakness in which the spermatic cord in men and the round ligament in women passes through the abdominal wall into the groin area; more common in men.
2. Femoral: protrusion of the intestine through the femoral ring; more common in women.
3. Umbilical: occurs most often in children when the umbilical opening fails to close adequately; occurs in adults when the abdominal muscle is weak.
4. Incisional: weakness in the abdominal wall due to a previous incision.
5. Classification.
a. Reducible: Hernia may be replaced into the abdominal cavity by manual manipulation.
b. Incarcerated: Hernia may not be replaced back into the abdominal cavity.
c. Strangulated: Blood supply and intestinal flow to the herniated area are obstructed; a strangulated hernia leads to intestinal obstruction.

Data Collection

A. Clinical manifestations.
1. Hernia protrudes over the involved area when the client stands or strains.

2. Severe pain occurs if hernia becomes strangulated or blood supply is compromised.
3. Strangulated hernia will cause symptoms associated with intestinal obstruction.
B. Diagnostics (Appendix 13-1).

Treatment

A. Preferably elective surgery (herniorrhaphy) to prevent complications of strangulation
B. Strangulated hernia involves an emergency surgery for resection of the involved bowel.

Nursing Interventions

❖   **Goal:** To prepare client for surgery if indicated (see Chapter 3).
❖   **Goal:** To maintain homeostasis and promote healing postoperative herniorrhaphy.
A. Follow general postoperative nursing care (see Chapter 3).
B. Assess male clients for development of scrotal edema (inguinal hernia).
C. Discourage coughing, but encourage deep breathing and turning.
D. When coughing occurs, teach client how to splint the incision.
E. Refrain from heavy lifting for approximately 6 to 8 weeks postoperatively.
F. Wound care
1. Keep wound clean and dry, may use a dressing or leave incision open to air.
2. On infants, change diapers frequently and prevent irritation and contamination of the incisional area.

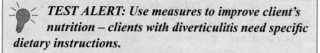 ## Inflammatory Bowel Disease

✳   **Crohn's disease is a chronic, nonspecific, inflammatory disease that extends through all layers of the bowel wall and occurs in patches throughout the distal ileum and colon.**
✳   **Ulcerative colitis is inflammation and ulceration of the mucosal layer of the colon and rectum; area of inflammation is diffuse and involves mucosa and submucosa of the intestinal wall. It frequently begins in the rectum, and spreads in a continuous manner up the colon; seldom is the small intestine involved.**

Data Collection

A. Risk factors/etiology.
1. May begin in adolescence; peak incidence occurs between ages 20 and 30 years, second peak of occurrence occurs in client 60 years and older.
2. Clients with long-standing ulcerative colitis have significant increase in cancer of the colon.
3. Clients with ulcerative colitis may have history of difficulty in handling stress.

B. Clinical manifestations.
1. Abdominal pain.
2. Diarrhea; more severe in colitis clients.
3. Steatorrhea due to poorly absorbed fats.
4. Nausea and vomiting.
5. Abdominal distention and tenderness.
6. Stool may contain occult blood or bright red blood.
7. Weight loss, nutritional deficiency, impaired absorption of vitamin B_{12}.
C. Diagnostics (Appendix 13-1).
1. Stool analysis to rule out bacterial or parasitic infection.
2. Even though the two conditions have distinctive criteria for diagnosis, frequently a clear differentiation cannot be made between them.

Treatment

A. Dietary modifications: low-residue and low-fiber diet; increased calorie intake; increased protein intake; increased vitamin and iron supplementation.
B. Medications.
1. Corticosteroids to reduce the inflammation (see Appendix 5-7).
2. Antidiarrheal medications (see Appendix 13-2).
3. Antibiotics (see Appendix 5-10).
C. Surgical intervention if fistulas, perforation, bleeding, or intestinal obstruction occurs; an ileostomy may be necessary in clients with wide spread disease.

Nursing Interventions

❖ **Goal:** (acute): To monitor inflammatory response and promote healing.
A. Observe number and character of stool.
B. Evaluate fluid status; record daily intake and output and body weight.
C. Perform good skin hygiene around anal area to prevent excoriation due to diarrhea.
D. Evaluate character of bowel sounds.
E. Monitor lab values for anemia and electrolyte imbalance.
F. Assess for development of anemia due to lack of absorption of vitamin B_{12}; may require replacement vitamin B_{12}.
G. Assist client to identify food that precipitate discomfort and diarrhea.
H. Promote comfort by assisting client to keep anal area clean and keeping room free of offensive odors.

> 💡 **TEST ALERT: Monitor client's nutritional status. Use measures to improve nutritional intake; identify signs and symptoms of fluid imbalance.**

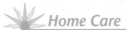 *Home Care*

A. Modify diet: encourage low-residue, bland foods that are high in calories and protein. Diet may progress as inflammation subsides.
B. Understand medication regimen.
C. Identify symptoms indicating reoccurrence of the problem, as well as when to call the physician.
1. Bleeding from the colon, or vomiting blood.
2. Significant increase in abdominal pain.
3. Increase in stools with decrease in body weight.
4. Chills, fever, increased lethargy.
D. Avoid smoking and alcohol.

 ## Gastritis and Gastroenteritis

✳ **Gastritis is an inflammatory process involving the mucosa of the stomach.**
✳ **Gastroenteritis involves the small bowel as well as the stomach.**

> ✓ **NURSING PRIORITY: Problem is usually self-limiting; fluid balance is of increased concern in the older adult and in the infant.**

Data Collection

A. Risk factors.
1. Ingestion of contaminated food (*Salmonella* and *Staphylococcus* bacteria).
2. Alcohol.
3. NSAIDs, aspirin.
4. Radiation therapy.
B. Clinical manifestations.
1. Epigastric tenderness with abdominal cramping.
2. Nausea, vomiting, and diarrhea.
C. Diagnostics: identify precipitating cause.

Treatment

Appropriate medication for causative agents.

Nursing Interventions

❖ **Goal:** To evaluate and maintain hydration and electrolyte balance, and to prevent spread of disease.
A. NPO until vomiting ceases.
B. Begin clear liquids (ORS) gradually after vomiting ceases.
C. Follow contact precautions until organism is identified; then follow appropriate precautions as indicated.
❖ **Goal:** To provide symptomatic nursing care for diarrhea, nausea, and vomiting.
A. See general intestinal disorders.

Hirschsprung's Disease
(Congenital Aganglionic Megacolon)

* **This disease is characterized by congenital absence of innervation in a segment of the colon wall.**

A. Precipitates a neurogenic bowel obstruction.
B. Most common site is the rectosigmoid colon; colon proximal to the area dilates (i.e., megacolon).

Data Collection

A. Clinical manifestations.
  1. Varies according to age and amount of colon involved.
  2. Newborn (first 24 to 48 hours).
    a. Failure to pass meconium.
    b. Bile-stained vomitus.
    c. Abdominal distention.
  3. Older infant.
    a. Failure to thrive.
    b. Abdominal distention.
    c. Chronic constipation and overflow diarrhea.
    d. Passage of "ribbon-like" stool.
B. Diagnostics - rectal biopsy.

Treatment

A. Surgery: usually done in two stages: first a temporary colostomy, then later more complete repair.

Nursing Interventions

❖ Goal: To promote normal attachment and prepare infant and parents for surgery.
A. Allow parents to vent feelings regarding congenital defect of infant.
B. Foster infant-parent attachment.
C. Follow general preoperative preparation of the infant.
D. Provide explanation of colostomy to parents, provide opportunity for parents to participate in care of infant's colostomy.
❖ Goal: To assist parents to understand and provide appropriate home care for the child postoperative colostomy.
A. Colostomy is generally temporary.
B. Parents should be actively involved in colostomy care before discharge (see Appendix 13-8).

Cancer of the Colon and Rectum

* **Colorectal cancer is the third most common cancer in the United States.**

Data Collection

A. Risk factors/etiology.
  1. Significant increase in clients over age 50 years.
  2. History of inflammatory bowel disease.
  3. Family history of colon cancer.
  4. Majority of malignant tumors are found in the rectal area.
B. Clinical manifestations.
  1. Symptoms are vague early in disease state, and condition may take years to be identified.
  2. Change in bowel habits: constipation and diarrhea.
  3. Rectal bleeding, bloody stools, melena (dark tarry) stools.
  4. Change in shape of stool (pencil-shaped or ribbon-shaped from sigmoid or rectal cancer).
  5. Weakness and fatigue from anemia and chronic blood loss.
  6. Constipation and distention, abdominal cramping.
  7. Tenesmus: ineffective, painful straining at stool.
  8. Pain is a late symptom.
  9. Bowel obstruction with perforation may occur.
C. Diagnostics: sigmoidoscopy and colonoscopy with biopsies.

Treatment

A. Surgical resection of tumor: a temporary or permanent colostomy may be performed.
B. Radiation therapy.
C. Chemotherapy.

> ✔ *OLDER ADULT PRIORITY: Abdominal pain, obstruction, and rectal bleeding are common symptoms in the older adult; older adults are at higher risk for complications.*

Nursing Interventions

❖ Goal: Provide information to high risk clients.
A. Increased fiber in diet, with decrease in fat and red meat.
B. Digital rectal exams yearly after age 40.
C. Annual fecal occult blood testing after age 50.
D. Flexible sigmoidoscopy/colonoscopy after age 50, subsequent exams depend on findings and risk factors.
❖ Goal: To provide preoperative care as indicated for abdominal laparotomy and colostomy (see Appendix 13-8).
A. Client must usually undergo extensive preoperative bowel preparation (see Appendix 13-2).
B. Determine extent of surgery to be performed, discuss implications and placement of ostomy if indicated.
❖ Goal: To provide appropriate wound care postoperative abdominal-perineal resection.
A. For rectal cancer, client will frequently have three incisional areas.
  1. Abdominal incision.
  2. Left abdominal incision for colostomy.
  3. Perineal incision.

> *TEST ALERT: Identify factors interfering with wound healing and or symptoms of infections.*

B.   Perineal wound may be closed with a Penrose drain inserted, or may be left open to heal by secondary intention.
1.   Drainage from wound should be serosanguineous.
2.   Drains are left in place until there is minimal (50mL or less) drainage.
3.   If wound is left open and packed, there may be profuse drainage initially after surgery. Check frequently, reinforce and or change dressing as necessary.
4.   Generally irrigate the perineal wound with saline.
5.   Use a warm sitz bath for 10-20 minutes to promote debridement, to increase circulation to the perineal area, and to promote comfort.
C.   Abdominal wound may need frequent dressing changes due to profuse serosanguineous drainage immediately postoperative.
D.   Usually the position of comfort is on the side, to prevent pressure on rectal area and to relax abdominal muscles.
E.   Keep room free of offensive odors, client may feel very self conscious about open wound and colostomy.

❖   **Goal:** To prevent complications of immobility postoperative abdominal-perineal resection (see Chapter 3).
❖   **Goal:** To maintain homeostasis and promote wound healing postoperative abdominal-perineal resection (see Chapter 3).
A.   Provide opportunity for client to participate in colostomy care early in recovery.
B.   Infections, hemorrhage, wound disruption and stoma problems are not uncommon in postoperative period.

Home Care

A.   Frequently for the older adult client, recovery period may be long; assist client and family to identify community resources.
B.   Provide instructions in care of perineal wound if it is not healed.
1.   Sitz baths – therapeutic bath, not a cleansing bath, always check temperature of water.
2.   Presence of continuous drainage could indicate a fistula.
B.   Assist client and family to perform colostomy care (see Appendix 13-8).
C.   Discuss importantance of returning for medical check ups.
D.   Understand symptoms to report to physician.
1.   Increased pain.
2.   Change in stool or bleeding.
3.   Weight loss.
4.   Sustained vomiting and diarrhea.

Celiac Disease (Malabsorption Syndrome)

＊   **Celiac disease is also known as sprue, gluten enteropathy, and malabsorption syndrome. Condition results from an immune reaction to rye, wheat, barley, and oat grains. An inflammatory response causes damage to the mucosa of the small intestines and resulting in the inability to absorb nutrients (malabsorption).**

A.   Previously considered a disease of childhood with symptoms beginning between the ages of 1 year and 5 years; celiac disease is now commonly seen at all ages with mean age of diagnosis being 40 years.
B.   Symptoms frequently begin in early childhood, but condition may not be diagnosed until client is an adult.
C.   Development of celiac disease is dependent on genetic predisposition, ingestion of gluten, and immune-mediated response.

Assessment

A.   Cause: congenital defect or an autoimmune response in gluten metabolism.
B.   Clinical manifestations.
1.   Symptoms may begin when child has increased intake of foods containing gluten: cereals, crackers, breads, cookies, pastas, etc.
2.   Foul-smelling diarrhea with abdominal distention and anorexia in infants and toddlers.
3.   Poor weight gain in children, failure to thrive.
4.   Constipation, vomiting, and abdominal pain may be the initial presenting symptoms in adults.
5.   Vitamin deficiency leads to central nervous system impairment and bone malformation.
C.   Diagnostics: biopsy of duodenum and small intestine.

Treatment

Primarily dietary management: gluten-free diet.

Nursing Interventions

❖   **Goal:** To help client and family understand diet therapy and promote optimal nutrition intake.
A.   Written information regarding a gluten-free diet; corn, rice, potato, and soy products may be substituted for wheat in diet.
B.   Diet should be well balanced and high in protein.
C.   Teach client and/or family how to read food labels for gluten content; thickenings, soups, instant foods may contain hidden sources of gluten.
D.   Important to discuss the necessity of maintaining a lifelong gluten-restricted diet; problems may occur in clients who relax their diet and experience an exacerbation of the disease state.
E.   Lack of adherence to dietary restrictions may precipitate growth retardation, anemia, and bone deformities.

Hemorrhoids

* Hemorrhoids are dilated veins of the anus and rectum; may be external (outside the external sphincter) or internal (above the internal sphincter).

Data Collection

A. Risk factors/etiology.
  1. By age 50, approximately 50% of people have them.
  2. May appear periodically depending on amount of anorectal pressure.
  3. Caused by conditions that increase anorectal pressure.
    a. Pregnancy.
    b. Prolonged constipation, obesity.
    c. Prolonged standing or sitting.
    d. Heavy lifting or straining.
    e. Portal hypertension.
B. Clinical manifestations.
  1. External hemorrhoids appear as reddish protrusions at the anus.
  2. Internal hemorrhoids may become constricted and painful, may bleed during defecation.
  3. Rectal bleeding.
C. Diagnostics: rectal examination.

Treatment

A. Ointments and topical anesthetics to shrink mucous membranes.
B. Stool softeners, increased fiber in diet.
C. Sitz bath, ointments for comfort.
D. Removal of the hemorrhoid by ligation, infrared coagulation of hemorrhoids, or surgical removal.

Nursing Interventions

❖ Goal: To provide appropriate information to assist client to manage problem at home.
A. Avoid prolonged standing or sitting.
B. Encourage sitz baths to decrease discomfort.
C. Apply over-the-counter ointments to decrease discomfort.
D. Use an ice pack followed by a warm sitz bath if severe discomfort occurs.
E. Avoid constipation and straining at stool.
F. Modify diet to prevent constipation (e.g., bulk laxatives).

❖ Goal: To maintain homeostasis and promote healing postoperative hemorrhoidectomy.
A. Rectal pain may be quite severe.
B. Assess for urinary retention.
C. Encourage taking a sitz bath 2 to 3 times a day after surgery; this promotes cleanliness, decreases pain, and increases healing.
D. Promote passage of normal stool.
  1. Encourage stool softeners and bulk-forming laxatives prior to surgery to prevent constipation (see Appendix 13-3).
  2. Teach client not to resist urge to defecate.
  3. Encourage activity to promote peristalsis.

Study Questions: Gastrointestinal System

1. A client has had extensive oral surgery for cancer of the mouth. What is an important nursing measure when providing oral care for this client?
  1 Gently cleanse the mouth with a lemon and glycerin swab.
  2 Assist the client to rinse his mouth with a weak bicarbonate solution
  3 Provide frequent oral care with a bactericidal mouthwash.
  4 Offer only cold foods that are nonirritating.

2. A client is placed on NPO status due to a bowel obstruction. A nasogastric tube is inserted. What is the purpose of this tube?
  1 Decrease gastric distention.
  2 Eliminate nausea and vomiting.
  3 Reduce pain postoperatively.
  4 Provide a route for tube feeding.

3. What type of stool can the nurse expect from a client who has a colostomy of the lower descending colon?
  1 Liquid.
  2 Bloody.
  3 Black.
  4 Formed.

4. A client has just had his nasogastric tube removed. What would be the best immediate nursing intervention?
  1 Check for the presence of bowel sounds.
  2 Assist client with oral hygiene.
  3 Offer the client some ice cream.
  4 Palpate the abdomen for distention.

5. A nurse is changing the ileostomy bag on a client the day after surgery. What is a normal characteristic of the stoma?
  1 Pitting edema around base.
  2 Dusky gray color.
  3 Red with some edema.
  4 Tissue sloughing in the area.

6. What is important for the nurse to assess and document in clients who have digestive tract problems?
1 Peripheral edema and urinary output.
2 Changes in bowel activity and weight fluctuation.
3 Decrease in appetite with blood glucose level of 110 mg/100 mL.
4 Alteration in appetite with a change in daily activities.

7. When attempting to auscultate bowel sounds that are decreased or not easily heard, how long should the nurse listen to each quadrant?
1 2 minutes.
2 5 minutes.
3 30 seconds.
4 1 minute.

8. While being prepared for gastroscopy, the client complains of excessive fatigue and says he does not want this procedure done. What is the best nursing management?
1 Wait 5 minutes; then return to prepare the client.
2 Explain to the client the importance of the procedure.
3 Stop the preparation and notify the charge nurse.
4 Call the nurse's station and ask for assistance.

9. The nurse is caring for a client who is being prepared for surgery for appendicitis. What is the preoperative preparation?
1 Ambulate to decrease problems with distention.
2 Administer meperidine (**Demerol**) for pain.
3 Allow position of comfort; maintain NPO.
4 Put a warm pad on abdomen; offer clear liquids.

10. A client has just returned to the nursing unit following a gastrectomy. A nasogastric tube is in place and the client begins to complain of nausea. What is the priority nursing action?
1 Gently irrigate the nasogastric tube with normal saline.
2 Clamp the tube for 30 minutes and reassess the client.
3 Measure gastric output to determine excessive acid production.
4 Determine if the nasogastric tube is patent and draining.

11. A client is receiving tube feedings via his nasogastric tube 3 days after surgery. What method of administration of the tube feeding would cause the client to experience the least problems with tolerance and absorption of the feeding?
1 Dilute formula infused via a continuous drip.
2 Full strength formula given at 50 mL/hour via continuous drip.
3 250 mL of dilute formula given as a bolus via gravity flow.
4 Bolus of 300 mL full-strength formula given via gravity flow.

12. What would be appropriate teaching for a client who is experiencing gastroesophageal reflux disease (GERD)?

1 Take an antacid after eating.
2 Lay down on your right side after eating.
3 Increase intake of fluids after eating.
4 Avoid eating within 3 hours of bedtime.

13. A client with nausea and vomiting would be placed in what position to prevent aspiration?
1 Supine with head turned to the right.
2 Prone with head of bed elevated 45 degrees.
3 Side-lying.
4 Trendelenburg.

14. What is the desired action of ranitidine (Zantac) in the treatment of a client with a gastric ulcer?
1 Increase gastric acid production.
2 Increase production of bile.
3 Neutralize hydrochloric acid production.
4 Decrease production of hydrochloric acid.

15. On the second day after gastric surgery, the client's nasogastric tube is draining a fluid that appears to contain coffee grounds. What is the nurse's interpretation of this drainage?
1 The fluid contains mucus and stomach contents.
2 The drainage probably contains old blood as a result of the surgery.
3 The client is actively bleeding and the tube should be irrigated.
4 There is an excessive amount of bile in the drainage.

16. The nurse is assessing a client who is 4-days postoperative for an exploratory surgery secondary to a ruptured appendix. What assessment finding would suggest the client is developing peritonitis?
1 Abdominal pain in the area of the incision; pain increases with coughing.
2 Temperature increase to 102° F; client has a rigid abdomen and decreased or absent bowel sounds.
3 Purulent drainage from the surgical wound; nausea and vomiting after clear liquid intake.
4 Absent bowel sounds, decreased white blood cell count, low-grade fever.

17. The nurse is caring for a client who is receiving tube feedings via a gastrostomy tube. The order is for $\frac{1}{2}$ strength formula at a continuous rate of 55 mL per hour. The formula comes in 250 mL cans. How many cans would the nurse anticipate using over an 8-hour period of time? Answer: _____ can(s)

18. Dietary modifications have not been successful in preventing constipation in an older client. What over-the-counter preparations would the nurse recommend to assist the client in the prevention of constipation?
1 Use laxatives that stimulate peristalsis and promote daily bowel movements.
2 Take a bulk laxative that contains psyllium with a full glass of water every morning.
3 Increase intake of raw fruits and vegetables.
4 Administer a tap water enema every other day.

Answers and rationales to these questions are in the section at the end of the book titled Chapter Study Questions: Answers and Rationales.

| Appendix 13-1 | GASTROINTESTINAL SYSTEM DIGNOSTICS |

X-Ray

Upper Gastrointestinal Series or Barium Swallow

X-ray examination using barium as a contrast material; used to diagnose structural abnormalities and problems of the esophagus and stomach.

Nursing Implications

1. Explain procedure to client (usually not done on client with undiagnosed abdominal pain until the pain is diagnosed and the possibility of perforation has been ruled out).
2. Maintain client's nothing by mouth (NPO) status at least 6 hours before procedure.
3. After examination, administer a laxative and encourage increased fluid intake to prevent constipation and to promote evacuation of barium.
5. Stool should return to normal color within 72 hours.

Lower Gastrointestinal Series or Barium Enema

X-ray examination of the colon in which barium is used as a contrast medium; barium is administered rectally.

Nursing Implications

1. Client may have clear liquids the evening before the test; maintain client's NPO status for 8 hours before test.
2. Colon must be free of stool; bowel evacuants are administered the day prior to the test, enemas may be administered the day of the test. (Appendix 13-2)
3. Explain to client that he or she may experience cramping and feel the urge to defecate during the procedure.
4. After the procedure, increase fluids and administer a laxative to assist in expelling the barium.

Endoscopy

Gastroscopy, Esophagogastroduodenoscopy (EGD), Colonoscopy, Sigmoidoscopy

Endoscopy is the direct visualization of the esophagus, stomach and duodenum through a flexible, lighted scope. Inflammation, ulcerations, tumors and esophageal varices may be identified. Biopsy specimens may be obtained and benign polyps may be removed.

Nursing Implications Before Procedure

1. Upper GI: NPO for up to 12 hours before procedure.
2. Lower GI: bowel prep—bowel evacuants and/or enemas, clear liquid diet for 24 hours prior to test.
3. Client should avoid aspirin, NSAIDs, iron supplements, and gelatin containing red coloring for several days prior to procedure.
4. May give preoperative medication for relaxation and to decrease secretions.
5. For upper GI studies, a topical anesthesia will be used to anesthetize the throat before insertion of the scope.
6. Upper GI studies: assess client's mouth for dentures and removable bridges.
7. Lower GI studies: help client into the left side-lying position, encourage the client to take a deep breath during the insertion of the scope; client may feel urge to defecate as scope is passed.
8. Conscious sedation frequently used for lower GI studies or colonoscopy.

Nursing Implications During Procedure

1. Immediately prior to procedure, verify informed consent and client identification.
2. Confirm NPO status for past 8 hours; for lower GI studies, confirm bowel preparation.
3. Maintain safety: airway precautions during sedation; positioning, monitor level of sedation (Chapter 3).

Nursing Implications After Procedure

1. Upper GI: maintain client's NPO status until the gag reflex returns; position client on his or her side to prevent aspiration until gag or cough reflex returns; use throat lozenges or warm saline solution gargles for relief of sore throat.
2. Monitor vital signs and O_2 saturation during recovery.
3. Observe for signs of perforation: upper GI bleeding—dysphagia, substernal or epigastric pain; lower GI bleeding—rectal bleeding, increasing abdominal distention.
4. Assist client to upright position: observe for orthostatic hypotension.
5. Warm sitz bath for any anal discomfort.

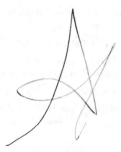

Continued

| Appendix 13-1 | GASTROINTESTINAL SYSTEM DIGNOSTICS—cont'd. |

ANALYSIS OF SPECIMENS

Paracentesis; Diagnostic Peritoneal Lavage

Procedure: A catheter is inserted into the peritoneal cavity, most often just below the umbilicus.

Purpose
1. To determine intra-abdominal bleeding.
2. To assess for presence and or drainage of ascites.
3. To identify cause of acute abdominal problems (e.g., perforation, hemorrhage).

Nursing Implications
1. A nasogastric tube may be used to maintain gastric decompression during procedure.
2. Have the client void before the procedure, if client has a full bladder at the time of insertion of the catheter, risk for bladder perforation and peritonitis is increased.
3. In clients with chronic liver problems, assess coagulation lab values before procedure.
4. Place client in semi-Fowler's position.
5. Maintain sterile field for puncture.
6. In clients with ascites, usually do not drain more than 1 L.

Complications
1. Perforation of bowel: peritonitis.
2. Introduction of air into abdominal cavity; client may complain of right referred shoulder pain (caused by air under the diaphragm).
3. Contraindicated in pregnancy and in clients with coagulation defects or possible bowel obstruction.

STOOL EXAMINATION

Stool is examined for form and consistency and to determine whether it contains mucus, blood, pus, parasites, or fat. Stool will be examined for presence of occult blood.

Nursing Implications
1. Collect stool in sterile container if examining for pathologic organisms.
2. A fresh, warm stool is required for evaluation of parasites or pathogenic organisms.
3. Collect the sample from various areas of the stool.
4. The result of the guaiac test for occult blood is positive when the paper turns blue.
5. Document medications and over-the-counter drugs client is taking when sample is obtained.

NURSING PROCEDURE: STOOL SPECIMEN

✔ KEY POINTS: Collecting the Specimen

- Always wear gloves during procedure.
- Use clean bedpan or bedside commode to collect stool; do not use stool that has been in contact with toilet bowl water or urine.
- Collect stool specimen in a clean, dry container. If stool is to be evaluated for organisms, use a sterile container. Use a tongue blade to obtain specimens from several areas of the stool and place in the stool collection container.
- The client collecting a stool specimen for an occult blood test needs to follow directions regarding diet restrictions (no red meat, beets, or foods that may cause the stool to turn red or lead to a false-positive result).
- Stool specimen should be approximately size of a walnut. If stool is liquid, approximately 30 mL is needed.
- Take the specimen to the laboratory. Do not allow it to remain in unit.

 TEST ALERT: Obtain specimen from client for laboratory tests.

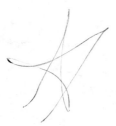

Appendix 13-2 GASTROINTESTINAL MEDICATIONS

ANTIEMETICS

Medications	Side Effects	Nursing Implications
Dopamine Antagonists: Depress or blocks dopamine receptors chemoreceptor trigger zone of the brain.		
Phenothiazines—suppress emesis Chlorpromazine hydrochloride (**Thorazine**): PO, suppository, IM Promethazine (**Phenergan**): PO, IM, suppository Prochlorperazine (**Compazine**): PO, suppository, IM Thiethylperazine maleate (**Torecan**): PO, suppository, IM	Central nervous system depression, drowsiness, dizziness, blurred vision, hypotension, photosensitivity	1. Subcutaneous injection or intravenous administration may cause tissue irritation and necrosis. 2. Use with caution in children – cause of nausea needs to be investigated. 3. **Thorazine** should be used only in situations of severe nausea or vomiting. Can also be used for intractable hiccups. 4. **Torecan**: used with caution in clients with liver and kidney diseases.
Prokinetics—stimulate motility Metoclopramide (**Reglan**): PO, IM, IV	Restlessness, drowsiness, fatigue, anxiety, headache	1. Used to decrease problems with esophageal reflux and nausea and vomiting associated with chemotherapy. 2. Use with caution in clients with undiagnosed abdominal pain; could precipitate a perforation.
Antihistamines: Depress the chemoreceptor trigger zone, block histamine receptors.		
Hydroxyzine (**Atarax, Vistaril**): PO, IM Dimenhydrinate (**Dramamine, Marmine**): PO, suppository, IM	Sedation; anticholinergic effects—blurred vision, dry mouth, difficulty in urination and constipation; paradoxical excitation may occur in children	1. Caution client regarding sedation: should avoid activities that require mental alertness. 2. Administer early to prevent vomiting. 3. Use with caution in clients with glaucoma and asthma. 4. Subcutaneous injection may cause tissue irritation and necrosis; use Z-track injection technique.

LAXATIVES

General Nursing Implications

- Laxatives should be avoided in clients who have nausea, vomiting, undiagnosed abdominal pain and cramping, and/or any indications of appendicitis.
- Dietary fiber should be taken for prevention of, and as first-line treatment for, constipation.
- Encourage increase in daily fluid intake.
- Increasing activity will increase peristalsis and decrease constipation.
- Narcotic analgesics and anticholinergics will increase problem with constipation.
- A laxative should be used only briefly and in the smallest amount necessary.
- Use laxatives with caution during pregnancy.

Continued

Appendix 13-2   GASTROINTESTINAL MEDICATIONS—cont'd.   ℞

Medications	Side Effects	Nursing Implications
Bulk laxatives—stimulate peristalsis and passage of soft stool Methylcellulose **(Citrucel)** Psyllium (**Metamucil, Perdiem**) Fibercon Bran **Surfactants**—decrease surface tension, allowing water to penetrate feces. Docusate (**Colace, Surfak**)	Esophageal irritation, impaction, abdominal fullness, flatulence Occasional mild abdominal cramping	1. Not immediately effective; 12 to 24 hours before effects are apparent. 2. Use with caution in clients with difficulty swallowing. 3. Administer with full glass of fluid to prevent problems with irritation and impaction.
Stimulants—stimulate and irritate the large intestine to promote peristalsis and defecation Bisacodyl (**Dulcolax**): suppository, PO	Diarrhea, abdominal cramping	1. Do not use concurrently with mineral oil. 2. Not recommended for children less than 6 years old.
Senna concentrate (**Senokot, Ex-Lax**): PO, suppository		1. Use for short period of time. 2. Do not use in presence of undiagnosed abdominal pain or GI bleeding.
Bowel evacuants—nonabsorbable osmotic agents that pull fluid into the bowel Polyethylene glycol (**GoLYTELY, Colyte**): PO, NG Magnesium citrate: PO	Nausea, bloating, abdominal fullness.	1. Primary use is in preparing the bowel for examination. 2. Clear liquids only (no red gelatin, or red drinks) after administration. 3. **GoLYTELY** requires the client to drink a large amount of fluid (4 L); provide 8 to 10 oz chilled at a time to increase client consumption and enhance taste. 4. Best if consumed over 3 to 4 hours. 5. Evacuants cause frequent bowel movements; advise client to plan accordingly.

ANTIEMETICS

Medications	Side Effects	Nursing Implications
Anhydrous morphine (**Paregoric**): **PO**	Lightheadedness, dizziness, sedation, nausea, vomiting, paralytic ileus, abdominal cramping	1. Opioid derivatives, suppress peristalsis. 2. Not recommended during pregnancy or breastfeeding. 3. Can produce dependence and mild withdrawal symptoms. 4. Encourage increased fluids. 5. Avoid activities that require mental alertness.
Diphenoxylate HCl Atropine (**Lomotil**): PO Loperamide HCl (**Imodium, Kaopectate II caplets**): PO Bismuth subsalicylate (**Kaopectate, Pepto-Bismol**): PO	May precipitate constipation and an impaction	1. May interfere with absorption of oral medications. 2. Cause of diarrhea should be identified prior to administering medications. 3. Should not be given to clients with fever greater than 101°. 4. Do not give in presence of bloody diarrhea.

Continued

Appendix 13-2   GASTROINTESTINAL MEDICATIONS—cont'd.

INTESTINAL ANTIBIOTICS AND ANTIINFLAMMATORY MEDICATIONS

Medications	Side Effects	Nursing Implications
Intestinal Antibiotics: Decrease bacteria in the GI tract; used to sterilize bowel before surgery.		
Kanamycin sulfate (**Kantrex**): PO Neomycin sulfate (**Mycifradin sulfate**): PO	Suprainfection of the bowel	1. Do not have side effects of parenterally administered aminoglycosides.
Paromomycin (**Humatin**): PO	Vomiting and diarrhea	1. Administer with meals. 2. Administer with caution in clients with ulcerative bowel disease.
5 Aminosalicylates (5 ASA): Antiinflammatory effect in small bowel and colon, used to treat client with inflammatory bowel disease (IBD).		
Sulfasalazine (**Azulfidine**): PO	Nausea, fever rash, arthalgia	1. Assess client for allergy to sulfur. 2. Should not be used with thiazide diuretics. 3. Monitor CBC, encourage fluids to maintain hydration. 4 May continue on medication to maintain remission.
Mesalamine (**Asacol**): PO, (**Pentasa**) PO enteric coated tablet (**Rowsa**) Suppository or enema	GI symptoms, headache	1. Suppository or enema has minimal systemic effects. 2. Rectal administration is usually at night.
Balsalazide (**Colazal**) PO	Abdominal pain, headache,	

GI, Gastrointestinal; *IM*, intramuscular; *IV*, intravenous; *NSAID*, nonsteroidal antiinflammatory drug; *PO*, by mouth (orally); *PUD*, peptic ulcer disease.

Appendix 13-3   ANTIULCER AGENTS

Medications	Side Effects	Nursing Implications
Antacid: An alkaline substance that will neutralize gastric acid secretions; nonsystemic. Some combination antacids also relieve gas, and some work as laxatives. Several antacids form a protective coating on the stomach and upper GI tract.		
Aluminum hydroxide (**Amphojel**)	Constipation, phosphorus depletion with long-term use	1. Avoid administration within 1 to 2 hours of other oral medications; should be taken frequently—before and after meals and at bedtime.
Aluminum hydroxide and magnesium salt combinations (**Gelusil, Maalox, Gaviscon**) Sodium preparations Sodium bicarbonate (**Rolaids, Tums**): PO	Constipation or diarrhea, hypercalcemia, renal calculi	2. Instruct clients to take medication even if they do not experience discomfort. 3. Clients on low-sodium diets should evaluate sodium content of various antacids. 4. Administer with caution to the client with cardiac disease, because indigestion may be characteristic of anginal pain and cardiac ischemia.
Sodium preparations Sodium bicarbonate (**Rolaids, Tums**): PO	Rebound acid production, alkalosis	1. Discourage use of sodium bicarbonate because of occurrence of metabolic alkalosis and rebound acid production.
Histamine H2 Receptor Antagonists: Reduce volume and concentration of gastric acid secretion.		
Cimetidine (**Tagamet**): PO, IV, IM	Rash, confusion, lethargy, diarrhea, dysrhythmias	1. Take 30 minutes before or after meals. 2. May be used prophylactically or for treatment of PUD. 3. Do not take with oral antacids.
Ranitidine (**Zantac**): PO, IM, IV	Headache, GI discomfort, jaundice, hepatitis	1. Use with caution in clients with liver and renal disorders. 2. Do not take with aspirin products. 3. Wait 1 hour after administration of antacids.
Nizatidine (**Axid**): PO Famotidine (**Pepcid**): PO, IV	Anemia, dizziness Headache, dizziness, constipation, diarrhea	1. Use caution in clients with renal or hepatic problems. 2. Dosing may be done without regard to food or to meal time. 3. Caution clients to avoid aspirin and other NSAIDs.
Proton Pump Inhibitors: Inhibit the enzyme that produces gastric acid.		
Omeprazole (**Prilosec**): PO Lansoprazole (**Prevacid**): PO	Headache, diarrhea, dizziness	1. Administer before meals. 2. Do not crush or chew; do not open capsules 3. Sprinkle granules of Prevacid over food; do not chew granules. 4. The combination of omeprazole (**Prilosec**) with clarithromycin (**Biaxin**) effectively treats clients with *Helicobacter pylori* infection in duodenal ulcer.
Cytoprotective Agents: Bind to diseased tissue; provides a protective barrier to acid.		
Sucralfate (**Carafate**): PO	Constipation, GI discomfort	1. Avoid antacids. 2. Used for prevention and treatment of stress ulcers, gastric ulceration, and PUD. 3. May impede the absorption of medications that require an acid medium.
Prostaglandin Analogues: Suppresses gastric acid secretion; increases protective mucus and mucosal blood flow.		
Misoprostol (**Cytotec**)	GI problems, headache	1. Contraindicated in pregnancy. 2. Indicated for prevention of NSAID-induced ulcers.

GI, Gastrointestinal; *IM*, intramuscular; *IV*, intravenous; *NSAID*, nonsteroidal antiinflammatory drug; *PO*, by mouth (orally); *PUD*, peptic ulcer disease.

Appendix 13-4   PARENTERAL NUTRITION

Parenteral Nutrition (PN or TPN for total parenteral nutrition): An intravenous (IV) delivery of highly concentrated nutrients and vitamins.

1. Goal is to provide adequate nutrition to promote healing and growth of new body tissue.
2. Utilized in conditions that interfere with the process of nutrition or in clients who require an extensive amount of nutrients for healing (burn clients).

Goal: To maintain client in positive nitrogen balance and promote healing.

Routes of Administration
1. **Peripheral:** Peripheral parenteral nutrition (PPN) is administered via a large peripheral vein or peripherally inserted central catheter (PICC) when nutritional support is indicated for a short period. May use IV fat (lipid) emulsions.
2. **Central:** Parenteral nutrition (PN or TPN) is administered via a parenteral line (PICC, Hickman, Broviac, central line) inserted in the antecubital, jugular or subclavian vein and threaded into the vena cava; used for nutritional support in the client who requires in excess of 2500 calories per day for an extended period. Solutions used are hypertonic with high glucose content and require rapid dilution.

Nursing Implications
1. Parenteral nutrition solution is customized in the hospital pharmacy specifically for the client's most recent blood analysis findings; nothing should be added to solution after it has been prepared in the pharmacy.
2. Orders are written daily, based on the current electrolyte and protein status; always check the doctor's order for correct fluid for the day.
3. Solution may be refrigerated for up to 24 hours, but solution should be taken out of refrigeration 30 minutes prior to infusion. If solution has been hanging for 24 hours, it should be discarded and a new bag of solution hung.
4. Do not randomly accelerate the infusion to "catch up" over an hour; parenteral nutrition must be carefully monitored and administered via an infusion pump.
5. Monitor serum blood glucose levels on a regular basis; some institutions require glucose testing every 4 to 6 hours. May be less frequent after first week of administration.
6. Infusion is initiated and discontinued on a gradual basis to allow the pancreas to compensate for increased glucose intake. If parenteral nutrition solutions is temporarily unavailable, *check with RN regarding fluid to hang until parenteral solution is available.*
7. Monitor intake and output and compare daily trends. Body weight is an indication of the adequacy of hydration. Tissue healing is an indication of adequacy of protein and positive nitrogen balance.
8. Check label on bag of solution against orders; check solution for leaks, clarity, or color changes.

Maintenance
1. A sterile occlusive dressing should be used at the catheter site, change site dressing every 48-72 hours or per facility protocol.
2. Change IV tubing every 24 hours or per facility protocol;
3. Do not draw blood or measure central venous pressure (CVP) from the PN line.
4. Maintain record of daily weight; desired weight gain is approximately 2 pounds per week.

 TEST ALERT: Monitor and provide for client's nutritional needs.

Complications
1. Hyperglycemia may be caused by too rapid infusion of solution. Blood glucose is monitored every 4 to 6 hours during initial infusion, and sliding scale insulin may be ordered.
3. Site infection: Monitor site and change dressing according to policy; important to follow sterile guidelines in dressing changes. Clients may be immunosuppressed and signs of infection may be masked. *If infection is suspected (erythema, tenderness, exudates), the RN should be notified immediately.*
5. Air embolus or risk for pneumothorax (central line): Increased tendency to occur during insertion of central catheter line and during dressing changes; place client in Trendelenburg position during insertion and during dressing changes.

Appendix 13-5   NURSING PROCEDURE: NASOGASTRIC TUBES

1. Levin tube: Single lumen.
   a. Suctioning gastric contents.
   b. Administering tube feedings.
2. Salem sump tube: Double lumen (smaller blue lumen vents the tube and prevents suction on the gastric mucosa; maintains intermittent suction, regardless of suction source).
   a. Suctioning gastric contents and maintaining gastric decompression.
   b. Do not clamp, irrigate, or apply suction to air vent tube.
   c. Connect to continuous low suction.

✔ KEY POINTS

Insert feeding/nasogastric

 TEST ALERT: *Insert nasogastric tube.*

- Before insertion, position the client in high-Fowler's position, if possible. (If client cannot tolerate high-Fowler's, place in left lateral position.)
- Use a water-soluble lubricant to facilitate insertion.
- Measure the tube from the tip of the client's nose to the earlobe and from the nose to the xiphoid process to determine the approximate amount of tube to insert to reach the stomach.
- Insert the tube through the nose into the nasopharyngeal area; flex the client's head slightly forward.
- Offer the client sips of water and ask the client to swallow; as the swallow occurs, progress the tube past the area of the trachea and into the esophagus and stomach. Withdraw tube immediately if client experiences respiratory distress (coughing or hoarse voice).
- Secure the tube to the nose; do not allow the tube to exert pressure on the upper inner portion of the nares.
- Validating placement of tube.
  a. Aspirate gastric contents.
  b. Measure pH of aspirated fluid (pH of gastric secretions is usually less than 4).
  c. It is *no longer recommended* to determine placement by injecting air and listening with a stethoscope for sound of air in the stomach.
  d. Always validate placement of a nasogastric tube prior to instilling anything into tube.
  e. After initial placement, request validation by x-ray.

 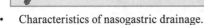 **TEST ALERT: *Check client feeding tube placement and patency.***

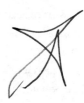

- Characteristics of nasogastric drainage.
  a. Normally is greenish yellow, with strands of mucus.
  b. Coffee-ground drainage: old blood that has been broken down in the stomach.
  c. Bright red blood: indicates bleeding in the esophagus, the stomach, or the lungs.
  d. Foul-smelling (fecal odor): occurs with reverse peristalsis in bowel obstruction; increase in amount of drainage with obstruction.
- If duodenal placement is required, have client lay in right lateral position for several hours. Provide enough excess in the tube to allow the tube to migrate down into duodenum.

Clinical Tips for Problem Solving

- Abdominal distention: Check for patency and adequacy of drainage, determine position of tube, assess presence of bowel sounds, and assess for respiratory compromise from distention.
- Nausea and vomiting around tube: Place client in semi-Fowler's position or turn to side to prevent aspiration; suction oral pharyngeal area. Attempt to aspirate gastric contents and validate placement of tube. Tube may not be far enough into stomach for adequate decompression and suction; try repositioning. If tube patency cannot be established, tube may need to be replaced.
- Inadequate or minimal drainage: Validate placement and patency; tube may be in too far and be past pyloric valve or not in far enough and in the upper portion of the stomach. Reassess length of tube insertion and characteristics of drainage, request x-ray for validation.

 TEST ALERT: *ALWAYS check the placement of a gastric tube before irrigating it or administering medications; placement should be checked each shift; do not adjust or irrigate the nasogastric tube on a client after a gastric resection or bariatric surgery.*

Appendix 13-6   NURSING PROCEDURE: ENTERAL FEEDING

Short-Term
1. **Nasogastric:** Provides alternative means of ingesting nutrients for clients.
2. **Nasointestinal:** A weighted tube of soft material is placed in the small intestine to decrease chance of regurgitation. A stylet or guide wire is used to progress the tube into the intestine. Do not remove stylet until tube placement has been verified via x-ray. Do not attempt to reinsert stylet while tube is in place; this could result in perforation of the tube.

Long-Term
1. **Percutaneous endoscopic gastrostomy (PEG):** A tube is inserted percutaneously into the stomach; local anesthesia and sedation are used for tube placement.
2. **Percutaneous endoscopic jejunostomy (PEJ):** A tube is inserted percutaneously into the jejunum.
3. **Gastrostomy:** A surgical opening is made into the stomach, and a gastrostomy tube is positioned with sutures.

> **TEST ALERT:** *Provide feeding and care for client with an enteral tube.*

Methods of Administering Enteral Feedings
- Continuous: Controlled with a feeding pump. Decreases nausea and diarrhea.
- Intermittent: Prescribed amount of fluid infuses via a gravity drip or feeding pump over specific time. For example, 350 mL is given over 30 minutes.
- Cyclic: Involves feeding solution infused via a pump for a part of a day, usually 12 to 16 hours. This method may be used for weaning from feedings.

Nursing Implications
- The client should be sitting or lying with the head elevated 30 to 45°. Head of bed should remain elevated for 30 to 60 minutes after feeding if intermittent or cyclic feeding is used.
- If feedings are intermittent, tube should be irrigated with water before and after feedings.
- Tube position should be validated every 4 to 6 hours for first 24 hours, then before each intermittent feeding, and then every 8 hours if on continuous feedings. Gastric contents are aspirated, and pH is checked. A pH of less than 4 indicates gastric contents.
- Aspirate gastric contents to determine residual. If residual is more than 200 mL, and there are signs of intolerance (nausea, vomiting, distention), hold next feeding for 1 hour and recheck residual or, if residual is greater than half of last feeding, delay next feeding for 1 to 2 hours.
- Return aspirated contents to stomach to prevent electrolyte imbalance.
- Flush the tube with 30 to 50 mL of water:
  a. After each intermittent feeding.
  b. Every 4 to 6 hours for continuous feeding.
  c. Before and after each medication administration.
- When a PEG or PEJ tube is placed, immediately after insertion measure the length of the tube from the insertion site to the distal end and mark the tube at the skin insertion site. This tube should be routinely checked to determine whether the tube is migrating from the original insertion point.
- Prevent diarrhea:
  a. Slow, constant rate of infusion.
  b. Keep equipment clean to prevent bacterial contamination.
  c. Check for fecal impaction; diarrhea may be flowing around impaction.
  d. Identify medical conditions that would precipitate diarrhea.
- For continuous feeding, change feeding reservoir every 24 hours.

> ✓ **NURSING PRIORITY:** *If in doubt of the placement of a nasogastric tube or an enteral feeding tube, stop or hold the feeding and obtain x-ray confirmation of location.*

Appendix 13-7	NURSING PROCEDURE: ENEMAS

Types of Enemas

Soap suds enema: Castile soap is added to tap water or normal saline. Dilute 5 mL of castile soap in 1 liter of water.

Tap water enema: Use caution when administering to adults with altered cardiac and renal reserve and to children and infants. Check with RN regarding specific amount of fluid to use.

Saline enemas: the safest enemas to administer; safe for infants and children.

Retention enema: An oil based solution that will soften the stool. Should be retained by client 30 to 60 minutes. Typically 150 to 200 mL. May be mineral oil or similar oil; or may include antibiotics or nutritive solution.

Hypertonic enema: Used when only a small amount of fluid is tolerated (120-180mL). Example is a commercially prepared Fleets enema.

Carminative enema: An agent used to expel gas from the GI tract. Example is magnesium sulfate/glycerin/water (MGW).

Harris flush or return flow enema: Mild colonic irrigation of 100 to 200 mL of fluid into and out of the rectum and sigmoid colon to stimulate peristalsis. Repeated multiple times by raising and lowering container until flatus is expelled and abdominal distention is relieved.

✔ KEY POINTS: Administering an Enema

- Fill enema container with warmed solution.
- Allow solution to run through the tubing before inserting into rectum so that air is removed.
- Place client on left lateral Sims' position.
- Generously lubricate the tip of the tubing with water-soluble lubricant.
- Gently insert tubing into client's rectum (3 to 4 inches for adults, 1 inch for infants, 2 to 3 inches for children), past the external and internal sphincters.
- Raise the solution container no more than 12 to 18 inches above the client.
- Allow solution to flow slowly. If the flow is slow, the client will experience fewer cramps. The client will also be able to tolerate and retain a greater volume of solution.

Clinical Tips for Problem Solving

If client expels solution prematurely:

- Place client in supine position with knees flexed.
- Slow the water flow and continue with the enema.

If the enema returns contain fecal material before surgery or diagnostic testing:

- Repeat enema.
- If after three enemas, returns still contain fecal material, notify health care provider.

If client complains of abdominal cramping during instillation of fluid:

- Slow the infusion rate by lowering the fluid bag.

 TEST ALERT: Assist and intervene with client who has an alteration in elimination.

Appendix 13-8 CARE OF THE CLIENT WITH AN OSTOMY

FIGURE 13-6 **Types of Ostomies** (From deWit, S, *Fundamental concepts and skills for nursing*, ed 3, St Louis, 2009, Saunders).

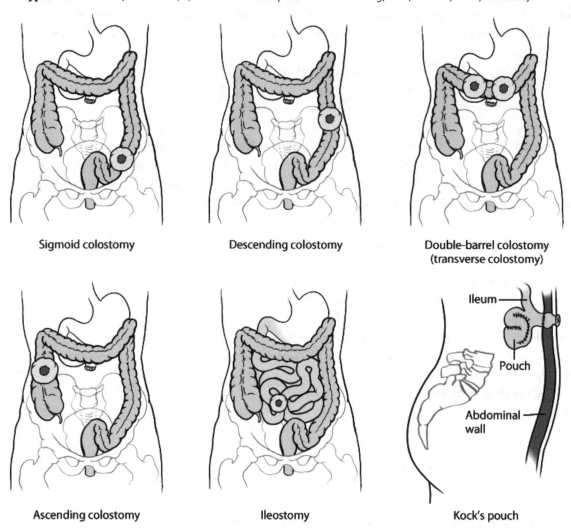

Sigmoid colostomy

Descending colostomy

Double-barrel colostomy
(transverse colostomy)

Ascending colostomy

Ileostomy

Kock's pouch

Colostomy: Opening of the colon through the abdominal wall; stool is generally semisoft and bowel control may be achieved.

Ileostomy: Opening of the ileum through the abdominal wall; stool drainage is liquid and excoriating; drainage is frequently continuous; therefore it is difficult to establish bowel control. Fluid and electrolyte imbalances are common complications.

Kock's ileostomy: May be referred to as a "continent" ileostomy; an internal reservoir for stool is surgically formed. Decreases problem of skin care caused by frequent irritation of stoma by drainage. Complications may include leakage at the stoma site and peritonitis.

✔ KEY POINTS: Nursing Implications—Initial Care

- Select a flat area of the abdomen, avoiding skin creases and folds; select site that does not interfere with clothing.
- Postoperatively evaluate stoma every 8 hours after surgery. It should remain pink and moist; dark blue stoma indicates ischemia.
- Measure the stoma and select an appropriately sized appliance. Mild to moderate swelling is common for the first 2 to 3 weeks after surgery, which necessitates changes in size of the appliance.
- Appliance should fit easily around the stoma and cover all healthy skin.
- Keep the skin around the stoma clean, dry, and free of stool and intestinal secretions. Prevent contamination of the abdominal incision.
- Change the skin appliance only when it begins to leak or becomes dislodged.
- Ostomy bags should be emptied when about one-third full to avoid weight of bag dislodging skin barrier.

Continued

Appendix 13-8   CARE OF THE CLIENT WITH AN OSTOMY —cont'd.

✔ KEY POINTS: Irrigation

- Do not irrigate an ileostomy or maintain regular irrigations in child with colostomy.
- Irrigate colostomy at same time each day to assist in establishing a normal pattern of elimination.
- Involve client in care as early as possible.
- In adults, irrigate with 500 to 1000 mL of warm tap water.

> ✔   **NURSING PRIORITY:**
> - *Use a cone tipped ostomy irrigator; do not use an enema tube/catheter.*
> - *Do not irrigate more than once a day.*
> - *Do not irrigate in the presence of diarrhea.*

- Place the client in a sitting position for irrigation, preferably in the bathroom with the irrigation sleeve in the toilet.
- Elevate the solution container approximately 12 to 20 inches and allow solution to flow in gently. If cramping occurs, lower fluid or clamp the tubing.
- Allow 25 to 45 minutes for return flow. Client may want to walk around before the return starts.
- Encourage client to participate in care of his or her own colostomy. Have client perform return demonstration of colostomy irrigation before leaving the hospital.
- Assist the client to control odors: diet and odor-control tablets.
- Kock's ileostomy is drained when client experiences fullness. A nipple valve is created in surgery and drained by insertion of a catheter.

Clinical Tips for Problem Solving

If water does not flow easily into colostomy stoma:
- Check for kinks in tubing from container.
- Check height of irrigating container.
- Encourage client to change positions, relax, and take a few deep breaths.

If client experiences cramping, nausea, or dizziness during irrigation:
- Stop flow of water, leaving irrigation cone in place.
- Do not resume until cramping has passed.
- Check water temperature and height of water bag; if water is too hot or flows too rapidly, it can cause dizziness.

If client has no return of stool or water from irrigation:
- Encourage ambulation, be sure to apply drainable pouch; solution may drain as client moves around.
- Have client increase fluid intake.
- Repeat irrigation next day.

If diarrhea occurs:
- Do not irrigate colostomy.
- Check client's medications; sometimes they may cause diarrhea.
- *If diarrhea is excessive and/or prolonged, notify RN.*

>   **TEST ALERT: Intervene to improve client elimination by instituting bowel management.**

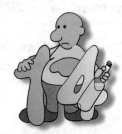

Hepatic and Biliary System

PHYSIOLOGY OF THE HEPATIC AND BILIARY SYSTEM

Organs of the Hepatic and Biliary System

A. Liver.
1. Located in the upper right portion of the abdominal cavity just under the diaphragm; vascular organ; protected by the rib cage.
2. Blood flow into the liver is from two sources.
   a. Portal vein carries venous blood from the stomach, intestines, pancreas, and spleen into the liver. The venous blood is rich in nutrients absorbed from the gastrointestinal (GI) system.
   b. The hepatic artery provides oxygenated blood to the liver.
   c. The portal vein and hepatic artery enter the liver via a common vessel and flow through the liver tissue; blood then leaves the liver via the hepatic vein and empties into the inferior vena cava.
3. Because of pressure differences in the hepatic and portal veins, the liver may normally store 200 to 400 mL of blood.
4. The liver produces approximately 600 to 1200 mL of bile daily.
   a. Bile drains from the liver via the common bile duct.
   b. The common bile duct enters the duodenum, either close to or in conjunction with the pancreatic duct.
5. It can sustain 90% damage with loss of tissue and still remain functional.
B. Gallbladder.
1. The gallbladder is capable of storing 20 to 50 mL of bile. When food enters the duodenum, the gallbladder contracts; the sphincter of Oddi, which controls the release of bile, relaxes; and bile enters the intestine via the common duct.
2. The primary function of the gallbladder is concentration and storage of bile.

Functions of the Liver

A. Synthesis of absorbed nutrients.
1. Serum glucose regulation.
2. Lipid (fat) metabolism.
3. Protein metabolism.

B. Synthesis of prothrombin for normal clotting mechanisms. Vitamin K is necessary for adequate prothrombin production.
C. Vitamin and mineral storage.
1. Produces and stores vitamins A and D.
2. Vitamin B_{12} and iron are stored in the liver.
D. Drug metabolism: barbiturates, amphetamines, and alcohol are metabolized by the liver.
E. Production of bile and bile salts.

System Data Collection

A. History.
1. History of liver, gallbladder, or jaundice problems.
2. History of bleeding problems.
3. History of reproductive problems.
4. Medication intake.
5. Recent association with anyone with jaundice.
6. Alcohol consumption.
B. Physical data collection.
1. Inspection.
   a. Skin.
      (1) Presence of vascular angiomas, skin lesions, or petechiae.
      (2) Hydration status.
      (3) Color of the skin (jaundiced).
      (4) Presence of peripheral edema.
   b. Abdomen.
      (1) Evidence of jaundice.
      (2) Contour of the abdomen.
      (3) Presence of visible abdominal wall veins.
2. Palpation of the abdomen.
   a. Pain, tenderness, presence of distention.
   b. Hepatomegaly, splenomegaly.
C. Nutritional assessment.
1. Weight gain or loss; dietary intake.
2. Problems of anorexia, nausea and vomiting.

Jaundice

A. Jaundice may begin so gradually that it is not noticed immediately.
B. The increased levels of bilirubin cause a yellowish discoloration of the skin. It may be first observed as a yellow color in the sclera of the eyes. Serum bilirubin levels must exceed 2 mg/dL for jaundice to occur. The yellow discoloration is due to deposits of bilirubin in the skin and body tissue.

C. Types of jaundice.
 1. Hemolytic jaundice.
   a. Occurs with an increase in the breakdown of red blood cells, which causes an increase in the amount of unconjugated bilirubin in the blood.
   b. The liver cannot handle the increased level of unconjugated bilirubin. The bilirubin is not water soluble; therefore it cannot be excreted. Unconjugated bilirubin is lipid soluble and is capable of entering nerve cells and causing brain damage.
   c. The increased production of urobilinogen will increase the amount of bilirubin excreted in the urine and feces.
   d. Causes of hemolytic jaundice.
     (1) Blood transfusion reactions.
     (2) Sickle cell crisis.
     (3) Hemolytic anemias.
     (4) Hemolytic disease of the newborn.
 2. Hepatocellular jaundice.
   a. Results from the inability of the liver to clear normal amounts of bilirubin from the blood.
   b. Increase in serum levels of unconjugated and conjugated bilirubin.
   c. Causes of hepatocellular jaundice.
     (1) Hepatitis.
     (2) Cirrhosis.
     (3) Hepatic cancer.
 3. Obstructive jaundice.
   a. Results from an impediment to bile flow through the liver and the biliary system.
   b. The obstruction may be within the liver, or it may be outside the liver.
   c. Causes of obstructive jaundice.
     (1) Hepatitis.
     (2) Liver tumors.
     (3) Cirrhosis.
     (4) Obstruction of the common bile duct by a stone.

Hepatitis

* **Widespread inflammation of the liver tissue is called hepatitis.**
A. Types of hepatitis (Table 14-1).
 1. Hepatitis A virus (HAV): infectious hepatitis.
   a. Primarily a disease of children because of mode of transmission and interaction of large numbers of children in daycare centers.
   b. The mortality rate is low, but there is an increase in fatalities in the older adult population.
   c. Administration of immune serum globulin (immunoglobulin G) to exposed individuals increases the immune resistance and/or decreases the severity of the illness (passive immunization).

 2. Hepatitis B virus (HBV): serum hepatitis.
   a. Identification of HBsAg (Australian antigen).
     (1) Identification of antigen in potential blood donors has significantly decreased transmission via blood transfusions.
     (2) Antigen is present in blood, vaginal secretions, menstrual fluid, semen, saliva, and respiratory secretions (see Table 14-1).
   b. Administration of hepatitis B immunoglobulin will provide some temporary immunity.
   c. HBV vaccine should be administered to everyone as a standard immunization (see Table 2-1).
 3. Hepatitis C (HCV).
   a. Transmission is very similar to that of HBV, with multiple causative agents; percutaneous inoculation (IV drug use), blood transfusions.
   b. Increased incidence occurs with crowded living conditions.
B. The inflammatory process causes hepatic cell degeneration and necrosis. Hepatitis A is generally self-limiting with liver regeneration and complete recovery. Hepatitis B and hepatitis C are more serious and can progress to total destruction of the liver.

> ✔ **NURSING PRIORITY:** *Follow infection control guidelines/protocols. Prevent transmission in the hospital in addition to teaching the importance of personal hygiene.*

Data Collection

Regardless of the type of hepatitis, the clinical picture is similar.
A. Risk factors/etiology and sources/spread of disease (see Table 14-1).
B. Clinical manifestations: all clients experience inflammation of the liver tissue and exhibit similar symptoms.
 1. Anorexia, nausea, malaise, headache.
 2. Upper right quadrant discomfort.
 3. Low-grade fever, hepatomegaly.
 4. Dark urine caused by increased excretion of bilirubin.
 5. Pruritus, stools light and clay colored.
 6. Liver remains enlarged and tender.
C. Diagnostics (see Appendix 14-1).
 1. Increased alanine aminotransferase, aspartate aminotransferase, and serum bilirubin levels.
 2. Presence of HBsAg in serum of client with hepatitis B.
 3. Presence of anti-HAV antibodies in blood with hepatitis A.

TABLE 14-1	HEPATITIS	
HEPATITIS A (HAV)	**HEPATITIS B (HBV)**	**HEPATITIS C (HCV)**
Transmission Modes		

Predominately fecal-oral
Poor personal hygiene
Oral-anal sexual practices
Contaminated food, water, and shellfish
  (commonly spread by infected food handlers)
Carriers are most contagious just before
  onset of symptoms (jaundice)
Transmission through sexual contact and
  percutaneous transmission are possible,
  but these are not primary modes of transmission
	Percutaneous inoculation with contaminated
	  needles or instruments is the primary mode
	Skin or mucous membrane break by inoculation
	  (needle-sticks, cuts, ear piercing, tattooing,
	  or contaminated drug paraphernalia)
	Blood and blood products
	Nonpercutaneous transmission—contact with
	  body fluids containing hepatitis B surface
	  antigen (HBsAg) (e.g., sexual contact)—
	  is the second most common mode
	Infants of mothers with HBV may contract
	  the disease in utero, at birth, or after delivery
	Infected asymptomatic carrier
	Hepatitis D (HDV) is very similar to HBV
		Percutaneous (parenteral)/mucosal
		  exposure to blood and blood
		  products
		High-risk sexual contact
		Perinatal contact
		Closely associated with HBV

Incubation Period		

2 to 6 weeks (average: 4 weeks);
  also the most contagious period
Virus is present in feces for 7 to 10 days
  before a person becomes ill
	6 weeks to 6 months (average: 12 weeks)
	Contagious as long as serum marker
	  (surface antigen; HBsAg) appears
		2 weeks to 6 months
		  (average: 8 weeks)
		Most contagious 1-2 weeks before
		  symptoms appear; infectivity
		  continues during clinical course
		Large number of cases (75%-85%)
		  develop chronic HCV

High-Risk Individuals		
Household contacts Sexual contacts Institutions, daycare centers, schools	Household contacts Sexual contacts Dental, laboratory, and medical personnel Multiple blood transfusion recipients IV drug users	Multiple blood transfusion recipients Sexual contacts IV drug users
Sources of Infection and Spread of Infection		

Crowded living conditions;
  poor hygiene and sanitation
Contaminated food, milk, water, and shellfish
Infected food handlers
Sexual contact
	Contaminated needles, syringes, and
	  blood products
	Sexual activity with infected partners
	Asymptomatic carriers
	Tattoo-body piercing with contaminated
	  needles; bites
		Blood and blood products, needles
		  and syringes
		Sexual activity with infected
		  partners

 TEST ALERT: *Follow infection control guidelines; standard precautions include blood and body fluids.*

IV, Intravenous.

Treatment

A. No specific medications for HAC, chronic HBV and
    HCV.
B. Encourage good nutrition; no specific dietary
    modifications; client will probably not tolerate a high-
    fat diet.
C. Decreased activity; promote rest.

Nursing Interventions

❖   **Goal:** To control and prevent hepatitis.
A. Understand characteristics of transmission and
    preventive measures for hepatitis A.

1. Good personal hygiene, especially handwashing.
2. Participate in community activities for health
    education, (e.g., environmental sanitation, food
    preparation, etc.).
3. Identify individuals at increased risk for exposure:
    those with household contact, intimate sexual
    contact, and/or institutional contact with those with
    active disease.
4. Administer immune serum globulin
    (immunoglobulin G) within 2 weeks of exposure, if
    they do not have presence of anti-HAV antibodies
    (antibody to HAV).

5. Preexposure prophylaxis: hepatitis A vaccine (single dose).
6. Implement standard precautions.
7. Client should abstain from sexual activity during periods of communicability.

> **OLDER ADULT PRIORITY:** *Older adult clients are at higher risk for liver damage and complications of hepatitis.*

B. Understand characteristics of transmission and preventive measures for hepatitis B.
1. Identify individuals at increased risk for exposure: those with oral or percutaneous contact with HBsAg-positive fluid and those who have had sexual contact with carriers within 4 weeks of the appearance of jaundice.
2. Administration of hepatitis B vaccine.
3. Postexposure prophylaxis: HBV vaccine series started and hepatitis B immune globulin (HBIG) given within 24 hours of exposure.
C. Understand characteristics of transmission and preventive measures for hepatitis C.
1. No vaccine for HCV.
2. Immunoglobulin G, antivirals, or α-interferon are not recommended.
D. Maintain strict contact-based standard precautions for hospitalized client with questionable diagnosis of hepatitis.
❖ **Goal:** To promote healing and regeneration of liver tissue.
A. Bed rest with bathroom privileges initially; progressive activity according to liver function test results.
B. Promote psychologic and emotional rest.
1. Strict bed rest may increase anxiety.
2. Frequently, young adults are very concerned about body image; encourage verbalization and emphasize temporary nature of symptoms.
3. Maintain communication and frequent contact.
C. Promote nutritional intake.
1. Anorexia and decreased taste for food potentiate nutritional deficits.
2. Small frequent feedings of favorite foods, good oral hygiene, and food served in a pleasant atmosphere.
D. Encourage increased fluid intake.

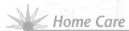 *Home Care*

A. Continued need for adequate rest and nutrition until liver function test results are normal.
B. Avoid alcohol and over-the-counter medications, especially those containing acetaminophen and phenothiazine.

> **TEST ALERT:** *Evaluate client's use of over- the-counter medications.*

C. Clients with hepatitis B should avoid intimate and sexual contact until antibodies to the HBsAg are present and the client is no longer contagious.
D. If possible, client should have his or her own bathroom.
E. Client and family must understand importance of personal hygiene and good handwashing.
F. Client should not donate blood.

Hepatic Cirrhosis

✳ **Hepatic cirrhosis is a chronic, progressive disease of the liver, characterized by degeneration and destruction of liver cells.**
A. Liver regeneration is disorganized and results in the formation of scar tissue, which in time, will exceed the amount of normal liver tissue.

Data Collection

A. Frequently, a combination of alcoholism and nutritional deficiency.
B. GI disturbances: anorexia, indigestion, change in bowel habits, weight loss.
C. Jaundice, pruritis.
D. Spider angiomas on the face, neck, and shoulders.
E. Palmar erythema: reddened areas on the palms that blanch with pressure.
F. Anemia, spontaneous bruising from thrombocytopenia.
G. Changes in sexual characteristics: gynecomastia, impotence in males; amenorrhea, vaginal bleeding in females.
H. Peripheral neuropathy: probably caused by inadequate intake of vitamin B complex.
I. Hepatomegaly, splenomegaly.
J. Portal hypertension.
1. Esophageal varices that bleed easily.
2. Hemorrhoids.
3. Veins visible on abdominal wall.
4. Development of edema and ascites.
K. Peripheral edema
1. Edema generally occurs in feet, ankles, and presacral area.
2. Severe abdominal distention and weight gain with ascites.
3. Portal-systemic encephalopathy.
   a. Changes in mental responsiveness.
   b. Memory problems.
   c. Asterixis (flapping tremors): clients with asterixis are unable to hold their hands out in front of them when asked; a flapping of the hands will occur.
   d. Fetor hepaticus: musty, sweet odor to breath due to inability of liver to degrade digestive products.

Treatment

A. Cirrhosis.
1. Rest.
2. Dietary modification: increase calories and carbohydrates; protein and fat may be consumed as tolerated.
3. Vitamin supplement, especially vitamin B complex.
4. Abstinence from alcohol.
B. Ascites.
1. IV albumin or other volume replacement after a high volume parancetesis.
2. Sodium restriction in diet.
3. Fluid restriction for cases of severe ascites.
4. Diuretics.
5. Paracentesis for temporary relief.
6. Peritoneovenous shunt (LaVeen shunt): a surgical procedure for reinfusion of ascitic fluid into venous system.
7. Surgical procedures to decrease portal hypertension by shunting portal blood flow: transjugular intrahepatic portosystemic shunt (TIPS).
C. Esophageal varices.
1. Blood transfusions to restore volume from bleeding varices.
2. Administration of IV vasopressin (**Pitressin**) for bleeding.
3. Endoscopic sclerotherapy: injection of a sclerosing agent directly into esophageal varices.
4. Endoscopic ligation or banding of the varices.
5. Balloon tamponade: mechanical compression of bleeding varices via esophageal gastric balloon tamponade (Minnesota or Sengstaken-Blakemore tube).
6. Shunting surgical procedures: decrease portal hypertension by shunting portal blood flow.
D. Decrease portal systemic encephalopathy.
1. Restriction of dietary protein intake.
2. Neomycin: decreases the normal flora in the intestines to reduce bacterial activity on protein.
3. Lactulose: used to reduce the amount of ammonia in the blood.

Nursing Interventions

❖ **Goal:** To promote health in the client with cirrhosis.
A. Proper diet: increased protein as tolerated, adequate carbohydrates, vitamin supplements.
B. Adequate rest.
C. Avoid potential hepatotoxic over-the-counter drugs (aspirin and acetaminophen).
D. Monitor body secretions for frank or occult blood.
E. Abstinence from alcohol.
F. Attention and care should be given the alcoholic client without being judgmental or moralizing.
G. Client should understand symptoms indicative of complications and when to seek medical advice.

H. Regular medical checkups.
❖ **Goal:** To maintain homeostasis and promote liver function.
A. Rest and activity schedule based on clinical manifestations and lab data.
B. Measures to prevent complications of immobility (see Chapter 3).
C. Assist client to maintain self-esteem.
1. Maintain positive, accepting atmosphere in the delivery of care.
2. Encourage ventilation of feelings regarding disease.
D. Assist in activities of daily living, as necessary, to prevent undue fatigue.
E. Promote nutritional intake.
1. Good oral hygiene; between-meal nourishment.
2. Provide food preferences when possible.
3. Administer antiemetic before meals, if necessary.
4. Iron and vitamin supplements, especially vitamin B complex.
5. Nasogastric or parenteral feeding, if client is unable to maintain adequate intake.
F. Decrease discomfort of pruritus caused by jaundice – cool rather than warm baths, avoid excessive soap.
G. Good skin care to prevent breakdown.
H. Evaluate serum electrolyte levels, especially potassium and sodium levels, because of the use of diuretics to decrease ascites and edema.
I. Monitor temperature closely because of increased susceptibility to infection.
J. Assess for bleeding tendencies and prevent trauma to the mucous membranes.
K. Measure abdominal girth to determine whether it is increasing from ascitic fluid (Figure 14-1).

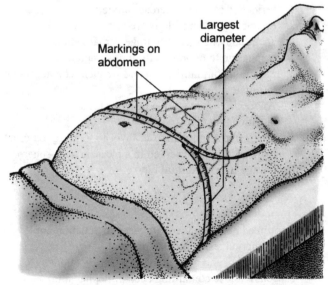

FIGURE 14-1 Measuring abdominal girth. (From Ignatavicius DD, Workman ML: *Medical-surgical nursing: patient-centered collaborative care*, ed 6, Philadelphia, 2010, Saunders.)

❖ **Goal:** To decrease risk for active bleeding, if esophageal varices are present.
A. Soft, nonirritating foods.
B. Discourage straining at stool.
C. Decrease esophageal reflux.
D. No salicylate compounds (aspirin).
E. Evaluate for active bleeding.
   1. Monitor vital signs.
   2. Assess for melena and hematemesis.
❖ **Goal:** To decrease bleeding from esophageal and gastric varices.
A. Gastric lavage with iced saline solution.
B. Assess and prevent complications associated with sclerotherapy.
   1. Client is sedated and the throat is anesthetized before the procedure.
   2. Bleeding from the varices should stop within minutes.
   3. Client may experience chest discomfort for 2 to 3 days; administer an analgesic.
   4. Observe for return of active bleeding.
C. *Notify RN immediately of any bright red vomiting (bleeding) or significant changes in vital signs.*
❖ **Goal:** To assess for and prevent complications associated with ascites.
A. Decrease sodium intake.
B. Administer diuretics, potassium supplements.
C. Daily measurements of abdominal girth.
D. Maintain semi-Fowler's position to decrease pressure on the diaphragm.
E. Assess weight daily.
F. Monitor pulse oximetry for indications of respiratory distress.
❖ **Goal:** To assess for and prevent complications of hepatic encephalopathy.
A. Frequent assessment of responsiveness and changes in level of orientation and for motor abnormalities (asterixis).
B. Decrease production of ammonia.
   1. Increase carbohydrates and fluids.
   2. Decrease activity, because ammonia is a by-product of metabolism.
   3. GI bleeding will increase ammonia levels as a result of the breakdown of red blood cells.
   4. Lactulose to promote excretion of ammonia in the stool, diarrhea may occur.
   5. Nonabsorbable intestinal antibiotics will decrease protein breakdown .
C. Prompt treatment of hypokalemia.
❖ **Goal:** To provide appropriate preoperative and post-operative care if surgical procedure is indicated (see Chapter 3).
A. Client is at increased risk for postoperative complications.
   1. Hemorrhage, electrolyte imbalance.
   2. Seizures, delirium tremens.

B. Surgical procedures do not alter course of progressive hepatic disease.

 ## Cancer of the Liver

✳ **Primary cancer of the liver is rare. Metastatic cancer is more common.**
A. Liver is a common site for metastases because of increased rate of blood flow and capillary network.
B. Metastases are found in the liver in approximately one-half of all clients with late-stage cancer.
C. Prognosis is poor.

Data Collection

A. Risk factors/etiology: malignancy elsewhere in the body.
B. Clinical manifestations.
   1. Anorexia, weight loss, fatigue, anemia.
   2. Right upper quadrant pain, ascites, jaundice.
C. Diagnostics (see Appendix 14-1).

Treatment

Treatment is primarily palliative.
A. Surgical excision of tumor, if it is localized.
B. Chemotherapy: very poor response.
C. Radiofrequency (RF) ablation uses heat to burn tumor (percutaneous approach).
D. Cryosurgery (cryoablation) uses liquid nitrogen to freeze liver tissue; not used for metastatic disease.
E. Percutaneous ethanol injection (PEI) or percutaneous acetic acid injection (PAI) used to treat unresectable liver cancer.

Nursing Interventions

Focused on maintaining comfort; nursing care is the same as that for the client with advanced cirrhosis.

 ## Liver Transplantation

Therapeutic option for clients with end-stage liver disease; not recommended for widespread malignant disease.

Data Collection

A. Rigorous prescreening process.
B. Rejection less common than with kidney transplants.

Treatment

A. Live liver transplant: portion of liver is donated.
B. Split liver transplant: donor liver is divided and given to two recipients.

Nursing Interventions

❖ **Goal:** To monitor for postoperative complications.
A. Rejection is not as common as it is with kidney transplants.

B. Assess neuro status, monitor for hemorrhage and common respiratory problems of pneumonia, atelectasis, and pleural effusion.
C. Monitor IV fluids, nasogastric tube drainage, Jackson-Pratt drain, and T-tube drainage.
D. Administer antibiotics and analgesics.
E. Critical to monitor for infection the first 2 months after surgery; fever may be the only sign.
❖ Goal: To provide nursing care of the immunocompromised client (see Chapter 5).

Cholelithiasis and Cholecystitis

✳ *Cholelithiasis* **is the presence of stones in the gallbladder; this is the most common form of biliary disease.**
✳ *Cholecystitis* **is an inflammation of the gallbladder, which is frequently associated with stones; this condition may be acute or chronic (Figure 14-2).**

Data Collection

A. Cholelithiasis: presence of gallstones.
  1. Increased incidence in females, especially during pregnancy.
  2. Increased incidence after age 40; obesity.
B. Cholecystitis: inflammation of the gallbladder.
  1. Associated with stones.
  2. *Escherichia coli* is common bacteria involved.
  3. May also be associated with neoplasms, anesthesia, or adhesions.

> ✔ *OLDER ADULT PRIORITY: Incidence of gallstone increases with age. Older adults are more likely to go from asymptomatic gallstones to serious complications of gallstones without biliary colic.*

C. Cholelithiasis: severity of symptoms depends on the mobility of the stone and whether obstruction occurs.
  1. Epigastric distress, feeling of fullness.
  2. Abdominal distention.
  3. Vague pain in the right upper quadrant after eating a meal high in fat.
  4. Biliary colic.
    a. Severe abdominal pain radiating to the back and shoulder.
    b. Nausea, vomiting, tachycardia, diaphoresis.
    c. Pain occurs 3-6 hours after eating a heavy meal, especially if high in fat.
  5. Jaundice may occur with obstruction of bile flow.
  6. Urine may become very dark, and stools may be clay colored.
D. Cholecystitis.
  1. Abdominal guarding, rigidity, rebound tenderness.
  2. Fever.
  3. Pain exacerbated by deep breathing.
  4. Onset may be sudden with severe pain.

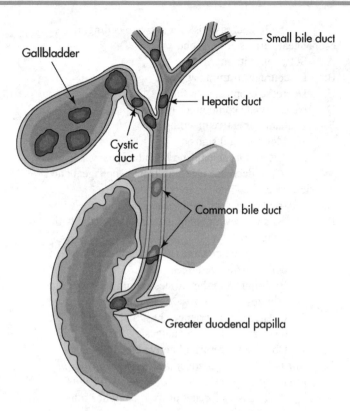

FIGURE 14-2 Common sites of gallstones. (From Monahan FD, et al: *Medical-surgical nursing: health and illness perspectives*, ed 8, St. Louis, 2007, Mosby.)

Treatment

A. Cholecystectomy for cholelithiasis: surgical removal of the stones.
B. Cholecystitis.
  1. Anticholinergics to decrease secretions and promote relaxation of the gallbladder.
  2. Analgesics: hydromorphone (**Dilaudid**) or morphine.
  3. Antibiotics.
  4. Atropine and dicyclomine (**Bentyl**) will relieve spasms and decrease pain.
  5. Ketorolac (**Toradol**) may be used to decrease spasms and pain in older adults.
C. Laparoscopic cholecystectomy.
  1. Three small incisions are made.
  2. Decreases risk to client; day surgery or overnight stay.
  3. Early ambulation and decreased pain.

> ✔ *NURSING PRIORITY: Common postoperative problem of referred pain to the shoulder due to CO_2 that was not released or absorbed by body, which can irritate the phrenic nerve and diaphragm causing difficulty breathing.*

D. Decrease dietary fat intake.

Nursing Interventions

❖ **Goal:** To decrease pain and inflammatory response.
A. Low-fat liquid diet during acute attack.
B. Low-fat solids added, as tolerated.
C. IV fluids and gastric decompression if nausea and vomiting are severe.
D. Antibiotics and analgesics.
E. Assess for indications of infection.

❖ **Goal:** To provide appropriate preoperative nursing care if surgery is indicated (see Chapter 3).

❖ **Goal:** To maintain homeostasis and prevent complications after cholecystectomy.
A. General postoperative care for clients having abdominal surgery (see Chapter 3).
B. Evaluate tolerance to diet and progress diet gradually to low-fat solids.
C. Penrose drain may be in place; client will frequently have large amounts of serosanguineous drainage; change dressing as indicated.
D. Sims' position to facilitate the movement of CO_2 gas pocket away from the diaphragm.
E. T-tube may be used to maintain patency of bile duct and to facilitate bile drainage until edema subsides (Figure 14-3).
1. Maintain tube to gravity drainage.
2. Observe amount and color of bile drainage.
3. Do not irrigate or clamp tube; do not raise tube above the level of the gallbladder.
4. Observe for bile drainage around the tube.
5. Observe and record drainage (bloody initially, then greenish-brown).
6. Drainage is usually around 500 mL per day for several days after surgery; drainage will gradually decrease, and the doctor will remove the tube.
7. Typically not placed or used after a laparoscopic cholecystectomy.

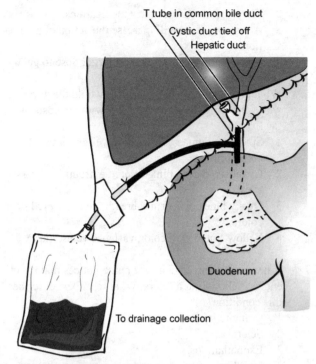

FIGURE 14-3 Placement of a T-tube. (From Black JM, Hawks JH: *Medical-surgical nursing: clinical management for positive outcomes,* ed 8, St. Louis, 2009, Mosby.)

F. Monitor urine and stool for changes in color.
❖ **Goal:** To assist client to understand implications of disease process and measures to maintain health after cholecystectomy.
A. Dietary teaching regarding low-fat diet.
B. Weight reduction, if appropriate.
C. Avoid heavy lifting.
D. *Report severe pain, increased distention, or leakage of bile from puncture sites to the charge nurse.*

Study Questions: Hepatic and Biliary System

1. Which client would be considered at an increased risk for developing hepatitis A?
   1 Older adult with daily alcohol consumption.
   2 Client required to have multiple blood transfusions.
   3 Client who regularly donates blood.
   4 Older client in long-term care facility.
2. Which nursing activity would put the nurse at the greatest increased risk for exposure to hepatitis B virus?
   1 Cleansing the client's anal area without wearing gloves.
   2 Recapping syringes and needles.
   3 Hand contact with client's blood.
   4 Spraying of blood into nurse's eyes.
3. A client is being discharged after treatment for hepatitis B. What is important to teach this client regarding over-the-counter medications?

1 Do not take acetaminophen products.
2 Increase your intake of vitamin A.
3 Do not take decongestive products.
4 Use cough medications with caution.
4. What are critical vaccinations for a person who is working in the health care field?
   1 Hepatitis B.
   2 Hepatitis A.
   3 Human immunodeficiency virus (HIV).
   4 Varicella.
5. Why is it important for a client with end-stage liver failure to be very cautious when taking any form of medication?
   1 The liver metabolizes many medications for utilization and excretion from the body.

2 The liver inactivates most medications.

3 A diseased liver will increase the action of medications.

4 The client will have to take a larger dose to get the actual therapeutic value.

6. What physiological characteristics would the nurse find while checking the skin of a client with cirrhosis of the liver?

1 Spider angiomas on the chest, yellow-tinted skin color, bruises.

2 Cyanosis, red- to pink-colored extremities, glassy eyes.

3 Dusky blue color, fruity breath, yellow-tinted skin color.

4 Yellow-tinted skin color, varicose veins, glassy eyes.

7. When evaluating a client, the nurse notices that the client has yellow-tinted sclera. What term best describes this condition?

1 Conjunctivitis.

2 Sclerosis.

3 Exophthalmos.

4 Jaundice.

8. A client being treated for ascites is placed on a strict low-sodium diet. Considering his diet, what foods would the nurse encourage the client to select?

1 Pasta and milk.

2 Whole wheat bread.

3 Slices of apple.

4 Peanut butter on crackers.

9. The nurse is caring for a client with advanced liver disease. What would the nurse expect to find while evaluating this client?

1 Client has difficulty maintaining normal blood pressure.

2 Urine output is significantly decreased.

3 Stools are black and tarry.

4 Client has a large abdomen with excessive free fluid.

10. The client is returning to his room following a laparoscopic cholecystectomy. What is the best position for this client?

1 Left Sims' position with knees flexed.

2 Semi-Fowler's to promote breathing.

3 Prone to decrease problems with aspiration.

4 Supine to decrease stress on the suture line.

11. In report the nurse is told that one of the assigned clients has advanced liver disease and has a high level of blood ammonia. What would the nurse expect to find with this client?

1 Increased breathing problems.

2 Altered level of consciousness.

3 Fragile skin and easy bruising.

4 Yellowish skin discoloration.

12. A client with chronic liver problems is to receive vitamin K before surgery. What is the purpose of this medication?

1 Decreases bleeding tendencies.

2 Increases healing after surgery.

3 Assists to maintain fluid balance.

4 Prevents nausea and vomiting.

13. The nurse is discharging a client after a laparoscopic removal of the gallbladder. What would be important discharge instructions?

1 Report any bile-colored drainage from the incisional areas.

2 Return the day after discharge for lab work.

3 Take a vitamin K supplement daily for the next 2 weeks.

4 Evaluate stools for the presence of steatorrhea.

14. A client is being discharged after a diagnosis of hepatitis B. What would be important to discuss with this client?

1 Use a condom during sexual intercourse.

2 Decrease alcohol intake.

3 Increase intake of green, leafy vegetables.

4 Take acetaminophen for pain or discomfort.

15. A client with advanced cirrhosis is diagnosed with esophageal varices. What would cause the nurse the most concern regarding complications associated with the varices?

1 Difficulty swallowing.

2 Coughing up bright red blood.

3 Decreased gag reflex.

4 Anorexia and dyspepsia.

16. A client is scheduled for laparoscopic removal of his gallbladder. The nurse is discussing the immediate postoperative care. What will the nurse tell the client?

1 There will be four small incisions, most often covered with light bandages.

2 A urinary retention catheter will be in place for the first 12 hours.

3 Right lower quadrant pain is the most common area of pain.

4 No food or fluid intake is allowed for the first 24 hours after surgery.

17. A client with cirrhosis is experiencing problem with hepatic encephalopathy. What would be severely restricted in the client's dietary intake?

1 Protein.

2 Carbohydrates.

3 Fats.

4 Cholesterol.

18. The nurse is caring for a client with severe ascites. In what position would the nurse anticipate the client to be most comfortable?

1 Semi-Fowler's.

2 Prone.

3 Supine.

4 Sims'.

Answers and rationales to these questions are in the section at the end of the book titled Chapter Study Questions: Answers and Rationales.

Laboratory Tests	Normal	Nursing Implications
SERUM LABORATORY TESTS		
Bilirubin		A rise in the serum level of bilirubin will occur if there is excessive destruction
Direct	0.1 to 0.3 mg/dL	of red blood cells or if the liver is unable to excrete normal amounts of bilirubin.
Indirect	0.1 to 1.0 mg/dL	
Total	0.2 to 1.3 mg/dL	
Protein studies		Proteins are responsible for maintaining the colloid oncotic pressure in the serum.
Total serum protein	6.0 to 8.0 g/dL	Synthesis of protein and normal serum protein levels are affected by various liver
Serum albumin	3.5 to 5.0 g/dL	impairments.
Serum globulin	2.0 to 3.5 g/dL	
Serum enzymes		
Lactic dehydrogenase (LDH)	50-150 units/L	Elevated in heart failure, hemolytic disorders, hepatitis, liver damage.
LDH_5		LDH_5 isoenzyme elevated in hepatitis.
Aspartate aminotransferase (AST)	10 to 26 units/L	Elevated in liver disease, acute hepatitis, myocardial infarction, pulmonary infarction.
Alanine aminotransferase (ALT)	10 to 35 units/L	Elevated in liver disease, shock.
Alkaline phosphatase (ALP)	30-120 units/L	Primary sources of ALP in body are bone and liver. Abnormally high readings may be associated with either liver or bone disease and must be correlated with presenting clinical symptoms.
Serum blood ammonia	30-70 mcg/dL	Increasing blood ammonia is indicative of the inability of the liver to convert ammonia to urea.
Hepatitis antigens and antibodies	Negative for antigens	Antigens indicate hepatitis (hepatitis B surface antigen [HBsAg] elevated in hepatitis B). Antibodies indicate exposure, current disease, or hepatitis B immunization.
BIOPSY		
Liver biopsy Percutaneous needle aspiration of liver tissue		1. Informed consent procedure. 2. Client's status is NPO for 6 hours before procedure. 3. Blood coagulation study results should be available on the chart before biopsy procedure. 4. Immediately before needle insertion, have client take a deep breath, exhale completely, and hold breath. This immobilizes the chest wall and decreases the risk for penetration of the diaphragm with the needle. 5. Keep client on bed rest for 12-14 hr. Client should be positioned on the right side for 2 hr postprocedure to apply pressure and decrease risk for hemorrhage. 6. Assess for complications of pneumothorax and hemorrhage immediately after biopsy; assess for right upper abdominal pain or referred shoulder pain; observe for development of bile peritonitis.

> **✔ NURSING PRIORITY:** *Monitor status of client after a procedure. Position the client on right side with a pillow under the costal margin to facilitate compression of the liver.*

CHOLANGIOGRAPHY		
Percutaneous transhepatic cholangiography (PTC) IV injection of radiopaque dye to visualize the biliary duct system		1. Client's status is NPO for 8 hr before the test. 2. Assess for sensitivity to iodine. 3. Evaluate for iodine reaction after the test. 4. Client should drink large amounts of fluid after test to increase excretion of dye.
NUCLEAR IMAGING SCANS (SCINTIGRAPHY)		
Hepatobiliary scintigraphy (HIDA) Shows size, shape and position of biliary system. Radionuclide (Tc-99m) injected IV; client positioned under a camera or counter to record distribution of tracer		1. Explain to client that traces of radionuclide pose minimal danger. 2. Needs to lie flat during scanning procedure

Continued

APPENDIX 14-1	DIAGNOSTICS OF THE HEPATIC AND BILIARY SYSTEM—cont'd.

Laboratory Tests	Nursing Implications

ULTRASOUND

Gallbladder ultrasound Uses high-frequency sound waves to examine the gallbladder; provides information about presence of tumors and patency of vessels and detects gallstones.	1. Client is NPO for 8-12 hours, since gas can reduce quality of images and food can cause gallbladder contraction. 2. Explain to client that a conductive gel (lubricant) will be applied to the skin and a transducer placed on the area.
Hepatobiliary ultrasound Detects abscesses, cysts, tumors, and cirrhosis.	

ENDOSCOPY

Endoscopic retrograde cholangiopancreatography (ERCP) Fiberoptic endoscope and fluoroscopy inserted orally, descended into duodenum, then into common bile duct and pancreatic ducts, where contrast medium is injected for visualization of the structures.	1. Client is NPO for 8 hours before procedure. 2. Explain that sedative will be given before and during procedure. 3. Check for allergy to contrast medium. 4. Informed consent must be signed. 5. Check vital signs—monitor for perforation or infection; pancreatitis is most common complication. 6. Check for return of gag reflex before giving fluids.

ALP, Alkaline phosphatase; *ALT*, alanine aminotransferase; *AST*, aspartate aminotransferase; *INR*, international normalized ratio; *IV*, intravenous; *NPO*, nothing by mouth.

Neurologic System

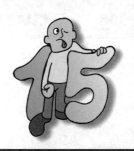

* The neurological or nervous system is composed of two primary areas: the central nervous system, which includes the brain and the spinal cord, and the peripheral nervous system, which includes the entire network of nerves extending from the central nervous system.

PHYSIOLOGY OF THE NEUROLOGICAL SYSTEM

Central Nervous System

The brain and the spinal cord within the vertebral column make up the central nervous system (CNS).

A. The brain and the spinal cord are protected by the rigid bony structure of the skull and by the vertebral column, respectively (Figure 15-1).

B. Meninges: the protective membranes that cover the brain and are continuous with those of the spinal cord.
1. Pia mater: covers the surfaces of the brain and the spinal column.
2. Arachnoid: waterproof membrane that encases the entire CNS; the subarachnoid space contains the cerebrospinal fluid.
3. Dura mater: a tough membrane that provides protection to the brain and spinal cord.

C. Cerebrospinal fluid (CSF) (Figure 15-2).
1. Serves to cushion and protect the brain and spinal cord; the brain literally floats in CSF.
2. CSF is clear, colorless, watery fluid; approximately 100- to 200-mL total volume, with a normal fluid pressure of 70 to 150 cm of water (average: 125 cm of water pressure).
3. Formation and circulation of CSF: CSF is formed continuously by the choroid plexus located in the ventricles of the brain. It is reabsorbed by the arachnoid villi in the ventricles at the same rate it is formed.

D. Brain: The basic brain anatomy consists of the cerebrum, the cerebellum, the brain stem, and the interior structures.
1. Cerebrum: the largest portion of the brain; separated into hemispheres. Each hemisphere is divided into four lobes: frontal, parietal, occipital, and temporal.
   a. Frontal: memory, language, personality, and emotions are primarily controlled here; highly vulnerable to traumatic brain injury.
   b. Parietal: integrates sensory information and interprets spatial relationships.

c. Occipital: center for visual perception and integration.
   d. Temporal: controls auditory, verbal, visual, memory, and personality functions.
   e. Some functions of the brain occur in more than one lobe.
2. Cerebellum: contains more neurons than the rest of the brain combined. It serves to interpret motor and mental dexterity, as well as sense of balance.
3. Brain stem: conduit for all information transmission between upper and lower nervous system. Consists of pons, midbrain, and medulla.
   a. Pons: responsible for alertness; relays sensory information between cerebellum and cerebrum.
   b. Midbrain: interprets auditory and visual reflexes.
   c. Medulla: lower portion of the brain stem. Controls autonomic functions.
      (1) Respiratory center for changes in rate and depth of breathing.
      (2) Controls heart rate.
      (3) Vomiting reflex center.
      (4) Swallowing reflex center.
4. Diencephalon: contains thalamus and hypothalamus.

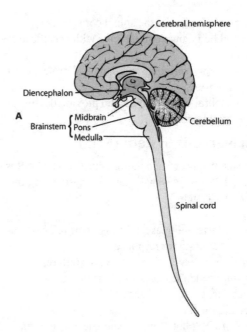

FIGURE 15-1 Major divisions of the central nervous system. (From Lewis SL et al: *Medical-surgical nursing: assessment and management of clinical problems,* ed 7, St. Louis, 2007, Mosby.)

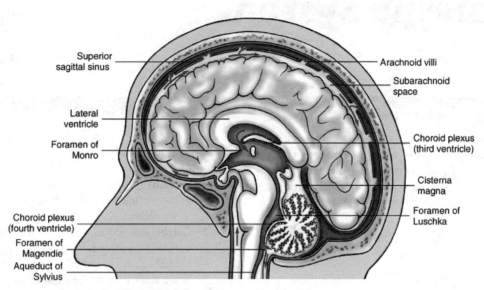

FIGURE 15-2 Cerebrospinal fluid circulation. Cerebrospinal fluid is produced by choroid plexus in lateral ventricles and flows around brain and spinal cord until it reaches arachnoid villi, from which it is absorbed into venous circulation. *Arrows* indicate major pathway of cerebrospinal fluid flow. *From From Monahan FD et al: Medical-surgical nursing: health and illness perspectives, ed 8, St. Louis, 2007, Mosby.*

a. Thalamus: receives and relays auditory, sensory, and visual signals.

b. Hypothalamus: controls body temperature regulation, sleep/wake cycles, and appetite; regulates the pituitary gland.

5. Limbic system: regulates emotions, drives, and appetite.

E. Spinal cord: a nerve bundle transmitting messages to and from the body.

1. Extends from medulla to first or second lumbar vertebra.

2. Nerves exit and enter the spinal cord at each vertebral body and communicate with specific areas of the body.

3. Rings of bony vertebrae surround and protect cord and nerve roots.

4. Intervertebral disks cushion and provide flexibility to the spinal column.

Peripheral Nervous System (PNS)

The PNS consists of sensory and motor neurons. The PNS is subdivided into the sensory/somatic nervous system and the autonomic nervous system.

A. Types of nerves.

1. Sensory (afferent or ascending) nerves relay sensations to the brain for response.

2. Motor components of cranial nerves (efferent or descending) send messages from the brain to muscles, glands, and specialized tissues (e.g., heart and lungs).

B. Functions of PNS: both sensory/somatic and autonomic responsibilities.

1. Sensory/somatic nervous system consists of cranial nerves and spinal nerves.

a. Cranial nerves: responsible for a variety of functions, from hearing and balance to regulation of chemoreceptors in the aortic body.

b. Spinal nerves: each pair of nerves is numbered according to the level of the spinal cord from which it originates.

2. Autonomic nervous system: regulates involuntary activity (e.g., cardiovascular, respiratory, metabolic, body temperature) (Table 15-1).

a. Parasympathetic division: maintains normal body functions.

b. Sympathetic division: prepares the body to meet a challenge or an emergency; "fight or flight."

c. Most of the organs of the body receive innervation from both the parasympathetic and the sympathetic divisions.

System Data Collection

A. History.

1. Neurological history.

2. Medical history.

a. Chronic, concurrent medical problems.

b. Medications (especially tranquilizers, sedatives, and narcotics).

c. If client is an infant or young child, a pregnancy and delivery history of the mother is obtained.

d. Sequence of growth and development.

3. Family history: presence of hereditary or congenital problems.

4. Personal history: activities of daily living; any change in routine.

5. History and symptoms of current problem.

a. Paralysis or paresthesia.

TABLE 15-1 AUTONOMIC NERVOUS SYSTEM

AREA AFFECTED	SYMPATHETIC (FIGHT OR FLIGHT)	PARASYMPATHETIC
Pupil	Dilates	Constricts
Bronchi	Dilates	Constricts
Heart	Increases rate	Decreases rate
Gastrointestinal	Inhibits peristalsis	Stimulates peristalsis
	Stimulates sphincter	Inhibits sphincters
Bladder	Relaxes bladder muscle	Contracts bladder muscle
	Constricts sphincter	Relaxes sphincter

b. Syncope, dizziness.
c. Headache.
d. Speech problems.
e. Visual problems.
f. Changes in personality.
g. Memory loss.
h. Nausea, vomiting.

B. Physical assessment.
1. General observation of client.
   a. Posture, gait.
   b. Position of rest for the infant or young child.
   c. Personal hygiene, grooming.
   d. Evaluate speech and ability to communicate.
      (1) Pace of speech: rapid, slow, halting.
      (2) Clarity: slurred or distinct.
      (3) Tone: high pitched, rough.
      (4) Vocabulary: appropriate choice of words.
   e. Facial features may suggest specific syndromes in children.

2. Mental status (must take into consideration the client's age, culture, and educational background) (Box 15-1, Box 15-2).
   a. General appearance and behavior.
   b. Level of consciousness.
      (1) Oriented to person, place, and time.
      (2) Appropriate response to verbal and tactile stimuli.
      (3) Memory, problem-solving abilities.
   c. Mood.
   d. Thought content and intellectual capacity.
   e. Judgment and abstract thinking.
   f. Perceptual distortion.
3. Assess pupillary status and eye movements.
   a. Size of pupils should be equal.
   b. Reaction of pupils.
      (1) Direct light reflex: constriction of pupil when light is shown directly into eye.
      (2) Accommodation: pupillary constriction to accommodate near vision.
   c. Evaluate eye movements.
      (1) Note nystagmus: fine, jerking eye movement.
      (2) Ability of eyes to move together.
      (3) Resting position should be at mid-position of the eye socket.
   d. PERRLA: Indicates that Pupils are Equal, Round, and Reactive to Light, and that Accommodation is present.
4. Evaluate motor function.
   a. Assess face and upper extremities for equality of movement and sensation; evaluate swallow reflex.
   b. Evaluate appropriateness of motor movement—spontaneous and on command.
   c. Movement of extremities should always be evaluated bilaterally, comparing tone, strength, and muscle movement of each side.
   d. Presence of inappropriate, nonpurposeful movement (e.g., posturing).
      (1) Decerebrate: extension and adduction of the arms; hyperextension of the legs.

BOX 15-1 OLDER ADULT CARE FOCUS
Assessing Neurologic Function in Older Adults

Signs of Cognitive Impairment
- Significant memory loss (person, place, and time).
- Person: Does client know who he or she is, and can client give you his or her full name?
- Place: Can client identify his or her home address and where he or she is now?
- Time: What was the most recent holiday; what month, time of day, day of the week is it now?
- Does client show a lack of judgment?
- Is client agitated and/or suspicious?
- As determined from client's appearance and family's response, does client have problems with ADLs?
- Short-term memory: Can the client recall your name, name of the President, or name of his or her doctor?
- Short-term recall: Ask the client to name three or four common objects; then ask client to recall them within the next 5 minutes.
- Does the client have sensory deficits (hearing and vision) of which he or she is not aware?

BOX 15-2 OLDER ADULT CARE FOCUS

Causes of Confusion in the Older Adult Client

Decreased Cardiac Output
- Myocardial infarction
- Dysrhythmias
- Congestive heart failure

Hypoxia/Respiratory Acidosis
- Pneumonia
- Infection
- Hypoventilation

Neurologic
- Vascular insufficiency
- Infections
- Cerebral edema

Metabolic – Altered Homeostasis
- Electrolyte imbalance
- Hypoglycemia/hyperglycemia
- Dehydration
- Urinary tract infections

Environmental
- Strange surroundings
- Hypothermia/hyperthermia

- (2) Decorticate: flexion, internal rotation of the arms; extension of the legs.
- (3) Presence of nonpurposeful involuntary movements such as tremors, jerking, twitching.
- (4) Opisthotonos position: rigid arching of the back.
- e. Ability of an infant to suck and to swallow.
- f. Asymmetrical contraction of facial muscles.
5. Evaluate reflexes.
   - a. Gag or cough reflex.
   - b. Swallow reflex.
   - c. Babinski reflex: Normal sign is negative in adults and children over 1 year; positive sign is dorsal flexion of the foot and large toe with fanning of the other toes.
6. Assess vital signs and correlate with other data; changes often occur slowly, and the overall trend needs to be evaluated.
   - a. Blood pressure and pulse rate: Intracranial problems precipitate changes: blood pressure may increase and pulse rate may decrease.
   - b. Respirations: Rate, depth, and rhythm are sensitive indicators of intracranial problems.
   - c. Temperature: Evaluate changes in temperature as related to a neurological control versus infection.
C. Bedside neurological checks: parameters for frequent nursing evaluation of neurological symptoms.
   1. Assess level of consciousness (LOC).

- a. Verbal and motor response to command.
- b. Appropriate conversation and speech.
- c. Appropriate behavior in infants and young children.
- d. Be explicit in describing LOC; may use a specific coma scale (Table 15-2).
2. Respiratory patterns: Evaluate current respiratory pattern and assess for changes in pattern.
3. Pupillary response.
   - a. Equality of pupils.
   - b. Presence of direct and accommodation reflexes.
   - c. Position of pupils at rest.
4. Motor function.
   - a. Ability to move all extremities with equal strength.
   - b. Presence of posturing.
   - c. Babinski reflex.
   - d. Presence of seizure activity.
   - e. Presence of gag and cough reflexes.
5. Vital signs.
   - a. Correlate blood pressure and pulse rate changes.
   - b. Assess respiratory pattern.
   - c. Assess temperature in regard to overall condition.
6. Assess for presence of pain, headache.
7. Presence of projectile vomiting not associated with nausea.
8. Infants: assess fontanel(s) and suture lines.
   - a. Size of fontanel(s) for growth and development level.
   - b. Fontanel(s) should be soft to touch, with slight pulsations.
   - c. Normal approximation of cranial suture lines.

Increased Intracranial Pressure

✳ **An increase in intracranial pressure (ICP) occurs any time there is an increase in the size or amount of intracranial contents.**

A. The cranial vault is rigid, and there is minimal room for expansion of the intracranial components.
B. An increase in any one of the components necessitates a reciprocal change in other cranial contents; this frequently results in ischemia of brain tissue. An increase in ICP results from one of the following:
   1. Increased intracranial blood volume (vasodilation).
   2. Increased CSF.
   3. Increase in the bulk of the brain tissue (edema).
C. Cerebral edema.
   1. Edema occurs when there is an increase in the volume of brain tissue caused by an increase in the permeability of the walls of the cerebral vessels.
      - a. Protein-rich fluid leaks into the extracellular space.
      - b. Edema is most often the cause of increased ICP in adults, which reaches maximum pressure in 48 to 72 hours.

TABLE 15-2	GLASGOW COMA SCALE		
CATEGORY OF RESPONSE	**APPROPRIATE STIMULUS**	**RESPONSE**	**SCORE**
Eyes open	Approach bedside Verbal command Pain	Spontaneous response	4
		Opening of eyes to name or command	3
		Lack of opening of eyes to previous stimuli but opening to pain	2
		Lack of opening of eyes to any stimulus	1
		Untestable	U
Best verbal response	Verbal questioning with maximum arousal	Appropriate orientation, conversant, correct identification of self, place, year, and month	5
		Confusion; conversant, but disorientated in one or more spheres	4
		Inappropriate or disorganized use of words (e.g., cursing), lack of sustained conversation	3
		Incomprehensible words, sounds (e.g., moaning)	2
		Lack of sound, even with painful stimuli	1
		Untestable	U
Best motor response	Verbal command (e.g., "raise your arm, hold up two fingers." Pain (pressure on proximal nail bed)	Obedience in response to command	6
		Localization of pain, lack of obedience but presence of attempts to remove offending stimulus	5
		Flexion withdrawal*, flexion of arm in response to pain without abnormal flexion posture	4
		Abnormal flexion, flexing of arm at elbow and pronation, making a fist	3
		Abnormal extension, extension of arm at elbow, usually with adduction and internal rotation of arm at shoulder	2
		Lack of response	1
		Untestable	U

A score of 7 or less indicates coma. The highest possible score is 15. Often reported as E4V3M6 - meaning eyes open to name or command, inappropriate or disorganized use of words, and obeys motor command.

From Lewis SL et al: *Medical-surgical nursing: assessment and management of clinical problems,* ed 7, St. Louis, 2007, *Mosby.*
*Added to the original scale by many centers.

2. Cytotoxic (cellular) edema occurs as a result of hypoxia. This results in abnormal accumulation of fluid within the cells (intracellular) and a decrease in extracellular fluid.
D. Poor ventilation will precipitate respiratory acidosis, or an increase in the Paco2.
 1. Carbon dioxide has a vasodilating effect on the cerebral arteries, which increases cerebrovascular blood flow and increases ICP.
 2. Clients should be adeaquately ventilated to prevent cyclic vasodilation, which increases intracranial pressure.
E. Regardless of the cause, increased ICP will result in progressive neurologic deterioration; the specific deficiencies seen are determined by the area and extent of compression of brain tissue.
F. If the infant's cranial suture lines are open, increased ICP will cause separation of the suture lines and an increase in the circumference of the head.

✓ **NURSING PRIORITY:** *There is no single set of symptoms for all clients with increased ICP; symptoms depend on the cause and on how rapidly increased ICP develops.*

Data Collection

A. Risk factors/etiology.
 1. Cerebral edema caused by some untoward event or trauma.
 2. Brain tumors.
 3. Intracranial hemorrhage (closed head injuries or ruptured blood vessels).
 4. Subarachnoid hemorrhage, hydrocephalus.
 5. Cerebral embolism and thrombosis.
 6. Encephalitis/meningitis.
 7. Reye's syndrome.
B. Clinical manifestations (bedside neurologic checks) (Figure 15-3).

> ✓ *NURSING PRIORITY: Determine change in a client's neurological status. Be able to rapidly evaluate the client and recognize neurologic signs that indicate an increase in ICP (Box 15-3).*

1. Assess for *changes* in level of consciousness, because change is the cardinal indicator of increased intracranial pressure.
   a. Any alteration in level of consciousness (early sign for both adults and children)— irritability, restlessness, confusion, lethargy, and difficulty in arousing—may be significant.

> ✓ *NURSING PRIORITY: The first sign of a change in the level of ICP is change in level of consciousness; this may progress to a decrease in level of consciousness.*

   b. Inappropriate verbal and motor response; delayed or sluggish responses.
   c. As the client loses consciousness, hearing is the last sense to be lost.
2. Changes in vital signs.
   a. Increase in systolic blood pressure with increase in pulse pressure.
   b. Decrease in pulse rate.
   c. Alteration in respiratory pattern (Cheyne-Stokes respiration, hyperventilation, ataxia).
   d. Assess temperature with regard to overall problems; temperature usually increases.
3. Pupillary response: normal pupils should be round, midline, equal in size, and equally briskly reactive to light and should accommodate to distance.
4. Decrease in motor and sensory function, unilateral or bilateral weakness or paralysis, failure to withdraw from painful stimuli, seizure activity.
5. Headache, photophobia.
6. Vomiting: projectile vomiting without prior nausea.
7. Infants.
   a. Tense, bulging fontanel(s).
   b. Separated cranial sutures.
   c. Increasing frontal-occipital circumference.
   d. High-pitched cry.
C. Diagnostics (see Appendix 15-1).

Treatment

A. Treatment of the underlying cause of increasing pressure.
B. Neurologic checks every hour or as ordered.
   1. May involve correlation of several variables including level of consciousness, vital signs, speech, facial symmetry, grasp strength, leg strength, and pupil responses.
   2. Careful comparison to previous assessment is critical to detect incremental changes.

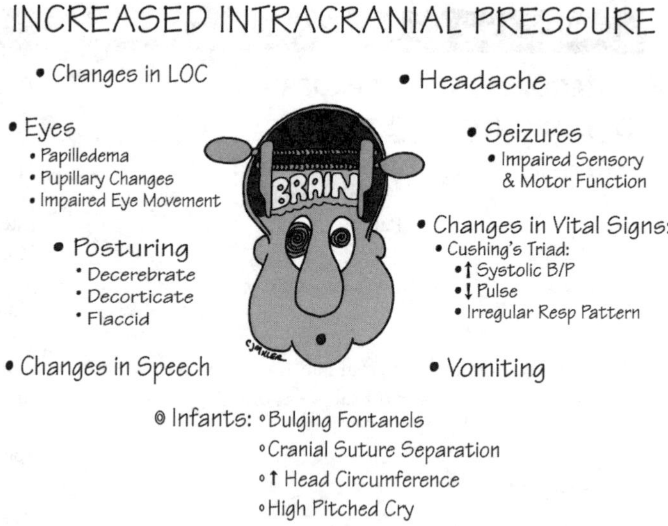

INCREASED INTRACRANIAL PRESSURE

- Changes in LOC
- Eyes
  - Papilledema
  - Pupillary Changes
  - Impaired Eye Movement
- Posturing
  - Decerebrate
  - Decorticate
  - Flaccid
- Changes in Speech
- Headache
- Seizures
  - Impaired Sensory & Motor Function
- Changes in Vital Signs:
  - Cushing's Triad:
    - ↑ Systolic B/P
    - ↓ Pulse
    - Irregular Resp Pattern
- Vomiting
- Infants:
  - Bulging Fontanels
  - Cranial Suture Separation
  - ↑ Head Circumference
  - High Pitched Cry

FIGURE 15-3 Increased intracranial pressure. (From Zerwekh J, Claborn J, Miller CJ: *Memory notebook of nursing, vol 1,* ed 4, Ingram, 2008, Nursing Education Consultants.)

C. Intravenous (IV) and oral fluids.
D. Medications.
   1. Osmotic diuretics, corticosteroids.
   2. Anticonvulsants, antihypertensives.
E. Maintain adequate ventilation by means of mechanical ventilation to lower $Paco_2$.
F. Placement of ventriculoperitoneal shunt during decompression surgery.

Complications

A. CSF leaks, may cause meningitis.
B. Herniation: shifting of the intracranial contents from one compartment to another.
   1. Brain compression occurs.
   2. Obstruction of the cerebrospinal fluid.
   3. Irreversible brain damage and death.
C. Permanent brain damage.

Nursing Interventions

❖ **Goal:** To identify and decrease problem of increased ICP.
A. Neurologic checks, as indicated by client's status.
B. Maintain head of bed in semi-Fowler's position (15-30 degrees) to promote venous drainage and respiratory function.

> ✓ *NURSING PRIORITY: Change client's position. If the client with increased ICP develops hypovolemic shock, do not place client in Trendelenburg position.*

C. Change client's position slowly; avoid extreme hip flexion and extreme rotation or flexion of neck. Maintain the head midline.

<table>
<tr><td>

BOX 15-3   **INCREASING INTRACRANIAL PRESSURE**

Adult
Early: Restless, irritable, lethargic
Intermediate: Unequal pupil response, projectile vomiting, vital signs changes
Late: Decreased level of consciousness, decreased reflexes, hypoventilation, dilated pupils, posturing

Infant/Child
Early: Poor feeding, tense fontanel, headache, nausea and vomiting, increased pitch of cry, unsteady gait
Intermediate (younger than 18 months): Increased head circumference, altered consciousness, bulging fontanel; shrill cry, severe headache, blurred vision, stiff neck
Late: Same as adult

</td></tr>
</table>

D. Monitor urine specific gravity.
E. Evaluate intake and output.
   1. In response to diuretics.
   2. As correlated with changes in daily weight.
F. Maintain intake evenly during therapeutic treatment.
G. Minimize respiratory suctioning and ensure hyperoxygenation before suctioning.
H. Sedatives and narcotics can depress respiration; use with caution because they mask symptoms of increasing ICP.
I. Client should avoid strenuous coughing, Valsalva maneuver, and isometric muscle exercises.
J. Avoid straining with stools (increases intrathoracic pressure sporadically).
K. In infants, measure frontal-occipital circumference to evaluate increase in size of the head.
L. Control hyperthermia.
M. Maintain head and spinal column in midline position.
❖   Goal: To maintain respiratory function.

> ✔ *NURSING PRIORITY: An obstructed airway is one of the most common problems in the unconscious client; position to maintain patent airway or use airway adjuncts.*

A. Prevent respiratory problems of immobility.
B. Evaluate patency of airway frequently; as level of consciousness decreases, client is at increased risk for accumulating secretions and airway obstruction by the tongue.
C. Suction secretions as necessary, but in short duration with rest periods.
D. Do not suction the nasopharyngeal area of a client when a cerebrospinal fluid leak is present (craniotomy, head injury, or basilar skull fracture).
❖   Goal: To protect client from injury.

A. Maintain seizure precautions (see Appendix 15-5).
B. Restrain client only if absolutely necessary; struggling against restraints increases ICP.
C. Do not clean the ears or nasal passages of a client with a head injury or a client who has had neurosurgery.
   1. Check for evidence of a CSF leak: CSF has glucose in it; test it with a dipstick.
   2. CSF also leaves a yellow "halo" stain.
D. Aspiration is a major problem in the unconscious client; place the client in semi-Fowler's position for tube feeding after ensuring correct tube placement by x-ray.
E. Maintain quiet, nonstimulating environment.
F. Inspect eyes and prevent corneal ulceration.
   1. Protective closing of eyes, if eyes remain open.
   2. Irrigation with normal saline solution or methylcellulose drops to restore moisture.
❖   Goal: To maintain psychologic equilibrium.
A. Neurologic checks should be done on a continual basis to detect potential problems.
B. Encourage verbalization of fears regarding condition.
C. Give simple explanation of procedures to client and family.
D. Altered states of consciousness will cause increased anxiety and confusion; maintain reality orientation.
E. If client is unconscious, continue to talk to him or her; describe procedures and treatments; always assume that client can hear.
F. Assist parents and family to work through feelings of guilt and anger.
❖   Goal: To prevent complications of immobility (see Chapter 3).
❖   Goal: To maintain elimination.
A. Urinary incontinence: may use condom catheter or indwelling bladder catheter.
B. Keep perineal area clean, prevent excoriation.
C. Monitor bowel function; evaluate for fecal impaction.

> ✔ *NURSING PRIORITY: Notify charge nurse or primary health care provider when client demonstrates signs of potential complications; interpret what data for a client need to be reported immediately.*

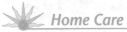 *Home Care*

A. Teach client and family signs of increased ICP.
B. Call the doctor if any of the following are observed:
   1. Changes in vision.
   2. Increased drainage from incision area or clear drainage in the ears.
   3. Abrupt changes in sleeping patterns or irritability.
   4. Headache that does not respond to medication.
   5. Changes in coordination, disorientation.
   6. Slurred speech, unusual behavior.
   7. Seizure activity, vomiting.
C. Review care of surgical incision, wounds, or drains.

Brain Tumors

✳ **Brain tumors may be benign, malignant, or metastatic; malignant brain tumors rarely metastasize outside the CNS. Regardless of the origin, site, or presence of malignancy, problems of increased ICP occur because of the limited area in the brain to accommodate an increase in the intracranial contents.**

Data Collection

A. Clinical manifestations: Symptoms correlate with the area of the brain initially involved.
1. Headache.
a. Recurrent. May vomit on arising and then feel better.
b. More severe in the morning.
c. Affected by position.
d. Headache in infant may be identified by persistent, irritated crying and head rolling.
2. Vomiting: initially with or without nausea; progressively becomes projectile.
3. Papilledema (edema of the optic disc).
4. Seizures (focal or generalized).
5. Dizziness and vertigo.
6. Mental status changes: lethargy and drowsiness, confusion, disorientation, and personality changes.
7. Localized manifestations:
a. Focal weakness: hemiparesis.
8. Sensory disturbances.
a. Language disturbances.
b. Coordination disturbances.
c. Visual disturbances.
9. Head tilt: child may tilt the head because of damage to extraocular muscles; may be first indication of a decrease in visual acuity.
10. Changes in vital signs indicative of increasing ICP.
11. Cranial enlargement in the infant younger than 18 months.
B. Diagnostics (see Appendix 15-1).

Treatment

A. Medical.
1. Dexamethasone (see Appendix 5-7).
2. Chemotherapy.
3. Anticonvulsants (see Appendix 15-2).
4. Complementary and alternative medicine.
B. Radiation: x-rays, gamma knife, stereotactic radiosurgery.
C. Surgical intervention: craniotomy/craniectomy, biopsy, shunt placement, reservoir placement, laser removal.

Complications

Complications include meningitis, brainstem herniation, diabetes insipidus. Residual effects include a wide array of complications such as seizures, dysarthria, dysphasia, disequilibrium, and permanent brain damage.

Nursing Interventions

❖   **Goal:** To provide appropriate preoperative nursing interventions.
A. General preoperative care with exceptions, as noted (see Chapter 3).
B. Carefully assess and discuss with surgeon the appropriateness of a preoperative enema.
C. Prepare client and family for appearance of the client after surgery, including partial or complete hair loss.
D. Encourage verbalization regarding concerns about surgery.
E. Skin preparation is usually done in the operating room.
❖   **Goal:** To monitor changes in ICP after craniotomy (see Box 15-3).
A. Obtain vital signs and perform neurologic checks and cranial nerve assessments as necessary.
B. Maintain pulmonary function and hygiene.
C. Anticipate use of anticonvulsants and antiemetics.
D. Discourage coughing.
E. Carefully evaluate level of consciousness; increasing lethargy or irritability may be indicative of increasing ICP.
F. Evaluate dressing.
1. Location and amount of drainage.
2. Clarify with surgeon whether the nurse or the surgeon will change dressing.
3. *Evaluate for CSF leak through the incision and report any drainage to charge nurse.*
G. Maintain semi-Fowler's position if there is a CSF leak from ears or nose.
H. Postoperative positioning for client who has had infratentorial surgery:
1. Bed should be flat.
2. Position client on either side; avoid supine position.
3. Maintain head and neck in midline.
4. Keep NPO for 24 hours to reduce edema around medulla and reduce vomiting.
I. Postoperative position for client who has had supratentorial surgery: semi- to low-Fowler's position.
J. Trendelenburg position is contraindicated.
K. Maintain fluid regulation.
1. After client is awake and the swallow and gag reflexes have returned, begin offering clear liquids by mouth.
2. Closely monitor intake and output.
L. Evaluate neurologic status in response to fluid balance and diuretics.
M. Evaluate changes in temperature: may be due to respiratory complications or to alteration in the function of the hypothalamus.

N. Provide appropriate postoperative pain relief.
1. Avoid narcotic analgesics.
2. Acetaminophen is frequently used.
3. Maintain quiet, dim atmosphere.
4. Avoid sudden movements.
O. Prevent complications of immobility (see Chapter 3).
P. Maintain seizure precautions (see Appendix 15-5).

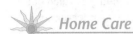 *Home Care*

See home care for client with increasing ICP.

 Head Injury

A. Classification.
1. Penetrating head injury: dura is pierced, as in stabbing or shooting.
2. Closed or blunt head injury: head is either drastically accelerated (whiplash) or decelerated (collision); most common head injury in civilian life.
B. Children and infants are more capable of absorbing direct impact because of the pliability of the skull.
C. Coup-contrecoup injury: damage to the site of impact (coup) and damage on the side opposite the site of impact (contrecoup) when brain "bounces" freely inside skull.
D. Primary injury to the brain occurs by compression and/or tearing and shearing stresses on vessels and nerves.
E. Although brain volume remains unchanged, secondary injury occurs from the cerebral edema in response to the primary injury and frequently precipitates an increase in ICP.
F. Types of head injuries.
1. Concussion: temporary interference in brain function; may affect memory, speech, reflexes, balance, and coordination.
   a. Only small number of victims actually "black out."
   b. Usually from blunt trauma including contact sports.
   c. Usually does not cause permanent damage.
   d. Transient, self-limiting.
2. Contusion (a bruise on the brain).
   a. Multiple areas of petechial hemorrhages.
   b. Headache, pupillary changes, dizziness, unilateral weakness.
   c. Blood supply is altered in the area of injury; swelling, ischemia, and increased ICP.
   d. May last several hours to weeks.
3. Intracranial hemorrhage.
   a. Epidural (extradural) hematoma: a large vessel (generally an artery) in the dura mater is damaged; a hematoma rapidly forms between the dura and the skull, precipitating an increase in ICP.
   (1) Momentary loss of consciousness, then free of symptoms (lucid period), and then lethargy and coma-seldom evident in children.
   (2) Symptoms of increasing ICP may develop within minutes after the lucid interval.
   b. Subdural hematoma: a collection of blood between the dura and arachnoid area filling the brain vault; usually the result of serious head injury.
   (1) May be acute (manifesting in less than 24 hours) or "chronic" (developing over days to weeks).
   (2) When neurologic compromise presents, subdural hematoma becomes an emergent event. Emergency neurosurgery may be required to relieve pressure.

Data Collection

A. Clinical manifestations.
1. Epidural hematoma: decreased GCS (Table 15-2), pupillary changes, unilateral weakness.
2. Subdural hematoma: headache, change in LOC, numbness, headache, slurred speech, or inability to speak.
B. Diagnostics (see Appendix15-1).

Complications

Complications include residual increased ICP, meningitis, diabetes insipidus, seizures, and permanent neurologic compromise.

Treatment

> ✔ **NURSING PRIORITY:** *The primary treatment objectives for the client with a head injury are to maintain a patent airway, to prevent hypoxia and acidosis, and to identify the occurrence of increased ICP.*

A. The majority of clients who experience concussion are treated at home.
B. A period of unconsciousness or presence of seizures is considered a serious indication of injury.
C. Surgical intervention.
1. Burr holes to evacuate the hematoma.
2. Craniotomy/craniectomy.

Nursing Interventions

❖ **Goal:** To provide instruction for care of the client in the home environment (Box 15-4).
A. Problems frequently do not occur until 24 hours or more after the initial injury.
B. Observe the client for increased periods of sleep; if client is asleep, awaken every 3 to 4 hours to determine whether client can be aroused normally.

BOX 15-4 **DISCHARGE INSTRUCTIONS FOR CLIENTS WITH HEAD INJURY**

- Arouse the client every 3 to 4 hours for the first 24 hours.
- Anticipate complaints of dizziness, headaches.
- Do not allow client to blow his nose; try to prevent sneezing.
- No alcohol or sedatives for sleep.
- Acetaminophen for headaches.
- No exercising over next 2 to 3 days.
  Call the doctor if any of the following is noted:
- Change in vision: Blurred or diplopia.
- Poor coordination: Walking, grasping.
- Drainage (serous or bloody) from the nose or ears.
- Forceful vomiting.
- Increasing sleepiness, more difficult to arouse.
- Slurred speech.
- Headache that does not respond to medication and continues to get worse.
- Occurrence of a seizure.

C. Maintain contact with physician for reevaluation if complications occur.
D. Health care provider should be notified when any of the following are observed:
   1. Any change in level of consciousness (increased drowsiness, confusion).
   2. Inability to arouse client, seizures.
   3. Bleeding or watery drainage from the ears or nose.
   4. Loss of feeling or sensation in any extremity.
   5. Blurred vision, slurred speech, vomiting.

☑ *NURSING PRIORITY: Written and oral instructions should be given to the client and to the family. Increased anxiety may affect comprehension of oral directions (see Box 15-4).*

❖ Goal: To maintain homeostasis and to monitor and identify early symptoms of increased ICP.
A. Bed rest and clear liquids initially.
B. Frequent neurologic checks for increased ICP.
   1. Change or decrease in level of consciousness is frequently the first indication.
   2. Instruct clients with head injury not to cough, sneeze, or blow nose.
C. *Notify nurse or PCP of any drainage from nose, ears, and mouth.*
   1. Do not clean out the ears: place loose cotton in the auditory canal and change when soiled.
   2. Check continuous clear drainage from the nose with Dextrostix; if glucose is present, it is indicative of a CSF leak, spinal fluid also dries with a yellow halo around edges of drainage.

3. If a CSF leak occurs, keep the head of the bed elevated and monitor for development of an infection (meningitis).
D. Seizure precautions (see Appendix 15-5).
E. Maintain adequate fluid intake by IV infusion or oral intake; do not overhydrate.
F. Assess for other undetected injuries; stabilize spine after head injury until spinal cord injury is ruled out.
❖ Goal: To provide appropriate nursing interventions for the client experiencing an increase in ICP (see nursing goals for increased ICP).
❖ Goal: To provide adequate nutritional and caloric intake for the client with a head injury (see Appendix 13-6).
A. Provide enteral feedings if client is unable to eat.
B. Assist client to take oral feedings once swallow reflex is normal; client is at increased risk for aspiration.

Hydrocephalus

✳ **Hydrocephalus is a condition caused by an imbalance in the production and absorption of CSF in the ventricles of the brain.**

Data Collection

A. Risk factors/etiology.
   1. Neonate: usually the result of a congenital malformation.
   2. Older child, adult.
      a. Space-occupying lesion.
      b. Preexisting developmental defects.
B. Clinical manifestations: infant.
   1. Head enlargement: increasing circumference in excess of normal 2 cm per month for first 3 months.
   2. Separation of cranial suture lines.
   3. Fontanel becomes tense and bulging.
   4. Dilated scalp veins.
   5. Frontal enlargement, bulging "sunset eyes."
   6. Symptoms of increasing ICP.
C. Clinical manifestations: older child, adult.
   1. Symptoms of increasing ICP.
   2. Specific manifestations related to site of the lesion.
D. Diagnostics (see Appendix 15-1).
   1. Increasing head circumference is diagnostic in infants.

Treatment

A. Ventriculoperitoneal shunt; CSF is shunted into the peritoneum.
B. Surgery: removal of the obstruction (cyst, hematoma, tumor).

Nursing Interventions

❖ Goal: To monitor for the development of increasing ICP.

A. Daily measurement of the frontal-occipital circumference of the head in infants.
B. Assess for symptoms of increasing ICP (see Box 15-3).
C. Infant is often difficult to feed; administer small feedings at frequent intervals because vomiting may be a problem.
❖ Goal: To maintain patency of the shunt and monitor ICP after shunt procedure.
A. Position supine, with head turned opposite side up to prevent pressure on the shunt valve and to prevent too-rapid depletion of CSF.
B. Position is not a problem with children who are having a shunt revision; they have not had an increase in ventricular pressure.
C. *Monitor for increasing ICP and notify charge nurse.*
D. Monitor for infection, especially meningitis or encephalitis.

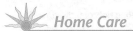

Home Care

A. Teach parents symptoms of increasing ICP.
B. Have parents participate in care of the shunt before client's discharge.
C. Encourage parents and family to ventilate feelings regarding client's condition.
D. Refer client to appropriate community agencies.

Reye's Syndrome

✳ **Reye's syndrome is a rare acute illness that occurs after a viral illness (frequently, after aspirin has been consumed) and results in liver problems and increased intracranial pressure.**

Data Collection

A. Clinical manifestations.
1. Primarily affects children from the age of 6 months to adolescence.
2. Frequently, the affected child has received salicylate (aspirin) for control of fever during the preceding viral infection.
3. Severe persistent vomiting, lethargy leading to irritability, and increased ICP.

Treatment

A. Measures to decrease ICP.

Nursing Interventions

❖ Goal: To monitor progress of disease state and maintain homeostasis.
A. IV fluids.
B. Monitor serum electrolytes and liver function studies.
C. Maintain respiratory status; prevent hypoxia.
D. Assess for problems of impaired coagulation due to liver problems.

E. Decrease stress, anxiety: child may not remember events before the critical phase.
❖ Goal: To monitor for and implement nursing actions appropriate for increasing ICP.

Stroke (Brain Attack)

✳ **Stroke or brain attack is the disruption of the blood supply to an area of the brain, resulting in tissue necrosis and sudden loss of brain function. It is the leading cause of adult disability in the United States.**
A. Atherosclerosis (see Chapter 11), resulting in cerebrovascular disease, frequently precedes the development of a stroke.
B. Types of stroke.
1. Ischemic stroke.
   a. Thrombotic stroke: formation of a clot that results in the narrowing of a vessel lumen and eventual occlusion; most common stroke.
      (1) Associated with hypertension and diabetes.
      (2) Produces ischemia of the cerebral tissue.
   b. Embolic stroke: occlusion of a cerebral artery by an embolus.
      (1) Common site of origin is the endocardium.
      (2) May affect any age group
2. Hemorrhagic stroke.
   a. Rupture of a cerebral artery caused by hypertension, trauma, or aneurysm.
   b. Bleeding compresses the brain and causes inflammation.
C. The area of edema resulting from tissue damage may precipitate more damage than the vascular damage itself.
D. TIA and RIND.
1. Transient ischemic attack (TIA, silent stroke).
   a. Brief episode, less than 24 hours, of neurologic dysfunction; usually resolves within 30-60 minutes.
   b. Should be considered a warning sign of an impending stroke.
   c. Neurologic dysfunction is present for minutes to hours, but no permanent neurologic deficit remains.
2. Reversible ischemic neurologic deficit (RIND).
   a. Symptoms similar to TIA.
   b. Neurologic symptoms last longer than 24 hours, but less than a week.
3. Stroke: client has neurologic deficits related to mobility, sensation, and cognition.
E. Neuromuscular deficits resulting from a stroke are due to damage of motor neurons of the pyramidal tract.
1. Damage to the left side of the brain will result in paralysis of the right side of the body (Figure 15-4).
2. Both upper and lower extremities of the involved side are affected.

Data Collection

A. Clinical manifestations.
1. Transient ischemic attack (TIA) and reversible ischemic neurologic deficit (RIND).
    a. Visual defects: blurred vision, diplopia, blindness of one eye, tunnel vision.
    b. Transient hemiparesis, gait problems.
    c. Slurred speech, confusion.
    d. Transient numbness of an extremity.
2. Complete stroke (occurs suddenly with an embolism, more gradually with hemorrhage or thrombosis); symptoms vary according to which cerebral vessels are involved.
    a. Hemiplegia: loss of voluntary movement; damage to the right side of the brain will result in left-sided weakness and paralysis.
    b. Aphasia: defect in using and interpreting the symbols of language; may include written, printed, or spoken words.
    c. May be unaware of the affected side; neglect syndrome.
    d. Cranial nerve impairment: chewing, gag reflex, dysphagia, impaired tongue movement.
    e. May be incontinent initially.
    f. Agnosia: a perceptual defect that causes a disturbance in interpreting sensory information; client may not be able to recognize previously familiar objects.
    g. Cognitive impairment of memory, judgment, proprioception (awareness of one's body position).
    h. Hypotonia (flaccidity) for days to weeks, followed by hypertonia (spasticity).
    i. Visual defects.
C. Diagnostics (see Appendix 15-1).

Treatment

A. Prophylactic.
1. Aspirin, platelet inhibitors.
2. Antihypertensives, anticoagulants.
B. Immediate treatment (differs depending on whether thrombotic or hemorrhagic stroke).
1. Medical.
    a. Medications to decrease cerebral edema.
        (1) Osmotic diuretics.
        (2) Corticosteroids (dexamethasone).
    b. Anticoagulants for thrombotic stroke (never administered to a client with hemorrhagic stroke).
    c. Anticonvulsants.
    d. Thrombolytic therapy or fibrinolytic therapy (such as recombinant tissue plasminogen activator (rtPA [**Retavase**]) considered for nonhemorrhagic strokes within 3 hours of first manifestation of stroke signs.
    e. Antihypertensives and antidysrhythmics.

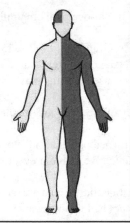
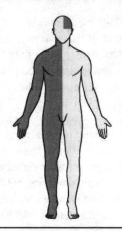

Right-brain damage (stroke on right side of the brain)	**Left-brain damage** (stroke on left side of the brain)
• Paralyzed left side: hemiplegia	• Paralyzed right side: hemiplegia
• Left-sided neglect	• Impaired speech/language aphasias
• Spatial-perceptual deficits	• Impaired right/left discrimination
• Tends to deny or minimize problems	• Slow performance, cautious
• Rapid performance, short attention span	• Aware of deficits: depression, anxiety
• Impulsive, safety problems	• Impaired comprehension related to language, math
• Impaired judgment	
• Impaired time concepts	

FIGURE 15-4 Manifestations of right-brain and left-brain stroke. (From Lewis SL et al: *Medical-surgical nursing: assessment and management of clinical problems,* ed 7, St. Louis, 2007, Mosby.)

2. Surgical.
    a. Carotid endarterectomy, especially for transient ischemic attack.
    b. Craniotomy for evacuation of hematoma.
    c. Extracranial-intracranial bypass for mild strokes.
C. Specific therapies to resolve physical, speech or occupational complications, including use of assistive devices.

Nursing Interventions

❖   **Goal:** To prevent stroke through client education (see Box 15-5).
A. Identification of individuals with reversible risk factors and measures to reduce them.
B. Appropriate medical attention for control of chronic conditions conducive to the development of stroke
C. Teach high risk clients early signs of TIA and RIND and to seek medical attention immediately if they occur.
❖   **Goal:** To maintain patent airway and adequate cerebral oxygenation.
A. Place client in side-lying position with head elevated.
B. Assess for symptoms of hypoxia; administer oxygen or assist with endotracheal intubation and mechanical ventilation as necessary (see Appendix 10-8).
C. Maintain patent airway; use oropharyngeal airway to prevent airway obstruction by the tongue.

BOX 15-5   RISK FACTORS ASSOCIATED WITH STROKE

Modifiable
- Smoking
- Obesity
- Increased salt intake
- Sedentary lifestyle
- Increased stress
- Oral contraceptives

Partially Modifiable
- Hypertension
- Cardiac valve disease
- Dysrhythmias
- Diabetes mellitus
- Hypercholesterolemia

Nonmodifiable
- Sex: Increased incidence in men
- Age
- Race: Increased incidence in the African-American population
- Hereditary predisposition

D. Client is prone to obstructed airway and pulmonary infection; have client cough and deep-breathe every 2 hours.

❖ **Goal:** To assess for and implement measures to decrease ICP (see nursing goals for increased ICP).

❖ **Goal:** To maintain adequate nutritional intake.

A. Before oral feedings, evaluate need for swallow studies.

B. Administer oral feedings with caution; start after first 24 hours; check for presence of gag and swallowing reflexes before feeding.

C. Place food on the unaffected side of the mouth; begin with clear foods (gelatins).

D. Select foods that are easy to control in the mouth (thick liquids) and easy to swallow; liquids often promote coughing, because client is unable to control them.

E. Maintain high-Fowler's position for feeding.

F. Maintain privacy and unrushed atmosphere.

G. If client is unable to tolerate oral intake, enteral feedings may be initiated.

 TEST ALERT: Identify potential for aspiration; assess client's ability to eat.

❖ **Goal:** To preserve function of the musculoskeletal system.

A. Passive range of motion (ROM) on affected side; begin early because the exercises are more difficult if muscles begin to tighten.

B. Active ROM on unaffected side.

C. Prevent foot drop: passive exercises; rigid boots; have client out of bed as soon as possible.

D. Legs should be maintained in a neutral position; prevent

external rotation of affected hip by placing a trochanter roll or rolled pillow at the thigh.

E. Reposition every 2 hours, but limit the period of time spent on the affected side.

✔ **NURSING PRIORITY:** *Protect the client's affected side: do not give injections on that side, watch for pressure areas when positioning, have client spend less time on affected side than in other positions.*

F. Assess for adduction and internal rotation of the affected arm; maintain arm in a neutral (slightly flexed) position with each joint slightly higher than the preceding one.

G. Restraints should be avoided because they often increase agitation.

H. Maintain joints in position of normal function to prevent flexion contractures.

I. Assist client out of bed on the unaffected side; this allows client to provide some stabilization and balance with the good side.

TEST ALERT: Mobility: Assist client to ambulate, perform active and passive ROM exercises, assess for complications of immobility, prevent DVT, prevent skin breakdown and encourage independence.

❖ **Goal:** To maintain homeostasis.

A. Evaluate adequacy of cardiac output.

B. Monitor hydration status: prevent fluid overload.
1. Carefully regulate IV fluid intake.
2. Evaluate response to diuretics.
3. Assess for the development of peripheral edema.
4. Restrict fluid intake, as indicated.
5. Assess respiratory parameters indicative of fluid overload.
6. Monitor daily weight.

C. Determine previous bowel patterns and promote normal elimination.
1. Avoid use of urinary catheter, if possible; if catheter is necessary, remove as soon as possible.
2. Offer bedpan or urinal every 2 hours; help establish a schedule.
3. Prevent constipation: provide increased bulk in diet, stool softeners, etc.
4. Provide privacy and decrease emotional trauma related to incontinence.

TEST ALERT: Assess and manage a client with an alteration in elimination. Establish a toileting schedule; the client who has had a stroke will need assistance in reestablishing a normal bowel and bladder routine.

D. Prevent problems of skin breakdown through proper positioning and good skin hygiene.

E. Assist client to identify problems of vision.

F. Maintain psychologic homeostasis.
   1. Client may be very anxious because of a lack of understanding of what has happened and because of his or her inability to communicate.
   2. Speak slowly and clearly and explain what has happened.
   3. Assess client's communication abilities and identify methods to promote communication.

Home Care

A. Encourage independence in ADLs.

B. Provide clothing that is easy to get in and out of.

C. Active participation in ROM; have client do his or her own ROM on affected side.

D. Physical, occupational, and speech therapy for retraining of lost function.

E. Assist client to maintain sense of balance when in the sitting position; client will frequently fall to the affected side (unilateral neglect syndrome).

F. Encourage participation in carrying out daily personal hygiene.

G. Teach client safe transfer from bed to wheelchair and provide assistance as needed.

H. Bowel and bladder training program.
   1. To promote bladder tone, encourage urination (with or without assistance) every 2 hours rather than allowing the client to void when he or she feels the urge.
   2. Teach client to perform Kegel exercises regularly.
   3. Advise client to avoid caffeine intake.
   4. Increased bulk in diet will help avoid constipation.
   5. Increase fluids to 2000 mL per day as tolerated.
   6. Administer stool softeners PRN.
   7. Establish regular daily time for bowel movements.

I. Encourage social interaction.
   1. Speech therapy.
   2. Frequent and meaningful verbal stimuli.
   3. Allow client plenty of time to respond.
   4. Speak slowly and clearly; do not give too many directions at one time. Use short sentences.
   5. Do not "talk down to" client or treat client as a child (elder speak).
   6. Client's mental status may be normal; do not assume it is impaired.
   7. Nonverbal clients do not lose their hearing ability.

J. Evaluate family support and the need for home health services.

> ✓ *NURSING PRIORITY: Assist family to manage care of a client with long-term care needs; determine needs of family regarding ability to provide home care after discharge.*

Cerebral Aneurysm, Subarachnoid Hemorrhage

❋ **A cerebral aneurysm occurs when a weakened saccular outpouching of the cerebral vasculature bulges from pressure on the weakened tissue. A Berry aneurysm is a cerebral aneurysm occurring in the arterial junction of the circle of Willis. A ruptured cerebral aneurysm often results in hemorrhagic stroke.**

A. A subarachnoid hemorrhage is a potentially fatal condition in which blood accumulates below the arachnoid mater in the subarachnoid space; most often occurs secondary to an aneurysm.

B. An aneurysm frequently ruptures and bleeds into the subarachnoid space.

C. Symptoms occur when an aneurysm enlarges, or when it ruptures. As blood collects in the subarachnoid space, it compresses and damages the surrounding brain tissue.

D. Subarachnoid hemorrhage may lead to neurologic compromise including seizures, stroke, permanent brain damage, and even death.

E. Often, symptoms do not appear until rupture has occurred.

Data Collection

A. Clinical manifestations.
   1. Rupture may be preceded by severe headache and nausea.
   2. Rupture frequently occurs without warning.
      a. Sudden severe headache, seizures.
      c. Nuchal rigidity, hemiparesis.
      d. Loss of consciousness.
      e. Symptoms of increasing ICP: nausea, vomiting, photophobia,
   3. Severity of symptoms depends on the site and amount of bleeding.

B. Diagnostics (see Appendix 15-1).

Treatment

A. Aminocaproic acid: inhibits fibrinolysis in life-threatening situations.

B. Osmotic diuretics, anticonvulsants.

C. Corticosteroids.

D. Calcium channel blockers: minimize vasospasm after hemorrhage.

E. Surgical intervention: ligation or "clipping" of the aneurysm to reduce the swelling and minimize the risk for re-bleeding.

Nursing Interventions

❖ **Goal:** To prevent further increase in ICP and possible rupture.

A. Immediate bed rest; bathroom privileges may be permitted.

B. Prevent Valsalva maneuver.
C. Client should avoid straining, sneezing, pulling up in bed, and acute flexion of the neck.
D. Elevate head of the bed 30 degrees to 45 degrees to promote venous return.
E. Quiet, dim, nonstimulating environment: disconnect telephone; promote relaxation.
F. Constant monitoring of condition to identify occurrence of bleeding, as evidenced by symptoms of increasing ICP.
G. Administer analgesics cautiously; the client should continue to be easily aroused so that neurologic checks can be performed.
H. No hot or cold beverages or food, no caffeine, no smoking.
I. Maintain seizure precautions (see Appendix 15-5).

> ✔ **NURSING PRIORITY:** *If the client survives the rupture of the aneurysm and re-bleeding occurs, it is most likely to occur within the next 24 to 48 hours.*

❖   **Goal:** To assess for and implement nursing measures to decrease ICP (see nursing goals for increased ICP).
❖   **Goal:** To provide appropriate preoperative nursing interventions (see nursing goals for brain tumor).
❖   **Goal:** To maintain homeostasis and monitor changes in ICP after craniotomy (see nursing goals for craniotomy).

Meningitis

✳   **Meningitis is an acute viral or bacterial infection that causes inflammation of the meningeal tissue covering the brain and spinal cord. Bacterial meningitis is less common but more severe than viral meningitis. Meningococcal meningitis is the only form that is readily contagious; transmitted by direct contact with droplets from the airway of an infected person.**

Data Collection

A. Clinical manifestations: older child and adult.
1. Rash, petechiae, purpura.
2. Nuchal rigidity.
3. Chills and high fever.
4. Severe and persistent headache.
5. Increasing irritability, malaise, changes in level of consciousness.
6. Respiratory distress.
7. Generalized seizures.
8. Nausea and vomiting.
9. Positive Kernig sign: resistance or pain at the knee and the hamstring muscles when client attempts to extend the leg after thigh flexion.
10. Positive Brudzinski sign: reflex flexion of the hips when the neck is flexed.
11. Photophobia.

C. Clinical manifestations: neonate and infant.
1. Fever.
2. Apneic episodes.
3. Bulging fontanel.
4. Seizures.
5. Crying with position change.
6. Opisthotonos positioning: a dorsal arched position.
7. Changes in sleep pattern, increasing irritability.
8. Poor sucking; may refuse feedings.
9. Poor muscle tone, diminished movement.
10. Irritability.
D. Diagnostics (see Appendix 15-1).
1. Lumbar puncture reveals increasing CSF pressure; if ICP is present, a CT scan may be done prior to procedure.
2. Elevated WBCs.
3. CSF and blood cultures positive for meningococcus bacteria.

Treatment

A. Droplet precautions until positive organism is identified.
B. IV antibiotics, steroids (see Appendices 5-9, 5-7).
C. Optimum hydration.
D. Anticonvulsant medications (see Appendix 15-2).
E. Antivirals.
F. Maintain ventilation.

Complications

A. Increasing ICP resulting in permanent brain damage.
B. Visual and hearing deficits, paralysis.
C. Subdural effusion; may be aspirated or allowed to absorb when meningitis treatment is started and protein leak stops.

Nursing Interventions

❖   **Goal:** To identify the causative organism, control spread, and initiate therapy.
A. Maintain respiratory droplet precautions until organism is identified; place client in a private room (Appendix 5-9).
B. Begin administration of IV antibiotics after lumbar puncture during which CSF sample was obtained.
C. Identify family members and close contacts who may require prophylactic treatment.
❖   **Goal:** To monitor course of infection and prevent complications.
A. Frequent nursing assessment for increased ICP (see Box 15-3).
B. Maintain adequate hydration; cerebral edema may require limiting fluid intake.
C. Monitor infusion site for complications of IV piggyback antibiotics.
D. Assess for side effects of high dosage of antibiotics.
E. Decrease stimuli in environment: dim lights, quiet environment, no loud noises.

F. Avoid movement or positioning that increases discomfort; client generally assumes a side-lying position.
G. Seizure precautions.
H. Prevent complications of immobility.
I. Good respiratory hygiene.
J. Measures to decrease fever.

Encephalitis

✳ **Encephalitis is an inflammatory process of the CNS, or "inflammation of the brain."**

Data Collection

A. Clinical manifestations.
  1. Severe headache, nuchal rigidity.
  2. Sudden fever.
  3. Seizures, irritability.
  4. Changes in level of consciousness.
  5. Motor involvement: ataxia, dysphasia, tremor, convulsions.
  6. Drowsiness, confusion, disorientation.
  7. Bulging fontanels in infants.
B. Diagnostics.
  1. Examination of the CSF.
  2. Viral studies to isolate the virus.
  3. EEG for seizure activity.
  4. Blood test for West Nile virus.

Treatment

A. Anticonvulsants.
B. Treatment to decrease ICP.
C. Hydration, bed rest, proper nutrition.

Nursing Interventions

Nursing interventions for encephalitis are the same as those for meningitis, with the exception of antibiotic therapy. Encephalitis is caused by a viral agent and is not responsive to antibiotic therapy; antibiotic therapy may be ordered to prevent bacterial infection.

> ✔ **NURSING PRIORITY:** *Identify changes in client's mental status; treat client with seizures.*

Spinal Cord Injury

✳ **Spinal cord injury (SCI) is damage to the spinal cord housed inside the spinal column. Most SCIs exist with the spinal cord intact yet compromised from injury or disease. SCI most often occurs as a result of direct trauma to the head or neck area.**

A. Initially after the injury, the nerve fibers swell, and circulation to the spinal cord is decreased; hemorrhage and edema occur, causing an increase in the ischemic process, which progresses to necrotic destruction of the spinal cord.
B. Consequences of SCI depend on the extent of damage, as well as the level of cord injury (Figure 15-5).
  1. The higher the lesion, the more severe the injury.
  2. Complete transection (complete cord dissolution, complete lesion): immediate loss of all sensation and voluntary movement below the level of injury; minimal, if any, return of function.
  3. Cord edema peaks in about 2 to 3 days and subsides within about 7 days after the injury.
D. Spinal cord shock (areflexia): temporary loss or dysfunction of spinal reflex activity; occurs predominantly in complete cord lesions; loss of communication with the higher centers of control results in flaccidity and loss of functional control below the level of injury.
  1. Interruption of nerve impulses leads to vasodilation, hypotension, and shock-like symptoms.
  2. Condition may persist for several weeks and reverse spontaneously; resolution of spinal shock will be evident by return of reflexes.
  3. Hyperreflexia will occur as recovery progresses; spastic movements may be precipitated by emotion and cutaneous stimulation.
E. Autonomic dysreflexia occurs in clients with an injury at T6 or higher.
  1. A noxious stimulus below the level of injury triggers the sympathetic nervous system, which causes a release of catecholamines (epinephrine, norepinephrine).
  2. Most common stimuli causing the response are a full bladder or bowel, UTI, pressure ulcers, and skin stimulation.

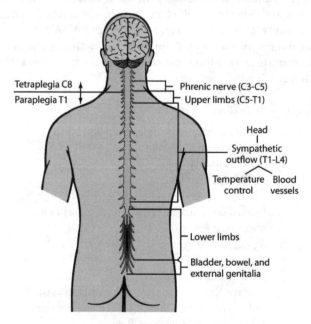

FIGURE 15-5 Spinal cord injury: areas of paralysis. (From Lewis SL, et al: *Medical-surgical nursing: assessment and management of clinical problems,* ed 7, St Louis, 2007, Mosby.)

3. Rapidly occurring severe hypertension, nausea, pounding headache, bradycardia, restlessness, flushing piloerection, and blurred vision are the most common body responses.

F. Bladder dysfunction will occur as a result of the injury; normal bladder control is dependent on the sensory and motor pathways and the lower motor neurons being intact.

G. Long-term rehabilitation potential depends on the amount of damage done to the cord, which may not be evident until several weeks after the injury.

Data Collection

A. Clinical manifestations: depend on level of SCI (see Figure 15-5).
   1. Injury at C3 through C5 will cause respiratory compromise.
   2. Depending on degree of injury, the degree of paralysis and amount of sensory loss below the level of injury will vary.
   3. Spinal shock.
      a. Generally occurs within 72 hours and may last for several weeks.
      b. Flaccid paralysis.
      c. Loss of sensation and absence of reflexes.
      d. Bowel and bladder dysfunction.
      e. Hypotension and bradycardia.
      f. After spinal shock, reflexes and autonomic activity return, as evidenced by development of spasticity.
   4. Autonomic dysreflexia in clients with injuries at T6 or higher.
      a. Severe hypertension, bradycardia.
      b. Complaints of headache.
      c. Flushing and diaphoresis above level of injury.
B. Diagnostics (see Appendix 15-1).
C. Complications.
   1. Respiratory stasis; pulmonary edema and emboli.
   2. Cardiovascular compromise from neurogenic shock, or autonomic dysreflexia.
   3. Skin breakdown resulting in localized and systemic infections.
   4. Immobility issues causing renal and gastrointestinal compromise.
   5. Psychologic, social, and body image issues.

Treatment

A. Emergency intervention required.
B. Corticosteroids within 8 hours of injury (methylprednisolone).
C. Immobilization of the vertebral column in cervical fracture.
   1. Cervical tongs (Crutchfield, Gardner-Wells) for cervical immobility.
   2. Halo vest/jacket traction to promote mobility.

3. Sterno-occipital mandibular immobilizer (SOMI) brace worn with cervical fusion.
D. Spinal surgery to remove bone fragments and assure spinal alignment.
E. Respiratory support as necessary.

Nursing Interventions

❖ **Goal:** To maintain stability of the vertebral column and prevent further cord damage.
A. Emergency care and treatment.
   1. Suspect SCI if there is any evidence of direct trauma to the head or neck area (contact sports, diving accidents, motor vehicle accident).
   2. Immobilize client and place on spinal board with the head and neck in a neutral position; do not allow the neck to flex.
   3. Airway, status of breathing and circulation are the primary concerns initially after injury.
   4. Neurogenic shock may occur within first 24 hours, observe for decreased B/P, severe bradycardia.

> ✔ *NURSING PRIORITY: Do not hyperextend the neck in a client with a suspected cervical injury. Airway should be opened by the jaw-lift method. Improper handling of the client often results in extension of the damaged area.*

   3. Maintain in extended position with no twisting or turning; do not remove cervical collar or spinal board until area of injury is identified.
   4. Maintain patent airway during transportation.
B. Maintain stability of the vertebral column as indicated by the level of injury.
   1. Prescribe and maintain bed rest on firm mattress with supportive devices (sandbags, skin traction, etc.); maintain alignment in the supine position; logroll without any flexion or twisting.
   2. Maintain cervical traction: tongs are inserted into the skull with traction and weights applied; do not remove weights; logroll to maintain spinal immobility.
   3. Halo vest/jacket traction: maintains cervical immobility but allows client to be mobile.
      a. If bolts or screws come loose, keep the client immobilized and call the doctor.
      b. Clean pin sites according to facility policy, observe for infection.
      c. Roll client onto his or her side at the edge of the bed and allow client to push up from the mattress to a sitting position. Never use the halo vest frame to assist the client to turn or sit up.
      d. Correct size of wrench should be kept at bedside to remove the anterior bolts in case of emergency.
      e. Assist client to maintain balance when standing; the traction is heavy for a person who is weak, and the client is at increased risk for falling.
   4. Maintain extremities in neutral, functional position.

TEST ALERT: *Apply, maintain, or remove orthopedic devices (e.g. traction, splints, braces, casts).*

C. Perform appropriate nursing intervention when surgery is indicated to stabilize the injury.
❖ **Goal:** To identify level of damage and changes in neurologic status.
A. Assess respiratory function: symmetrical chest expansion, bilateral breath sounds, presence of retractions or dyspnea.
B. Motor and sensory evaluation.
1. Ability to move extremities; strength of extremities.
2. Sensory examination, including touch and pain.
3. Presence of deep tendon reflexes.
C. Ongoing assessment and status of:
1. Bladder, gastric, bowel function.
2. Psychologic adjustment to the injury.
D. Evaluate history of how injury occurred; obtain information regarding how client was transported.
E. Determine status of pain.
❖ **Goal:** To maintain respiratory function.
A. Frequent assessment of respiratory function during the first 48 hours.
1. Changes in breathing pattern.
2. Observe breathing pattern for use of sternocleidomastoid and intercostal muscles for respiration.
3. Evaluate arterial blood gas values and pulse oximetry.
4. Determine development of hypoxia.
B. Maintain adequate respiratory function, as indicated.
1. Chest physiotherapy.
2. Incentive spirometry.
3. Changing position within limits of injury.
4. Assess for complications of atelectasis, pulmonary emboli, and pneumonia.
5. Nasopharyngeal or endotracheal suctioning based on airway and level of injury.
❖ **Goal:** To maintain cardiovascular stability.
A. Spinal shock.
1. Monitor vital signs and evaluate changes.
2. Vagal stimulation, hypothermia, and hypoxia may precipitate spinal shock.
3. Assess deep tendon reflexes and muscle strength as resolution of shock occurs.
B. Assess for development of autonomic dysreflexia; if it occurs:
1. Elevate the head of the bed, and check the client's blood pressure.
2. Assess for sources of stimuli: distended bladder (check urinary tubing), fecal impaction, constipation, tight clothing.
3. Relieve the stimuli, and dysreflexia will subside.
4. Maintain cardiovascular support during period of hypertension.

5. A hypertensive crisis from dysreflexia will require immediate intervention.
C. Evaluate cardiovascular responses when turning or suctioning client.
D. Apply antiembolism stockings or elastic wraps to the legs to facilitate venous return. (Lack of muscle tone and loss of sympathetic tone in the peripheral vessels result in decreases in both venous tone and venous return, which predispose client to deep vein thrombosis.)
E. Implement measures to promote venous return.

TEST ALERT: *Prevent complications of immobility; prevent venous stasis: identify symptoms of deep venous thrombosis, apply compression stockings, and change client's position.*

❖ **Goal:** To maintain adequate fluid and nutritional status.
A. During the first 48 hours, evaluate gastrointestinal function frequently; decrease in function may necessitate use of a nasogastric tube to decrease distention.
B. Prevent complications of nausea and vomiting.
C. Evaluate bowel sounds and client's ability to tolerate oral fluids.
D. Increase protein and calories in diet; may need to decrease calcium intake.
E. Evaluate for presence of paralytic ileus.
F. Increase roughage in diet to promote bowel function.
❖ **Goal:** To prevent complications of immobility (see Chapter 3).
❖ **Goal:** To promote bowel and bladder function.
A. Urine is retained as a result of the loss of autonomic and reflexive control of the bladder.
1. Intermittent catheterization or indwelling catheter may be used initially to prevent bladder distention.
2. Perform nursing interventions to prevent urinary tract infection; avoid urinary catheterization, if possible.
B. Determine type of bladder dysfunction based on level of injury.
C. Assess client's awareness of bladder function.
D. Initiate measures to institute bladder control.
1. Establish a schedule for voiding; have client attempt to void every 2 hours.
2. Use the Credé method (in adults) for manual expression of urine.
3. May be necessary to teach client self-catheterization.
4. Record output and evaluate for presence of residual urine.
E. Evaluate bowel functioning.
1. Incontinence and paralytic ileus frequently occur with spinal shock.
2. Incontinence and impaction are common later.

F. Initiate measures to promote bowel control (after spinal shock is resolved).
    1. Identify client's bowel habits before injury.
    2. Maintain sufficient fluid intake and adequate bulk in the diet.
    3. Establish specific time each day for bowel evacuation.
    4. Assess client's awareness of need to defecate.
    5. Teach client effective use of the Valsalva maneuver to induce defecation.
    6. Induce defecation by digital stimulation, suppository, or as a last resort, enema.

> ✔ **NURSING PRIORITY:** *Assess and manage a client with alteration in elimination; initiate a toileting schedule; the client with SCI may need bowel and bladder retraining, depending on level of the injury.*

❖   **Goal:** To maintain psychologic equilibrium.
A. Provide simple explanations of all procedures.
B. Anticipate outbursts of anger and hostility as client begins to work through the grieving process and adjusts to changes in body image.
C. Anticipate and accept periods of depression in client.
D. Encourage independence whenever possible; allow client to participate in decisions regarding care and to gain control over environment.

> 💡 **TEST ALERT:** *Plan measures to deal with client's anxiety and promote client's adjustment to changes in body image; assist client and significant others to adjust to role changes.*

E. Encourage family involvement in identifying appropriate diversional activities.
F. Avoid sympathy and emphasize client's potential.
G. Initiate frank, open discussion regarding sexual functioning.
H. Assist client and family to identify community resources.
I. Assist client to set realistic short-term goals.

Myasthenia Gravis

✳ **Myasthenia gravis is a sporadic, progressive neuromuscular disease characterized by a decrease in the acetylcholine level at the receptor sites in the neuromuscular junction. This results in a disturbance in nerve impulse transmission, causing progressive weakness in skeletal muscles. Myasthenia gravis literally means "grave muscle weakness."**

Data Collection

A. Risk factors/etiology.
    1. Autoimmune disease.
    2. More common in women younger than 40 and men older than 60 but may occur at any age.
B. Clinical manifestations.
    1. Primary problem is skeletal muscle fatigue with sustained muscle contraction; symptoms are predominantly bilateral.
        a. Muscular fatigue increases with activity.
        b. Ptosis (drooping of the eyelids) and diplopia (double vision) are frequently the first symptoms.
    c. Impairment of facial mobility and expression.
        d. Impairment of chewing and swallowing.
        e. Speech impairment (dysarthria).
        f. No sensory deficit, loss of reflexes, or muscular atrophy.
        g. Poor bowel and bladder control.
    2. Course is variable.
        a. May be progressive.
        b. May stabilize.
        c. May be characterized by short remissions and exacerbations.
    3. Myasthenic crisis: an acute exacerbation of symptoms that may require intubation and mechanical ventilation to support respiratory effort; caused by major muscular weakness and inability to maintain respiratory function.
        a. Severe respiratory distress and hypoxia.
        b. Increased pulse and blood pressure.
        c. Decreased or absent cough or swallow reflex.
    4. Cholinergic crisis: a toxic response to the anticholinesterase medications; anticholinesterase medications must be withheld—this response is rare with proper dosing of **Mestinon**.
        a. Nausea, vomiting, and diarrhea.
        b. Weakness with difficulty in swallowing, chewing, and speaking.
        c. Increased secretions and saliva.
        d. Muscle fasciculation, constricted pupils.
C. Diagnostics (See Appendix 15-1).
    1. Electromyography: shows a decreasing response of muscles to stimuli.
    2. Ice pack test: assess clients with ptosis; muscles improve with cold application; place pack on closed lids for 2 minutes to see whether ptosis improves.
    3. Tensilon test.
        a. Used for diagnosing myasthenia gravis.
        b. Used to differentiate cholinergic crisis from myasthenic crisis.
        c. IV injection of neostigmine or edrophonium causes immediate, although short-lived, relief of muscle weakness.

Treatment

A. Anticholinesterase (cholinergic) medications (see Appendix 15-3).
   1. Neostigmine (**Prostigmin**).
   2. Pyridostigmine (**Mestinon**).
B. Corticosteroids (see Appendix 5-7)
C. Plasma electrophoresis (plasmapheresis): separation of plasma to remove autoantibodies from the bloodstream.
D. Immunosuppressive therapy.
E. Surgical removal of the thymus (thymectomy).

Nursing Interventions

Client may be hospitalized for acute myasthenic crisis or for respiratory tract infection.

❖ **Goal:** To maintain respiratory function.

A. Assess for increasing problems of difficulty breathing. Measure forced vital capacity frequently to assess respiratory status.
B. Determine client's medication schedule. When was medication last taken?
C. Assess ability to swallow; prevent problems of aspiration.

> ✔ **NURSING PRIORITY:** *Identify clients at high risk for aspiration; do not give the client experiencing a myasthenic crisis anything to eat or drink.*

D. Evaluate effectiveness of cough reflex.
E. Be prepared to intubate or provide ventilatory assistance.

❖ **Goal:** To distinguish between a myasthenic crisis and a cholinergic crisis.

A. Maintain adequate ventilatory support during crisis.
B. Assist in administration of **Tensilon** test to differentiate crisis.
   1. Myasthenic crisis: client's condition will improve.
   2. Cholinergic crisis: client's condition will temporarily worsen.
C. If myasthenic crisis occurs, neostigmine may be administered.
D. If cholinergic crisis occurs, atropine may be administered, and cholinergic medications may be reevaluated.
E. Avoid use of sedatives and tranquilizers, which cause respiratory depression.
F. Provide psychologic support during crisis.

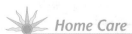 Home Care

A. Teach client importance of taking medication on a regular basis; peak effect of the medication should coincide with mealtimes.
B. If ptosis becomes severe, client may need to wear an eye patch to protect cornea (alternate eye patches if problem is bilateral).

C. Emotional upset, severe fatigue, infections, and exposure to extreme temperatures may precipitate a myasthenic crisis.

 Multiple Sclerosis

✳ **Multiple sclerosis (MS) is characterized by multiple areas of demyelination from inflammatory scarring of the neurons in the brain and spinal cord (CNS).**

A. The progression of the disease results in total destruction of the myelin, and the nerve fibers become involved.
   1. Loss of myelin sheath causes decreased impulse conduction, destruction of the nerve axon, and a blockage of the impulse conduction.
   2. The demyelination occurs in irregular scattered patches throughout the CNS.
B. The condition is chronic with unpredictable remissions and exacerbations.

Data Collection

A. Risk factors/etiology: cause is unknown; possible auto immune or exposure to viruses.
   1. More common in women.
   2. Problem of young adults.
   3. More common in cooler climates.
B. Clinical manifestations.
   1. Signs and symptoms vary from person to person, as well as within the same individual, depending on the area of involvement.
   2. Cerebellar dysfunction: nystagmus, ataxia, dysarthria, dysphagia.
   3. Motor dysfunction: weakness of eye muscles, weakness or spasticity of muscles in extremities.
   4. Sensory: vertigo, blurred vision, decreased hearing, tinnitus.
   5. Bowel and bladder dysfunction.
   6. Sexual dysfunction.
   7. Psychosocial.
      a. Intellectual functioning remains intact.
      b. Emotional lability: increased excitability and inappropriate euphoria.
      c. Emotional effects of the chronic illness and changes in body image.
C. Diagnostics: no definitive diagnostic test.

Treatment

A. No cure; medical treatment is directed toward slowing of the disease process and relief of symptoms.
B. Medications to decrease edema and inflammation of the nerve sites.
   1. Antiinflammatory agents.
   2. Immunosuppressive agents: interferons.
   3. Adrenocorticotropic hormone for acute exacerbations.

Nursing Interventions

Client may be hospitalized for diagnostic workup or for treatment of acute exacerbation and complications.

❖   Goal: To maintain homeostasis and prevent complications during an acute exacerbation of disease symptoms.

A.   Maintain adequate respiratory function.
1. Prevent respiratory tract infection.
2. Good pulmonary hygiene.
3. Prevent aspiration; sitting position for eating.
4. Evaluate adequacy of cough reflex.

B.   Maintain urinary tract function.
1. Prevent urinary tract infection.
2. Increase fluid intake, at least 3000 mL/24 hr.
3. Evaluate voiding: assess for retention and incontinence.

> **TEST ALERT: Monitor client's elimination pattern. Use alternative methods to promote client voiding.**

C.   Maintain nutrition.
1. Evaluate coughing and swallowing reflexes.
2. Provide food that is easy to chew.
3. If client is experiencing difficulty swallowing, observe client closely during fluid intake.

❖   Goal: To prevent complications of immobility (see Chapter 3).

❖   Goal: To promote psychologic well-being.

A.   Focus on remaining capabilities.
B.   Encourage independence and assist client to gain control over environment.
C.   If impotence is a problem, initiate sexual counseling.
D.   Assist client to work through the grieving process.
E.   Identify community resources available.

 Home Care

A.   Medical regimen and side effects of the medications.
B.   Physical therapy to maintain muscle function and decrease spasticity.
C.   Measures to maintain voiding; may need to perform self-catheterization.
D.   Safety measures because of decreased sensation.
1. Check bath water temperature.
2. Wear protective clothing in the winter.
3. Avoid heating pads and clothing that is constrictive.
E.   Client should understand that relapses are frequently associated with an increase in physiologic and psychologic stress.

 Guillain-Barré Syndrome

✳   **Guillain-Barré syndrome is an acute, rapidly progressing motor neuropathy involving segmental demyelination of nerve roots in the spinal cord and medulla. This causes inflammation, decreased nerve conduction, and rapidly ascending paralysis. Both sensory and motor impairment occur.**

Data Collection

A.   Clinical manifestations.
1. Progressive weakness and paralysis begin in the lower extremities and ascend bilaterally.
2. Paralysis ascends the body symmetrically.
a. Paralysis of respiratory muscles.
b. Cranial nerve involvement, most often facial nerve (CN VII), produces difficulty talking and swallowing.
3. Loss of sensation and function of bowel and bladder.
4. Manifestations may progress rapidly over hours or may occur over 2 to 4 weeks.
5. Muscle atrophy is minimal.
6. Paralysis decreases as the client begins recovery; most often, there are no residual effects.

> ✓ **NURSING PRIORITY:** Of the neuromuscular disorders, Guillain-Barré syndrome is the most rapidly developing and progressive condition. It is potentially fatal if unrecognized.

B.   Diagnostics (see Appendix 15-1).
1. Elevated protein concentration in CSF.

Treatment (Supportive)

A.   Respiratory support, possibly mechanical ventilation.
B.   Corticosteroids.
C.   Immunosuppressives and immunoglobulins.
D.   Plasmapheresis: plasma exchange.

Nursing Interventions

❖   Goal: To evaluate progress of paralysis and initiate actions to prevent complications.

A.   *Evaluate rate of progress of paralysis; carefully assess changes in respiratory pattern and report to charge nurse.*
B.   Frequent evaluation of cough and swallow reflexes.
1. Remain with client while client is eating; have suction equipment available.
2. Maintain NPO (nothing by mouth) status if reflexes are involved.
C.   If ascent of paralysis is rapid, prepare for endotracheal intubation and respiratory assistance.
D.   Prevent complications of immobility during period of paralysis (see Chapter 3).
E.   Assess for involvement of the autonomic nervous system.
1. Orthostatic hypotension.
2. Hypertension.
3. Cardiac dysrhythmias.
4. Urinary retention and paralytic ileus.

❖ **Goal:** To prevent complications of hypoxia if respiratory muscles become involved (see Chapter 10).

❖ **Goal:** To maintain psychologic homeostasis.

A.   Simple explanation of procedures.

B.   Complete recovery is anticipated.

C.   Provide psychologic support during period of assisted ventilation.

D.   Keep client and family aware of progress of disease.

 ## Amyotrophic Lateral Sclerosis

✳   **Amyotrophic lateral sclerosis (ALS), also known as Lou Gehrig's disease, is a rapidly progressive, invariably fatal degeneration of nerves controlling voluntary muscles.**

Data Collection

A.   Clinical manifestations.
1.   Twitching, cramping, and muscle weakness.
2.   Dysarthria and dysphagia.
3.   Fatigue; asymmetrical muscle atrophy and weakness.
4.   Progressive muscle weakness.
  a.   Begins with upper extremities and progressively involves muscles of neck and throat.
  b.   Trunk and lower extremities are involved late in course of disease.
5.   Most often fatal within 2 to 5 years after onset.
6.   Intellectual functioning and all five senses are usually unaffected.

B.   Diagnostics: electromyography and nerve conduction studies.

Nursing Interventions

❖   **Goal:** To provide ongoing assessment in assisting client to deal with progressive symptoms.

A.   Promote independence in ADLs.
1.   Conserve energy; space activities.
2.   Avoid extremes of hot and cold.
3.   Use of appliances to prolong independence in ambulation and ADLs.

B.   Promote nutrition.
1.   Small frequent feedings.
2.   Have client sit upright with head slightly flexed forward while eating.
3.   Keep suction equipment easily available during meals.

C.   Encourage family and client to talk about losses and the difficult choices they face.

D.   Assist family and client to identify need for advanced directives and to complete them.

 ## Muscular Dystrophy

✳   **Muscle dystrophy (MD) is a group of genetic diseases characterized by progressive weakness and skeletal** muscle degeneration affecting a variety of muscle groups. **The term *pseudohypertrophy* describes the characteristic muscle enlargement (caused by fatty infiltration) that occurs in muscular dystrophy.**

A.   Duchenne's muscular dystrophy is the most common and most severe form of MD.

B.   Condition is characterized by gradual degeneration of muscle fibers and progressive symmetrical weakness and wasting of skeletal muscle.

Data Collection

A.   Risk factors/etiology.
1.   Genetic: sex-linked disorder primarily affecting males, females are carriers.
2.   Onset generally occurs between the ages of 3 and 5 years.

B.   Clinical manifestations.
1.   History of delay in motor development, particularly a delay in walking.
2.   Abnormal waddling gait.
  a.   Child falls frequently and develops characteristic manner of rising.
  b.   Gower's sign: from sitting or squatting position, the child assumes a kneeling position and pushes the torso up by "walking" his or her hands up the thighs.
3.   Progressive muscle weakness, atrophy, and contractures.
  a.   Ambulation is frequently impossible by the age of 9 to 11 years.
  b.   Ultimately destroys essential muscles of respiration; death occurs from respiratory tract infection or cardiac failure.

C.   Diagnostics.
1.   Electromyography, muscle biopsy.
2.   Serum enzymes: creatinine phosphokinase level is increased in neonate, then gradually declines.

Treatment

A.   Steroids administered to boys older than 5 years of age.

Nursing Interventions

Child is frequently cared for at home and hospitalized only when complications occur.

❖   **Goal:** To maintain optimal motor function as long as possible.

A.   Regular physical therapy for stretching and strengthening muscles; ROM exercises.

B.   Maintain child's independence in ADLs.

C.   Assist family to identify resources, to adapt physiologic barriers within the home, and to promote mobility of the child in a wheelchair.

D.   Assist family to identify methods of preventing respiratory tract infection; assess for respiratory problems.

E.   Provide braces, splints, and assistive devices as needed.

❖ **Goal:** To assist parents and child to maintain psychologic equilibrium and to adapt to chronic illness.
A. Assist parents to understand importance of independence and self-help skills; frequently, parents are overprotective of the child.
B. Counseling to assist parents and family members to identify family activities that can be modified to meet child's needs.
C. Mother may feel particularly guilty because of transmission of disease to her son.
D. Identify available community resources.
E. Counseling to assist family and child with chronic illness and child's eventual death.

Cerebral Palsy

✻ **Cerebral palsy is a nonprogressive, lifelong neuromuscular genetic disorder resulting from damaged motor centers of the brain that cause nerve impulses to be incorrectly sent and/or received. The overall result is impairment of muscle control with poor muscle coordination.**

Data Collection

A. Risk factors/etiology.
1. May result from existing prenatal brain abnormalities (kernicterus, hemolytic disease of newborn).
2. Prematurity is single most important determinant of cerebral palsy.
B. Clinical manifestations.
1. Delayed achievement of developmental milestones.
2. Increased or decreased resistance to passive movement.
3. Abnormal posture.
4. Presence of infantile reflexes (tonic neck reflex, exaggerated Moro reflex).
5. Associated disabilities.
   a. Mental retardation, seizures.
   b. Attention-deficit problems.
   c. Vision and hearing impairment.
6. Muscle tightness and spasms.
C. Diagnostics.
1. Frequently difficult to diagnose in early months; condition may not be evident until child attempts to sit alone or walk.
2. Neurologic exam and contributing history.

Treatment

A. Maintain and promote mobility with orthopedic devices and physical therapy.
B. Skeletal muscle relaxants.
C. Anticonvulsants, as indicated.

Nursing Interventions

Child is frequently cared for at home and on an outpatient basis unless complications occur.

❖ **Goal:** To assist child to become as independent and self-sufficient as possible.
A. Physical therapy program designed to assist individual child to gain maximum function.
B. Bowel and bladder training may be difficult because of poor control.
❖ **Goal:** To maintain physiologic homeostasis.
A. Maintain adequate nutrition.
1. May experience difficulty eating because of spasticity; may drool excessively; use of manual jaw control when feeding.
2. Encourage independence in eating and use of self-help devices.
3. Provide a balanced diet with increased caloric intake to meet extra energy demands.
B. Maintain safety precautions to prevent injury.
C. Increased susceptibility to infections, especially respiratory tract infections, because of poor control of intercostal muscles and diaphragm.
D. Increased incidence of dental problems; schedule frequent dental checkups.
❖ **Goal:** To promote a positive self-image in the child and provide support to the family.
A. Assist parents to set realistic goals.
B. Encourage play activity.
C. Utilize principles in caring for chronically ill pediatric client (Chapter 2).

Parkinson's Disease (Paralysis Agitans)

✻ **Parkinson's disease is a progressive neurologic disorder with gradual onset that causes destruction and degeneration of nerve cells in the basal ganglia; results in damage to the extrapyramidal system, causing difficulty in control and regulation of movement.**

Data Collection

A. Risk factors/etiology.
1. In general, onset occurs after age 60.
2. More common in males.
B. Clinical manifestations (Figure 15-6).
1. Tremor.
   a. Affects the arms and hands bilaterally: often, the first sign.
   b. Tremors usually occur at rest; voluntary movement may decrease tremors; tremors during voluntary movement are not as common.
   c. Described as "pill-rolling" tremor.
   d. Exacerbated by emotional stress and increased concentration.
2. Muscle rigidity.
   a. Increased resistance to passive movement.
   b. Movement may be described as "cog-wheel rigidity" because of jerky movement of extremities.
3. Bradykinesia: slow activity.
   a. Decreased blinking of the eyelids.

b. Loss of ability to swallow saliva.

c. Facial expression is blank or "mask-like."

d. Loss of normal arm swing while walking.

e. Difficulty initiating movement.

4. Stooped posture, shuffling propulsive gait.

5. May exhibit mental deterioration similar to that associated with Alzheimer's disease.

6. Depression occurs in two-thirds of clients.

C. Diagnostics: no specific diagnostic test.

Treatment

A. Medications (see Appendix 15-4).

B. Surgical therapy: aim is to decrease symptoms.

1. Ablation (destruction of tissue).

2. Deep brain stimulation (DBS).

Nursing Interventions

❖ **Goal:** To maintain homeostasis.

A. Encourage independence in ADLs with use of self-help devices.

B. Maintain nutrition.

1. Increase calories and protein; provide more easily chewed foods.

2. Frequent small meals.

3. Allow ample time for eating.

4. Monitor weight loss.

5. Provide pleasant atmosphere at mealtime; client frequently prefers to eat alone because of difficulty swallowing and inability to control saliva.

6. Increase fluid intake with increased bulk in the diet to decrease problem with constipation.

C. Maintain muscle function.

1. Full ROM to extremities to prevent contracture.

2. Decrease effects of tremors.

3. Exercise and stretch daily.

4. Physical therapy, as indicated.

D. Closely monitor response to or changes in response to medications.

❖ **Goal:** To promote a positive self-image.

A. Encourage diversional activities.

B. Assist client to set realistic goals.

C. Explore reasons for depression; encourage client to discuss changes occurring in lifestyle.

D. Assist client in gaining control of ADLs and environment.

E. Assist client to identify and avoid activities that increase frustration levels.

F. Encourage good personal hygiene.

📋 Headache

✳ **Headache is a very common symptom of various underlying pathologic conditions in which pain-sensitive nerve fibers respond to unacceptable levels of stress and tension, muscular contraction in the upper body, pressure from a tumor, or increased ICP.**

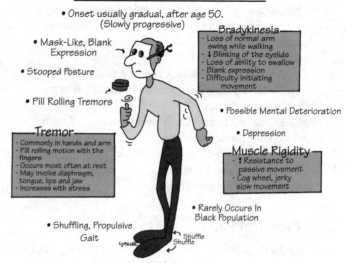

FIGURE 15-6 **Parkinson's disease.** (From Zerwekh J, Claborn J, Miller CJ: *Memory notebook of nursing, vol 1*, ed 4, Ingram, 2008, Nursing Education Consultants.)

Data Collection

A. Types of headaches.

1. Tension headache (muscle contraction headache): most common of all headaches; feeling of tightness like a band around the head; onset is gradual; may be accompanied by dizziness, tinnitus, or lacrimation; associated with stress and premenstrual syndrome.

2. Migraine: constriction of intracranial vessels leading to an intense throbbing pain when vessels return to normal; prodromal or aura; crescendo quality; unilateral pain, often beginning in eye area; nausea, vomiting, photophobia—migraines are seriously debilitating and may require lifestyle and occupational changes.

3. Cluster headache: rare headache that is more common in men; occurs in numerous episodes or clusters; no aura; unilateral pain often arising in nostril and spreading to forehead and eye; often occurs at same time of day.

Treatment

A. Migraine: sumatriptan (**Imitrex**); dihydroergotamine mesylate (**Migranal**).

B. Nonsteroidal antiinflammatory drugs.

C. Relaxation, yoga, stress management.

D. Cluster headaches treated with high flow oxygen.

Nursing Interventions

A. Prevention: recognize triggers, decrease stress, adjust medications during menstrual cycle.

B. Watch for signs of ominous headache: new-onset unilateral headache in person older than 35 years; vomiting not accompanied by nausea; pain that awakens client.

C. Encourage client to keep a "headache diary" for best management and treatment.

 Trigeminal Neuralgia

* **Trigeminal neuralgia is a fleeting unilateral sensory disturbance of cranial nerve V, causing brief, paroxysmal pain and facial spasm; also known as tic douloureux.**

Data Collection

A. Risk factors/etiology.
 1. Onset generally occurs between 20 and 40 years of age.
 2. Increased frequency with aging.
B. Clinical manifestations.
 1. Abrupt onset of paroxysmal intense pain in the lower and upper jaw, cheek, and lips.
 a. Tearing of the eyes and frequent blinking.
 b. Facial twitching and grimacing.
 c. Pain is usually brief; ends as abruptly as it begins.
 d. Pain may be described as severe, stabbing, and shock-like.
 2. Recurrence of pain is unpredictable.
 3. Pain is initiated by cutaneous stimulation of the affected nerve area.
 a. Chewing.
 b. Washing the face.
 c. Extremes of temperature: either on the face or in food.
 d. Brushing teeth.

Treatment

A. Medical management of pain (see Appendix 15-2): carbamazepine (**Tegretol**) and gabapentin (**Neurotin**).
B. Surgical intervention.
 1. Local nerve block.
 2. Surgical intervention to interrupt nerve impulse transmission.

Nursing Interventions

❖ **Goal:** To control pain.
A. Assess the nature of a painful attack.
B. Identify triggering factors; adjust environment to decrease factors.
 1. Keep room at an even, comfortable temperature.
 2. Avoid touching client.
 3. Avoid jarring the bed.
 4. Allow client to carry out own ADLs as necessary.
C. Administer analgesics to decrease pain.
❖ **Goal:** To maintain nutrition.
A. Frequently, client does not eat because of reluctance to stimulate the pain.
B. Provide lukewarm food that can be easily chewed.
C. Increase protein and calories.

Home Care

A. Identify presence of corneal reflex; provide protective eye care if reflex is absent.
B. If there is loss of sensation to the side of the face, client should:
 1. Chew on the unaffected side.
 2. Avoid temperature extremes in foods.
 3. Check the mouth after eating to remove remaining particles of food.
 4. Maintain meticulous oral hygiene.
 5. Have frequent dental checkups.

 Bell's Palsy

* **Bell's palsy is a transient cranial nerve disorder affecting the facial nerve (cranial nerve VII), characterized by a disruption of the motor branches on one side of the face, which results in muscle weakness or flaccidity on the affected side.**

Data Collection

A. Clinical manifestations.
 1. Lag or inability to close eyelid on affected side.
 2. Drooping of the mouth.
 3. Decreased taste sensation.
 4. Upward movement of the eyeball when the eye is being closed.
B. Diagnostics (see Appendix 15-1).

Treatment

A. Corticosteroids: administration should be started immediately after symptoms arise.
B. Antivirals.
C. Moist heat may relieve pain, if present.

Nursing Interventions

❖ **Goal:** To assess nerve function and prevent complications.
A. Analgesics to decrease pain.
B. Evaluate ability of client to eat.
C. Meticulous oral hygiene.
D. Prevent drying of the cornea on the affected side.
 1. Instill methylcellulose drops frequently during the day.
 2. Ophthalmic ointment and eye patches may be required at night.
E. As function returns, active facial exercises may be performed.
❖ **Goal:** To assist client to maintain a positive self-image.
A. Changes in physical appearance may be dramatic.
B. Tell client that the condition is usually self-limiting with minimal, if any, residual effects.
C. Client may require counseling, if change in facial appearance is permanent.

Study Questions: Neurologic System

1. An older adult client, diagnosed with Parkinson's disease, has been prescribed levodopa (l-dopa). What nursing observations would indicate the medication is working?
   1 Decrease in tremors in upper extremities.
   2 Blood pressure changes from 180/90 to 140/80 mm Hg.
   3 Urine output increases to 60 mL per hour.
   4 Increased strength on affected side.

2. The nurse is assisting a client with right-sided paralysis to get out of bed and into the wheelchair. What is an important safety principle for this transfer?
   1 Position client supine close to the edge of the bed.
   2 Position the wheelchair on the nonaffected side.
   3 Assist the client to stand and pivot to the wheel chair.
   4 Assist the client to sit, while two people move the client to the wheelchair.

3. The nurse is concerned about aspiration in a client who has had a stroke. What is the best nursing action to determine whether the client can begin oral intake of fluids safely?
   1 Touch the back of the client's throat with a tongue depressor to determine if this elicits the gag reflex.
   2 Place a few drops of water in the client's mouth and determine if this stimulates a swallowing reflex.
   3 Place the client in semi-Fowler's position and suction the airway; if this causes gagging and coughing, the client can take PO fluids.
   4 Wait until the client is fully responsive, place the client in semi-Fowler's position, and offer water through a straw.

4. The nurse is caring for a client who has just returned to his room from the recovery area after a craniotomy. What observation would the nurse report immediately to the RN or nursing supervisor?
   1 Confused and disoriented on awakening.
   2 Pupillary changes from equal and reactive to unequal and reactive only on right side.
   3 Urine output increased to 150 mL per hour for past 2 hours.
   4 Decreased breath sounds bilaterally and cough with no sputum production.

5. A client had a lumbar puncture, and the nurse is assessing the client after the procedure. What nursing observation would cause the nurse the most concern?
   1 Client complains of a headache.
   2 Clear fluid is observed to be oozing from the puncture site.
   3 Client complains of muscle weakness in upper extremities.
   4 Difficulty voiding from a supine position.

6. After a lumbar puncture, the client's post-treatment care plan states to keep him in a flat position for 3 to 6 hours. What is the purpose of this position?
   1 To decrease effects of hypertension.
   2 To increase the rate of replacement of spinal fluid.
   3 To increase ventilation and lung expansion.
   4 To prevent a headache from withdrawal of the spinal fluid.

7. The nurse enters the client's room as he begins to experience a generalized seizure. What is a priority nursing action?
   1 Hyperextend the neck to open the airway.
   2 Put a padded tongue depressor between the teeth.
   3 Record all events during seizure activity.
   4 Remain with the client and prevent injury.

8. A client is admitted to the nursing unit after a motor vehicle accident in which he sustained a head injury and now has a slow cerebrospinal fluid (CSF) leak. What would be important nursing interventions for this client?
   1 Frequent assessment and gentle cleaning of the nose and ears.
   2 Maintain client in a prone position to prevent aspiration.
   3 Maintain complete bed rest and low Fowler's position.
   4 Gently suction the nasopharynx area to promote pulmonary hygiene.

9. The nurse is caring for a postoperative craniotomy client. What nursing assessment data would be most important for the nurse to report?
   1 A pulse rate decrease from 90 to 70 beats per minute.
   2 A decrease in blood pressure from 140/90 to 120/80.
   3 Orientation change from alert and oriented to lethargic and confused.
   4 Decrease in bilateral breath sounds at the base of the lungs.

10. How can the nurse reliably assess the mental status of a client?
   1 Determine sensory function.
   2 Assess level of consciousness.
   3 Evaluate vital signs.
   4 Perform reality checks every 2 hours.

11. A client is experiencing increased intracranial pressure. Which response would be a characteristic change in the client's pupils?
   1 Reactive to light and pinpoint.
   2 Dilated and reactive to light.
   3 One is larger than the other.
   4 Fixed and pinpoint.

12. What is the best nursing measure to prevent constipation in clients after a stroke or a cerebrovascular accident?
    1 Encourage mobility and fluids.
    2 Offer an enema every other day.
    3 Administer laxatives three times a week.
    4 Use a glycerin suppository to stimulate defecation.
13. What nursing activities would assist in the prevention of complications in a client who is recovering from a stroke?
    1 Use a soft toothbrush and do not floss.
    2 Evaluate hourly urine output.
    3 Perform hourly neurological checks.
    4 Encourage mobility and deep breathing.
14. The nurse is caring for a client who has suffered a severe closed head injury from a motor vehicle accident. In report the nurse is told that the client has a Glasgow Coma Scale of 4. What would the nurse expect to find on the assessment of this client?
    1 Alert and responding appropriately to verbal commands.
    2 Lethargic, but arouses to verbal and physical stimulation.
    3 Responds to painful stimuli, no response to verbal stimuli.
    4 No intentional movement or response to stimuli.
15. In what position would the nurse place the stroke client to prevent tongue obstruction and/or aspiration in the airway?
    1 Side lying.
    2 Prone.
    3 Full-Fowler's.
    4 Semi-Fowler's.
16. What is the focus of nursing care immediately after a client has experienced a brain accident?
    1 Make sure there is adequate urinary output.
    2 Maintain a patent airway.
    3 Prevent contractures in arms and legs.
    4 Prevent skin break down on bony prominences.
17. The nurse is caring for a client who has had a stroke or brain accident affecting his right side. What activities will be important for the nurse to include in the care of this client?
    1 Passive range-of-motion exercises to the right side and active range-of-motion exercises on the left side.
    2 When assisting the client to eat, place the food on the affected side of the mouth.
    3 Turn every 2 hours and maintain position on the right side for 2 hours.
    4 Administer all intramuscular injections on the right side to decrease discomfort.
18. A client is scheduled for a computed tomography (CT) scan of the head. The nurse would explain to the client that:
    1 He will have to swallow a small amount of iodine for contrast studies.
    2 He will be asked to try to avoid moving during the test.
    3 After the test, he will have to remain on his back for 8 hours.
    4 He will have electrodes attached to his head.
19. The nurse is assigned a client who is described as being quadriplegic. What would the nurse expect to find on the evaluation of this client?
    1 One side of the client's body is paralyzed.
    2 The client is paralyzed with no sensation from the waist down.
    3 The client experiences no sensation to pain below the waist.
    4 There is minimal voluntary muscle response from the client's arms down.
20. Immobilization of a client with a spinal cord injury puts the client at increased risk for what complication?
    1 Bradycardia.
    2 Hypoglycemia.
    3 Peripheral edema.
    4 Skin breakdown.

Answers and rationales to these questions are in the section at the end of the book titled Chapter Study Questions: Answers and Rationales.

Appendix 15-1 NEUROLOGIC SYSTEM DIAGNOSTICS

Skull and Spine X-Ray Studies: Simple x-ray films are obtained to determine fractures, calcifications, etc.

Electroencephalography (EEG): A recording of the electrical activity of the brain to physiologically assess cerebral activity; useful for diagnosing seizure disorders; used as a screening procedure for coma; also serves as an indicator for brain death. May also be used to assess sleep disorders, metabolic disorders and encephalitis.

Nursing Implications
1. Explain to client that procedure is painless and there is no danger of electrical shock.
2. Determine from physician if any medications should be withheld before test, especially tranquilizers and sedatives.
3. Frequently, coffee, tea, cola, and other stimulants are prohibited before examination.
4. Client's hair should be clean before the examination; after the exam, assist client to wash electrode paste out of hair.

Carotid Doppler Ultrasonography: A noninvasive ultrasound scan to estimate blood flow in carotid.

Magnetic Resonance Imaging (MRI): Cell nuclei have magnetic properties; the MRI machine records the signals from the cells in a manner that provides information to evaluate soft tissue structures (tumors, blood vessels).

Nursing Implications
1. Procedure will take approximately 1 hour.
2. All metal objects should be removed from the client (hearing aids, hair clips, jewelry, buckles, etc.).
3. The client will be placed in a long magnetic tunnel for the procedure.
4. Poor candidates for MRI include the following.
    a. Clients with pacemakers (the magnetic field interferes with the function of the pacemaker and interferes with the test as well).
    b. Clients with implanted insulin pumps, or joint replacements.
    c. Pregnant clients, obese clients.
    d. Any client who requires life-support equipment (the equipment will malfunction in a magnetic field).

Computerized Axial Tomography (CAT) Scan: Computer-assisted x-ray examination of thin cross-sections of the brain to identify hemorrhage, tumor, edema, infarctions, and hydrocephalus. Machine is large donut-shaped tube with table through the middle.

Nursing Implications
1. Explain appearance of scanner to client and explain importance of remaining absolutely still during the procedure.
2. Remove all objects from client's hair; for 4 to 6 hours before test, client receives fluids only.
3. Dye will be injected via venipuncture; assess for iodine allergy and advise the client that he/she may experience a flushing or warm sensation when the dye is injected.
4. Contrast dye may discolor urine for about 24 hours.
5. Dye may be injected into spinal cord for assessment of intervertebral disks and bone density.

Brain Scan: A scanner traces the uptake of radioactive dye in the brain tissue. The dye is concentrated in the damaged tissue; it will take approximately 2 hours after dye is injected for the scan to be completed.

Nursing Implications
1. Determine whether medications need to be withheld before procedure.
2. Client will be asked to change positions during the test in order to visualize the brain from different angles.
3. The client should not experience any pain.

Caloric Testing: Test is performed at bedside by introducing cold water into the external auditory canal. It is contraindicated in the client with a ruptured tympanic membrane and is not done on the client who is awake. If the 8th cranial nerve is stimulated, nystagmus rotates toward the irrigated ear. If no nystagmus occurs, a pathologic condition is present.

Continued

Appendix 15-1 NEUROLOGIC SYSTEM DIAGNOSTICS—cont'd.

Lumbar Puncture: A needle is inserted into the lumbar area at the L4-L5 level; spinal fluid is withdrawn, and spinal fluid pressure is measured; contraindicated in presence of increased intracranial pressure. Normal spinal fluid values: opening pressure, 60 to 150 mm water; specific gravity, 1.007; pH, 7.35; clear fluid; protein concentration, 15 to 45 mg/dL; glucose concentration, 45 to 75 mg/dL; no microorganisms present.

Nursing Implications
Before test
1. Have client empty bladder.
2. Explain position (lateral recumbent with knees flexed) to client (Figure 15-7).
3. Advise physician if there is a change in the client's neurologic status before the test; increased intracranial pressure is a contraindication to a lumbar puncture.

After test
1. Keep client flat at least 3 hours, and sometimes up to 12 hours, to decrease occurrence of headache.
2. Encourage high fluid intake.
3. Observe for spinal fluid leak from puncture site; if leakage occurs, it may precipitate a severe headache.
4. Wear a surgical mask when placing a catheter or injecting material into the spinal column or subdural space (myelogram, lumbar puncture, spinal or epidural anesthesia).

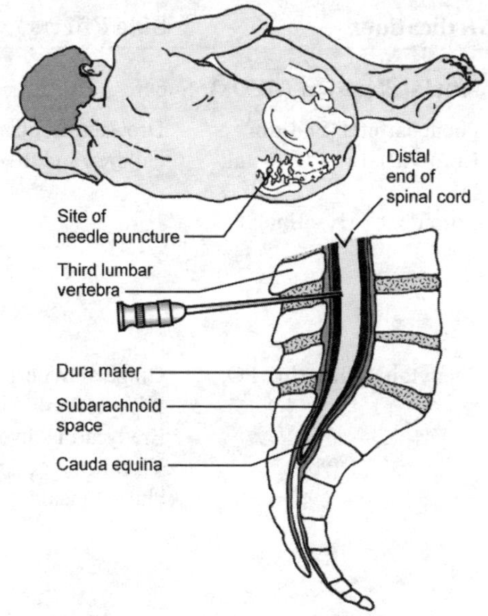

Myelogram: An outpatient procedure in which dye is injected into the subarachnoid space and x-ray films of the spinal cord and vertebral column are obtained to identify spinal lesions.

Nursing Implications
Before test
1. Same as for lumbar puncture.
2. Check whether client has any allergies to dye.

After test
1. Keep the head of the bed elevated 30 to 50 degrees to decrease dispersion of the dye in the CSF and to the brain.
2. Headache may occur as a result of irritation of the central nervous system.
3. Client should not receive any of the phenothiazines before or immediately after the examination.

FIGURE 15-7 **Lumbar puncture** (From deWit, S, *Medical-surgical nursing: Concepts and practices, ed 7*, St Louis, 2009, Saunders).

Cerebral Angiogram: Injection of contrast material into the cerebral circulation; series of x-rays films is taken to study the cerebral blood flow; dye is usually injected via a soft catheter that is inserted and threaded through the femoral artery.

Nursing Implications
Before test
1. Client should be well-hydrated, but should receive nothing by mouth for 6 to 8 hours before the test; client should void before procedure.
2. Determine if client has any allergies to iodine or to shellfish.
3. Inform client that he or she should remain very still during the procedure.
4. A feeling of warmth in the face and mouth and a metallic taste in the mouth are common when dye is injected.

After test
1. Evaluate client's neurologic status; complications involve occlusion of cerebral arteries.
2. Observe injection site for hematoma formation.
3. Posttest complications include continuous bleeding at injection site, rash, dizziness, and tingling in an extremity.
4. Check circulation distal to area of puncture.

Electromyography (EMG): Measures electrical discharge from a muscle. Flat electrodes or small needles are placed in the muscle. The client may be asked to move and perform simple activities; the electrical stimulus for the muscle will be recorded. Useful for diagnosis in spinal cord deformity, muscular dystrophy, myasthenia gravis or amyotrophic lateral sclerosis.

Nursing Implications
Before test
1. May determine pretest serum muscle determinations.
2. Explain to the client that small needles will be inserted into the skin.

After test
1. Client may need something for pain because of muscle stimulation.
2. Assess needle sites for areas of hematomas; apply ice pack to prevent and/or relieve.

Appendix 15-2 ANTIEPILEPTICS

Medications	Side Effects	Nursing Implications
Antiepileptics (AEDs): Suppress discharge of neurons within a seizure focus to reduce seizure activity.		
Phenobarbital (**Sodium Luminal**): IM, PO, rectal, IV Primidone (**Mysoline**): PO	Drowsiness, ataxia, excitation in children and the older adult	1. Client should avoid potential hazardous activities requiring mental alertness. 2. Sudden withdrawal from chronic use may precipitate symptoms. 3. Closely observe response in children and older adult. 4. Used to treat grand mal and focal seizures. 5. See Appendix 15-5 for care of client with seizures.
Phenytoin (**Dilantin**): PO, IV	Gingival hyperplasia, skin rash, hypoglycemia Bradycardia, hypotension Visual changes: nystagmus, diplopia, blurred vision	1. Administer PO preparations with meals or milk to decrease gastric irritation. 2. Frequently used with phenobarbital for control of grand mal seizures. 3. IM injection is not recommended. 4. Do not mix with any other medications when administering IV solution. 5. Promote good oral hygiene; gum hyperplasia is a problem with long-term use. 6. See Appendix 15-5 for care of client with seizures. 7. AEDs should be withdrawn slowly over 6 weeks to several months when medication therapy is discontinued.
Divalproex sodium (**Depakote**): PO	GI disturbances, rash, weight gain, hair loss, tremor, blood dyscrasias GI, dermatologic effects, blood dyscrasias	1. Should not be given to clients with severe liver dysfunction. 2. Potentiates action of phenobarbital, phenytoin, diazepam. 3. *Uses*: seizures, bipolar disorder, migraine.
Carbamazepine (**Tegretol**): PO, suspension	Drowsiness, dizziness, headache; visual disturbances common during first few weeks of treatment	1. Wean client from medication as soon as seizures are controlled. 2. Antimanic properties as well.
Clonazepam (**Klonopin**): PO	CNS depression, ataxia	1. Antianxiety effects may assist with seizure control. 2. Monitor results of liver function tests.

CNS, Central nervous system; *GI*, gastrointestinal; *IM*, intramuscular; *IV*, intravenous; *PO*, by mouth (orally).

Appendix 15-3	CHOLINERGIC (ANTICHOLINESTERASE) MEDICATIONS	

Medications	Side Effects	Nursing Implications
Cholinergic: Intensify transmission of impulses throughout the CNS, where acetylcholine is necessary for transmission.		
Neostigmine bromide (**Prostigmin**): PO, subQ, IM Pyridostigmine bromide (**Mestinon**): PO, IM, IV Edrophonium chloride (**Tensilon**): IV, IM	Excessive salivation, increased GI motility, urinary urgency, bradycardia, visual problems	1. Primary group of medications used for treatment of myasthenia gravis. 2. Atropine is the antidote for overdose. 3. In treatment of myasthenia gravis, medication is frequently administered 30 to 45 minutes before meals. 4. Mestinon is given as maintenance therapy for the client with myasthenia gravis. 5. Tensilon is used for diagnostic purposes; not recommended for maintenance therapy. 6. Teach client symptoms of side effects and advise client to call the doctor if they are present.

CNS, Central nervous system; *GI*, gastrointestinal; *IM*, intramuscular; *IV*, intravenous; *PO*, by mouth (orally); *subQ*, subcutaneous.

Appendix 15-4	ANTIPARKINSONISM AGENTS	

Medications	Side Effects	Nursing Implications
Anticholinergics: Inhibit action of acetylcholine at sites throughout the body and CNS. Decrease synaptic transmissions in the CNS.		
Benztropine mesylate (**Cogentin**): PO, IM, IV Trihexyphenidyl hydrochloride (**Artane**): PO, IM, IV Procyclidine (**Kemadrin**): PO	Paralytic ileus, urinary retention, cardiac palpitations, blurred vision, nausea and vomiting, sedation, dizziness Minor side effects such as dry mouth, jitteriness, and nausea	1. Administer PO preparations with meals to decrease gastric irritation. 2. Medications have cumulative effect. 3. Should not be used in clients with glaucoma, myasthenia gravis, GU or GI tract obstruction or in children younger than 3 years. 4. Monitor client carefully for bowel and bladder problems. 5. May be used to treat side effects of Thorazine.
Dopaminergics: Assist to restore normal transmission of nerve impulses.		
Levodopa (**L-DOPA, Larodopa**): PO	*Early:* Anorexia, nausea and vomiting, abdominal discomfort, postural hypotension *Long-term:* Abnormal, involuntary movements, especially involving the face, mouth, and neck; behavioral disturbances involving confusion, agitation, and euphoria	1. Administer PO preparations with meals to decrease GI distress. 2. Almost all clients will experience some side effects, which are dose related; dosage gradually increased according to client's tolerance and response. 3. Onset of action is slow; therapeutic response may require several weeks to months. 4. Vitamin B_6 (pyridoxine) is antagonistic to the effects of the medication; decrease client's intake of multiple vitamins and fortified cereals.
Carbidopa/levodopa (**Sinemet**): PO	Same as for levodopa	1. Same as for levodopa. 2. Use of carbidopa significantly decreases the amount of levodopa required for therapy. 3. Prevents inhibitory effects of levodopa on vitamin B_6.
Amantadine hydrochloride (**Symmetrel**): PO	Orthostatic hypotension, dyspnea, dizziness, drowsiness, blurred vision, constipation, urinary retention (side effects are dose related)	1. Less effective than levodopa; produces a more rapid clinical response.

CNS, Central nervous system; *GI*, gastrointestinal; *GU*, genitourinary; *IM*, intramuscular; *IV*, intravenous; *PO*, by mouth (orally).

| Appendix 15-5 | SEIZURE DISORDERS |

A seizure disorder is the interruption of normal brain functioning by uncontrolled paroxysmal discharge of electrical stimuli from the neurons.

Classification of Seizures

Simple Partial Seizures (remains conscious throughout seizure)

Rarely last longer than 1 minute; an aura may occur before the seizure.
1. Confined to a specific area (hand, arm, leg), client may experience unusual sensations.
2. One-sided movement of an extremity.
3. Autonomic changes – skin flushing, change in heart rate, epigastric discomfort.

Complex Partial Seizures (may have impairment of consciousness)
1. May loose consciousness for 1-3 minutes.
2. May produce automatisms (lip smacking, grimacing, repetitive hand movements).
3. Client may be unaware of environment and wonder at the beginning of the seizure.
4. In the period after the seizure, client may experience amnesia and confusion.
5. Also called temporal lobe seizures or psychomotor.

Generalized Seizures (bilaterally symmetric and without local onset)

No warning or aura, as client loses consciousness for a few seconds to several minutes.
1. Absence (petit mal): Characterized by a short period of time when the client is in an altered level of consciousness. Staring, blinking period (followed by resumption of normal activity) is characteristic. May occur more than 100 times per day; may go unnoticed; in general, onset is in childhood between the ages of 4 and 12 years.
2. Tonic-clonic seizures: May last 2-5 minutes. Full recovery may take several hours; client may be confused, amnesic, and irritable during this recovery period.
    Tonic phase: Loss of consciousness with stiffening and rigidity of muscles. Apnea and cyanosis are common during this period; phase generally lasts for about 1 minute.
    Clonic phase: Hyperventilation, with rapid jerking movements. Tongue biting, incontinence, and heavy salivation may occur during this period.

Seizure Etiology

Acute Disorders

Rarely last longer than 1 minute; an aura may occur before the seizure.
- Increased intracranial pressure, metabolic alterations
- Infections, febrile episodes in children (generally between 6 months and 3 years)

Chronic (Recurrent, Epilepsy)
- Brain injury at birth, trauma, vascular disease
- Brain tumors, genetic factors, idiopathic

Nursing Assessment
1. Identify any activities that occurred immediately before the seizure.
2. Was the client aware a seizure was going to occur? If so, how did client know?
3. Describe type of movements that occurred and the body area affected (e.g., jaw clenched, tongue biting).
4. Presence of incontinence.
5. Period of apnea and cyanosis.
6. Presence of automatisms (lip smacking, grimacing, chewing).
7. Duration of seizure: time the seizure.
8. Changes in level of consciousness.
9. Condition of client after seizure: oriented, level of activity, any residual paralysis or muscle weakness.

> ✔ *NURSING PRIORITY: Airway management and ventilation cannot be performed on a client who is experiencing a tonic-clonic seizure. After the seizure is over, evaluate the airway and initiate ventilations as necessary.*

Continued

Appendix 15-5   SEIZURE DISORDERS—cont'd.

Nursing Management

1. Remain with the client who is having a seizure; note the time the seizure began and how long it lasted.
2. Do not attempt to force anything into the client's mouth if the jaws are clenched shut.
3. If the jaws are not clenched, place an airway in the client's mouth. This protects the tongue and also provides a method of suctioning the airway, should the client vomit.
4. Protect the client from injury (risk for falling out of bed or striking self on bedrails, etc).
5. Loosen any constrictive clothing.
6. Do not restrain client during seizure activity; allow seizure movements to occur, but protect client from injury.
7. Evaluate respiratory status; if vomiting occurs, be prepared to suction the client to clear the airway and prevent aspiration.
8. Maintain calm atmosphere and provide for privacy after the seizure activity.
9. Reorient client.

> **TEST ALERT:** *Report characteristics of a client's seizure; determine changes in client's neurologic status.*

Client Education

1. Identify activities/events that precipitate the seizure activity.
2. Avoid alcohol intake, fatigue, and loss of sleep.
3. Take medications as directed.
4. Counseling for the family and for the client to assist them in maintaining positive coping mechanisms.
5. Wear medical alert bracelet or have identification card.

Appendix 15-6   APHASIA

Aphasia is a total loss of comprehension and use of language. The most common cause of aphasia is vascular. The speech center is located in the dominant side of the cerebral hemisphere. A stroke affected the left cerebral hemisphere of the brain commonly affects the area of language. Clients with aphasia are often frustrated and irritable. Emotional lability is common. Accept the behavior in a manner that prevents embarrassment for the client.

Types of Aphasia

Sensory aphasia (receptive or fluent, Wernicke's area): Cannot understand oral or written communication. Client cannot interpret or comprehend speech or read.

Motor aphasia (expressive, Broca's aphasia): Inability to speak or to write. However, the client can comprehend incoming speech and can read.

Mixed: Most aphasia involves both the sensory and motor aspects of speech. Rarely is aphasia only sensory or only motor.

Global aphasia: All communication and receptive function is lost.

Dysarthria: A disturbance in the muscular control of speech. Does not affect the meaning of communication or comprehension, just the mechanics of speech—pronunciation, articulation, and phonation.

Nursing Implications

1. Stand in front of the client; speak clearly and slowly.
2. Do not shout or speak loudly; the client can hear.
3. Be patient; give the client time to respond; do not press him or her for immediate answers.
4. Use nonverbal communications such as touch, smiles, and gestures.
5. Assist the client with motor aphasia to practice repeating simple words such as yes, no, and please.
6. Listen carefully, try to understand, and try to communicate; this conveys to the client that you care.
7. Involve family members in practice and assist them to identify ways they can support the client.

> **TEST ALERT:** *Assist client to communicate effectively.*

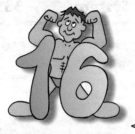

Musculoskeletal and Connective Tissue System

✗ Read every line!

PHYSIOLOGY OF THE MUSCULOSKELETAL SYSTEM

Skeletal System

A. Bone structure.
  1. Periosteum: dense fibrous membrane covering the bone; periosteal vessels supply bone tissue.
  2. Epiphysis: a widened area found at the end of a long bone.
  3. Epiphyseal plate (growth plate): a cartilaginous area in children's bones that provides for longitudinal growth of the bone.
  4. Red bone marrow: primary function is production of red blood cells.

B. Bone maintenance and healing.
  1. Regulatory factors determining bone formation and resorption.
     a. Weight-bearing stress stimulates local bone resorption and formation; therefore in states of immobility where weight bearing is prevented, calcium is lost from the bone.
     b. Vitamin D promotes absorption of calcium from the gastrointestinal (GI) tract and accelerates mobilization of calcium from the bone to increase or maintain serum calcium levels.

C. Musculoskeletal changes in the older adult (Box 16-1).

Connective Tissue: Joints and Cartilage

A. Joints.
  1. The action of joints permits bones to change position and facilitate body movement.
  2. Synovial joints contain synovial fluid, which lubricates the joints and facilitates joint mobility.
  3. Cartilage is rigid fibrous tissue that forms a capsule over the end of the bone and joins the end of each bone together.

B. Ligaments and tendons are tough fibrous connective tissue that provides stability while continuing to permit movement.
  1. Tendons attach muscles to the bone.
  2. Ligaments attach bones to joints.

Skeletal Muscle

A. Muscles are attached to tendons, bones, and connective tissue.
B. Lower motor neurons control the activity of skeletal muscle.

C. Energy is consumed when skeletal muscles contract in response to a stimulus.
D. Muscle contraction.
  1. Muscles accomplish movement only by contraction.
     a. Flexion: bending at a joint.
     b. Extension: straightening of a joint.
     c. Abduction: action moving away from the body.
     d. Adduction: action moving toward the body.

> ✓ **NURSING PRIORITY:** *When caring for clients with orthopedic or musculoskeletal problems, it is essential to know the terms used for referring to movement of the joints.*

  2. Hypertrophy, or increased muscle mass, will occur if muscle is exercised repeatedly.
  3. Atrophy, or decreased muscle mass, will occur with muscle disuse.

 ### System Data Collection

A. History.
  1. History of musculoskeletal injuries, neuromuscular disabilities, inflammatory and metabolic conditions directly or indirectly affecting the musculoskeletal system.
  2. Familial predisposition to orthopedic problems.

BOX 16-1 | **OLDER ADULT CARE FOCUS**
Musculoskeletal Changes

- Decreased bone density leads to more frequent fractures.

- Decrease in subcutaneous tissue results in less soft tissue over bony prominences.

- Degenerative changes in the spine alter posture and gait; disk compression causes a loss in height.

- Degenerative changes in cartilage and ligaments result in decreased joint movement as well as causing joint stiffness and pain.

- Decreased range of motion of extremities; older adult may need increased assistance with activities of daily living.

- Slowed movement and decreased muscle strength lead to decreased response time.

3. Level of normal activity.
   a. Occupation, exercise, recreation.
   b. Level of normal activity, ability to maintain own ADLs.
4. Existence of other chronic health problems.

B. Physical assessment.
1. Initial inspection for gross deformities, asymmetry, swelling, and edema.
2. Nutritional status: appropriateness of client's weight and body frame.
3. Joints
   a. Movement: active and passive; examine active movement first; compare movement and range of motion to opposite side.
   b. Inflammation and tenderness: with or without movement.
   c. Presence of joint deformities or dislocations.
   d. Palpate joints for the presence of crepitus.
4. Evaluate client's spinal alignment, posture, and gait.
5. Evaluate skeletal muscle.
   a. Muscle strength bilaterally.
   b. Coordination of movement.
   c. Presence of atrophy or hypertrophy.
   d. Presence of involuntary muscle movement.
6. Assess peripheral pulses and peripheral circulation; capillary refill should normally take about 2 to 3 seconds.
7. Assess for presence of and characteristics of pain.
   a. Most musculoskeletal pain is relieved by rest.
   b. Identify precipitating activities and/or precipitating factors.
   c. Type of pain and location.
8. Assess for any alteration of normal sensation in extremities.
9. Assess for use of proper body mechanics (Box 16-2).
10. Assess for changes in musculoskeletal system related to aging (Box 16-1).
11. Principles of body mechanics for health care personnel (Box 16-2, Appendix 3-1).

> **TEST ALERT: Orthopedic questions may be based on concepts of immobility, nursing assessment of an extremity, compromised circulation, and/or general perioperative care. Pay close attention to the direction of the question.**

Developmental Dysplasia of the Hip

* **Malformations of the hip that occur as a result of imperfect development of the femoral head, the acetabulum, or both.**

BOX 16-2   BODY MECHANICS

- The wider the base of support, the greater the stability. Position your feet wide apart.
- The lower the center of gravity, the greater the stability. Flex the knees; let the strong muscles of the legs do the work.
- Position yourself close to object and/or client.
- Face the client; keep back, pelvis, and knees aligned; avoid twisting.
- Balance activity between arms and legs.
- Avoid bending to lift; this decreases strain on the back.
- Encourage client to assist.
- Pivoting, turning, rolling, and leverage require less work.
- Person with heaviest load should coordinate team efforts.
- Obtain assistance with heavy or difficult transfers or lifts.
- Teach clients proper body mechanics.

> **TEST ALERT:** *Use good body mechanics when providing care – use assistive devises when possible.*

Data Collection (Newborn)

A. Ortolani sign: With the infant supine, knees flexed, and hips fully abducted, a click is heard or felt as the hip is abducted.
B. Asymmetrical gluteal and thigh folds.
C. Shortening of the leg on the affected side.
D. Limited hip abduction on affected side.

Treatment

A. Treatment should be initiated as soon as condition is identified.
B. Abduction devices.
   1. Pavlik harness is a fabric harness that maintains the legs in the flexed, abducted position at the hip, it will hold the affected hip in an abduction position, and prevent extension and adduction. It may be removed for bathing but the infant will wear it fulltime until the hip is stable.
   2. Hip spica cast may be used when an adduction contracture is present.
C. Surgery may be done if the correction is not feasible with abduction devices.

Nursing Interventions

❖ **Goal:** To identify problem in the newborn before discharge.
❖ **Goal:** To assist parents to understand mechanism to maintain reduction.

A. Pavlik harness.

1. Put an undershirt on the infant and place the brace on the outside of the shirt; always place the brace straps on the outside of the diaper.
2. Check the skin under the harness for irritation or pressure areas.
3. Do not apply oils or lotions under the harness.
4. Evaluate peripheral circulation and maintain cleanliness.

B. Teach parents cast care if hip spica cast is applied.

> ★ **TEST ALERT: Apply or remove immobilizing equipment.**

❖ **Goal:** To facilitate developmental progress and adapt nurturing activities to meet needs of infant and parents.
A. Provide appropriate stimuli and activity for developmental level.
B. Encourage parents to hold and cuddle child.
C. Maintain normal home routine.

Herniated Intervertebral Disk

✳ **The intervertebral disk forms a cushion between the vertebral bodies of the spinal column. As stress on an injured or degenerated disk occurs, the cartilage material of the disk (nucleus pulposa) herniates inward toward the spinal column, causing compression or tension on the spinal nerve root.**

Data Collection

A. The problem most commonly occurs in the lumbosacral area.
B. May be caused by an injury or stress to the lower back.
C. Clinical manifestations.
1. Low back pain radiating down one buttock and the posterior thigh (sciatica pain).
2. Coughing, straining, sneezing, bending, twisting, and lifting aggravate the pain.
3. Lying supine and raising the leg in an extended position will precipitate the pain.
D. Diagnostics: Appendix 16-1.

Treatment

A. Medical.
1. Analgesics, muscle relaxants, antiinflammatory medications.
2. Weight reduction if appropriate.
3. Cool therapy (ice) may be used for the first 24 to 48 hours after an injury, and then moist heat is applied.
4. Physical therapy.
5. Bed rest with good body alignment when pain is acute, then activity modification using good body mechanics.

B. Surgical.
1. Laminectomy: removal of the herniated portion of the disk.
2. Microlaminectomy (diskectomy): removal of the herniated disk with the use of a microscope to minimize the incision. There is less trauma in the disk area, improved hemostasis, minimal nerve root involvement, and quicker recovery using this procedure.

Nursing Interventions

❖ **Goal:** To relieve pain via conservative measures and prevent recurrence of problem.
A. Decrease muscle spasms with bed rest and medications.
B. Begin ambulation slowly and avoid having client bend, stoop, twist, sit, or lift.
C. Instruct the client regarding the principles of proper body mechanics (Box 16-2) and any prescribed mobility limitations.
D. The client will need a firm mattress; client should not sleep or lie in the prone position.
E. Encourage correct posture; avoid prolonged standing.
F. Sit in straight-backed chairs with firm seat and arm rests.

❖ **Goal:** To prepare client for laminectomy.
A. Follow general preoperative nursing interventions.
B. Have client practice logrolling preoperatively.
C. Have a male client practice voiding from supine position.
D. Explain to client that postoperative pain is very similar to preoperative pain, due to temporary inflammation and edema of the area around the spinal cord.
E. Evaluate bowel and bladder function.
F. Record specific characteristics of pain to include in a database so that preoperative pain can later be compared with postoperative pain.
G. Establish a baseline neurologic assessment for postoperative reference.

❖ **Goal:** To maintain spinal alignment postoperative laminectomy.
A. Keep the bed in a flat position.
B. Logroll client when turning.
C. Keep pillows between the legs when positioned on the side; do not place pillow under the knees.
D. Elastic stockings or pneumatic compression devices may be used to increase venous return.
E. Encourage good pulmonary hygiene (e.g., increase fluid intake; perform coughing, deep breathing, and spirometry exercises).
F. The client with microdisk surgery will have fewer limitations on mobility. Generally, the client may assume a position of comfort.

❖ **Goal:** To maintain homeostasis and assess for complications postoperative laminectomy.

> ✔ *NURSING PRIORITY: A hematoma at the incisional area may cause swelling and pressure resulting in neurological deficits in the lower extremities.*

A.   Evaluate incision area for possible leakage of spinal fluid and bleeding.

> ✔ *NURSING PRIORITY: Notify RN or surgeon if clear fluid is leaking from incision.*

B.   Evaluate characteristics of pain, administer analgesics.
C.   Perform neurovascular checks on extremities.
　1.   Evaluate sensation of extremities.
　2.   Evaluate ability to move feet and toes.
　3.   Evaluate vascular status of legs and feet.
D.   Assess for urinary retention and loss of sphincter control. *Need to notify RN or physician immediately; it may be an indication of cord compression.* Normal bladder function usually returns in 24-48 hours.
E.   Ambulate as soon as indicated (frequently on first postoperative day if no fusion was done). Client who has a microdisk laminectony will have fewer limitations on movement.
F.   If fusion was performed, often need to apply a back brace or body brace before ambulation.
G.   The client with the microlaminectomy generally experiences less pain, is frequently out of bed the day of surgery, and has fewer complications.

> ✔ *NURSING PRIORITY: The laminectomy client frequently has difficulty voiding after surgery. Palpate the suprapubic area to make sure the bladder is not full.*

Scoliosis

＊   **Adolescent idiopathic scoliosis is a lateral curvature of the spine. Without treatment, it will severely affect the shape of the thoracic cavity and impair ventilation.**

Data Collection

A.   Most frequently identified at beginning of growth spurt; more common in females.
B.   Visible curvature of the spinal column; head and hips are not in alignment.
C.   When client bends forward from the waist, there is visible difference in the level of the shoulders. The ribs and shoulder are more prominent on one side.
D.   Waistline is uneven, one hip is more prominent.
F.   Defect is progressive if not treated.

Treatment

A.   Brace if spinal curvature progresses, Cotrel's traction used for early correction; Milwaukee brace used for high thoracic curvatures.
B.   Surgery: spinal fusion and placement of a rod or instrument to maintain alignment of the fused segment. The rod may be left in place permanently unless it becomes displaced or causes discomfort.

Nursing Interventions

❖   **Goal:** To identify defects early and promote effective conservative therapy.
A.   Promote health programs in schools to identify condition.
B.   Assist client and parents to properly use braces.
　1.   Ensure brace is properly fitted and does not inadvertently rub bony prominences.
　2.   May put light T-shirt under brace for comfort.
　3.   Initially the brace is worn 20 to 23 hours per day.
　4   Brace is regularly adjusted to promote correction.
　5.   If progress is good, child is weaned from the brace during the daytime and wears it only at night.
　6.   Supplemental exercises may be prescribed.
❖   **Goal:** To maintain spinal alignment postoperative correction (see preceding postoperative laminectomy goal).
❖   **Goal:** To maintain homeostasis and assess for complications postoperative correction (see preceding postoperative laminectomy goal).

Fractures

＊   **A disruption or break in the continuity of a bone; generally occurs from a traumatic injury.**
A.   Pathological fractures occur secondary to a disease process.
B.   Classification of fractures.
　1.   Type.
　　a.   Comminuted: fracture with multiple bone fragments; more common in adults.
　　b.   Greenstick: an incomplete fracture with bending and splintering of the bone; more common in children.
　　c.   Complete: fracture line extends through the entire bone; the periosteum is disrupted on both sides of the bone.
　　d.   Impacted: complete fracture with bone fragments being driven into each other.
　2.   Classified according to location on the bone: proximal, middle, or distal.
　3.   Simple, closed fracture: does not produce a break in the skin.
　4.   Complex, open, or compound: fracture involves an open wound through which the bone has protruded.

Data Collection

A. Clinical manifestations.
   1. Edema, swelling of soft tissue around the injured site.
   2. Pain: immediate and often severe.
   3. Abnormal positioning of extremity; deformity.
   4. Loss of normal function due to disruption of bone integrity.
   5. False movement; movement occurs at the fracture site.
   6. Crepitation: palpable or audible crunching as the ends of the bones rub together.
   7. Discoloration of the skin around the affected area.
   8. Sensation may be impaired if there is nerve damage.
B. Diagnostics - Clinical manifestations and history. (Appendix 16-1).

Treatment

A. Immediate immobilization of suspected fracture area.
B. Fracture reduction.
   1. Closed reduction: nonsurgical, manual realignment of the bones; injured extremity is usually placed in a cast for continued immobilization until healing occurs.
   2. Open reduction and internal fixation (ORIF): surgical correction to maintain bone alignment with steel plates and screws.
   3. External fixation: application of a rigid external device consisting of pins placed through the bone and held in place by a metal frame (Figure 16-1).
      a. May be used to treat open complicated fractures.
      b. Requires meticulous care of pin insertion site to prevent infection.
      c. Provides early mobility for the client
C. Traction (Figure 16-2).
   1. Purposes.
      a. Immobilization of fractures until surgical correction is performed; immobilization or alignment of fracture until edema is decreased enough to permit casting.
      b. Decrease, prevent, or correct deformities associated with muscle diseases and bone injury.
      c. Decrease or prevent muscle spasms.
   2. Types.
      a. Skeletal: wire or metal pin is inserted into or through the bone and a system of weights and pulleys are used to maintain an external force of pull to the bone for immobilization of fracture site (e.g., Crutchfield tongs).
      b. Skin: force of pull is applied directly to the skin and indirectly to the bone at the fracture site to maintain fracture reduction.
D. Cast application to maintain immobility of affected area above and below the injured area.

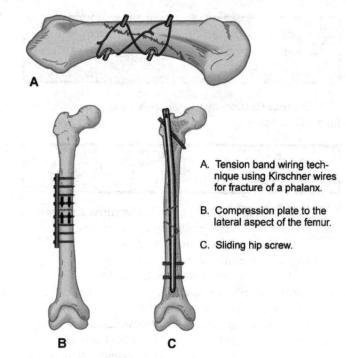

A. Tension band wiring technique using Kirschner wires for fracture of a phalanx.

B. Compression plate to the lateral aspect of the femur.

C. Sliding hip screw.

FIGURE 16-1 **External fixation.** (From deWit, S. *Medical surgical nursing: concepts and practices,* St Louis, 2009, Saunders/Elsevier.)

Complications

A. Infection
   1. Osteomylitis: infection in the bone
      a. Most often has a sudden onset.
      b. Tenderness and pain at the site.
      c. More common in older adults with open wounds that have caused a break in the periosteum.
   2. Infection at site of wound or incision, may progress to osteomyelitis.
      a. Infection may occur under the cast, around pin sites or in the incision.
      b. Unpleasant odor.
      c. Purulent drainage, either through the cast, or at incision or pin sites.
      d. Elevated body temperature.
      e. Increased warmth on cast over injured area.
B. Compartment syndrome.
   1. Caused by internal pressure within or around the compartments of tissue lined by fascia; the fascia does not expand in response to an increase in the contents of the compartment (Figure 16-3).
   2. Any increase in the size of the compartment due to bleeding or swelling will put pressure on the structures (nerves and vessels) within that compartment.
   3. May be caused by external pressure from a cast or dressing that is too tight.
   4. Either external or internal pressure may cause permanent damage if not relieved as soon as possible – it is possible for permanent damage to occur within hours.

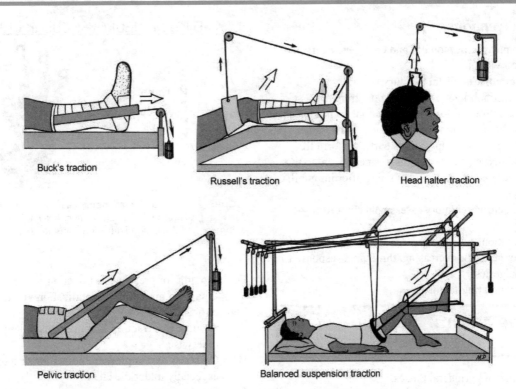

FIGURE 16-2 Examples of common types of traction (From deWit, S. *Medical surgical nursing: concepts and practices*, St Louis, 2009, Saunders/Elsevier).

5. An early sign of compartment syndrome is paresthesia; weak pulse or pulselessness is a late sign. Clients may complain of a throbbing, severe pain unrelieved by analgesics.
6. Evidence of decreased circulation distal to the involved area.
   a. Decreased quality of pulses distal to the injury.
   b. Pain and edema.
   c. Pale, cool, dusky extremity.
   d. Decreased capillary refill time.
7. Evidence of pressure on a nerve.
   a. Decreased sensation to touch.
   b. Paresthesia, tingling.
   c. Impaired motion.
8. Treatment is directed toward immediate release of pressure. If the client has a cast, the cast may be "bivalved." The cast is split in half, and the halves are secured around the extremity by a wrap such as an elastic bandage.
9. Volkmann's contracture: a type of compartment syndrome that occurs when pressure is exerted on the radial or ulnar nerves at the wrist, causing a flexion contraction of the hand. Most commonly occurs with fractures to the elbow and forearm. The flexion contraction may be permanent.
C. Venous stasis and thrombus formation related to immobility (see Chapter 11).
D. Fat embolism.
   1. Often associated with fractures of long bones; primarily occurs in adults.

2. Clinical manifestations most often occur within the first 48 hours of injury.
3. Fat globule moves through the venous system to the lungs.
   a. Change in mental status.
   b. Respiratory distress – tachypnea, tachycardia, petechiae over upper torso.
   c. Anxiety and decreasing pulse oximetry.

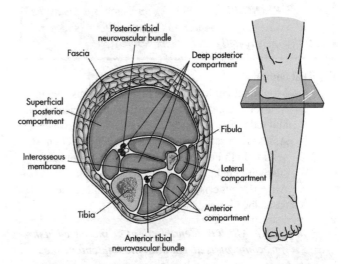

FIGURE 16-3 Compartment syndrome. (From Monahan: Phipp's W. *Medical-surgical nursing: Health and illness perspectives*, ed 8, St Louis, 2007, Mosby.)

Nursing Interventions

❖ **Goal:** To provide immobility and emergency care before transporting victim.
A. Evaluate circulation distal to injury.
B. Splint and immobilize extremity before transfer.
C. If traction is initiated for immobilization, do not release it until further evaluation and treatment is available.
❖ **Goal:** To identify complications early, perform frequent peripheral nerve and vascular assessment distal to the area of injury (before treatment and ongoing after immobilization of injury).
A. Five Ps of neurocirculatory assessment (Figure 16-4).
   1. **Pain.**
       a. Location.
       b. Increasing or decreasing, throbbing, response to analgesics.
       c. Precipitating factors.

> ✔ **NURSING PRIORITY:** *Immediately report pain that is unrelieved by analgesics.*

   2. **P**resence of peripheral **P**ulses.
   3. **P**allor of skin.
       a. Skin pale and cool to touch.
       b. Nail beds: normal capillary refill occurs within 3 seconds.
   4. **P**aresthesia (nerve compression).
       a. Decreased sensation.
       b. Numbness, tingling.
   5. **P**aralysis (nerve compression).
B. Evaluate for presence of compartmental syndrome – if any symptoms are present, obtain assistance immediately.

> ✔ **NURSING PRIORITY:** *It is important for the nurse to be aware of the symptoms of compartment syndrome, identify it early and report it immediately.*

C. Fat emboli.
   a. Monitor client for changes in mental status – change in level of consciousness, confusion, disorientation, and lethargy.
   b. Assess respiratory status, if hypoxic place client in semi to high Fowler's position, begin oxygen and stay with client.
   c. An emergent crisis, stay with client and request assistance immediately.

> 💡 **TEST ALERT:** *Identify client at increased risk for compromised circulation; implement measures to prevent neurovascular complications; recognize client at increase risk for complications.*

5 P's OF NEUROVASCULAR CHECKS

P Pain
P Paresthesia
P Paralysis
P Pulse
P Pallor

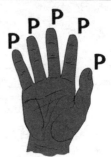

FIGURE 16-4   **5 P's of neurovascular assessment**   (From Zerwekh J, Claborn J, Miller CJ: *Memory notebook of nursing,* vol 2, ed 3, Ingram, 2007, Nursing Education Consultants.)

D. Monitor for presence of infection.
❖ **Goal:** To maintain immobilization via traction (see Figure 16-2).
A. Assume that traction is continuous unless designated otherwise.
B. Carefully assess pressure points for skin breakdown, especially under the client.
C. Do not change or remove traction weights on a client with continuous traction.
D. The traction ropes and weights should hang free from any obstructions.
E. Traction applied in one direction requires an equal counter traction to be effective; client's weight is the countertraction.
   1. Do not let the client's feet touch the end of the bed; it will cause the counter traction to be lost.
   2. Do not allow the traction weights to rest on any thing at the end of the bed; this negates the pull of the traction.
F. Carefully assess the pin sites for evidence of infection in clients with skeletal traction, or with external fixation.
G. Position the client in the center of the bed with the traction pull in a straight line.

> **TEST ALERT: Maintain client traction devices; implement measures to promote venous return.**

❖ **Goal:** To maintain immobilization via cast.
A. Allow plaster cast to dry adequately before handling or moving the client.
   1. Do not cover the cast with a blanket.
   2. Encourage cast to dry by using fans and maintaining adequate circulation.
   3. Synthetic casts dry in about 20 minutes; cast will feel warm during the drying process.
   4. Plaster casts take several hours to dry completely; the cast will also feel warm during drying.
   5. Avoid handling a wet cast to prevent indentions, which may cause pressure areas inside the cast.

6. Reposition client every 2 hours to facilitate the drying of all cast surfaces.
7. "Petaling" a cast is done to cover the rough, crumbling edges of a plaster cast. Small strips of waterproof adhesive are used to cover the cast edges.

B. Continue to assess for compartment syndrome.
C. Body jacket cast and hip spica cast.
   1. Evaluate for abdominal discomfort due to cast compression of mesenteric artery against duodenum.
   2. Relief of gastric distention: may be necessary to relieve gastric distention by a nasogastric tube and gastric suction.
   3. Evaluate for pressure areas over iliac crest.
D. Do not allow cast to become excessively damp or to get wet.
E. Elevate casted extremity, especially during the first 24 hours after application.
F. Apply ice packs directly over the area of injury during the first 24 hours, being careful not to allow the cast to become wet.

> ✔ *NURSING PRIORITY: Do not apply any type of heat to a cast to enhance drying.*

G. Assess for evidence of infection.
❖ **Goal:** To provide care to a client with an external fixation device.
A. Assess for neurovascular complications.
B. Inspect exposed skin and pin insertion sites for signs of infection.
C. Do not use frame to pull or lift client.
D. Frame will be removed when fracture has healed.
❖ **Goal:** To prevent complications of immobility (see Chapter 3).

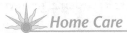 *Home Care*

A. Client should not:
   1. Bear weight on the cast until instructed to do so.
   2. Allow the plaster cast to get wet; discuss alternatives for bathing.
   3. Insert anything under or in the cast.
   4. Remove any of the padding under the cast.
B. Client should report any symptoms associated with swelling or increased pain.

> ✔ *NURSING PRIORITY: Check for complications caused by cast, traction, external fixation device or other immobilizing equipment.*

BOX 16-3   OLDER ADULT CARE FOCUS
Musculoskeletal Nursing Implications

• It is more difficult to maintain immobility in these clients after fractures; therefore surgical intervention (e.g., ORIF) is frequently used for treatment.

• The older client heals more slowly, so use of the affected extremity and weight bearing are frequently delayed.

• Complications of immobility occur more frequently; mobilize hospitalized clients as early as possible.

• Do not rely on fever as the primary indication of infection; decreasing mental status is more common.

• Contractures are more common. Encourage use of assistive devices (canes and walkers).

 Specific Fractures

A. Colles' fracture.
   1. Fracture of the distal radius.
   2. Primary complication is compartmental syndrome.
B. Fractured pelvis.
   1. Frequently occurs in older adults and is associated with falls.
   2. May cause serious intraabdominal and urinary tract injury.
   3. Bed rest is prescribed for treatment of stable fractures.
   4. Combination of external fixation and ORIF may be used to treat complex fractures.
   5. Turn client only on specific orders.
C. Fractured hip.
   1. Common in women over 60 years of age, increased risk in clients with osteoporosis.
   2. Clinical manifestations.
     a. External rotation and adduction of the affected extremity.
     b. Shortening of the length of the affected extremity.
     c. Severe pain and tenderness.
   3. Treatment.
     a. Initially, Buck's or Russell's traction with sand bags and trochanter roll to immobilize fracture, decrease muscle spasms, and control external rotation (see Figure 16-2).
     b. Surgical repair when client's condition allows (permits earlier mobility and prevents complications of immobility).
   4. Nursing interventions postoperatively (Box 16-3).
     a. Circulatory and neurological checks distal to area of injury/surgery.
     b. Position to prevent flexion, adduction, and internal rotation, which may cause dislocation of the prosthesis.

(1) Do not adduct the affected leg past the neutral (midline) position.

(2) Maintain the affected leg in an abducted position; initially with an A-frame pillow or by keeping pillows between the knees.

(3) It is important to prevent internal or external rotation and/or adduction of the operative hip by the use of sandbags, pillows, or trochanter rolls at each thigh.

(4) Avoid greater than 90-degree flexion of the operative hip, when out of bed position client in a chair that provides support, but not sitting at a 90-degree angle of flexion.

(5) Do not allow legs to cross at the knees or the feet.

> ✓ *NURSING PRIORITY: Check with the RN regarding the positioning for clients with fractured hip; positioning for these clients is critical.*

c. Evaluate blood loss.
(1) Check under the client for hemorrhage.
(2) Measure the diameter of the thigh to evaluate the presence of internal bleeding.
d. Client is frequently mobilized on first or second postoperative day to prevent complications of immobility.
e. The client is prone to complications of immobility; use thigh-high anti-embolism stockings or pneumatic compression devices on legs; encourage foot flexion; low-dose heparin may be used prophylactically.

D. Rib fractures.
1. Usually heal in 3 to 6 weeks with no residual impairment.
2. Painful respirations cause clients to breath more shallow and refrain from coughing, thus increased problems of atelectasis.
3. Chest taping or strapping is not usually done because it prevents thoracic excursion and deep breathing.
4. Multiple rib fractures may precipitate the development of a pneumothorax or a tension pneumothorax (see Chapter 10).

E. Mandible fracture.
1. Wiring of jaws (intermaxillary fixation) is common treatment.
2. Postoperative problems: airway obstruction and aspiration of vomitus.
3. Wire cutters at bedside in case of emergency
a. Suction client via nasopharyngeal and or oral methods if vomiting occurs.
b. Cut the wires only as last resort in an emergency (cardiac or respiratory arrest).

c. Wire cutters should remain with the client at all times.
4. Oral hygiene is very important – use normal saline rinses after eating and a soft catheter or water pik for a more thorough oral cleansing.
5. Tracheostomy set at bedside.
6. Establish system for communication - a pad/pencil or picture board to communicate post-op.
7. Discharge teaching: oral hygiene, techniques for handling secretions, diet (problems with constipation due to low fiber in diet), always keep wire cutters with them.

Hip Replacement

A. Hip replacement surgery may be performed to correct a pathological fracture or as treatment for a disease process such as rheumatoid arthritis.
B. Preoperative care.
1. Encourage client to practice using either crutches or a walker, whichever is anticipated to be used post operatively (see Appendix 16-4).
2. Encourage client to practice moving from the bed to the chair in the same manner client will perform this transfer postoperatively.
3. Client should discontinue use of NSAID's and or aspirin about a week prior to surgery.

Nursing Implications

A. Postoperative care (see Chapter 2).
1. Position client to prevent complications.
a. Supine with head slightly elevated, maintain abduction of affected leg, do not use knee gatch on bed.
b. Do not allow the client's hip to flex greater than 90 degrees; therefore do not elevate the bed greater than 60 degrees.
c. Maintain abduction and prevent external rotation of extremity.
d. When sitting, keep client's knees below level of hip.
e. Legs should not be crossed, either at the knee or the ankle.
2. Client may be out of bed to stand at the bedside on the first postoperative day.
3. Encourage postoperative exercises to maintain muscle tone and prevent DVT.
4. Perform neurovascular assessment with vital sign checks.
5. Monitor wound drainage; frequently this client will have a portable wound suction device.
6. Prevent complications of immobility
a. Carefully monitor skin for areas of pressure.
b. Keep client's heels off the bed to prevent skin breakdown.

c. Client is usually out of bed on first or second postoperative day.

d. Antiembolism stockings and/or sequential compression pumps on lower extremity to prevent venous stasis.

e. Low-molecular-weight heparin (see Appendix 11-3) may be given to prevent thrombophlebitis and deep vein thrombosis.

> ✓ **NURSING PRIORITY:** *After surgery, do not allow the repaired hip to flex greater than 90 degrees; avoid adduction and internal rotation of extremity. Flexion and adduction will dislocate the hip prosthesis (use raised toilet seats, reclining wheelchairs).*

7. Observe for signs of possible hip dislocation.
   a. Increased hip pain.
   b. Shortening of affected leg.
   c. External leg rotation.
   d. *If these symptoms are observed, contact the RN immediately.*
8. Pain management.
   a. Pain control is frequently difficult secondary to age, respiratory status, and need to mobilize client.
   b. Evaluate pain using a pain scale.
   c. Epidural or intraspinal analgesia, or a PCA may be used; client frequently on oral pain medication on the 2nd or 3rd postoperative day.
   d. Utilize non-pharmacologic methods for pain relief (see Chapter 3).
9. Closely observe the incisional area for evidence of infection; fever is not a common sign of infection in the older adult, assess for change in orientation status and confusion.

Total Knee Replacement

A. This surgery is often performed to treat joint complications of arthritis.

B. Postoperative care
   1. Client usually returns from surgery with a compression dressing; monitor neurovascular status of extremity distal to the operative site.
   2. Apply cold packs to incision site to decrease edema and bleeding.
   3. Client may have a portable wound suction device to remove drainage from wound.
   4. A continuous passive motion (CPM) device may be used; it promotes healing by increasing circulation and movement of joint.
      a. Check settings for schedule of designated hours and for degree of flexion.
      b. Make sure joint is positioned correctly on equipment.

c. Assess client's tolerance of motion.
d. Turn machine off for meals in bed.
e. Provide padding to prevent pressure points.
5. When client is out of bed in a chair, the knee-immobilizing device may be applied; elevate the extremity.
6. Client has weight-bearing limitations postoperatively; weight bearing gradually increases with healing.
7. Pain management
   a. Provide comfort; promote increased activity and joint mobility.
   b. Manage pain control for total hip replacement, may also use peripheral nerve blocks.
   c. Evaluate pain using a pain scale.
8. Maintain knee in a neutral position, do not allow external or internal rotation.
9. Assess for development of anemia, infection, and DVT.
10. Client is frequently ambulatory at discharge with use of assistive devices. (Appendix 16-4)

 ## Osteoporosis

* **A metabolic bone disease that involves an imbalance between new bone formation and bone resorption.**

A. Primary osteoporosis is most common type; occurs most often in women after menopause.

B. Bone loss occurs predominantly in the vertebral bodies of the spine and the femoral neck in the hip. As bone mass declines, the bone becomes brittle and weak.

> ✓ **OLDER ADULT PRIORITY:** *Aging is the major risk factor; protect older adult clients from falls.*

Data Collection

A. Clinical manifestations (Figure 16-5).
   1. May be asymptomatic until x-rays demonstrate skeletal weakening. Bone loss in excess of 25% occurs before osteoporosis can be identified on standard x-rays.
   2. Spinal deformity and "dowager's hump."
      a. May be diagnosed after a fracture or a vertebral compression fracture.
      b. Gradual loss of height.
      c. Increase in spinal curvature (kyphosis).
   3. Vertebral fractures may occur spontaneously or as a result of minimal trauma.
   4. Chronic low thoracic and midline back pain.
   5. Height loss may precipitate thoracic problems, such as a decrease in deep breathing and exercise tolerance.
   6. Hip fractures and vertebral compression are frequent complications.

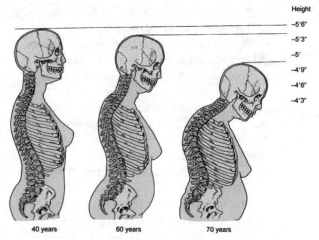

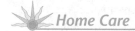

FIGURE 16-5 Progression of osteoporosis. (From Black JM, Hawks JH: *Medical-surgical nursing: Clinical management for positive outcomes,* ed 7, Philadelphia, 2005, Saunders.)

B. Diagnostics.
   1. Serum lab values of calcium, phosphorus, and alkaline phosphatase are usually normal.
   2. Computed tomography to evaluate bone loss.
   3. Bone scan to identify bone density.

Treatment

A. Dietary: increased intake of protein, calcium, and vitamin D.
B. Calcium supplements, and medications to increase bone density (see Appendix 16-2).
C. Vitamin D supplements to enhance utilization of calcium.
D. Exercise: activities that place moderate stress on bones by working them against gravity. Weight-bearing exercise is believed to decrease the development of osteoporosis and possibly increase new bone formation.
   1. Swimming and yoga may not be as beneficial because of lack of stress on bone mass.
   2. Walking for 30 minutes 3-5 times a week is most effective exercise, along with lifting weights.
F. Compression fractures of the vertebrae usually heal without surgical intervention.

Complications

Bone fractures occurring in the vertebral bodies, distal radius, or the hip.

Nursing Interventions

❖ **Goal:** To decrease pain and promote activities to diminish the progress of the disease.
A. Encourage pain relief measures.
   1. Bed rest initially with a firm mattress.
   2. Narcotic analgesics initially followed by NSAIDs.
B. Assess bowel and bladder function; client will be prone to constipation and paralytic ileus if vertebrae are involved.

C. Encourage regular, daily weight-bearing exercise; encourage outdoor exercises because sunlight increases utilization of vitamin D.
D. Discourage use of caffeine, alcohol, and cigarettes.

Home Care

A. Decrease falls and injury by maintaining a safe home environment; use assistive devices.
B. Understand need to continue medications, even if they do not make the client feel better. Important for client to understand that the calcium supplements are to prevent further damage.
C. Do not exercise if pain occurs.
D. Avoid heavy lifting, stooping, and bending. Review and demonstrate good body mechanics with the client (Box 16-2).

Osteomyelitis

✳ **An infection of the bone, bone marrow, and surrounding tissue. The most common causative organism is Staphylococcus.**

Data Collection

A. Tenderness, swelling, and warmth in affected area.
B. Drainage from infected site or wound.
C. Fever, chills.
D. Constant pain in affected area – gets worse with activity.
E. May be a chronic process with persistent problems and exacerbations.

Diagnostics

A. Wound and/or blood cultures.

Treatment

A. Prevention is primary goal.
B. Intensive intravenous (IV) antibiotics.
C. Immobilization of affected area.
D. Surgical debridement may be necessary.

Nursing Interventions

❖ **Goal:** To decrease pain, promote comfort, and decrease spread of infection.
A. Maintain correct body alignment.
   1. Move affected extremity gently and with support.
   2. Prevent contractures by encouraging joint mobility, especially of affected extremity.
   3. Apply warm, moist soaks to increase circulation and healing.
B. If there is an open wound, maintain wound contact precautions (see Chapter 5).
C. Client is usually discharged with antibiotics and should maintain close follow-up care.

D. Condition may become chronic with reoccurrence after primary infection.

> **TEST ALERT:** *Monitor client' wounds for infection; identify signs and symptoms of infection.*

Malignant Bone Tumors

A. The most common primary bone cancer is osteogenic sarcoma; it advances very rapidly with metastasis to the lungs via the blood (see Chapter 2). Bones may be a primary site or a metastatic cancer site.
 1. Most commonly affects the long bones, especially the distal end of the femur.
 2. Primary malignancy most often occurs in males 10 to 25 years old.
B. Metastatic bone cancer occurs when there is a malignancy in another part of the body that has metastasized to the bone (e.g., breast and prostate cancer).

Data Collection

A. Clinical manifestations: generally nonspecific.
 1. Localized pain and swelling.
 2. Tender, palpable bony mass.
B. Diagnostics. (See Appendix 16-1)

Treatment

A. Primary site: extensive resection of area around tumor; amputation may be necessary.
B. Metastatic site: identify and treat primary site if possible.
C. Chemotherapy and radiation may be used. (Chapter 2)

Nursing Interventions

❖ **Goal:** To maintain homeostasis and prevent complications after surgery.
A. An extensive pressure dressing with wound drains/suction may be present.
B. ROM is usually begun immediately; continuous passive motion may be used immediately or on first postoperative day for both upper and lower extremity surgery.
C. Muscle toning is important before weight bearing.
D. Frequent neurovascular assessment is necessary because of resection of nerves and vessels in area; extremity may also be casted or splinted for support.
❖ **Goal:** To prevent complications and promote mobility after amputation (see Appendix 16-3).
❖ **Goal:** To assist the client/child and family to cope with the diagnosis and build basis for rehabilitation.
A. Provide honest, straightforward information to client and family regarding the situation.
B. Allow opportunity for client and family to express concerns and fears.
C. Anticipate sense of loss of control and anger over changes in body.

D. Encourage normal growth and developmental activities as appropriate; allow client to be as independent as possible.
❖ **Goal:** To assist the client and family to cope with the side effects of chemotherapy and radiation (see Chapter 2).

Rheumatoid Arthritis

✳ **A systemic autoimmune disease that affects all areas of the body. It produces a chronic inflammatory process involving connective tissue, especially synovial joints.**

A. Exacerbations and remissions occur. Condition tends to be progressive with each exacerbation. Seldom does the client return to the previous level of functioning before the exacerbation.
B. Early diagnosis may prevent or delay permanent damage.
C. May occur in children as juvenile rheumatoid arthritis.

Data Collection

A. Clinical manifestations.
 1. Gradual onset.
 2. Stiffness and pain worse in the morning; generally decrease during the day with moderate activity.
 3. Joint involvement is bilateral and symmetrical, most frequently involves the hands and feet.
   a. Warm, tender, red, painful joints.
   b. Decrease in range of motion.
   c. Decrease in strength.
 4. Subcutaneous nodules on the fingers.
 5. Systemic effects.
   a. Low fever.
   b. Malaise and weakness.
   c. Anorexia and weight loss.
   d. Depression.
   e. Easily fatigued.
 6. Chronic deformities develop most often in the hands and feet.
 7. Exacerbation of symptoms may be associated with physical or emotional stress.
B. Diagnostics (Appendix 16-1).

Treatment

A. Nonsteroidal antiinflammatory drugs (NSAIDs).
B. Corticosteroids.
C. Disease-modifying antirheumatic drugs (DMARDs) (see Appendix 16-2).
D. Heat and/or cold applications.
E. Physical and rehabilitative therapy.
F. Surgery: joint replacements.

Nursing Interventions

❖ **Goal:** To relieve pain and preserve joint mobility and muscle strength.

A. Use warm, moist compresses to relieve pain and stiffness of muscle spasms associated with chronic stiffness.

B. If acute inflammation is present, cold compresses may provide relief.

C. Acutely inflamed joints may be immobilized in a device that maintains a functional position.

D. Position client to maintain correct body alignment and prevent contractures, especially flexion contractures.

E. Perform range of motion (ROM) exercises to maintain joint mobility and to decrease pain.

F. Antiinflammatory medications should be taken with meals or food to decrease gastric upset.

G. If client is taking corticosteroids, medical identification should be worn.

✓ **NURSING PRIORITY:** *Nursing care of the client with arthritis is directed toward decreasing pain and maintaining joint function.*

❖ **Goal:** To assist client to understand implications of the disease process and measures to prevent joint deformity, relieve pain, and reduce inflammation (Box 16-4).

A. Encourage regularly scheduled rest periods to relieve fatigue and pain; amount of rest varies with the individual and the disease process.

B. Protect small joints.
1. Maintain joint alignment; avoid positions that precipitate joint contraction (e.g., do not use pillow under the knees; encourage activities that involve pressing down the fingers).
2. Change position frequently; maintain good body alignment.
3. Use large muscle groups instead of smaller ones; avoid repetitive movements in small joints.
4. Modify home routine to decrease or avoid stress on joints: modify dressing activities and other activities of daily living (ADLs) as needed.

C. If joint becomes painful during exercise, and the pain persists for 2 hours after the exercise, the activity should be evaluated.

D. Discuss with client importance of identifying false advertising regarding claims of cure and relief of chronic pain.

E. Encourage client to be independent in ADLs as long as possible – focus on what client can do.

Osteoarthritis

❋ **A progressive degenerative joint disease that primarily affects the synovial joints of weight-bearing long bones. It is nonsystemic and noninflammatory.**

A. Frequently involves joint that have excessive use – knees in athletes, feet in gymnast and dancers.

B. Hips and knees are common disease sites.

BOX 16-4   OLDER ADULT CARE FOCUS
Protecting Joints

• If pain lasts longer than 1 hour after exercise, need to change exercises that involve that joint.

• Plan activity and work schedule to conserve energy: do important tasks first.

• Alternate activities; do not complete all heavy tasks at one time.

• Minimize stress on joints: sit rather than stand, avoid prolonged repetitive movements, move around frequently, avoid stairs or prolonged grasping.

• Use larger muscles rather than smaller ones: use shoulders or arms rather than hands to push open doors; pick up items without stooping or bending, use leg muscles; women can carry purses on their shoulders rather than in their hands.

• Painful, acutely swollen inflamed joints should not be exercised beyond basic ROM.

• Regularly exercise even when joints are slightly painful and stiff: swimming and bike riding maintain mobility without weight bearing.

Data Collection

A. Clinical manifestations.
1. Joints involved.
   a. Primarily involves weight-bearing joints.
   b. May be unilateral and involve a single joint.
   c. Joints of hands may be involved.
2. Pain, swelling and tenderness, stiffness of the joint.
3. Pain occurs on motion and with weight-bearing activity.
4. Pain increases in severity with activity – pain becomes worse as day progresses.

B. Diagnostics – (Appendix 16-1).

Treatment

A. NSAIDs may be effective in pain relief.
B. Methotrexate to decrease swelling and pain.
C. Activity balanced with adequate rest.
D. Joint injection with corticosteriods.
E. Physical therapy and exercise.
F. Surgical intervention with joint replacement.

Nursing Interventions

❖ **Goal:** To relieve pain, prevent further stress on the joint, and maintain function.

A. Maintain functional joint alignment; desired position may not be position of comfort.

B. Plan ADLs to prevent stress on involved joints and provide adequate rest periods.

C. Use warm compresses and hot showers to reduce stiffness and pain.

D. Cold compresses may be used if the joint is acutely inflamed.

E.   Acutely inflamed joint may be immobilized with a splint or brace.

F.   Maintain regular exercise program, decrease activity in affected joints.

❖   **Goal:** To assist client to understand measures to maintain health. (Box 16-4)

A.   Identify activities requiring increased stress on involved joints.

B.   Encourage regular exercise program to preserve muscle strength and joint mobility, protect affected joints (activities that do not cause joint stress, such as swimming).

C.   Encourage independence in ADLs.

> 💡   *TEST ALERT: maintain correct body alignment; monitor client response to interventions to prevent complications; implement measures to maintain range of motion.*

Gout

✳   **An arthritic condition resulting from a defect in the metabolism of uric acid (hyperuricemia).**

Data Collection

A.   Clinical manifestations.
1.   Characterized by remissions and exacerbations of acute joint pain.
2.   Onset is generally rapid.

3.   Intense pain and inflammation of one or more small joints, especially the joint in the large toe.

4.   Presence of tophi or uric acid crystals on the big toe or the outer ear.

B.   Diagnostics: persistent high serum uric acid levels.

Treatment

A.   Antigout medications (see Appendix 16-2).

B.   Decrease dietary intake of purine (see Chapter 3).

C.   Avoid aspirin, alcohol, and diuretics, as they may precipitate an attack.

Nursing Interventions

❖   **Goal:** To prevent acute attack, promote comfort, and maintain joint mobility.

A.   Medications should be taken early in the attack to decrease the severity.

B.   Protect affected joint.
1.   Immobilize the joint.
2.   Elevate the joint.
3.   No weight-bearing activity on the joint.

C.   Cold packs may decrease pain.

D.   Provide client with information regarding a low-purine diet.

E.   Encourage high fluid intake to increase excretion of uric acid and to prevent the development of uric acid kidney stones.

F.   Frequently requires pain medication.

Study Questions: Musculoskeletal and Connective Tissue System

1.   What nursing observations would cause the nurse the most concern for a client who is 3 days postoperative for a below-the-knee amputation?
   1   Warmth at the end of the stump.
   2   Serosanguineous drainage on the dressing.
   3   Bright red blood on the dressing.
   4   Bilateral femoral pulses of 80 beats per minute.

2.   A client is admitted with a fractured hip. Before surgery the client is placed in Buck's traction. What is an important nursing intervention for this client?
   1   Remove the traction boot every 4 hours to check circulation.
   2   Check the pin sites for infection and clean them three times a day.
   3   Check for adequate circulation at the fracture site.
   4   Make sure the client's feet are not touching the end of the bed.

3.   The nurse is checking a client for capillary refill. What is the normal time for the nail bed to return to its pink color?
   1   1 minute.
   2   2 to 3 seconds.

   3   10 seconds.
   4   15 seconds.

4.   The client tells the nurse that he is feeling pain in the area where his leg has been removed. What is the best nursing response?
   1   Because there was severe pain in that area previously, this is a subconscious pain.
   2   The pain is referred from another area that is injured.
   3   The injured nerve endings do not accurately reflect the area of the pain.
   4   This is pain that is actually occurring at the stump.

5.   A client is being treated with a long leg cast for his leg fracture. What are important nursing measures while the cast is still wet?
   1   The fingertips should be used when handling the cast.
   2   Support the cast on a pillow with a plastic cover.
   3   Apply a heat lamp and a fan to accelerate the drying time.
   4   Do not reposition the client until the cast is dry.

6. A client has a comminuted fracture of the right tibia and fibula. An external fixation device has been applied to the leg for fracture immobilization. This client is at increased risk for what postoperative complication?
    1   Osteomyelitis.
    2   Poor bone realignment.
    3   Hip flexion contraction.
    4   Venous stasis and pulmonary emboli.

7. An older adult client had a fractured hip repaired. The client returns to the unit with a wound drainage system that is connected to low suction. Over the next 4 hours, the client has 75 mL of bright red bloody drainage. What is the best nursing action?
    1   Notify the physician of the abnormal amount of bleeding in the container.
    2   Empty the drainage container, record the amount, and continue to observe.
    3   Apply pressure at the incisional area and evaluate for increase in drainage.
    4   Check the operative record for the placement of the drain.

8. The nurse is checking a child in a left hip spica cast and suspects an infection. What findings would validate the nurse's conclusion?
    1   Increased complaints of pain and a hot spot found over the incision area.
    2   Complaints of itching and discomfort inside the cast.
    3   Dusky colored toes with weak pedal pulses.
    4   Tingling of the leg with a 3-second capillary refill.

9. A client has a compound fracture of his left femur. He has required an increased amount of pain medication, but without therapeutic results. What complication should the nurse assess for in this client?
    1   Infection.
    2   Compartment syndrome.
    3   Deep vein thrombosis.
    4   Muscle cramping.

10. A client complains that the plaster cast on his leg is rubbing his skin raw. What is the best nursing action?
    1   Call the physician to have the cast cut back.
    2   Apply aloe vera lotion to the irritated area.
    3   Petal the edges of the cast.
    4   Increase the client's pain medication.

11. The nurse is caring for a client who is experiencing an exacerbation of her rheumatoid arthritis. Her hands and fingers are painful, swollen, and inflamed. What is an important nursing measure for this client?
    1   Assist with active range-of-motion exercises in the affected extremity.
    2   Place client's hands in a position of comfort and apply cold packs.
    3   Apply warm packs to increase circulation to the area.
    4   Explain the importance of therapeutic joint exercises to increase mobility.

12. An adolescent is placed in Buck's traction for temporary reduction of a femoral fracture. The client is scheduled for an open reduction and internal fixation of the fracture. Before surgery, what would be an important nursing intervention?
    1   Evaluate the quality of the pulses proximal to the temporary cast.
    2   Check the client's feet to make sure they are not touching the end of the bed.
    3   Evaluate under the client for skin breakdown.
    4   Check the pin sites for inflammation and purulent drainage.

13. The nurse is caring for a client in the immediate postoperative period following a lumbar laminectomy. What nursing observations would cause the nurse the most concern?
    1   Complaints of pain when moving either leg.
    2   Pain radiating down the hip and thigh.
    3   Bilaterally delayed capillary refill on the lower extremities.
    4   Complaints of numbness and tingling in the client's right foot.

14. What is the nursing management for a client in balanced suspension traction?
    1   Position client with his feet against the end of the bed to prevent foot drop.
    2   Remove the weights to allow the client to reposition himself.
    3   Adjust the weights every 8 hours to improve quality of circulation.
    4   Check the weights to make sure they are hanging freely in place.

15. A client is learning to use crutches. What is important for the nurse to teach the client?
    1   When going up stairs, advance the affected leg first.
    2   The axillary bar on the crutches should be firmly in the axillary area for full weight bearing.
    3   Always keep arms and elbows straight when walking.
    4   The axillary bar on the crutches should be two fingers width below the axillary area.

16. A woman is going to be taking alendronate (**Fosamax**) for treatment of her osteoporosis. The nurse is discussing with the woman how she should take the medication. What is very important to include in this discussion?
    1   The medication must be taken on an empty stomach, and no food must be eaten for at least 30 minutes after the medication is taken.
    2   The medication should be taken with a minimal amount of water, and the client should lie down after taking it.
    3   The client should take the medication every night at bedtime, and she should not suddenly stop taking it.
    4   Orthostatic hypotension may be a potential side affect, so she should stand up slowly and make sure she has her balance.

Answers and rationales to these questions are in the section at the end of the book titled Chapter Study Questions: Answers and Rationales.

Appendix 16-1	DIAGNOSTIC STUDIES

Serum Diagnostics

Rheumatoid factor (RF): Used to determine presence of autoantibodies (rheumatoid factor) found in clients with connective tissue disease; if antibody is present, it is suggestive of rheumatoid arthritis; the higher the antibody titer, the greater the degree of inflammation.
Antinuclear antibody (ANA): Identifies the presence of antibodies that destroy the nucleus of body tissue cells (i.e., those seen in connective tissue diseases); a positive test result is associated with systemic lupus erythematosus.
Creatine kinase (CK): Elevated levels found in muscular dystrophy and traumatic skeletal muscle injury.

Invasive Diagnostics

Arthroscopy: Involves the use of an arthroscope inserted into a joint for visualization of the joint structure; procedure is usually conducted in the operating room and performed with either local or general anesthesia; frequently used to diagnose structural abnormalities of the knee.

Nursing Implications
1. Perform preoperative nursing interventions, appropriate for the level of anesthesia to be used.
2. After procedure, wound is covered with a sterile dressing.
3. A compression bandage may be applied for 24 hours after the test.
4. Teach client symptoms of vascular compromise, mobility restrictions, and dressing change procedure.
5. Weight bearing may be limited, walking is permitted; however, excessive exercise should be avoided for a few days.
6. Teach the client signs of infection (increased temperature, local inflammation, and drainage at site).

Arthrocentesis: Incision of a joint capsule to obtain samples of synovial fluid; local anesthesia, and aseptic preparation is done before fluid aspiration. Synovial fluid is examined for infection and bleeding into the joint and to confirm specific types of arthritis.

Nursing Implications
1. Explain procedure to client.
2. May be done at bedside or in an examination room.
3. Compression dressing is usually applied, and joint is rested for several hours after test.
4. Observe dressing for leakage of blood or fluid.
5. Assess the puncture site for evidence of infection.

Myelogram and CT scan: Used to determine status of vertebral disk. See Appendix 15-1.
Bone biopsy: May be performed in client's room or in a treatment room. Local anesthesia is used and a long needle is inserted into the bone, or a small incision is made to obtain bone tissue.

Nursing Implications
1. Plan for analgesic to be administered before procedure.
2. If an incision was made, maintain a pressure dressing over the site.
3. Extremity is elevated to decrease edema and may be immobilized for about 12 to 24 hours.
4. Assess the puncture site or incision for evidence of infection.

Electromyelogram (EMG): Evaluates the electric potential of the muscle with muscle contraction. Small needles are inserted into the muscle and recording of electrical activity is performed.

Nursing Implications
1. Explain to client that there is discomfort with procedure.
2. No stimulants (caffeine) or sedatives 24 hours before the procedure.

Noninvasive Diagnostics

X-ray films: The most common diagnostic procedure to determine musculoskeletal problems.
1. Identify musculoskeletal problems.
2. Determine progress of disease or condition.
3. Evaluate effectiveness of treatment.

Bone scan: Radioisotopes may be injected intravenously, and bone is scanned to determine where the isotopes are "taken up." May be used to determine presence of malignancies, arthritis, and osteoporosis. No special precautions before or after test; need to encourage fluid intake to increase excretion of dye.
Computerized axial tomography (CAT scan): See Appendix 15-1.
Magnetic resonance imaging (MRI): See Appendix 15-1.

| Appendix 16-2 | MEDICATIONS | |

Medications	Side Effects	Nursing Implications

ANTIGOUT AGENTS : Decrease the plasma uric acid levels either by inhibiting the synthesis of uric acid or increasing the excretion of uric acid.

Colchicine: PO	Nausea, vomiting, diarrhea Toxic effects: bone marrow depression	1. Take medication at earliest indication of impending gout attack. 2. Take medication with food. 3. Encourage high fluid intake to promote uric acid excretion. 4. In acute attack, administer 1 tablet every hour until symptoms subside, until GI problems occur, or until a total of 8 mg has been taken.
Allopurinol (**Zyloprim**): PO	Rash, GI distress, fever, headache	1. Administer with food to decrease gastric upset. 2. Discontinue medication if rash occurs. 3. Use with caution in clients with renal insufficiency. 4. May be used to decrease serum uric acid levels in clients receiving chemotherapy.
Probenecid (**Benemid**): PO	GI disturbances, headache, skin rash, fever	1. Urate tophi deposits should decrease in size with therapy. 2. Give with food.

SKELETAL MUSCLE RELAXANTS: Relax skeletal muscle by depressing synaptic pathways in the spinal cord.

Methocarbamol (**Robaxin**): PO, IM, IV	Drowsiness, dizziness, GI upset, rash, blurred vision	1. Used to treat muscle spasms. 2. Caution clients to avoid activities that require mental alertness for safety (driving, using power tools, etc.). 3. Advise client to avoid CNS depressants (e.g., alcohol, opioids, antihistamines). 4. Administer with meals to decrease GI distress.
Cyclobenzaprine (**Flexeril**): PO Carisoprodol (**Soma**): PO	Drowsiness, dizziness, headache, GI upset, orthostatic hypotension	
Baclofen (**Lioresal**): PO	Drowsiness, weakness, fatigue, confusion	
Dantrolene (**Dantrium**): PO, IV	Hepatotoxicity, muscle weakness, drowsiness	1. Teach clients symptoms to report any yellowing skin or eyes, it may indicate a problem with liver function. 2. Acts directly to relax skeletal muscle.

CALCIUM MEDICATIONS: Hormones that enhance bone density by preventing the reabsorption of calcium in bone and kidneys.

Calcitonin-salmon (**Calcimar, Miacalcin**): subQ, IM, nasal spray	GI upset, local inflammation at injection site, flushing	1. Monitor levels of serum calcium. 2. Treatment of established postmenopausal osteoporosis.
Bisphosphonates— alendronate (**Fosamax**), ibandronate, (**Boniva**): PO, nasal spray	Esophagitis, GI flushing, rash, musculoskeletal pain, fever, chills, jaw pain	1. Have client swallow tablet whole; it should not be chewed. 2. Take in morning on an empty stomach with large glass of water (6 to 8 oz) and wait at least 30 minutes before eating or lying down. 3. Encourage client to take supplemental vitamin D. 4. Used for prevention and treatment of postmenopausal osteoporosis.

CORTICOSTEROIDS: See Appendix 5-7.

Continued

Appendix 16-2   MEDICATIONS—cont'd.

Medications	Side Effects	Nursing Implications

DISEASE-MODIFYING ANTIRHEUMATIC DRUGS (DMARDs): Antimetabolite, antirheumatic, and antimalarial drugs that act to decrease inflammation.

Methotrexate (**Rheumatrex**): PO	*Toxic effects:* hepatotoxicity, bone marrow depression Nausea, vomiting, stomatitis	1. Caution women of childbearing age to avoid pregnancy. 2. Monitor CBC regularly. 3. Avoid alcohol during therapy. 4. Administer with food.
Hydroxychloroquine (**Plaquenil**): PO	*Toxic effects:* retinopathy, skeletal muscle myopathy or neuropathy Headache, anorexia, dizziness	1. Recommend eye exams every 3 months. 2. Not recommended for children. 3. Therapeutic effect may not be evident for 3 to 6 months.
Leflunomide (**Arava**): PO	*Toxic effects:* hepatotoxicity, diarrhea, teratogenesis	1. Not recommended for women who may become pregnant. 2. May slow the progression of joint damage caused by rheumatoid arthritis and improves physical function.

BIOLOGICAL THERAPY: Agents that bind TNF to decrease inflammatory and immune responses; used in cases of severe arthritis.

Etanercept (**Enbrel**): subQ	Increased risk for infections, injection site reactions, heart failure, headache, nausea, dizziness	1. Use cautiously in clients with heart disease. 2. Rotate injection sites at least 1 inch apart. 3. Advise clients that injection site reaction generally decreases with continued therapy. 4. Do not administer to clients with chronic or localized infections. 5. Have client report signs of infection, bruising, or bleeding.
Infliximab (**Remicade**): IV Adalimumab (**Humira**): subQ	Increased risk for opportunistic infections, abdominal pain, nausea/vomiting, headache, rash, injection site reactions	1. Avoid in clients with heart disease. 2. Assess clients for infections; administer TB skin test and chest x-ray before starting medication. 3. Rotate injection sites at least 1 inch apart. 4. Perform periodic CBCs to monitor for blood dyscrasias.

NONSTEROIDAL ANTIINFLAMMATORY MEDICATIONS (NSAIDS): See Appendix 5-8.

CBC, Complete blood count; *CHF,* congestive heart failure; *CNS,* central nervous system; *GI,* gastrointestinal; *IV,* intravenous; *PO,* by mouth (orally); *subQ,* subcutaneous; *TNF,* tumor necrosis factor.

Appendix 16-3	AMPUTATIONS

Removal of all or part of an extremity. The precipitating problem determines if the amputation is an elective or an emergency procedure.

POSTOPERATIVE CARE

Residual limb wound care

1. The residual limb may be elevated for approximately 24 hours; after that time, keep the joint immediately above the limb in an extended position. Flexion contracture hinders the use of a prosthesis.
2. Discuss the phenomenon of phantom limb pain; it does not help for the nurse to point out to the client that the extremity is gone.
3. Administer analgesics; assist the client to differentiate between incisional pain in residual limb and phantom limb pain; phantom limb pain is very real to the client.
4. The residual limb may be elevated for a short time postoperatively to decrease edema; the skin flap should be pink and the area should be warm with minimum drainage.
5. A rigid compression dressing (plaster molded over the wound dressing) may be applied to prevent injury and to decrease swelling. Controlling the edema will enhance healing and promote comfort.
6. If the client is not fitted with a rigid compression dressing, the residual limb will be shaped with a compression bandage.
7. Compression wrapping with elastic bandage should be applied in a distal to proximal direction. To protect circulation a figure 8 wrapping should be used with decreasing pressure while wrapping from the distal to the proximal area.
8. For client with above the knee (AKA), or below the knee amputations (BKA), encourage range of motion exercises, especially to the knee and the hip. Discourage prolonged time in semi-Fowler's position in the client with above-the-knee amputation; this position encourages flexion contraction at the hip.
9. For clients with a AKA, encourage resting in a prone position for 30 minutes every 3-4 hours.

> ✔ *NURSING PRIORITY: Be familiar with the nursing management of a client with an amputated extremity, especially regarding positioning to prevent contractures.*

Residual limb care after wound has healed

1. Continually assess for skin breakdown; visually inspect the residual limb daily.
2. The residual limb should be washed, carefully rinsed, and dried daily. Soap and moisture contribute to skin breakdown.
3. Do not apply anything to the residual limb (alcohol increases skin dryness and skin cracking; lotions keep skin soft and hinder prosthetic use).
4. Client should put the prosthesis on when he/she gets up and it should be worn all day. The residual limb tends to become edematous if the prosthesis is not applied. The more the client wears the prosthesis; the less edema will occur.

> 💡 *TEST ALERT: Provide support to client with changes in body image. Maintain correct body alignment of client. Monitor client mobility, gait, and strength.*

Appendix 16-4   ASSISTIVE DEVICES FOR IMMOBILITY

Crutches

Measuring a Client (Figure 16-6)

- Measurement may be taken with client supine, or standing.
- **Supine** - measure the distance from the client's axilla to a point 6 inches lateral to the heel.
- **Standing** – measure the distance from the client's axilla to a point 4 - 6 inches to the side and 4-6 inches in front of the foot.
- Adjust hand bars so that client's elbows are flexed approximately 30 degrees.
- If client was measured while supine, assist client to stand with crutches. Check the distance between client's axilla and arm pieces. You should be able to put two of your fingers between client's axilla and the crutch bar.

Three-Point Alternate Crutch Gait

- Most common gait for clients with musculoskeletal injuries.
- The client must be able to bear the total body weight on one foot; the affected foot or leg is either partially or totally non-weight-bearing.
- In this gait both crutches are moved forward together with the affected leg while the weight is being borne by the client's hands on the crutches. The unaffected leg is then advanced forward.

Crutch Walking

- **Up stairs:** Unaffected leg moves up first, followed by the crutches and the affected leg.
- **Down stairs:** While bearing weight on unaffected leg, crutches are moved to lower stair and client transfers weight to crutches and moves affected leg first, body weight is transferred to the crutches, and the unaffected leg is moved down.

 TEST ALERT: Assess client's use of assistive devices; evaluate correct use; assist client to ambulate with an assistive device.

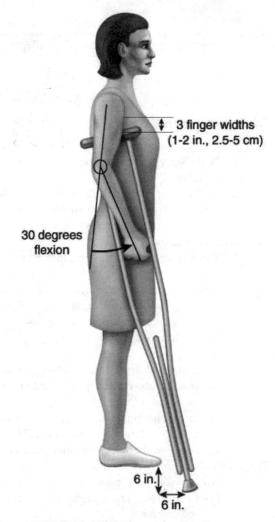

3 finger widths
(1-2 in., 2.5-5 cm)

30 degrees
flexion

6 in.

6 in.

FIGURE 16-6 Crutch measurement
(From Harkreader H, Hogan MA: Fundamentals of nursing: Caring and clinical judgment, ed 2, Philadelphia, 2004, Saunders).

Canes

- The cane is used on the side opposite the affected leg and the elbow should be flexed no more than 30°.
- The cane and the affected leg move together.
- The top of the cane should be parallel to the greater trochanter of the femur.

Walkers

- Lift the walker and place it approximately 12-18 inches in front; make sure all 4 feet of walker are resting on the floor. While resting on walker, step forward with weaker leg first, take alternating small steps toward walker.
- Gain balance before moving walker forward again; balance provides stability and equal weight bearing.

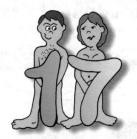

Reproductive System

PHYSIOLOGY OF THE REPRODUCTIVE SYSTEM

Study T.U.R.P. especially

Male Reproductive System

A.   External genitalia.
1.   Penis: serves both reproductive and urinary function.
2.   Scrotum: wrinkled double pouch of skin that protects testes and sperm by maintaining temperature lower than that of the body.

B.   Internal genitalia.
1.   Testes (gonads): sperm formation and production of testosterone.
2.   Epididymis: a tubular, coiled segment of the spermatic duct that stores spermatozoa until they are mature and then transports sperm from the testis to the vas deferens.

C.   Accessory glands.
1.   Seminal vesicles: sac-like structures posterior to the prostate that secrete nearly one-third of the volume of semen; also prostaglandin.
2.   Prostate gland: produces a slightly alkalotic substance that contains high levels of acid phosphatase and serves as the vehicle for spermatozoa.

D.   Semen.
1.   Average volume of ejaculate: 2.5 to 4 mL; may vary from 1 to 10 mL; repeated ejaculation leads to decreased volume.
2.   Sterility: sperm count less than 20 million per milliliter (normal sperm count = 100 million per milliliter).
3.   Storage of sperm: varies from a period of several hours to 40 days, depending primarily on the frequency of ejaculation.

Female Reproductive System

A.   External genitalia.
1.   Labia majora: contain an extensive venous blood supply, which leads frequently to edema and varicosities in pregnancy.
2.   Perineum: are of fibromuscular tissue located between the vagina and anal opening.

B.   Internal genitalia.
1.   Vagina: a thin-walled, muscular membranous canal that connects the external genitalia with the center of the pelvis.

2.   Cervix: protrudes into the vagina.
a.   Provides an alkaline environment to shelter sperm from the acidic vagina.
b.   Cervical mucus pH increases (alkaline) and becomes clear and more viscous at ovulation, similar to egg white consistency.
3.   Uterus: a hollow, pear-shaped, muscular pelvic organ; located between the bladder and the rectum.
a.   Uterine wall: endometrium is the inner mucosal lining; undergoes cyclic changes as a result of hormonal levels.
b.   Uterine ligaments: maintain upright position of uterus in pelvic cavity.
4.   Fallopian tubes: attached to the upper, outer section of the uterus.
a.   Distal tubules are fimbriated (fringed) and bell shaped.
b.   By their peristaltic and ciliary action, they move the ovum (egg) into the uterine cavity.
5.   Ovaries: located behind and below the fallopian tubes, produce ova, estrogen, and progesterone.

C.   Breasts: divided into lobes and lobules arranged in a radial pattern, separated by fibrous tissue called Cooper's ligaments.

D.   Menstrual cycle.
1.   The cyclical hormonal changes occurring from menarche to menopause.
2.   Phases.
a.   Menstrual phase: shedding of the superficial two thirds of the endometrium; initiated by periodic vasoconstriction of the spiral arteries.
b.   Proliferative phase: a period of rapid growth; extends from day 5 to ovulation.
c.   Secretory phase: follows ovulation; large amounts of progesterone are produced; uterine lining is prepared to receive and nourish a fertilized ovum if one is present.
3.   Fertilization: generally occurs in the outer third of the fallopian tube; a single ejaculation deposits 2.5 to 4.0 mL of semen, containing approximately 200 to 400 million spermatozoa.
4.   Implantation: The zygote (fertilized ovum) is propelled by ciliary action of the fallopian tube into the uterine cavity; implants in the endometrium about 7 to 10 days after fertilization.

System Assessment

A. External assessment.
1. Assess vulvar area for discharge, erythema, swelling, or growths.
2. Assess penis for growths, masses, erosions, ulcers, or vesicles.
3. Inspect breasts for nipple inversion, retraction, secretions, nodules, lumps, color changes, erythema or masses.
4. Determine whether there is any abdominal pain or tenderness on palpation.

B. History.
1. Menstrual history.
   a. Age at onset.
   b. Last menstrual period.
   c. Duration of cycle, amount of flow, number of cycles per year, and use of birth control methods.
2. Obstetrical history.
3. Urinary system.
   a. Pattern of voiding: dysuria, urgency, nocturia, frequency.
   b. Difficulty starting stream, stopping stream, or changing the force of stream; a feeling of incomplete emptying of bladder.
   c. Hematuria, incontinence, color, odor.
4. Sexual function.
   a. Ability to achieve erection and ejaculation.
   b. Problems with intercourse.
   c. Bleeding after intercourse.
   d. Exposure to sexually transmitted diseases (STDs).
   e. Change in sex drive, libido.
   f. Lubrication for estrogen status.

Prostate Disorders

* **Benign prostatic hypertrophy (BPH) or hyperplasia: enlargement of prostate gland tissue. (Figure 17-1)**
* **Cancer of the prostate: a malignancy of the prostate gland.**
Both conditions encroach on the urethra and decrease the diameter of the bladder opening. Both conditions can eventually cause bladder obstruction.

Assessment

A. Risk factors/etiology.
1. BPH: very common in men older than 50 years.
2. Prostatic carcinoma: rarely found in men younger than 60 years; usually found in the posterior lobe of the prostate gland.

B. Clinical manifestations.

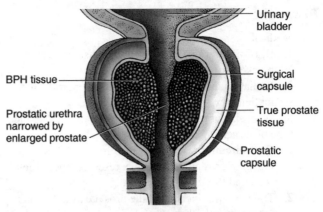

FIGURE 17-1 Benign prostatic hyperplasia (BPH) grows inward, causing narrowing of the urethra (From Ignatavicius, DD, Workman, ML: *Medical Surgical Nursing Patient-Centered Collaborative Care*, ed 6, St Louis, 2010, Saunders).

> ✔ *NURSING PRIORITY: Prostate problems occur in the majority of men over 60 years of age.*

1. Common to both disorders.
   a. Urinary hesitancy, frequency, urgency, and dribbling.
   b. Nocturia, hematuria, urinary retention, and a sensation of incomplete emptying of the bladder.
   c. Urinary retention may cause overflow urinary incontinence and dribbling after voiding.
   d. Acute retention may cause hydroureter and pressure in the kidney.
   e. Increased incidence of urinary tract infection due to residual urine.
2. Prostatic cancer.
   a. Tumor grows slowly and is confined to capsule; therefore prostate may appear normal, thus delaying the diagnosis.
   b. On digital rectal exam, unilateral prostatic enlargement; prostate is described as "stony hard" and fixed.
   c. Obstruction is rare unless BPH is also present.
   d. Pain in the hip or back may be presenting symptom as a result of metastasis.

C. Diagnostics.
1. Digital rectal examination.
2. Cystoscopy and bladder scan.
3. Urinalysis with culture and sensitivity.
4. Transrectal and/or transabdominal ultrasound.
5. Rule out or diagnose cancer.
   a. Prostate-specific antigen (normal PSA 0-4 mcg/L) for cancer.
   b. Tumor markers for diagnosis, staging, and monitoring progress.
   c. Needle biopsy of prostate.

Treatment

A. Medical
   1. BPH: finasteride (**Proscar**) and alpha adrenergic blockers to shrink prostatic tissue.
   2. Radiation, hormonal therapy, and chemotherapy for malignancy.
B. Surgical: size of prostate and general health dictate the type of surgery.
   1. Transurethral resection of the prostate (TURP): removal of prostatic tissue via a resectoscope, which is passed through the urethra.
   2. Transurethral incision of the prostate (TUIP): making transurethral slits or incisions into prostate to relieve obstruction; effective with minimally enlarged prostate (BPH).
   3. Prostatectomy: removal of the prostate via suprapubic, retropubic, or perineal approach, may be done by incision or laproscopically; most often for removal of malignancy.
   4. Transurethral microwave therapy (TUMT) and transurethral needle ablation (TUNA): microwaves are delivered directly to the prostate; heat causes necrosis of tissue; both procedures are done on an outpatient basis.
   5. Internal radiation therapy (brachytherapy) involves the placement of tiny radioactive "seeds" into the prostate for treatment of cancer.
   6. Hormone therapy (anti-androgen medications - **Lupron**): depriving the cancer cells of testosterone may help slow the growth of prostatic cancer.
   7. Cryotherapy (cryablation) Liquid nitrogen is applied to the prostate via a transrectal ultrasound probe, dead cells are absorbed by the body.

Complications

A. BPH.
   1. Preoperative.
   a. Urinary tract infection (UTI).
   b. Rupture of overstretched blood vessels in the bladder and hematuria.
   c. Hydroureter (distention of the ureter) and hydronephrosis (enlargement of kidney caused by postrenal obstruction) with resultant renal failure.
   2. Postoperative.
      a. Hemorrhage: especially in the first 24 hours.
      b. Urinary incontinence.
      c. Bladder spasms.
      d. Retrograde ejaculation: semen passed into the bladder rather than out through the penis.
      e. Infection.
B. Prostatic cancer.
   1. Preoperative.
      a. Complications are similar to BPH.
      b. Cancer may spread via the perineal lymphatic system to the regional lymph nodes; from the

veins of the prostate, it may metastasize to the pelvic bones, bladder, lungs, and liver.
   2. Postoperative.
      a. Increased problems with deep venous thrombosis caused by lithotomy position during open perineal resection.
      b. Change in sexual functioning: impotence and failure to ejaculate.
      c. Incontinence assessment.

Nursing Interventions

❖ **Goal:** To promote elimination, to treat UTI, and to provide client education (Box 17-1)
A. Evaluate adequacy of voiding and presence of urinary retention and infection.
B. Teach client to avoid bladder distension, which results in loss of muscle tone.
   1. Do not postpone the urge to void; it is important to prevent overdistention of the bladder, which further complicates the problem.
   2. Avoid drinking a large amount of fluid in a short period of time.
   3. Avoid alcohol because of the diuretic effect.
C. Encourage annual digital rectal examination of the prostate for all men older than 40 years.
D. Examination is recommended every 6 months for clients who have BPH or who have had a prostatectomy.
❖ **Goal:** To maintain closed irrigation after surgery in the client who has undergone TURP or suprapubic prostatectomy.
A. Continuous bladder irrigation (CBI) with sterile, antibacterial, isotonic irrigating solution (Murphy drip, closed bladder irrigation). (Figure 17-2)

BOX 17-1 **OLDER ADULT CARE FOCUS**
Benign Prostatic Hypertrophy (BPH)

General

- All men over 50 years of age should be assessed for urinary retention and adequacy of bladder emptying.
- Increased problem with urinary stasis; increased straining to urinate; increased incidence of infections.

After Surgery

- Closely evaluate for presence of infection, especially UTI and respiratory.
- Assess fluid balance; confusion and agitation may be symptoms of fluid overload.
- Help the client ambulate as soon as possible—increased risk for pooling of blood in pelvic cavity and pulmonary emboli from immobility.
- Client is at increased risk for falls.
- Determine psychologic response to physical stress (confusion, disorientation); orient to surroundings frequently.

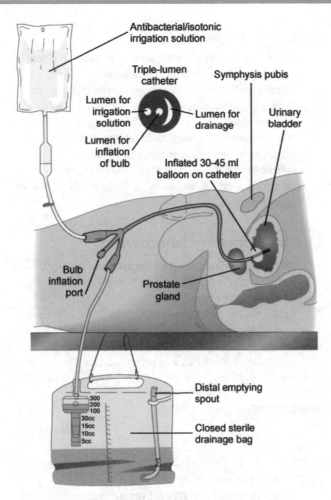

FIGURE 17-2   A closed bladder irrigation system. (From Black, J. & Hawks. J.: *Medical-Surgical Nursing*, ed 8, 2009, St. Louis, Mosby.)

1. Closed bladder irrigation is done with a triple-lumen catheter: one lumen for inflating the balloon (30 to 50 mL of water), one for maintaining outflow of urine, and one for the instillation of the continuous irrigating solution.
2. Provides continuous irrigation to prevent infection and to flush the bladder of tissue and clots after TURP.
3. If clots occur, the catheter may be irrigated, or the rate of flow may be increased until the drainage outflow clears.
4. Calculate intake and output carefully; a large amount of bladder irrigation fluid must be subtracted from total output to determine client's true urinary output.
5. Monitor/titrate CBI so the outflow is light pink without clots; notify surgeon of any increase in bleeding.
6. If catheter is occluded and does not drain properly, turn off the CBI until catheter patency is reestablished. *Notify charge nurse or PCP.*

B. Blood clots and pieces of tissue are normal for the first 24 hours after TURP.
C. If client has excessive bleeding, the physician may increase the size of the balloon on the indwelling catheter and put traction on the catheter to compress the area of bleeding.
D. Client should void within 6 hours of removal of catheter.

> ✔ **NURSING PRIORITY:** *Maintain continuous bladder irrigation for the client who has undergone TURP; prevent overdistention of the bladder. If client complains of pain, check the urinary drainage and make sure it is patent. Obstruction most commonly occurs in the first 24 hours as a result of clots in the bladder.*

E. Bladder spasms: belladonna and opium suppositories or antispasmodics are administered as needed; spasms often occur because of the presence of clots in the catheter – check the catheter for patency.
F. The sensation of a full bladder is common while the irrigating catheter is in place; explain (repeatedly) about the urinary catheter and advise the client to avoid bearing down in an attempt to void.
❖ **Goal:** To provide postoperative care. (Figure 17-3)
A. After client is ambulatory, encourage walking, rather than sitting for prolonged periods.
B. Teach client exercises to control urinary stream and maintain continence.
   1. Have client contract perineal muscles (Kegel exercises) by squeezing buttocks together.
   2. Instruct client to practice starting and stopping the stream several times while voiding.
C. Assure client that TURP does not usually cause problems relating to sexual functioning; provide an opportunity for open discussion of sexual concerns.
D. Dribbling after voiding is a common problem, which often subsides within a few weeks.
E. Teach client to avoid straining during bowel movement; encourage diet high in fiber, and administer stool softeners as needed.
F. Discuss with the client the importance of maintaining a high fluid intake to prevent UTIs.
G. Encourage client to minimize use of caffeine-containing products, which may cause bladder spasms.
❖ **Goal:** To provide postoperative care for a client after radical open prostatectomy.
A. Maintain adequate pain control, frequently with patient-controlled analgesia.
B. As a result of the surgical position and postoperative immobility, client is at high risk for deep venous thrombosis.
   1. Monitor sequential compression devices.
   2. Apply antiembolism stockings.
   3. Administer low-dose prophylactic heparin.

TURP
(Transurethral Resection of the Prostate)

- Continuous or Intermittent Bladder Irrigation (C.B.I.)
  Murphy Drip
- Close observation of drainage system-
  (↑ Bladder Distention Pain & Bleeding).
- Maintain Catheter Patency

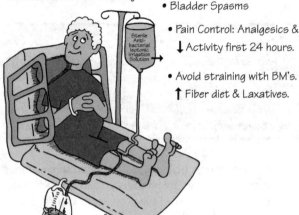

- Bladder Spasms
- Pain Control: Analgesics &
  ↓ Activity first 24 hours.
- Avoid straining with BM's.
  ↑ Fiber diet & Laxatives.

- Complications:
  - Hemorrhage - Bleeding should gradually ↓
    to light pink in 24 hrs.
  - Urinary Incontinence - Kegal Exercises
  - Infections - ↑ Fluids
  - Prevent deep vein thrombosis
    - Sequential compression stockings
    - Low dose heparin
    - Discourage sitting for prolonged periods

FIGURE 17-3 Transurethral resection of the prostate. (From Zerwekh J, Claborn J: (From Zerwekh J, Claborn J, Miller CJ: *Memory notebook of nursing, vol 1*, ed 4, Ingram, 2008, Nursing Education Consultants.)

> *TEST ALERT: Identify symptoms of deep venous thrombosis.*

C. Perineal prostatectomy and total prostatectomy for cancer frequently result in erectile dysfunction and urinary incontinence.
D. Record output from drains.
E. Emphasize importance of not straining against catheter to relieve bladder pressure.
F. Urinary retention.

 NURSING PRIORITY: Explain procedure to client and family. It is important to clarify for the client the information the doctor gives him; however, it is the doctor's responsibility to advise the client regarding any complications he may experience with sexual functioning.

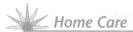 *Home Care*

A. If client is discharged with urinary catheter in place, teach him how to care for the catheter.
B. Client should avoid use of suppositories and enemas.
C. Primary care provider should be contacted if signs of UTI are noted.
D. After removal of urinary catheter, teach client Kegel exercises to increase urinary control (see BPH).
E. Instruct client to continue high fluid intake, avoid strenuous exercise, and avoid prolonged sitting; encourage walking.

Inflammatory Disorders

A. Prostatitis: inflammation of the prostate, usually caused by bacteria (*Escherichia coli, Proteus spp.*) or by a sudden decrease in sexual activity.
B. Epididymitis: inflammation of epididymis, often associated with prostatitis or a UTI; often develops as a complication of gonorrhea; in men younger than 35 years, the primary cause is infection with *Chlamydia trachomatis.*

Assessment

A. Clinical manifestations.
  1. Prostatitis.
    a. Fever, chills, dysuria, urethral discharge.
    b. Perineal, rectal, and/or back pain.
    c. Prostate is enlarged, firm, and tender when palpated.
    d. May be acute or chronic with exacerbations.
    e. Increased risk with catheterizations, bladder infection, or alternative sexual activity.
  2. Epididymitis.
    a. Pain and tenderness in the inguinal canal.
    b. Painful swelling in the scrotum and groin.
    c. Fever, chills, pyuria and bacteriuria.
B. Diagnostics.
  1. Rectal examination.
  2. Urine and semen culture and sensitivity.
  3. Screen for STDs.

Treatment

A. Prostatitis - antibiotics, analgesics, stool softeners, and sitz baths.
B. Epididymitis.
  1. Bed rest with elevation of the scrotum (scrotal support or scrotal bridge).
  2. Antibiotics, if indicated.
  3. Treatment of client's sexual partners (for gonorrhea infection).
  4. Cold compresses; NSAIDs.

Complications

A. Chronic prostatitis can lead to recurrent UTIs and epi didymitis.
B. May cause chronic reoccurring infections.

Nursing Interventions

❖ Goal: To assist client to understand measures to maintain health.
A. Encourage early treatment to prevent complications.
B. For chronic prostatitis, encourage activities that drain the prostate, including intercourse, masturbation, and prostatic massage.
C. Antibiotics may not be effective because it is difficult to obtain therapeutic levels in prostatic secretion.
D. Encourage treatment of sexual partners when epididymitis is caused by chlamydia or gonorrhea.

Undescended Testes (Cryptorchidism)

✳ **Cryptorchidism is a condition of failure of one or both testes to descend into the scrotal sac.**

Assessment

A. Inability to palpate the testes in the scrotal sac.
B. Testicle may be absent or small or may be located in the abdomen.

Treatment

A. Condition may be observed for a year, most cases descend spontaneously; if undescended by 1 year old, surgery may be required.
B. Surgical intervention-orchiopexy: testis is brought into the scrotal sac and secured.
　1. Prevents damage to the undescended testicle by body heat.
　2. Usually done between the ages of 6 and 24 months of age; fewer complications are encountered if repair is done before 5 years of age.

Nursing Interventions

 Home Care

A. Long-term follow-up regarding fertility.
B. Prevent infection by careful cleansing after defecation and urination because of the close proximity of the scrotum.
C. Teach parents to show the child how to do testicular self-examinations when he is old enough.

Testicular Tumors (Cancer)

✳ **Tumors of the testicles are often malignant and tend to metastasize quickly.**

Assessment

A. Most common cancer in men ages 15 to 35 years.
B. More common in clients who have had cryptorchidism and infections.
C. A painless lump (typically, pea-sized) is palpated in the scrotum.
D. Most men experience "heaviness" in the scrotum.
E. A significant enlargement of or shrinking of one testicle.

Treatment

A. Surgical intervention: orchiectomy (removal of the testicle) is performed as soon as possible to remove the tumor and/or retroperitoneal lymph node dissections.
B. Medical.
　1. Radiation therapy.
　2. Multiple chemotherapy medications.

Nursing Interventions

❖ Goal: To detect any abnormality of the testes through self-examination by client (Box 17-2).
A. Teach clients, especially those between the ages 15 and 35 years, to self-examine monthly while showering or bathing to detect any abnormality of the testes.
B. Emphasize importance of follow-up for clients with a history of undescended testes or a previous testicular tumor.
❖ Goal: To assist the client to understand the implications of surgery.

BOX 17-2 TESTICULAR SELF-EXAMINATION

- Examine the testicles at same time every month, to help you remember to do it.
- Visually inspect scrotum in front of a mirror observing for swellings.
- Perform the examination after a bath or shower because this is when the scrotal sac is relaxed.
- Examine each testicle individually by placing index and middle fingers of both hands under one testicle at a time with thumbs on top of testicle. Roll the testicle between the thumbs and fingers. This should NOT cause pain. The tissue should feel smooth.
- Locate the epididymis which is a tubular sac behind the testicle. This sac should not be confused with a lump.
- Also assess for any "heaviness" or dull ache in the groin or abdomen or significant increase or decrease in size of either testicle.
- If there is any lump or irregularity on either testicle, report it to the doctor as soon as possible.

Hydrocele and Varicocele

A. *Hydrocele:* a collection of fluid around the testicle or along the spermatic cord. Client usually does not experience any pain. If circulation becomes impaired, then client experiences more discomfort.

B. *Varicocele:* a cluster of dilated veins in the scrotal sac, often just above the testes; occurs most often in young adults.
   1. Does not experience severe pain, but a chronic dull ache in the scrotal area.
   2. May contribute to infertility because sperm temperatures may be too high which affects sperm formation and motility.

C. Treatment.
   1. Hydrocele: needle aspiration or surgical aspiration and drainage.
   2. Varicocele: surgical intervention only if there are complications with fertility; otherwise, a scrotal support is used.

D. Nursing intervention: provide preoperative and postoperative care (see Chapter 3).

Erectile Dysfunction (ED)

Inability to attain or maintain an erect penis.

Assessment

A. Risk factors/etiology.
   1. Physiologic (organic): diabetes, hypertension, prostatectomy.
   2. Psychologic (functional): stress, depression, low self-esteem.

B. Clinical manifestations.
   1. Inability to attain or maintain an erection.
   2. Gradual onset with physiologic ED and abrupt onset with psychologic ED.

Treatment

A. Medical: ED medications (Appendix 17-1).

B. Vacuum constriction devices (VCD): applying a suction device to the penis to pull blood up into the corporeal bodies, then placing a penile ring or constrictive band to trap the engorgement.

C. Intraurethral devices: medicated urethral system for erection (MUSE)—administration of medications as a topical gel, injection into penis, or insertion of medication pellet into urethra.

D. Penile implants: surgical insertion of an implant.

Nursing Interventions

❖ Goal: To help the client understand the implications of the medications or devices used to treat ED and assist to obtain counseling.

A. Teach client about how ED medications can potentiate

hypotensive effects of nitrates and should not be taken at the same time.

B. Client should abstain from alcohol if taking ED medications.

Cystocele and Rectocele

✱ **Cystocele is a weakened support between the vagina and bladder allowing the bladder to bulge into the vagina. Rectocele is a weakened support between the vagina and rectum allowing the rectum to bulge into the vagina.**

Assessment

A. Risk factors/etiology.
   1. Obesity and childbearing.
   2. Genital atrophy caused by aging.

B. Clinical manifestations.
   1. *Cystocele:* protrusion of the bladder into the vagina.
      a. Stress incontinence: occurs during coughing, lifting, or sneezing.
      b. Frequency, urgency, difficulty emptying bladder.
   2. *Rectocele:* protrusion of the rectum through the vaginal wall.
      a. Constipation.
      b. Incontinence of gas or liquid feces.

Treatment

A. Medical: Kegel exercises for mild stress incontinence (tighten and release perineal muscles several times during the day); client can also practice stopping urination in midstream and holding it for a few seconds.

B. Surgical.
   1. Cystocele: anterior colporrhaphy.
   2. Rectocele: posterior colporrhaphy.
   3. Procedure is usually called "A and P repair."

Nursing Interventions

❖ Goal: To help the client understand the implications of, and be prepared for, surgery.

A. Preoperative teaching.

B. Postoperative period.
   1. Prevent wound infection.
   2. Warm compresses to abdomen may relieve discomfort.
   3. Assess for urinary retention and excessive vaginal bleeding.

C. Perineal care after each voiding or defecation.

Home Care

A. Encourage the use of mild laxatives to prevent straining at stool.

B. Prevent constipation.

C. Certain activities are restricted until area has healed: lifting objects heavier than 5 pounds; intercourse; prolonged standing, walking, and sitting.

D. Call the doctor if there is persistent pain or purulent, foul-smelling vaginal discharge.

Vaginal Inflammatory Conditions

Common Predisposing Factors

A. Excessive douching.
B. Oral contraceptives, steroids.
C. Antibiotics: especially broad-spectrum, which wipe out normal vaginal flora (vagina is protected by an acidic pH and the presence of *Döderlein's bacilli*).
D. Improper cleaning after voiding and defecating.
E. Assess for recurrent chronic infection; there may be an underlying condition (prediabetic state, HIV infection) that should be further evaluated.

Bacterial Vaginosis

A. Characteristics.
 1. Causative organisms: *E. coli, Haemophilus vaginalis*, and *Gardnerella vaginalis*.
 2. Profuse yellowish discharge, "fishy smell."
 3. Itching, redness, burning, and edema.
B. Treatment: antibacterial/antiprotozoal medication.
C. Complications: Bacterial vaginosis may increase susceptibility to STDs and HIV infection if woman is exposed to either.
D. Factors associated with bacterial vaginosis include multiple sex partners, douching, smoking but may occur in non-sexually active women.

Candidiasis

A. Characteristics.
 1. Organism: *Candida albicans* (fungus).
 2. Internal itching, beefy red irritation, inflammation of vaginal epithelium.
 3. White, cheese-like, odorless discharge that clings to the vaginal mucosa.
 4. Occurs frequently and is difficult to cure.
 5. Increased risk in women with diabetes and women taking birth control pills, during pregnancy, and after treatment with antibiotics.
B. Treatment.
 1. Antifungal vaginal medication.
 2. Oral antifungals.

Trichomoniasis

A. Characteristics.
 1. Organism: *Trichomonas vaginalis* (protozoan).
 2. May be asymptomatic.
 3. Itching, burning, dyspareunia (painful intercourse).
 4. Frothy, green-yellow, copious, malodorous vaginal discharge; strawberry spot on cervix.
 5. Sexual partners must be treated also because of cross-infection; men are usually asymptomatic.
B. Treatment: antibacterial/antiprotozoal medication.

C. Prevention: avoid extended time in synthetic or tight-fitting undergarments; use of condoms may reduce incidence of STDs.

Postmenopausal Vaginitis (Atrophic Vaginitis)

A. Characteristics.
 1. Lack of estrogen (this is also the cause).
 2. Itching and burning.
 3. Loss of vaginal tissue folds and epithelial covering.
B. Treatment: estrogen vaginal cream.

Nursing Interventions

❖ **Goal:** To teach client to prevent infection by performing appropriate personal hygiene, to decrease inflammation, and to promote comfort.
A. Appropriate cleansing from front of vulva to back of perineal area.
B. Frequently a postmenopausal problem.
C. Client should not douche; douching removes normal protective bacteria from vaginal cavity, and other bacteria are introduced.
D. If infection is chronic, it may be necessary to have sexual partner tested; partner may be reinfecting the woman.
E. Discourage use of feminine hygiene sprays because they cause increased irritation.
F. Discourage client from wearing constricting clothing and synthetic underwear (encourage use of cotton underwear).
❖ **Goal:** To educate the woman regarding correct use of medication.
A. Vaginal suppositories, ointments, and creams are often used.
 1. Handwashing before and after insertion of suppository or application of cream.
 2. Remain recumbent for 30 minutes after application to promote absorption and prevent loss of the medication from the vaginal area.
 3. Wear a perineal pad to prevent soiling of clothing with vaginal drainage.

Dysfunctional Uterine Bleeding

✳ **Dysfunctional uterine bleeding is bleeding that is excessive or abnormal in amount or frequency without regard to systemic conditions; occurs when the hormonal events responsible for the balance of the cycle are interrupted.**

Amenorrhea

A. Absence of menses.
 1. Primary: no menstruation has occurred by age 16 years.
 2. Secondary: woman previously had menses.
B. May be indicative of menopause.
C. May be first indication of pregnancy.

D. Occurs when woman has lost a critical fat percentage (e.g., athletes, clients with anorexia).

Menorrhagia

A. Excessive vaginal bleeding.
B. Single episode of heavy bleeding may indicate a spontaneous abortion.
C. May be associated with an intrauterine device (IUD).
D. Causes: hypothyroidism, uterine fibroids, hormone imbalance.

Metrorrhagia

A. Vaginal bleeding between periods.
B. May be normal menopause.
C. Ectopic pregnancy.
D. Breakthrough bleeding from oral contraceptives.
E. Cervical polyps.

> ✔ **NURSING PRIORITY:** *Vaginal bleeding after menopause or surgical hysterectomy is a symptom of a problem that needs to be evaluated.*

Nursing Interventions

A. Help determine most likely cause of problem.
B. Report excessive bleeding, abdominal pain, fever.
C. Treatment.
  1. Dilation and curettage (D&C) for diagnostic purposes in older women.
  2. Endometrial ablation.
  3. Removal of fibroids.
     a. Often done on outpatient basis with either general regional or local anesthesia.
     b. Spotting and vaginal drainage are common for several days; if amount is more than a normal period or if it lasts longer than 2 weeks, client should call the doctor.
     c. Client should report any signs of infection: fever; foul, purulent discharge; increasing abdominal pain.
     d. Nonsteroidal antiinflammatory drugs are often used for pain control.
     e. Client should avoid sexual intercourse and use of tampons for about 2 weeks.
D. Assess and treat for anemia.
  1. Encourage diet high in iron.
  2. Administer iron preparations, if required.

Endometriosis

✳ **Endometriosis is the presence of endometrial tissue outside of the uterus. The tissue responds to hormonal stimulation by bleeding into areas within the pelvis, causing pain and adhesions.**

Assessment

A. Risk factors/etiology.
  1. Small pieces of endometrial tissue back up through the fallopian tubes into the abdomen during menstruation.
  2. Most common in women in their late 20s and early 30s who have never been pregnant.
B. Clinical manifestations.
  1. Dysmenorrhea: deep-seated aching pain in the lower abdomen, vagina, posterior pelvis, and back occurring 1 to 2 days before menses.
  2. Abnormal excessive uterine bleeding and dyspareunia; painful defecation.

Treatment

A. Medical: androgenic agents may be given over a 6- to 8-month period; or oral contraceptives may be prescribed; if a woman desires more children, she is encouraged to get pregnant, because the condition recedes during pregnancy.
B. Surgical intervention.
  1. Laser treatment of endometrial tissue in the extrauterine sites.
  2. Hysterectomy (usually carried out in women close to menopause).

Nursing Interventions

❖ **Goal:** To help client minimize the pain and discomfort associated with endometriosis.

A. Warm baths or moist heat packs may reduce discomfort.
B. Encourage client to explore alternative sexual positions that may minimize discomfort during intercourse.
C. Encourage client to discuss abstinence with partner if intercourse is painful.

❖ **Goal:** To assist client to understand measures to maintain health.

A. Teach client about disease process; clarify any false ideas.
B. Provide emotional reassurance; discuss potential for infertility.
C. Initiate preoperative and postoperative teaching if surgery is elected.

 ## Pelvic Inflammatory Disease

✳ **Pelvic inflammatory disease (PID) is an infectious condition of the pelvic cavity that involves the fallopian tubes, the ovaries, and/or the peritoneum.**

Assessment

A. Risk factors/etiology.
  1. Complication of gonorrhea and Chlamydia trachomatis.
  2. IUDs are correlated with an increased incidence of PID.

3. Increased number of sexual partners increases incidence of PID.
4. Increased risk for repeat cases after previous episode of PID.

B. Clinical manifestations.
1. General malaise, fever, chills, nausea, and vomiting.
2. Leukocytosis and pain on urinating.
3. Dull tenderness or bilateral lower abdominal pain.
4. Vaginal discharge that is heavy and purulent.
5. Painful intercourse.
6. Chronic PID: persistent pelvic pain, secondary dysmenorrhea, dysfunctional uterine bleeding, and periodic episodes of acute symptoms.

C. Complications.
1. Sterility.
2. Ectopic pregnancy.

Treatment

A. Medical: broad-spectrum antibiotics, analgesics.
B. Surgical: incision and drainage of abscesses with or without a laparotomy.

Nursing Interventions

❖ Goal: To prevent the spread and extension of the infection.

A. Maintain semi-Fowler's position to promote drainage of the pelvic cavity by gravity.
B. Strict medical asepsis when in contact with discharge; wound and skin precautions.
C. Encourage oral fluids and maintain adequate nutrition.
D. Client should avoid sexual activity and douching.
E. Strongly encourage sexual partner(s) to seek medical treatment.

❖ Goal: To provide psychologic support.

A. Encourage expression of feelings related to guilt and possibility of sterility.
B. Explain factors relating to the long-term management of PID and the importance of medical supervision.

SEXUALLY TRANSMITTED DISEASES

✳ **Infectious diseases transmitted most commonly through sexual contact.**

A. Characteristics
1. Transmitted by sexual activity, including oral and rectal activities between people of the same or opposite sex.
2. One person can have more than one STD at a time.
3. All sexual partners need to be evaluated.

B. Nursing role is to recognize and provide factual information.
1. Mode of transmission.
2. Prevention of transmission.
3. Importance of contacts being identified and treated.
4. Information provided in accepting, nonjudgmental manner.

5. Oral contraceptives do not provide any protection.
6. Clients with STDs should be tested for HIV.
7. Hepatitis B (HBV) and Hepatitis C (HCV) are considered STDs (see Chapter 14).

> ✔ *NURSING PRIORITY: Consider all oral, genital, and rectal lesions to contain pathologic organisms until documented otherwise.*

 ## Syphilis

✳ **Syphilis is caused by the spirochete, *Treponema pallidum* that is transmitted by direct contact with primary chancre lesion, body secretions (saliva, blood, vaginal discharge, semen); also transmitted transplacentally to the fetus.**

Data Collection

A. Primary stage.
1. Chancre: small, hard painless lesion found on the penis, vulva, lips, vagina, or rectum.
2. Usually heals spontaneously within 2 to 3 weeks, with or without treatment.
3. Regional lymphadenopathy.
4. Will progress without treatment.
5. Highly infectious during primary stage.

B. Secondary stage.
1. Client may be asymptomatic; secondary stage usually begins anywhere from 2 weeks to 6 months after the chancre has healed.
2. Maculopapular rash on the palms of the hands and soles of the feet, sore throat, and headache.
3. Lymphadenopathy; gray mucous patches in the mouth.
4. Condylomata lata: flat lesions that may appear in moist areas; are most infectious of any syphilitic lesion (not to be confused with *condylomata acuminata* in genital warts).
5. Symptoms will disappear within 2 to 6 weeks.

C. Latent stage.
1. Absence of clinical symptoms, noninfectious after 1 year during the latent stage.
2. Results of serologic tests for syphilis remain positive.
3. Transmission can occur through blood contact.
4. The majority of clients remain in this stage without further symptoms.

D. Congenital syphilis.
1. Maculopapular rash over face, genital region, palms, and soles.
2. Snuffles: a mucopurulent nasal discharge indicative of some degree of respiratory obstruction.
3. After the age of 2 years: Hutchinson's teeth (notched central incisors with deformed molars and cusps).

E. Diagnostics.
1. Serologic screening tests: Venereal Disease Research Laboratories (VDRL).
2. Rapid plasma reagin test (PRP and RPR): may produce false-negative results in early stages.
3. Fluorescent treponemal antibody absorption (FTA-ABS) test.
4. VDRL and fluorescent treponemal antibody absorption tests are based on presence of antibodies, and results are not positive until about 4 weeks after the appearance of the chancre.
F. Complications: development of late (tertiary) syphilis and the resultant systemic involvement of the cardiovascular and central nervous systems.

Nursing Interventions

A. Administration of parenteral penicillin is treatment of choice. Tetracycline or doxycycline is administered if client is allergic to penicillin.
B. If pregnant mother is treated before the 18 weeks' gestation, the fetus will usually be born unaffected.
C. Preventive education regarding sexual exposure, adequate case finding, and treatment of contacts.
D. All cases are reported to local public health authorities.

Gonorrhea

✳ **Gonorrhea is an STD that may also affect the rectum, pharynx, and eyes that is caused by the bacteria, *Neisseria gonorrhoeae* and is transmitted by direct contact with exudate via sexual contact or transmission to the neonate during passage through the birth canal.**

Data Collection

A. Men.
1. Urethritis, epididymitis, dysuria, and purulent urethral discharge.
2. Increased evidence of asymptomatic disease or a chronic carrier state in males.
B. Women.
1. Initial urethritis or cervicitis that is often mild enough to remain undetected by client.
2. Vulvovaginitis, vaginal discharge, dysuria.
3. If untreated, may result in PID.
C. Both men and women; arthralgias, joint pain from disseminated gonococcus.
D. Neonate: ophthalmia neonatorum.
E. Diagnostics.
1. Positive Gram stain smear of discharge or secretion.
2. Positive culture.
F. Complications.
1. Men: prostatitis, urethral strictures, urethritis, and sterility.
2. Women: PID, Bartholin's abscess, ectopic pregnancy, infertility.

Nursing Interventions

A. Prophylactic antibiotic treatment for gonorrhea eye infection in the neonate (ophthalmia neonatorum).
B. Encourage follow-up cultures in 4 to 7 days after treatment and again at 6 months.
C. Teach importance of abstinence from sexual intercourse until cultures are negative.
D. Urge client to inform sexual partner so that he or she may be treated for infection.
E. Important to take the full course of antibiotics.

Herpes Genitalis

✳ **Herpes genitalis is an infection caused primarily by herpes simplex virus 2 (HSV-2) that is characterized by recurrent outbreaks, which are usually less severe than the original outbreak of lesions.**
* HSV-1 causes infection above the waist, involving the gingivae, dermis, and upper respiratory tract.
* HSV-2 lesions characteristically occur below the waist, generally in the genital area and perineum; however, it is possible for HSV-2 to cause oral lesions, and HSV-1 can cause genital lesions.
* Virus enters a latent phase and may be harbored by the individual for an indefinite period of time; virus may be reactivated by stress, sunburn, sexual activity, and fever.

A. Transmission: by direct contact with the vesicles; asymptomatic shedding and transmission of virus is well documented.
B. Communicability: highly contagious.

Assessment

A. Initial sensation of tingling and itching before rupture of the lesion.
B. Signs of primary infection usually consist of local inflammation, pain, lymphadenopathy, and systemic symptoms.
C. Initial systemic malaise, fever, headache, and muscle aches.
D. Irritation of the genitals.
E. Genitals may become reddened with painful blisters, which burst into lesions that gradually heal.
F. During asymptomatic period when there are no lesions present, there may be virus shedding and client is infectious.

Nursing Interventions

A. Teach importance of genital hygiene and avoidance of unprotected sexual contact.
B. Teach good hygiene practices. Explain that the fluid inside the lesions contains the virus. If a lesion breaks open, the virus can be spread by contact with the fluid and cause a lesion in any area of the body.

> ✔ *NURSING PRIORITY: Always wear gloves when cleaning the perineal area of a client with HSV-2 to prevent herpetic whitlow, a herpes lesion around the nail bed. Nurses are at risk for developing this because of local contact with the HSV on broken skin areas around the nails.*

C. If administration of oral antiviral agent is started at the first sign of a lesion, the duration of the outbreak may be decreased.
D. Symptomatic treatment: sitz baths, wet compresses, and analgesics for relief of pain.

 ## Cytomegalovirus

* **Cytomegalovirus is a virus belonging to the herpes family, which leads to very mild illnesses but can cause a wide range of serious congenital deformities in the fetus or newborn (known as congenital cytomegalovirus).**

Data Collection

A. The mother is usually asymptomatic or has mononucleosis-type symptoms.
B. Effect on the neonate: serious hematologic and central nervous system consequences; high mortality rate in severely affected neonates.
C. Diagnostics.
   1. **TORCH** screening: **T**oxoplasmosis, **O**ther (hepatitis), **R**ubella, **C**ytomegalovirus infection, **H**erpes simplex.
   2. Increased lymphocyte count and abnormal liver function test results.

Nursing Interventions

A. Prevention is the primary goal. Pregnant women should avoid being around affected individuals and congenitally infected infants.
B. Prevention of exposure is almost impossible, because the primary infection is asymptomatic.

 ## Chlamydia Infection

* **An infectious disease caused by *Chlamydia trachomatis* (most common STD).**

Data Collection

A. Males.
   1. Urethritis, epididymitis, proctitis.
   2. Primary reservoir is the male urethra.
B. Females.
   1. Mucopurulent cervicitis, postpartal endometritis, salpingitis, vaginitis.
   2. Primary reservoir is the cervix.
C. Newborns.
   1. Inclusion conjunctivitis.

   2. Pneumonia.
   3. Hepatomegaly and splenomegaly.
D. Both males and females are frequently asymptomatic and often do not seek medical attention until a complication arises (PID, epididymitis).
E. Diagnostics: isolation of the organism in a tissue culture or serologic complement fixation testing.
F. Complication: reactive arthritis (can also be a primary symptom).

Nursing Interventions

A. Urge client to have sexual partner treated.
B. Emphasize the importance of long-term drug therapy because of the pathogen's unique life cycle, which makes it difficult to eliminate.
   1. Antibiotics: doxycycline and azithromycin are primary antibiotics for treatment.
   2. Penicillin and its derivatives are not effective against these organisms; consequently, this usually explains the persistence of infection in clients who are treated for gonorrhea and do not respond.

 ## Genital Warts

* **Genital warts is characterized by cluster of warts caused by the human papilloma virus (HPV): condylomata acuminata. It is continually shed from the surface, and re-infection may occur.**

Data Collection

A. Warts are found in areas subject to trauma during sexual activity: penis, urethra, perianal area, anal canal, vulva, cervix, vaginal canal.
B. Diagnosed by observation and biopsy of lesions.
C. The cervix and anal canal may be involved if there are lesions on the vaginal or anal area.
D. Lesions are raised, skin-toned, damp, cauliflower-like growths.
E. Genital itching.
F. May cause nonmenstrual bleeding after intercourse.

Nursing Interventions

A. Education regarding transmission.
B. Close follow-up with Pap smears in women; genital warts are associated with an increased incidence of cervical cancer.
C. Increased incidence of squamous cell cancer of penis in men.
D. **Podophyllin**, applied topically once or twice a week.
E. Transmission is by direct contact with a person who has lesions present.
F. Vaccination with **Gardasil** may reduce or prevent genital warts.

Cervical Cancer

Assessment

A. Risk factors/etiology.
   1. Multiple sex partners, first intercourse at early age.
   2. History of STDs, HSV-2.
   3. Genital warts (HPV-positive), abnormal Pap smears.
B. Clinical manifestations.
   1. Clients are asymptomatic until late in disease state.
   2. Thin and watery drainage that becomes dark and foul smelling as the disease progresses.
   3. Abnormal vaginal bleeding or discharge.
   4. Low back pain.
   5. Painful sexual intercourse.
C. Diagnostics.
   1. Pap smear.
      a. Initial Pap smear at age 21 or 2-3 years after first sexual intercourse.
      b. Pap smears are continued after menopause and hysterectomy.
   2. Classification of Pap test results: Bethesda Classification System (2001) replaced older system, which had 5 classes.
      a. The adequacy is assessed as satisfactory or unsatisfactory.
      b. The findings are described as negative or having epithelial cell abnormalities (either squamous cell or glandular cell).

> ✔ **NURSING PRIORITY:** *If cancer of the cervix is identified before it becomes invasive (or in the in situ stage), there is virtually a 100% cure rate.*

   3. Cervical biopsy (office procedure)—after the test, the client should:
      a. Avoid strenuous activity for 24 hours.
      b. Leave vaginal packing in for about 24 hours.
      c. Abstain from sexual intercourse for approximately 24 hours.
      d. Avoid using tampons and douching.

Treatment

A. Surgical intervention.
   1. Conization (cryosurgery): used for carcinoma in situ.
   2. As treatment for cervical cancer, the following procedures may be done:
      a. Vaginal hysterectomy: removal of the uterus; fallopian tubes and ovaries remain intact.
      b. Hysterectomy: total abdominal hysterectomy with bilateral salpingo-oophorectomy (TAH-BSO); includes removal of fallopian tubes and ovaries.
      c. Radical hysterectomy: a panhysterectomy plus a partial vaginectomy and removal of lymph nodes.
      d. Pelvic exoneration: radical hysterectomy plus total vaginectomy, removal of bladder with urinary diversion, bowel resection, and colostomy.
   3. Radiation therapy, either internal (radium implant) or external for invasive cancer.
   4. **Gardasil** vaccine for prevention of cervical cancer.

Nursing Interventions

❖ **Goal:** To provide health teaching to help clients detect premalignant cervical dysplasia.
A. Warning signs of cancer.
B. Importance of yearly Pap smears.
C. Encourage verbalization of feelings related to the surgery and diagnosis of cancer.

❖ **Goal:** To provide preoperative and postoperative teaching in preparation for a total abdominal hysterectomy.
A. General preoperative care.
B. After surgery, assess for complications, such as backache or decreased urine output, because these symptoms can indicate accidental ligation of the ureter.
C. Urinary retention may occur as a result of bladder atony and edema; explain to client the necessity for a urinary retention catheter.
D. Early ambulation is encouraged to prevent postoperative thrombophlebitis.

❖ **Goal:** To provide psychologic support.
A. Encourage verbalization of concerns related to body image.
B. Teach that sexual activity should be avoided until checkup to determine wound healing (about 4 to 6 weeks).
C. Client should avoid heavy lifting.
D. Client who has had a pelvic exoneration will have many concerns regarding sexual function, because the vagina will be lost. Menopause will occur, and there may be a urinary or bowel diversion to the abdominal wall (an ileal conduit or colostomy).

Breast Carcinoma

Assessment

A. Risk factors/etiology.
   1. Leading cause of cancer death in women ages 14 to 54 years.
   2. Family history of breast cancer; however, 85% of women with breast cancer have a negative family history.
   3. Nulliparity or parity after the age of 30 years.
   4. Early menses, late menopause; removal of the ovaries before the age of 35 years significantly decreases the risk for breast cancer.

5. The incidence of recurrence of breast cancer is significant.
6. Presence of other cancer: endometrial, ovarian, colon, rectal.

B. Clinical manifestations.
1. Asymmetry of the breasts.
2. Skin dimpling, flattening, and nipple deviation are suggestive of a lesion.
3. Skin coloring and thickening, large pores, sometimes called peau d'orange (orange peel appearance).
4. Changes in the nipple; discharge from the nipple.
5. Mass is painless, nontender, hard, irregular in shape, and nonmobile.
6. Majority of malignant lesions are found in the upper outer quadrant of the breast (tail of Spence).

C. Diagnostics.
1. Mammography; ultrasound.
2. Breast biopsy.
3. Serum tumor markers: carcinoembryonic antigen (CEA), human chorionic gonadotropin (hCG).

D. Complications:
1. Metastases via the lymphatic system to bone, lungs, brain, and liver.
2. Postmastectomy pain syndrome: pain persisting past 3 months.
3. Sentinel lymph node dissection (SLND).

Treatment

A. Surgical.
1. Modified radical mastectomy (most common): removal of all breast tissue and axillary lymph nodes.
2. Local excision (lumpectomy): removal of lump or tumor with preservation of the breast.
3. Breast reconstruction: may be delayed until after radiation therapy is completed or may be done at the time of the mastectomy.

B. Radiation: combined with surgery and chemotherapy.

C. Hormonal therapy: breast cancers that are classified as "estrogen receptors" are less invasive tumors and respond to changes in estrogens; hormone therapy is being used in conjunction with surgical intervention to prevent/decrease recurrence.

D. Chemotherapy: a combination of drugs will be used to treat the malignancy.

Nursing Interventions

❖ Goal: To promote early detection of breast cancer through mammography, clinical breast exam, and breast self-examination (BSE);

A. Screening mammography should begin at age 40.

B. Teach client how to perform breast self-examination. (see Box 17-3).

C. Clinical breast exam should begin with clients in their 20s and 30s, and every year for asymptomatic woman age 40 or older.

BOX 17-3	BREAST SELF-EXAMINATION

- Evaluate risk factors; educate woman about increased risk factors.

- Woman should perform breast self-examination (BSE) on a regular basis; once a month about a week after her period or at the same time each month if the woman has no periods.

- It is important for the BSE to be done on a regular basis; this makes it easier to detect abnormalities when they occur.

- The BSE should include the following three steps:

STEP 1: Inspection before a mirror to determine asymmetry or changes in size. Breast should be evaluated from three positions: with the arms relaxed at the sides; with the arms over the head pressing on the back of the head; with the hands on the hips, palms pressing inward to flex the chest muscles. Look for dimpling, differences in sizes of the breast, ulcerations, nipple retraction, and increased vascularity.

STEP 2: Breast should be palpated while lying down; flatten the right breast by placing a pillow under the right shoulder. With the fingers flat, use the sensitive pads of the middle three fingers of the left hand. Feel for lumps or changes using a rubbing motion. Press firmly enough to feel the different breast tissues. Examine the entire breast from the collarbone to area on which the base of your bra rests and the axillary area. Pay particular attention to the upper outer quadrant of each breast. Gently squeeze the nipple to determine presence of any drainage.

STEP 3: In the shower or bath examine your breasts; hands glide easier over wet skin.

- Women older than 40 years should have a mammogram every year; women with increased risk factors should maintain regular follow-up with a physician.

- The American Cancer Society provides excellent teaching opportunities for nurses, as well as extensive information for women regarding early detection of breast cancer and rehabilitation after a mastectomy.

D. American Cancer Society recommends a yearly MRI and a mammography for women age 30 or older who have a family history of breast cancer.

❖ Goal: To prepare the client physiologically and psychologically for surgery (normal preoperative and postoperative care; see Chapter 3).

A. Assist woman to decrease emotional stress and anxiety; encourage use of spiritual and social resources.

B. Provide emotional support; encourage verbalization.

C. Anticipate concerns related to sexuality and fear of rejection by husband or sex partner after the mastectomy (see the section on Body Image in Chapter 6).

> **TEST ALERT: Plan measures to assist client to cope with anxiety; assess client's response to illness; identify coping mechanisms of client and family.**

D. Determine whether any plans for reconstructive surgery have been discussed.

❖ Goal: To recognize and prevent postoperative complications (Figure 17-4).
A. There may be one or more drains in the incisional area. Jackson-Pratt drains are commonly used.

> **TEST ALERT: Empty and reestablish negative pressure of portable wound suction devices.**

B. Assess wound for infection.
C. Position client in semi-Fowler's and arm on affected side so that each joint is elevated and positioned higher than the more proximal joint; this promotes gravity drainage via the lymphatic and venous circulations.
D. Do not take blood pressure or perform any injections or venipuncture on the arm of the affected side.
E. Arm exercises are usually started on the first postoperative day.
   1. Assist/teach the woman to perform flexion and extension exercises with the wrist and elbow frequently throughout the day. Squeezing a ball is good exercise at this time.
   2. The affected arm should not be abducted or externally rotated in initial exercises. Encourage movement of the arm in activities of daily living (brushing her hair, eating, washing her face).

F. Approximately 2 to 3 weeks after surgery and with good wound healing, more active exercises are initiated.
   1. Pendulum arm swings.
   2. Pulley-type rope exercise to promote forward and lateral movement of the arms.
   3. "Wall climbing" with the fingers.

> **TEST ALERT: Identify factors interfering with wound healing. The arm on the affected side will be at increased risk for developing problems of edema and infection. The arm should be protected throughout rehabilitation and during activities of daily living for an indefinite period of time.**

Home Care

❖ Goal: To promote the client's return to homeostasis and to help her understand implications of modified lifestyle; to identify measures to maintain health.
A. Discuss symptoms of recurrence and importance of making regular visits to the physician to monitor recovery and to detect changes.
B. Promote a positive self-image and reintegration with family and loved ones.
C. Discuss with client plans for obtaining a breast prosthesis.
D. Encourage the woman to participate in the Reach to Recovery program through the American Cancer Society. Check with the physician to see whether representatives may visit with the client before the surgery.
E. Compression arm sleeves used to minimize swelling from lymphedema.

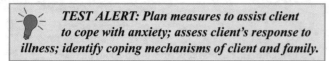

POST MASTECTOMY
NURSING CARE

- Elevate affected side with distal joint higher than proximal joint.
- No BP, injections or venipunctures on affected side.
- Watch for S & S of edema on affected arm. (edema may occur post op or years later)
- Lymphedema can occur any time after axillary node disection.
- Limited arm exercises 24 hrs post op.
- Abduction and external rotation arm exercises after wound has healed.
- Assess dressing for drainage.
- Assess wound drain for amount and color.
- Provide privacy when client looks at incision.
- Chemotherapy.
- Radiation therapy.
- Psychological concerns:
  Altered body image
  Altered sexuality
  Fear of disease outcome

FIGURE 17-4 Postmastectomy nursing care. (From Zerwekh J, Claborn J, Miller CJ: *Memory notebook of nursing, vol 1,* ed 4, Ingram, 2008, Nursing Education Consultants.)

Study Questions: Reproductive System

1. A client is 1-day postoperative from a suprapubic pros-tatectomy. The nurse notices pink-tinged urine in the client's urine bag. What is the best nursing interpre-tation of this finding?
   1. This is a normal occurrence at this time after this type of surgery.
   2. There is increased bleeding and the client should be kept on bed rest.
   3. This is probably due to an infection; a urinalysis needs to be performed.
   4. The continuous bladder irrigation should be in-creased to flush the bladder.

2. The nurse is evaluating her teaching with a client who has herpes genitalis (HSV-2). How would the nurse know her teaching was effective?
   1. Client understands that after blisters break, she is no longer contagious.
   2. Client understands the importance of washing her hands after touching her perineal area.
   3. Client understands the need to take **Zovirax** for the rest of her life to prevent additional outbreaks.
   4. Client understands that after the initial outbreak she will be immune and have no further lesions.

3. Why are all sexually transmitted diseases (STDs) re-ported to the public health department?
   1. To slow transmission by informing all who may have had contact with the client.
   2. To help the bureau of statistics study characteristics and decrease the incidence.
   3. So the public health department will know whom to treat.
   4. To develop educational programs for the infected client and their sexual partners.

4. A client is 48 hours after surgery for a left mastectomy. What would be included in a teaching plan for this client?
   Select all that apply:
   _____ 1. Massage the wound site with essentials oils once incision has healed.
   _____ 2. Avoid needle sticks in the left arm.
   _____ 3. Begin active exercises immediately, such as pendu-lum arm swings.
   _____ 4. Keep affected arm close to the body.
   _____ 5. Elevate the arm on pillows to prevent edema.
   _____ 6. Take blood pressure measurements from the right arm.

5. A client has a painless lesion on the side of his penis. What is the nurse's best interpretation of this finding?
   1. The presence of a chancre lesion is characteristic of syphilis.
   2. The lesion is characteristic in clients with long-term gonorrhea.
   3. The lesion may indicate the outbreak of herpes sim-plex virus.
   4. The area should be cultured for the presence of papilloma virus.

6. The nurse is preparing a client for a pelvic examination. What is important for the nurse to do before the exami-nation?
   1. Make sure the client had a bowel prep and cleansing enema.
   2. Carefully document the menstrual cycle; client should not be in last third of cycle.
   3. Question the client regarding her last period and the possibility of pregnancy.
   4. Make sure the client voids before the procedure.

7. The nurse is caring for a client the first postoperative day after a left-sided mastectomy. What observations would cause the nurse the most concern?
   1. Temperature of 100.6° F, pulse of 110 beats per minute.
   2. Moderate amount of serosanguineous drainage on dressing.
   3. Left forearm and hand swollen, palpable radial pulse.
   4. Urine output of 40 mL per hour, slight increase in blood glucose level.

8. An older adult client complains of vaginal itching and burning. What would be the best nursing management?
   1. Douche daily with a weak vinegar solution.
   2. Apply estrogen vaginal cream.
   3. Wash the perineal area well with soap and water.
   4. Encourage the use of petroleum jelly during inter-course.

9. The nursing assessment of a client with prostatic hyper-trophy would identify which symptom?
   1. Pain when voiding.
   2. Urinary frequency.
   3. Distended bladder.
   4. Scrotal edema.

10. What equipment will be needed by the primary care provider to check a client's prostate?
    1. Straight catheter tray.
    2. Urethral stints and gloves.
    3. A lubricant and gloves.
    4. A stethoscope and a rectal tube.

11. A client is postoperative after a transurethral resection of the prostate (TURP). He is receiving a continuous bladder irrigation. The nurse notices that the fluid is not draining into the urinary catheter bag. The nurse attempts to irrigate to clear the catheter line, but is unsuccessful. What action should the practical nurse take next?
    1. Notify the primary care provider.
    2. Irrigate again, increasing the pressure.
    3. Observe for 30 minutes before irrigating again.
    4. Replace the current catheter.

Answers and rationales to these questions are in the section at the end of the book titled Chapter Study Questions: Answers and Rationales.

Appendix 17-1 MEDICATIONS USED IN REPRODUCTIVE SYSTEM DISORDERS

Medications	Side Effects	Nursing Implications

BENIGN PROSTATIC HYPERPLASIA MEDICATIONS: Act by decreasing the size of the prostate, therefore decreasing pressure on the urinary tract in clients with BPH or by promoting smooth muscle relaxation (alpha adrenergic blockers).

Medications	Side Effects	Nursing Implications
Alpha Adrenergic Blocker (Nonselective) Doxazosin (**Cardura**): PO Tamsulosin (**Flomax**): PO Terazosin (**Hytrin**): PO	Dizziness, fatigue, orthostatic hypotension, dyspnea, headache.	1. Advise client of possible problems of decreased blood pressure and orthostatic hypotension. 2. Prostatic cancer should be ruled out before medications are started. 3. Medication should decrease problems of urination associated with BPH. 4. Monitor blood pressure closely if taking antihypertensive medications.
Finasteride (**Proscar**): PO	Erectile dysfunction, decreased libido	1. Client should take contraceptive precautions or not have sexual intercourse with women who could become pregnant. 2. Women who may be or are pregnant should not handle the tablets.

ANTIFUNGAL/PROTOZOAL MEDICATIONS: Used to treat vaginal fungal infections.

Medications	Side Effects	Nursing Implications
Clotrimazole (**Gyne-Lotrimin**): intravaginally (OTC) Miconazole (**Monistat 3**): intravaginally Fluconazole (**Diflucan**): PO Terconazole (**Terazol**): intravaginally Metronidazole (**Flagyl**): PO	Nausea, vomiting, headache, vaginal irritation	1. Creams are not recommended to be used with tampons or diaphragms. 2. Not recommended for use during pregnancy or lactation. 3. **Flagyl** is used to treat trichomoniasis; instruct client to avoid alcohol because it can lead to serious side effects of throbbing headaches, nausea, excessive vomiting, hyperventilation, and tachycardia. 4. Suppositories or applicators are used to place medication in the vagina. 5. If client does not see improvement within 3 days, she should return to her health care provider. 6. **Diflucan** can be given as a single dose for vaginal candidiasis.

ERECTILE DYSFUNCTION MEDICATIONS: Promote an increase in arterial pressure and inflow of blood into the penis and reduce the venous outflow causing engorgement and producing an erection.

Medications	Side Effects	Nursing Implications
Sildenafil (**Viagra**): PO Vardenafil (**Levitra**): PO Tadalafil (**Cialis**): PO	Hypotension can be a serious SE Headache, flushing, visual changes	1. Should not be taken concurrently with nitrates. 2. Alpha blockers (used for treatment of BPH) are contraindicated in the client taking tadalafil and vardenafil, should be used with caution in client taking sildenafil. 3. Vardenafil can cause prolonged QT interval on ECG, should not be used in combination with antidysrhythmic medications. 4. Primary differences in the medications is the onset and duration of action. 5. Priapism, painful erection, or erection lasting over 4 hours may require medical intervention to prevent penile damage.

> ✓ **NURSING PRIORITY:** *Always inquire if a client is taking an ED medication before treating chest pain with any nitrate medication.*

BPH, Benign prostatic hypertrophy; *IV*, intravenous; *OTC*, over the counter; *PO*, by mouth (oral).

Appendix 17-2	HORMONE REPLACEMENT	

Medications	Side Effects	Nursing Implications
Conjugated estrogen (**Premarin, Ortho-est, Prempro**): PO, intravaginally Micronized estradiol (**Estrace, Vagifem**): PO, IM, intravaginally Estradiol (**Estraderm, Ortho Tri-Cyclen Lo**): transdermal patches	Nausea, vomiting, breakthrough bleeding, weight gain, swollen tender breasts, increased blood pressure Increased risk for uterine cancer	1. Important for menopausal women to continue with 1200 to 1500 mg/day calcium intake and weight-bearing exercises along with estrogen replacement to prevent osteoporosis. 2. Should not be used by women who have known or suspected cancer of the breast, undiagnosed vaginal bleeding, or possible pregnancy. 3. Used with precaution—or not at all—in women with clotting disorders or history of DVT/PE. 4. Report any unusual bleeding to primary care provider. 5. Research data changed the practice of treating perimenopausal women's symptoms with HRT. It is their decision to take it or not, but use should be short-term and lowest effective dose with risks outlined. 6. *Use:* Replacement hormone to treat symptoms associated with menopause—hot flashes, atopic vaginitis (local vaginal application of low-dose estrogen—**Vagifem**) prevention of postmenopausal osteoprosis..
Medroxyprogesterone acetate (**Provera, Depo-Provera**): PO, IM	Menses may become more irregular	1. *Use:* Provera—for menopausal women who still have a uterus, significantly decreased risk for uterine cancer when used with estrogen therapy. **Depo-Provera**—birth control injection given every 3 months. 2. Women should continue with increased calcium intake and weight-bearing exercises to prevent osteoporosis; should have yearly Pap smears, mammograms, and cholesterol test.

IM, intramuscular; *IV*, intravenous; *PO*, by mouth (oral).

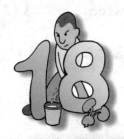

Urinary-Renal System

PHYSIOLOGY OF THE KIDNEY AND URINARY TRACT

A. Kidney function.
   1. Excretory.
      a. Rid the body of metabolic wastes.
         (1) Regulate fluid volume; normally, 125 mL of fluid is filtered each minute (glomerular filtration rate [GFR]); however, *only* 1 mL is excreted as urine; average urine output is about 1440 mL per day.
         (2) Regulate the composition of electrolytes.
         (3) Assist in maintaining acid-base balance.
      b. Regulation of blood pressure.
         (1) Juxtaglomerular cells are located in the afferent arteriole just before it enters the glomerulus.
         (2) The cells respond to a decrease in the blood flow (decrease in blood pressure) by increasing the secretion of renin.
         (3) Renin acts on angiotensin I and converts it to angiotensin II, which is a powerful vasoconstrictor. Peripheral resistance is increased; therefore, blood pressure is increased.
         (4) Kidneys receive 20-25% of total cardiac output with a renal blood flow rate of 600-1300 mL/min.
   2. Endocrine.
      a. Aldosterone production is stimulated by the increase in angiotensin I; therefore sodium and water are retained to increase circulating volume and increase blood pressure.
      b. Regulates red blood cell production through synthesis of erythropoietin; released in response to hypoxia and reduced renal blood flow.
      c. Aids in calcium metabolism by activating vitamin D, which allows for absorption of calcium from the gastrointestinal tract.

B. Nephron function.
   1. Filtration: occurs in the glomerulus via a semipermeable membrane. The membrane does not normally allow large protein molecules to be filtered out of the blood.
      a. GFR is the amount of blood filtered by the glomeruli in a given time (approximately 120-140 mL/min).
      b. Changes in GFR occur when the pressure gradi-

ents from the glomerular capillaries across the semipermeable membrane to the glomerulus are altered.
   (1) Pressure gradient changes occur when there is a variation in the systemic blood pressure (hypotension), a significant change in the pressure in Bowman's capsule in the glomerulus (edema) occurs, and when ureteral obstruction occurs.
   (2) The kidneys' response to changes in pressures is buffered by an autoregulatory mechanism to maintain a stable range of blood pressure. The autoregulatory mechanism maintains renal blood flow and the GFR within wide fluctuations of blood pressure. When the pressure range is outside the autoregulatory mechanism (hypotension/hypertension), the GFR will fluctuate with the systemic blood pressure.

> ✔ **NURSING PRIORITY:** *Determine whether client has a decreased urinary output (below 30 mL per hour in an adult, 20 mL per hour in a child, and 1 mL/kg/hr in an infant); urinary output should be carefully evaluated regarding blood pressure level; blood pressure must provide renal perfusion to maintain adequate urinary output. The level of blood pressure to maintain renal perfusion varies greatly from one client to another.*

   (3) If the glomerular membrane is damaged, plasma proteins will escape. A decrease in serum proteins decreases the normal serum oncotic pressure; this results in water retention and edema formation.
   2. Tubular reabsorption: after the glomerulus has filtered the blood, the tubules separate the water and solutes by osmosis and diffusion. Water moves across the semipermeable membrane and is reabsorbed or excreted in response to the concentration gradient of the solutes (sodium, potassium, chloride, urea, etc.). Only a small amount of the total water filtered out of the kidneys is excreted as urine. Solutes are also reabsorbed according to the concentration gradient.
   3. Tubular secretion: regulates the potassium level and maintains the acid-base balance with other regulatory mechanisms.

C.   Urinary tract (Figure 18-1).
1.   Ureters.
a.   Muscular tubes through which urine flows from the kidneys to the bladder.
b.   Ureterovesical valve: located at the opening of the ureter into the bladder (ureterovesical junction); prevents backflow of urine into the ureters when the bladder contracts.
2.   Bladder.
a.   As the bladder fills, the stretch receptors are stimulated. In the adult, the first urge to void will occur when 100 mL to 150 mL has collected; approximately 400 mL to 600 mL of urine will initiate a feeling of bladder fullness.
b.   Bladder capacity varies from 600 mL to 1000 mL.
3.   Voiding: stimulation is sent to the sacral area of the spinal column where the micturition reflex, or voiding reflex, is initiated; after toilet training, the cerebral cortex (via the spinal column) allows for voluntary control of bladder contractions that initiate urination.
4.   Urethra: a small, membranous tube that conveys urine from the bladder to the exterior of the body.
a.   Female urethra is 1 to 2 inches long.
b.   Male urethra is 8 to 10 inches.

System Assessment

A.   External assessment.
1.   Inspect skin for changes in color, turgor, texture (urate crystals), bruising, and excoriations.
2.   Assess face, abdomen, and extremities for edema.
3.   Determine weight gain or loss.
4.   Palpate kidneys and bladder.
a.   Landmark: for kidney palpation, the landmark is the costovertebral angle, formed by the rib cage and the vertebral column.
b.   Bladder is palpated just above the suprapubic area (or symphysis pubis bone).
c.   Kidney and bladder should be nonpalpable with no discomfort on palpation.
5.   General: fatigue, lethargy, level of alertness.
B.   History.
1.   Presence of renal or urologic congenital defect.
2.   Determine whether client has ever been exposed to chemicals, especially carbon tetrachloride, phenol, and ethylene glycol, because these are nephrotoxic. Determine smoking history: cigarette smoking is a risk factor for bladder cancer.
3.   Determine whether client has received antibiotics that may be nephrotoxic: aminoglycosides, amphotericin B, and sulfonamides.

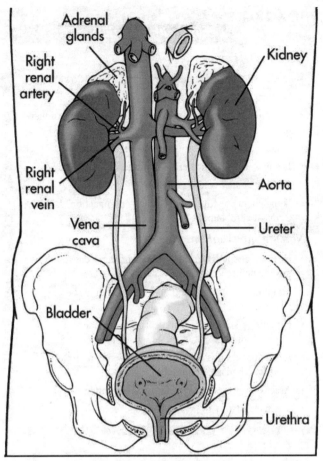

FIGURE 18-1 Structure of the Urinary System (Monahan: *Phipps' Medical-Surgical Nursing*, ed 8, 2007, Mosby.)

4.   Assess dietary intake: Determine increased levels of calcium. Anorexia and nausea and vomiting may cause dehydration or be the result of altered renal function.
5.   Determine level of activity: immobility leads to demineralization of the bones, which can predispose to infection and calculus formation.
6.   Evaluate complaints of pain: dysuria; flank, costovertebral, or suprapubic pain.
7.   Assess changes in pattern of urination: frequency, nocturia, urgency, enuresis, incontinence (Box 18-1 and Table 18-1).
8.   Assess changes in urine output: polyuria, oliguria, anuria.
9.   Assess changes in urine consistency: hematuria, pyuria, diluted, concentrated, change in color.
10. Determine whether client is taking any medications that may affect urinary or renal function.
11. Determine whether client has any chronic health care problems that affect renal and urinary tract structures (diabetes mellitus, hypertension, allergies, or multiple sclerosis).

BOX 18-1   OLDER ADULT CARE FOCUS
Dealing with Incontinence

Need to Determine:

- Does client have difficulty initiating urinary flow?
- Is client aware of need to void?
- Can client empty bladder completely, or is there residual urine?
- Is there bladder distention and overflow dribbling?
- Is stress incontinence present or urge incontinence?
- What are usual voiding times?
- Is the client constipated or is there an impaction? Is this a chronic problem?

Nursing Interventions

- Help the client determine when he or she needs to urinate before an accident occurs.
- Maintain adequate fluid intake but limit fluids before bedtime.
- Establish a voiding schedule: offer assistance and encourage voiding.
- Assess the client's access to the bathroom; determine need for a bedside commode.
- Assess for presence of urinary tract infection.
- Teach client how to perform Kegel exercises.

Urinary Tract Infections

✱   **Stasis of urine in the bladder and reflux of urine back into the original reservoir are the primary causes of urinary tract infections (UTIs).** *Escherichia coli* **is the most common pathogen leading to UTIs.**

A.   Upper UTIs: *pyelonephritis*, an inflammation of the renal pelvis and the parenchyma of the kidney(s).
B.   Lower UTI.
   1.   *Cystitis:* inflammation/infection of the bladder.
   2.   *Urethritis:* inflammation of the urethra.
C.   UTIs occur in an ascending route up the urinary tract system.

> **TEST ALERT: Use alternative measures to promote voiding; promote bowel and bladder control.**

Data Collection

A.   Factors contributing to UTI.
   1.   Adult female urethra is short and close to the rectum and vagina, which predisposes it to contamination from fecal material.
   2.   Ureterovesical reflux: the reflux of urine from the urethra into the bladder; this causes a constant residual of urine in the bladder after voiding and precipitates UTI.

TABLE 18-1   TYPES OF URINARY INCONTINENCE

TYPE OF URINARY INCONTINENCE (UI)	DEFINITION	SYMPTOMS AND SIGNS
Urge	Involuntary loss of urine associated with a strong sensation of urinary urgency.	Loss of urine with an abrupt and strong desire to void; involuntary loss of urine (without symptoms). Nocturia is common.
Stress	Involuntary loss of urine, usually associated with increased intra-abdominal pressure.	Small amount of urine loss during coughing, sneezing, laughing, or other physical activities; continuous leak at rest or with minimal exertion (e.g., postural changes).
Mixed	Combination of urge and stress UI.	Combinations of urge and stress UI symptoms (as listed above).
Overflow	Bladder overdistention.	Frequent or constant dribbling or urge or stress incontinence symptoms, as well as urgency and frequent urination.
Functional	Chronic impairment of physical and/or cognitive functioning.	Residual urine after voiding is common. Urge incontinence or functional limitations or environmental factors.
Unconscious or reflex	Neurologic dysfunction secondary to nerve damage.	Postmicturitional or continual incontinence; severe urgency with bladder hypersensitivity (sensory urgency).

From Fantl J et al: *Managing acute and chronic incontinence: clinical practice guideline: quick reference guide for clinicians,* No. 2, Rockville, MD, 1996, U.S. Department of Health and Human Services, Public Health Service, Agency for Health Care Policy and Research, AHCPR Pub. No. 96-0686.; Lewis SM et al: *Medical-surgical nursing: assessment and management of clinical problems,* St. Louis, 2007, Mosby.

3. Vesicoureteral reflux (ureterovesical reflux): the reflux of urine from the bladder into one or both of the ureters and possibly into the renal pelvis.
4. Instrumentation: catheterization or cystoscopic examination.
5. Stasis of urine in the bladder leading to urinary retention for any reason (clients with prostate disease).
6. Obstruction of urinary flow: congenital anomalies, urethral strictures, ureteral stones, contracture of the bladder neck, tumor, fibrosis, or fecal impaction.
7. Bladder hypotonia: mechanical compression of the ureters; hormone changes predispose pregnant and postmenopausal women to more frequent UTIs.
8. Metabolic disorders such as diabetes.
9. Sexual intercourse promotes development of UTI.
10. Fecal contamination of the urethral meatus.

 TEST ALERT: Identify an infection and be able to assess and to identify pertinent data indicating a urinary tract and/or kidney infection.

B. Clinical manifestations.
1. Cystitis (lower UTI) (Figure 18-2).
a. Frequency, urgency, dysuria (classic triad of symptoms).
b. Hematuria.
c. Nocturia, incontinence, hesitancy, weak stream.
d. Often asymptomatic with bacteriuria.
e. Low back pain or suprapubic pain.
2. Pyelonephritis (upper UTI).
a. Fever, chills, malaise, flank pain on affected side.
b. Symptoms of cystitis.
c. Older adults may not have a fever, and those older than 80 years may have a decrease in temperature and exhibit confusion (Box 18-2).
3. Urosepsis: a urinary tract infection that has become systemic and is life-threatening.
C. Diagnostics (see Appendix 18-1).
D. Complications.
1. A lower UTI may progress to an upper UTI.
2. Chronic pyelonephritis may develop after repeated bouts of acute pyelonephritis.

Treatment

A. Medical (see Appendix 18-2).
1. Broad-spectrum antibiotics, especially the sulfonamides for lower urinary tract infections; fluoroquinolones for upper urinary tract infections.
2. Urinary analgesics.
3. Antispasmodics.
4. Antipyretics.

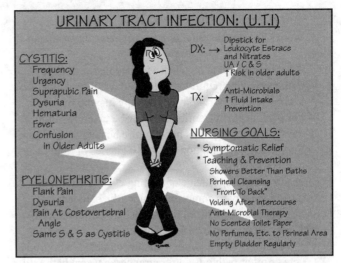

FIGURE 18-2 **Urinary tract infection.** (From Zerwekh J, Claborn J, Miller CJ: *Memory notebook of nursing, vol 1,* ed 4, Ingram, 2008, Nursing Education Consultants.)

B. Dietary.
1. Encourage fluid intake of 3000 mL per day.
a. Dilute urine causes less irritation.
b. The increase in flow of urine through the urinary tract decreases the movement of bacteria up the urinary tract.
c. Discourage consumption of carbonated beverages and foods or drinks containing baking powder or baking soda. Caffeine, alcohol, citrus fruits, and highly spiced foods can cause bladder irritation.
d. Daily intake of cranberry juice or cranberry essence tablets is helpful for some clients, as it appears to decrease the ability of bacteria to adhere to the epithelial cells lining the urinary tract.

BOX 18-2 **OLDER ADULT CARE FOCUS**
Urinary Tract Infection

- First symptom may be increased confusion.
- A sudden onset of incontinence or an increase in frequency of incontinence should be investigated.
- A client with fever, chills, and tachycardia in the absence of urinary tract symptoms should be evaluated for septicemia from a urinary tract origin.
- Avoid use of indwelling urinary catheters.
- Encourage clients to void every 2 hours even if they do not feel a need; decreases residual urine and incontinence.
- Cleanse perineal area after each voiding and prevent fecal contamination of the urinary meatus.
- Women should wear cotton underwear and avoid tight, restrictive clothing.

Nursing Interventions

❖   **Goal:** To provide relief of pain, urgency, dysuria, and fever.

A.   Antibiotics need to be taken as scheduled. Initially, therapy may be required for 1 to 3 days; if problem is recurrent, 10 to 14 days of therapy may be required. For pyelonephritis, antibiotics may be taken for 14 to 21 days; severe symptoms may require hospitalization.

B.   Encourage consumption of 8 to 10 glasses of fluids daily (3000 mL).

C.   Teach client importance of voiding every 2 to 3 hours during the day to completely empty the bladder.

D.   Sitz baths may be taken to decrease irritation of urethra.

❖   **Goal:** To prevent recurrence of infection.

A.   Avoid sitting in a bathtub with added bubble bath products or other bath oils and fragrances; a warm bath will decrease symptoms, but nothing should be added to the water.

B.   Explain importance of cleansing the perineal area from front to back after voiding and after each bowel movement. Avoid use of perineal sprays and powders.

C.   If intercourse seems to predispose to infection, encourage voiding immediately before and after intercourse. A female client with recurrent UTIs may need to temporarily stop using a diaphragm and spermicidal creams/jelly.

D.   Teach importance of long-term therapy if recurrent infections are a problem.

E.   Encourage and explain the need for follow-up care to prevent complications of chronic UTIs.

F.   Caffeine, alcohol, citrus juices, and carbonated beverages should be avoided.

 Urinary Calculi

✳   **Stones may form anywhere in the urinary tract; the most common location for stones is in the pelvis of the kidney. If the stones are small, they may be passed into the bladder.**

A.   Stones in the bladder may increase in size if urinary stasis and alkaline pH are present.

B.   Types of urinary calculi.
   1.   Calcium oxalate or phosphate stones: tend to be small; account for 40% to 50% of all upper urinary tract calculi.
   2.   Struvite stones: contain bacteria and tend to be large; more common in women than men.
   3.   Uric acid stones: occur most often in clients with primary or secondary problems of uric acid metabolism (gout); high incidence in men, particularly Jewish men.

Data Collection

Regardless of the type of stone formed, the clinical manifestations, diagnostics, and treatment are essentially the same.

A.   Risk factors/etiology.
   1.   Infection, urinary stasis, immobility.
   2.   Hypercalcemia and hypercalciuria (hyperparathyroidism, renal tubular acidosis).
   3.   Excessive intake of dietary proteins, which increases uric acid production.
   4.   Excessive consumption of tea or fruit juice, which elevates urinary oxalate levels.
   5.   Low fluid intake.
   6.   Majority of clients are between the ages of 20 and 55. Stones occur more often in the summer months.
   7.   Increased incidence of family history with stone formation due to inherited metabolic risk factors.

B.   Clinical manifestations.
   1.   Sharp, sudden, severe abdominal or flank pain.
      a.   May be described as "colic," either ureteral or renal.
      b.   Pain may be intermittent, depending on the movement of the stone; spasm in the ureter occurs as it attempts to move the stone toward the bladder.
      c.   Pain may radiate around the flank area, down into the bladder, the genitalia, and the thigh.
   2.   Hematuria may be present as a result of the traumatic effects of the stone on the ureter and the bladder.
   3.   Oliguria or anuria suggest urinary obstruction and must be treated immediately.
   4.   Nausea and vomiting are common.
   5.   May be associated with fever and infection.

C.   Diagnostics (see Appendix 18-1).

D.   Complications.
   1.   Recurrent stone formation.
   2.   Infection.
   3.   Renal failure.

Treatment

A.   Medical.
   1.   Increase fluid intake to 3000 mL/day to decrease urine concentration.
   2.   Medications that prevent the absorption of calcium (thiazide diuretics and phosphates).
   3.   Medications to increase urinary flow: tamsulosin (**Flomax**).
   4.   Spasmolytic agents (anticholinergics).
   5.   For uric acid stones, allopurinol (**Zyloprim**).
   6.   Opioids for pain relief.
   7.   Dietary.
      a.   Sodium may also be restricted, because sodium increases the excretion of calcium in the urine.
      b.   Decrease in protein intake or an alkaline-ash diet for clients with uric acid stones.
      c.   Decrease intake of cola, coffee, and tea, which tend to increase the risk for calculi formation.

B.   Surgical.
   1.   Nephrolithotomy: incision into the kidney and removal of the stone.

2. Ureterolithotomy: incision into the ureter to locate a stone and remove it.
3. Stenting: insertion of a small tube (stent) into ureter via ureteroscopy to dilate ureter to enlarge passageway for expulsion of stone or stone fragments.
C. Lithotripsy: cystoscopic, percutaneous ultrasonic, laser, or extracorporeal shock-wave lithotripsy (ESWL).
1. For ESWL, client is anesthetized and placed in a water bath. Some lithotripters do not require submersion.
   a. Sound waves travel through the water and are directed to the stone. The force of the sound wave shatters the stone, and the remains are excreted in the urine.
   b. It is essential that the client remain absolutely motionless during the procedure, which lasts about 30 to 45 minutes. Therefore some form of sedation or analgesia is necessary during the procedure.
   c. A ureteral stent is often placed after lithotripsy procedures to promote passage of stone fragments and left in place for 2 weeks.
2. Hematuria is common after the procedure.

Nursing Interventions

❖ Goal: To relieve pain.
A. Administer analgesics as prescribed: morphine or hydromorphone (**Dilaudid**).
B. Hot baths or moist heat applied to flank area.
C. Encourage increased fluid intake (3000 mL/day) to prevent dehydration.
D. Strain all urine and inspect for blood clots and passage of stone.
E. If stone is passed, it should be saved and sent to the lab for analysis to determine the type of stone so appropriate therapy can be maintained.
❖ Goal: To promote understanding of health care regimen.
A. Dietary restrictions, depending on type of stone.
B. Discuss rationale, dose, frequency, and important information relating to medication administration.
C. Teach symptoms of recurring stone formation, such as hematuria, flank pain, and signs of infection.
D. Instruct client to continue high fluid intake.
E. Promote periodic medical follow-up visits to evaluate for symptoms of infection and recurring stone formation.

Hypospadias and Epispadias

✳ *Hypospadias:* **the urethral opening is located behind the glans penis or along the penile shaft; this is a common anomaly.**
✳ *Epispadias:* **the urethral opening is located on the dorsal or upper side of the penis; this is a rare problem.**

Data Collection

A. Clinical manifestations.
1. Visualization of defect.
2. Chordee: ventral curvature of the penis, which gives it a crooked appearance (hypospadias).
3. Stream of urine does not come out the end of the penis.
4. Hypospadias is associated with cryptorchidism in severe cases.
5. Bladder exstrophy is a severe form of epispadias.

Treatment

A. Surgical correction of the defect.
1. *Hypospadias:* recommended repair by 6 to 18 months of age.
2. *Epispadias:* more complex and frequently associated with other genitourinary system defects; repair may be very involved and require multiple staged surgical procedures.

Nursing Interventions

❖ Goal: To provide emotional support and to promote normal growth and development.
A. Frequently the infant is not circumcised until the repair of the hypospadias.
B. The infant with epispadias may be discharged home before repair is done.
C. The preferred time for repair is between 6 and 12 months; it is important not to delay repair of hypospadias beyond the time for toilet training.
D. A diaper and a sterile nonadherent dressing are applied over the exposed bladder when the infant has a bladder defect.
E. Teach parents signs of UTI.
F. Help parents understand realistic expectations of the outcome of surgery (epispadias and/or bladder exstrophy).

Nephrotic Syndrome

✳ **A problem with glomerular permeability to plasma proteins results in massive urinary protein loss. The most common type is a primary condition, minimal change nephrotic syndrome.**
A. Changes occur in the basement membrane of the glomeruli that allow the large protein molecules to pass through the membrane and be excreted. The loss of albumin from the serum decreases the oncotic pressure in the capillary bed and allows fluid to pass into the interstitial tissues and the abdominal cavity (ascites) and interstitial spaces (edema).
B. The interstitial fluid shift causes hypovolemia. The renin-angiotensin response is stimulated. Aldosterone secretion is increased, and the tubules begin to conserve sodium and water to increase the circulating volume.

C. In the majority of children with the syndrome, the cause is unknown; it may be congenital, idiopathic, or secondary to another disease; frequently, there is no evidence of renal dysfunction or systemic disease.

Data Collection

A. Risk factors/etiology.
1. Usual history is a well child who begins to gain weight and exhibits pallor and fatigue.
2. Majority of children affected are male and between the ages of 2 and 4 years; uncommon in infants younger than 1 year.
3. May occur in adults secondary to systemic disease (e.g., SLE, diabetes) or may be idiopathic.

B. Clinical manifestations.
1. Hallmarks: edema, proteinuria, hypoalbuminemia, and hyperlipidemia in the absence of hypertension and hematuria in children.
   a. Facial edema, especially periorbital edema; may be more pronounced in the morning and subside during the day.
   b. Generalized edema of the lower extremities; may increase during the day.
   c. Labia or scrotum may become very edematous.
   d. Edema may progress to the level of severe generalized edema (anasarca).
   e. Ascites and pleural effusion.
2. Gradual increase in weight.
3. Volume of urine is decreased, and urine may be foamy and tea colored.
4. Irritability, fatigue, lethargy.
5. Malnourishment: child is malnourished as a result of decreased intake and loss of protein in the urine but may not appear so because of edema.
6. Infection can result in significant morbidity or mortality.

C. Diagnostics (see Appendix 18-1).
1. Decreased serum protein levels: hypoalbuminemia.
2. Urinalysis: increased specific gravity, massive proteinuria (greater than 3+ as determined by dipstick test).
3. Creatinine clearance may be decreased, with normal serum creatinine levels.

D. Potential complications.
1. Compromised immune system leading to an increase in infections (e.g., pneumonia, bronchitis, peritonitis).
2. Circulatory insufficiency caused by hypovolemia, with severe edema.
3. Thromboembolism secondary to hypercoagulability.

Treatment

A. Medical.
1. Corticosteroids: prednisone/prednisolone.
2. Diuretics: used when edema progresses despite sodium restriction.

3. Salt-poor human albumin is used for treatment of vascular insufficiency and severe edema.
4. Prophylactic broad-spectrum antimicrobial agents.
5. Immunosuppressant therapy is prescribed for children who are not responsive to steroid therapy.

B. Dietary.
1. Decreased sodium intake.
2. Proteins consumed should have high biologic value (low to moderate protein diet).
3. Usually, fluid is not restricted.

Nursing Interventions

❖ **Goal:** To monitor disease progress and reduce edema.
A. Support edematous areas such as scrotum.
B. Provide and encourage a salt-restricted diet.
C. Administer salt-poor albumin; monitor closely for circulatory overload during and after administration.
D. Provide meticulous skin care and keep opposing skin surfaces dry; change position frequently, and monitor good body alignment.
E. Determine weight daily, maintain accurate intake and output record, measure abdominal girth daily.
F. Test urine with dipstick for protein; check specific gravity.
G. Monitor cardiac function for complications of fluid balance (marked edema but hypovolemic).

❖ **Goal:** To prevent infection.
A. Child is susceptible to infection because of a compromised immune state, as well as steroid therapy.
B. Protect child from upper respiratory tract infections; provide good pulmonary hygiene; check breath sounds.
C. Prevent skin excoriation and breakdown; assess carefully for indications of infection.

❖ **Goal:** To promote nutrition.
A. Encourage low to moderate protein intake of high biologic value.
B. Serve frequent small quantities of food to child.
C. Encourage input from child in selection of foods from prescribed diet.

Home Care

A. Inform child and parents about medical regimen: steroids, diuretics, antibiotics.
B. Reassure parents that the prognosis is good; there may be relapses that will require therapy, but few children progress to chronic disease.
C. Obtain medical assistance if relapse occurs; relapse is indicated by edema, proteinuria, fever.
D. Encourage normal growth and development activities; try to prevent social isolation.
E. Teach parents how to perform dipstick urine test for protein; may need to keep a daily diary to evaluate level of proteinuria.

Glomerulonephritis

✻ **Glomerulonephritis is an inflammatory reaction in the glomerulus most commonly as a result of an antigen-antibody response to beta-hemolytic streptococci. An immune complex is formed as a result of the antigen-antibody formation; the complex becomes trapped in the glomerulus. As a result of the edema in the glomeruli, the GFR is significantly decreased. It is the third leading cause of renal failure in the United States.**

Data Collection

A. Risk factors/etiology.
1. The stimulus of the antigen-antibody reaction is most often group A beta-hemolytic *Streptococcus* infection of the throat (tonsillitis, pharyngitis) or skin (impetigo), which ordinarily precedes the onset of the condition by about 10 to 21 days.
2. Most common in children, but all age groups can be affected; males are more frequently affected than females.
B. Clinical manifestations.
1. Acute glomerulonephritis.
   a. Disease may be mild with proteinuria and/or asymptomatic hematuria.
   b. Tea- or cola-colored urine caused by hematuria.
   c. Facial and periorbital edema.
   d. Decrease in urine output (oliguria).
   e. Mild to moderate increase in blood pressure; hypertension is more severe in adults.
   f. Azotemia: presence of nitrogenous waste products in the blood.
2. Chronic glomerulonephritis: symptoms reflect progressive renal failure; more common in adults.
C. Diagnostics (see Appendix 18-1): reduced complement (C3) levels in early stages and elevated antistreptolysin O titer.
D. Complications.
1. Chronic renal failure.
2. Circulatory overload (pulmonary edema) and congestive heart failure (CHF).
3. Hypertensive episodes.

Treatment

A. Medical.
1. Diuretics for severe edema and fluid overload.
2. Antihypertensives.
3. Antibiotics, if the streptococcal infection is still present.
4. Plasmapheresis for filtering out immune complexes (antigens & antibodies).
B. Dietary.
1. Decrease sodium intake.
2. Protein restriction if client is azotemic; however, the anorexia that a child experiences frequently limits protein intake sufficiently.

3. Foods containing large amounts of potassium are often restricted during the oliguric phase.
C. Children with normal blood pressure, adequate urine output, and mild symptoms are cared for at home.
D. Fluid restriction may be implemented if urinary output is decreased.

Nursing Interventions

❖ **Goal:** To protect client's kidneys by preventing secondary infections.
A. Antibiotic therapy if cultures are positive.
B. Child usually experiences fatigue and malaise and will voluntarily restrict activity.
C. Avoid medications that are nephrotoxic.
❖ **Goal:** To maintain fluid balance.
A. Monitor intake and output; maintain diet and fluid restrictions.
B. Monitor renal function: check proteinuria, specific gravity, and color of urine; weigh client daily; if client has hypertension, check blood pressure every 2 to 4 hours.
C. Monitor serum potassium levels.
D. Frequently, the first sign of improvement is an increase in the urine output, which may progress to profuse diuresis.
❖ **Goal:** To prevent complications and promote comfort.
A. Encourage verbalization of fears.
B. Decrease anxiety by explaining treatments and reassuring client and family that the majority of clients recover fully.
C. Most children recover spontaneously, and recurrences are uncommon.

Home Care

A. Teach parent or client symptoms to be reported to physician: nausea, fatigue, vomiting, decrease in urinary output, and symptoms of infection.
B. Explain the need for rest, good nutrition, and avoidance of people with respiratory tract infections.
C. Teach measures to prevent UTIs.
D. Instruct client in regard to diet, fluid needs, and medication therapy.
E. Teach client to perform dipstick urine test to monitor for protein.

Wilms' Tumor (Nephroblastoma)

✻ **Nephroblastoma (Wilms' tumor) is one of the most common intraabdominal tumors of childhood and is associated with congenital anomalies, especially those of the genitourinary tract. The treatment and survival rate are based on the stage of the tumor at the time it is diagnosed.**
A. Risk factors/etiology.
1. Associated with genitourinary anomalies.
2. Majority of children (80%) are younger than 5 years; peak incidence at 3 years.

B. Clinical manifestations.
1. Swelling or mass within the abdomen: firm, confined to one side of the abdomen, causing vague or no pain.
2. Abdominal pain as tumor enlarges.
3. Hematuria, pallor, anorexia, weight loss, and malaise occur as condition progresses.
4. Hypertension (63%).
C. Diagnostics (see Appendix 18-1).

Treatment

The survival rate greatly depends on the stage of the tumor at the time of diagnosis. If the tumor is diagnosed and treated in the early stages, there is a high survival rate.
A. Surgery.
1. Surgery is frequently scheduled within 24 to 48 hours after the diagnosis.
2. Nephrectomy: kidney is removed, but the adrenal gland may be spared, depending on the invasiveness of the tumor.
3. If both kidneys are involved, the less affected kidney is retained, and the more involved one is removed. Bilateral nephrectomy is a last resort.
B. Medical.
1. Preoperative and postoperative radiation therapy for large tumors.
2. Postoperative chemotherapy.

Nursing Interventions

❖ **Goal:** To provide safe preoperative care.

> ✔ *NURSING PRIORITY: Post a sign above the bed that reads "Do Not Palpate Abdomen."*

A. Handle child carefully to prevent trauma to the tumor site.
B. Prepare child and family for the surgery, including anticipation of a large incision and dressing. ICU care immediately after surgery.
C. Assess vital signs, especially blood pressure, for indications of hypertension. If adrenal gland is removed, blood pressure may be labile.
❖ **Goal:** To assess kidney function and to prevent infection.
A. Usual postoperative care for abdominal surgery.
B. Monitor for GI complications.
C. Provide good pulmonary hygiene because child is at increased risk for pulmonary infections postoperatively.
D. Vincristine is frequently used in chemotherapy; closely observe the child for the development of a paralytic-ileus.
E. Child is at risk for intestinal obstruction from the vincristine-induced adynamic ileus, edema caused by radiation, or postsurgical adhesions.

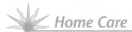 *Home Care*

A. Teach parents effects of chemotherapy.
B. Child has only one kidney; teach parents how to protect renal function.
1. Signs and symptoms of UTI.
2. Methods to prevent UTIs.
3. Advise all health care providers of compromised renal function.
4. Prompt treatment of other infections.

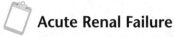 **Acute Renal Failure**

✳ **A clinical syndrome with abrupt loss of renal function that may occur over several hours or days, characterized by uremia. The most common cause is hypotension and prerenal hypovolemia or exposure to a nephrotoxin.**

Phases of Acute Renal Failure

A. Oliguric phase.
1. Urinary output decreases to less than 400 mL per 24 hours.
2. Increase in BUN, creatinine, uric acid, potassium, and magnesium levels and presence of metabolic acidosis.
3. Duration is 1-3 weeks; the longer it lasts, the less favorable the recovery.

> ✔ *OLDER ADULT PRIORITY: The older adult client loses the ability to concentrate urine; therefore urinary output may not be significantly reduced in this stage of renal failure.*

4. Nonoliguric renal failure: referred to as *high output failure;* urine is dilute and renal disease is present. These clients usually recover quicker and have fewer complications.
B. Diuretic phase.
1. Often has a sudden onset within 2-6 weeks after oliguric phase. Diuresis up to 10 L/day; urine is very dilute.
2. Hypovolemia and hypotension may occur due to massive fluid losses.
3. BUN level stops increasing. Urinary creatinine clearance stabilizes.
4. Client must be monitored for hypokalemia and hyponatremia.
5. May last for 1 to 3 weeks.
C. Recovery (convalescent) phase.
1. Begins when the GFR increases. May take up to 12 months for renal function to stabilize.
2. There is usually some permanent loss of renal function, but remaining renal function is sufficient to maintain healthy life. The older adult is less likely to experience a return to full kidney function.

3. Complications: secondary infection, which is the most common cause of death.

Data Collection

A. Risk factors/etiology.
1. Prerenal (renal ischemia).
   a. Circulatory volume depletion: caused by hemorrhage, dehydration.
   b. Decreased cardiac output: pump failure and/or CHF, especially in older adults.
   c. Decreased peripheral resistance: caused by septic shock, anaphylaxis, antihypertensives.
   d. Volume shifts: third spacing of fluid, gram-negative sepsis, hypoalbuminemia.
   e. Vascular obstruction: renal artery occlusion, dissection abdominal aneurysm.
2. Intrarenal (kidney tissue disease).
   a. Acute tubular necrosis: caused by hemolytic blood transfusion reactionnephrotoxic chemicals (carbon tetrachloride, arsenic, lead, mercury), nephrotoxic medication (aminoglycoside antibiotics, amphotericin B, and streptomycin), radiology contrast material.
   b. Infections: acute glomerulonephritis, pyelonephritis, CMV, candidiasis.
   c. Diseases that precipitate vascular changes (e.g., atherosclerosis, diabetes mellitus, hypertension).
3. Postrenal (obstructive problems).
   a. Urinary and renal calculi.
   b. Benign prostatic hypertrophy.
   c. Urethral stricture.
   d. Trauma resulting in obstruction.
   e. Bladder cancer, neuromuscular disorders.

> **NURSING PRIORITY:** *Many disorders across the life span can precipitate acute renal failure. It is important to know who is at increased risk for developing renal failure and the initial symptoms. Renal failure is frequently incorporated into a test question as a complication of a variety of conditions.*

B. Clinical manifestations (multiple body systems affected).
1. Urinary: decreased urinary output (oliguria, less than 400 mL/day; in older adults, may be 600 to 700 mL/day).
   a. Intrarenal and postrenal failure: fixed specific gravity, increased sodium in the urine; proteinuria with glomerular membrane alteration, "muddy brown" casts.
   b. Prerenal failure: history of precipitating event; urine specific gravity may be high; high urinary sodium concentration and proteinuria.
   c. High output renal failure: the kidney no longer filters the urine; high urinary output, but the

urine is dilute and does not contain waste products from filtering.
2. Cardiovascular.
   a. Pericarditis, pericardial effusion.
   b. Dysrhythmias caused by acidosis or hyperkalemia.
   c. CHF, hypotension followed by hypertension.
3. Respiratory.
   a. Pulmonary edema caused by fluid overload.
   b. Kussmaul respiration caused by metabolic acidosis.
   c. Pleural effusions.
4. Hematologic.
   a. Anemia caused by impaired erythropoietin.
   b. Leukocytosis, increased susceptibility to infection.
   c. Altered platelet function leading to bleeding tendencies.
5. Neurologic.
   a. Decreased seizure threshold caused by uremia.
   b. Altered mentation, memory impairment, lethargy.
6. Fluid and electrolyte imbalances.
   a. Fluid retention.
   b. Hyperkalemia.
   c. Hyponatremia (usually dilution).
   d. Metabolic acidosis from accumulation of acid waste products.

C. Diagnostics (see Appendix 18-1).

Treatment

A. Medical.
1. Identify and treat precipitating cause of acute renal failure (management varies according to whether disorder is prerenal, intrarenal, or postrenal).
2. Diuretic therapy may be used with fluid challenges.
3. Decrease serum potassium level.
   a. Sodium polystyrene sulfonate (**Kayexalate**): a cation exchange resin given by mouth or retention enema.
   b. Sorbitol: an osmotic cathartic; may be given with exchange resins to induce diarrhea to eliminate potassium ions.
   c. IV hypertonic glucose and regular insulin may be administered to move potassium into the intracellular space; used for severe hyperkalemia.
4. IV administration of sodium bicarbonate: corrects metabolic acidosis and causes electrolyte shift.
5. IV dopamine to enhance renal perfusion.

B. Dietary.
1. Fluid restriction; intake may be carefully calculated with output.
2. Intake of protein, potassium, and sodium is regulated according to serum plasma levels.
3. Increased intake of carbohydrates and protein of high biologic value.

BOX 18-3   TYPES OF DIALYSIS

Hemodialysis
Circulation of the client's blood through a compartment that contains an artificial semipermeable membrane surrounded by dialysate fluid, which removes excess body fluid by creating a pressure differential between the blood and the dialysate solution.

Continuous Renal Replacement Therapy (CRRT)
An alternative measure for treating acute renal failure. The uremic toxins are removed slowly and continuously. This allows for constant maintenance of acid-base and electrolyte balance in an unstable client. Can be used in conjunction with hemodialysis. There are two types: continuous arteriovenous hemofiltration (CAVH) and continuous venovenous hemofiltration (CVVH).

Peritoneal Dialysis
Utilization of the peritoneal cavity and the peritoneum as the semipermeable membrane that removes excess fluid.

Continuous Ambulatory Peritoneal Dialysis
The dialysate is infused into the abdomen and remains there for a specified time (2 to 6 hours). The dialysate is removed by gravity drainage after the prescribed time.

Automated Peritoneal Dialysis
Uses a peritoneal dialysis cycling machine. It can be done continuously, intermittently, or nightly. Most clients prefer to have the dialysis done at night.

C.   Dialysis (see Box 18-3): indications are volume overload, BUN level greater than 120 mg/dL, metabolic acidosis, increased potassium with electrocardiographic changes, pericardial effusion, and cardiac tamponade.

Nursing Interventions

❖   **Goal:** To maintain client in functional homeostasis and monitor renal function.

A.   Identify and monitor high-risk clients (any client with a transient or significant decrease in blood pressure, regardless of the precipitating cause).

B.   Maintain accurate intake and output record.

C.   Determine weight daily (client may lose 0.2 to 0.3 kg/day during oliguric phase).

D.   Assess fluid balance (hypervolemia or hypovolemia), urine specific gravity, pulmonary status, cardiac output, mental status changes.

E.   Assess status of electrolytes and renal parameters: serum potassium, BUN, creatinine, phosphate levels; evaluate fluctuations of serum sodium levels.

F.   Evaluate for hypertension or hypotension.

G.   Support involved body systems.
  1.   Cardiac dysrhythmias.
  2.   Pulmonary function.

H.   Avoid nephrotoxic medications, including NSAIDs.

❖   **Goal:** To maintain nutrition.

A.   Maintain dietary restrictions on sodium, potassium, and protein.

B.   Encourage intake of carbohydrates and fats for energy source. Caloric needs are 30 to 35 kcal/kg.

C.   Offer small frequent feedings; limit fluids.

D.   Total parenteral or enteral nutrition may be necessary to promote healing if caloric intake cannot be maintained.

❖   **Goal:** To prevent infection.

A.   Avoid use of indwelling urinary catheter, if possible.

B.   Assess for development of infectious processes (local or systemic). Client is at increased risk because of compromised immune system; may not have an elevated temperature.

C.   Assess for and prevent UTI.

❖   **Goal:** To prevent skin breakdown.

A.   Frequent turning and positioning; inspect the skin for problem areas.

B.   Beds and protective devices are used to prevent pressure areas (see Pressure Ulcers section in Chapter 19).

C.   Frequent range of motion and activities to increase circulation.

❖   **Goal:** To provide emotional support.

A.   Always explain procedures.

B.   Provide honest information regarding progress of condition.

C.   May take 3 to 12 months for recovery.

D.   Encourage client to express fears and concerns regarding condition.

 ## Chronic Renal Failure

✳   **Chronic renal failure is a progressive, irreversible reduction in renal function such that the kidneys are no longer able to maintain the body environment. The GFR gradually decreases as the nephrons are destroyed. The nephrons left intact are subjected to an increased workload, resulting in hypertrophy and inability to concentrate urine.**

A.   End-stage renal failure (uremia).
  1.   Severe azotemia.
      a.   Hyperkalemia, hypernatremia, and hyperphosphatemia.
      b.   Metabolic acidosis.
  2.   Urinary system: specific gravity of urine fixed at 1.010; proteinuria, casts, pyuria, hematuria; oliguria eventually leads to anuria less than 100 mL/24 hr.
  3.   Endocrine system.
      a.   Hypocalcemia and hyperphosphatemia resulting in demineralization of the bones (renal osteodystrophy).
      b.   Hypothyroidism.
  4.   Hematologic system: anemia and bleeding, infection.
  5.   Cardiovascular system: hypertension, CHF, uremic pericarditis, pericardial effusion, atherosclerotic heart disease.
  6.   Gastrointestinal system: anorexia, nausea, vomiting, ammonia odor (uremic fetor) to the breath, gastrointestinal bleeding, peptic ulcer disease, gastritis.

7. Metabolic system: hyperglycemia, hyperlipidemia, gout, hypoproteinemia, carbohydrate intolerance.
8. Neurologic system: general central nervous system depression and peripheral neuropathy, headaches, seizures, sleep disturbances.
9. Musculoskeletal system: renal osteodystrophy, tissue calcification.
10. Integumentary system: yellow/gray discoloration, pruritus, uremic frost, ecchymosis.
11. Psychologic changes: emotional lability, withdrawal, depression, and psychosis, personality and behavioral changes.

Data Collection

A. Risk factors/etiology.
   1. Chronic hypertension and poorly controlled diabetes.
   2. Chronic glomerulonephritis and pyelonephritis.
B. Diagnostics (see Appendix 18-1).
   1. Elevated blood sugar and triglyceride levels.
   2. Increased serum potassium level.
   3. Decreased hemoglobin and hematocrit.

Treatment

A. Medical.
   1. Measures to reduce serum potassium level (see discussion under acute renal failure).
   2. Antihypertensives (see Appendix 11-4).
   3. Diuretics: thiazide and loop diuretics may be used early in the course of disease.
   4. Erythropoietin (**Epogen**, **Procrit**) or **Aranesp** for treatment of anemia.
   5. Phosphate binders and supplemental vitamin D for renal osteodystrophy.
B. Dietary.
   1. Problems with the client losing body weight, both adipose tissue and muscle mass.
   2. Restricted protein intake; may vary from just a decrease in protein intake to a specific restriction of 20 to 40 g/day.
   3. Fluid restriction: 600 to 1000 mL, adjusted according to urinary output and/or dialysis.
   4. Sodium and potassium restriction: based on laboratory values.
C. Dialysis (see Box 18-3).
D. Surgical: kidney transplantation—the primary limiting factor in the number of transplantations done is the availability of kidneys.

Nursing Interventions

❖ **Goal:** To assist the client to maintain homeostasis in early chronic renal failure.
A. Evaluate adequacy of fluid balance.
   1. Determine weight daily.
   2. Control hypertension.
   3. Discuss with the client how to monitor fluid intake

and plan for the allocated amount to be distributed over the day.

> ✔ *NURSING PRIORITY: Monitor hydration status, identify signs of fluid and electrolyte imbalance, and identify interventions to correct any imbalance.*

B. Encourage nutritional intake within dietary guidelines.
   1. Relieve gastrointestinal dysfunctions before serving meals.
   2. Plan diet according to client's preferences, if possible.
   3. Advise client that most salt substitutes contain potassium and should not be used.
C. Prevent problem of constipation.
   1. Include bran/fiber in diet.
   2. Stool softeners.
D. Avoid use of sedatives and hypnotics; increased sensitivity to these medications is caused by decreased ability of kidney to metabolize and excrete them.
E. Monitor electrolyte balance, especially levels of potassium and calcium.

> ✔ *NURSING PRIORITY: Hypocalcemia and hyperkalemia are critical problems and may cause fatal dysrhythmias.*

F. Assess cardiovascular status.
G. Assess client for bleeding tendencies. Encourage intake of folic acid (1 mg daily) for red blood cell production and integrity.
H. Evaluate client for pruritus and assist with measures to decrease skin irritation and itching.
I. Avoid products containing magnesium (antacids).
J. Assess client's activity tolerance in relation to anemia.
❖ **Goal:** To provide emotional support and to promote psychologic equilibrium.
A. Encourage client to express concerns.
B. Recognize that the long-term management of a chronic disease may lead to anxiety and depression.
C. Encourage ventilation of feelings regarding lifestyle changes.
D. Encourage client and family members to seek out support groups and community resources, as well as other clients with renal failure who are undergoing the same types of treatment.

Renal Transplant

✳ **The transplantation of a kidney from a compatible-blood-typed deceased donor, blood relative, or a live donor. Transplanted kidney is usually placed extraperitoneally in the iliac fossa (usually right side to facilitate anastomoses and decrease occurrence of ileus).**

Data Collection

A. Types of transplant rejection.
  1. Hyperacute: not common.
    a. Occurs within minutes to hours after transplant.
    b. No treatment; transplanted kidney removed.
  2. Acute rejection.
    a. Can occur within days; 3 months is most common time, but can be as late as 2 years; it is common to have at least one rejection episode.
    b. Increased white blood cell count, fever.
    c. Deteriorating renal function: increasing serum creatinine and BUN levels, increasing blood pressure.
    d. Tenderness over graft site—often an early sign, along with malaise.
    e. Hypertension.
    f. Treatment is increased immunosuppressive therapy: usually high-dose steroids, polyclonal or monoclonal antibody therapy.
  3. Chronic rejection.
    a. Occurs over months or years and is due to gradual occlusion of the renal blood vessels. It is irreversible, and the client will again require dialysis and/or be placed back on the transplant list.
    b. Hypertension, increasing serum creatinine and BUN levels, and proteinuria.
    c. Graft tenderness, malaise, and signs of early end-stage renal disease.
    d. Treatment is supportive - immunosuppressive therapy and corticosteroids.

Nursing Interventions

❖ Goal: To provide preoperative care for client scheduled for kidney transplantation.

A. Maintain client's metabolic state as close to homeostasis as possible; continue with dialysis.
B. Immunosuppressant drugs: may be started prior to surgery.
C. Conduct routine preoperative procedures, including labeling the arm with vascular access for dialysis, because the client may require dialysis in the immediate postoperative period.

❖ Goal: To provide postoperative care for the kidney transplant recipient.

A. Immunosuppressant therapy is continued indefinitely.
B. Assess for renal graft function.
  1. Maintain fluid and electrolyte balances because of early diuresis. Avoid dehydration.
  2. *Report to RN any sudden decrease or change in urine output.*
C. Monitor for rejection symptoms.
D. Prevent and monitor for infection (UTI, pneumonia, and sepsis are biggest threats in the early posttransplantation period; fungal and viral infections are also common).

E. Atherosclerotic cardiovascular disease is common in transplant recipients. It is the leading cause of death in these clients.
F. Promote adaptation and psychologic support for the client who has undergone successful transplantation.

Dialysis

❋ **Dialysis is the passage of particles (ions) from an area of high concentration to an area of low concentration across a semipermeable membrane.**

A. Indications.
  1. GFR less than 15 mL/min.
  2. Fluid volume overload.
  3. Serum potassium level greater than 6 mEq/L.
  4. BUN level greater than 120 mg/dL.
  5. Uremia, uncontrolled hypertension, and metabolic acidosis.
B. Types of dialysis (Box 18-3). Note that dialysis solutions are High-Alert Medications.

Nursing Interventions

❖ Goal: To remove waste products of metabolism and excess fluid; to maintain a safe concentration of blood components.

A. Peritoneal dialysis.
  1. Masks and sterile gloves should be used when accessing the catheter to change the tubing. Remember the catheter is an open conduit to the peritoneal cavity.
  2. Check the tubing for patency and keep drainage bag below the level of the abdomen.
  3. Turn client from side to side or put client in semi-Fowler's position to increase abdominal pressure.

> ✔ *NURSING PRIORITY: If dialysate is left in the peritoneal cavity too long, then hyperglycemia may occur. Heparinization is not required for peritoneal dialysis, as it is for hemodialysis.*

B. Hemodialysis.

> ✔ *NURSING PRIORITY: Do not take blood pressure, obtain blood samples, or infuse fluids or medications in the access site or the extremity that has a vascular access site. Report immediately any decrease of absence of pulsations or indications of decreased blood flow through the vascular access site.*

❖ Goal: To provide emotional support and to promote psychologic equilibrium.

A. Encourage client to express feelings of anger and depression. An increased rate of suicide exists among clients undergoing dialysis.

B. Encourage appropriate coping skills.

C. Clients undergoing chronic dialysis are in limbo; they know they are probably not going to get better and that they may or may not receive a transplant. Frequently, they have ambivalent feelings about dialysis; it maintains life but severely restricts lifestyle.

 Renal Tumors

✳ **The majority of renal tumors are malignant and occur more frequently in men between the ages of 50 and 70 years. The most common areas of metastasis are the liver, lungs, and bone, especially the mediastinum.**

Data Collection

A. Clinical manifestations.
1. Palpable abdominal mass.
2. Hematuria, flank pain.
3. Weight loss, weakness, anemia, hypertension.

B. Diagnostics (see Appendix 18-1).

Treatment

A. Medical.
1. Palliative radiation therapy.
2. Biologic therapy with alpha interferon and interleukin-2.

B. Surgical: nephrectomy.

Nursing Interventions

❖ Goal: To provide preoperative nursing care (see Chapter 3).

A. Inform client that flank incision will be on affected side and that surgery will be performed in a hyperextended, side-lying position.

B. Often, client experiences postoperative muscle aches and discomfort as a result of surgical positioning.

C. Radiation, biologic therapy, or both after surgery.

❖ Goal: To provide postoperative care.

A. Urinary output is important to assess; catheters should be labeled, and drainage should be recorded accurately.

B. Because of the level of the incision, respiratory complications are common; encourage coughing and deep breathing, as well as incentive spirometry, every 2 hours while client is awake.

C. Assess for abdominal distention and paralytic ileus.

D. Monitor for unstable blood pressure after surgery; may be caused by removal of adrenal gland.

E. Provide adequate pain control.

❖ Goal: To provide supportive nursing care in relation to malignancy.

Study Questions: Urinary-Renal System

1. A female client is diagnosed with recurrent cystitis and is asking for information about self-care. What practice would the nurse discourage?
1   Drink as much fluid as possible throughout the day.
2   Take a shower rather than bathing in a tub.
3   Refrain from voiding to reduce the concentration of the urine.
4   Immediately void and wash after intercourse.

2. What finding would be noted on an assessment of a client who has an acute lower urinary tract infection?
1   Gross painless hematuria.
2   Low back pain.
3   Polyuria.
4   Dysuria.

3. At 10 am the nurse begins a 24-hour urine collection. What are the guidelines for collection of this specimen?
1   Collect a specimen now, add it to the container, and collect all urine until 10 am the next day.
2   Ask client to void now and discard the specimen; then collect all urine for 24 hours, ask client to void at 10 am the next day, and add to specimen container.
3   Collect specimen now and discard it; then collect urine for 24 hours, ask client to void at 10 am the following morning, and discard specimen.
4   Ask client to void now and discard specimen; then collect all urine for next 24 hours at 2-hour intervals and save in sterile containers.

4. The nurse is caring for a group of clients in a long-term care facility. What nursing measure will promote continence?
1   Plan schedule to facilitate assisting everyone to the bathroom every 2 to 3 hours.
2   Decrease the amount of PO fluids to increase bladder control.
3   Record all clients' intake and output to evaluate adequacy of intake.
4   Assess for bladder distention in clients who are increasingly restless.

5. A client has a shunt in his left arm for dialysis. How will the nurse check the patency of the shunt?
1   Palpate above the forearm for a rushing sound.
2   Check the pulse site distal to the shunt.
3   Palpate the shunt site for presence of a thrill.
4   Check the shunt site for warmth and color.

6. An infant is born with hypospadias. The mother asks the nurse when circumcision should be done. What is the best nursing response?
1   There is no problem with circumcision; it can be done whenever the parents desire it.
2   Circumcision will probably be delayed until there can be further diagnostic studies of the problem.
3   Circumcision is most often done when the congenital condition is repaired.
4   Voiding studies will have to be completed before circumcision can be done.

7. Kidney transplant clients are frequently placed on immunosuppressant drugs. What nursing measure would not be appropriate in caring for these clients?
    1   Keep all irrigation fluids sterile.
    2   Maintain aseptic technique.
    3   Give all medications by injection.
    4   Screen all visitors for infections.

8. The nurse is caring for a client in renal failure. What observations would indicate the development of a complication of uremia in this client?
    1   Anorexia, nausea, and vomiting.
    2   Pneumonia and respiratory depression.
    3   Tachycardia and stupor.
    4   Restlessness and diuresis.

9. Which client would be at the highest risk for the development of acute renal failure?
    1   Client with placenta previa with hemorrhage controlled.
    2   Client with cardiac disease and frequent problems of tachycardia.
    3   Hypertensive client who forgets to take his medication.
    4   Older adult client with a 20-year history of type II diabetes.

10. Why is it important for the nurse to monitor the red blood cell count in a chronic renal failure client?
    1   Granulocytopenia could occur, which can cause infection.
    2   Production of erythropoietin will be affected due to renal failure.
    3   Blood cell production could increase due to the increased production of renin.
    4   An increase in waste products could cause thrombocytopenia.

11. A client has had a kidney stone removed by nephrolithotomy. A nephrostomy tube has been placed in the right kidney. What would be important nursing care for this client?
    1   Clamp the nephrostomy tube and drain every 2 hours.
    2   Irrigate the nephrostomy tube with 30 mL normal saline to maintain patency.
    3   Remove the tube at approximately 1 inch every hour.
    4   Maintain the drainage collection dependent to the client's position.

12. What is the best description of the pain that a client experiences when beginning to pass a renal calculus?
    1   Intermittent sharp pain that radiates down the left leg.
    2   Intermittent dull but hot pain in the upper thighs.
    3   Dull flank pain that only occurs with voiding.
    4   Sharp pain in the shoulder and chest that radiates.

13. When providing instructions to geriatric clients on the prevention of urinary tract infections, what would the nurse instruct the clients to avoid?

    1   Taking any medications containing acetaminophen.
    2   Increasing fluid intake to 3000mL daily.
    3   Cleansing the perineal area from back to front.
    4   Increasing intake of fruit juices.

14. A cystoscopy is going to be performed on a client. What is important for the nurse to tell the client?
    1   A local anesthetic and a sedative will be given; if he is awake during the procedure, he should not experience severe pain.
    2   A sedative will be given, but it is important for him to remain fully awake in order to cooperate with the physician during the procedure.
    3   A long black tube will be inserted through the wall of the bladder for 15 minutes to view the bladder wall and interior.
    4   A three-way Foley will be inserted, and dye will be injected into the urinary tract through the cystoscope.

15. What would the nurse anticipate finding when performing a skin assessment on a chronic renal failure client?
    1   Warm, moist, pink-colored skin.
    2   Cool, clammy, dusky-colored skin.
    3   Warm, edematous, copper-colored skin.
    4   Bruised, dry, yellow-colored skin.

16. The nurse is caring for a client in acute renal failure. What nursing observations would indicate the development of a complication associated with the problem of fluid volume excess in this client?
    1   Decreased sensation and tingling in the extremities.
    2   Increased incidence of bleeding gums and epistaxis.
    3   Increasing peripheral edema and moist breath sounds.
    4   Serum potassium above 4 mEq/L.

17. The nurse is assessing a client in acute renal failure. What is an indication the client is progressing into the oliguric stage?
    1   Hematuria of 600 mL/24 hours.
    2   Increasing urine specific gravity.
    3   Serum potassium level of 3.5 mEq/L.
    4   Urine output of 400 mL/24 hours.

18. A female client is being catheterized. The nurse advances the catheter into an opening 5 to 6 inches with no urine return. What is the best interpretation of this situation?
    1   The catheter is too small for urine to flow without pressure.
    2   There must be a defect in the catheter.
    3   The client was catheterized after she had voided.
    4   The catheter is not in the urinary meatus and is probably in the vagina.

Answers and rationales to these questions are in the section at the end of the book titled Chapter Study Questions: Answers and Rationales.

Appendix 18-1 DIAGNOSTICS OF THE URINARY-RENAL SYSTEM

Laboratory Tests	Normal	Clinical and Nursing Implications
BUN level	10-20 mg/dL	Common test used to diagnose renal problems; may be affected by an increase in protein intake or tissue breakdown.
Creatinine level	0.5-1.5 mg/dL	End product of protein and muscle catabolism; more accurate determinate of renal function than the BUN level; values are higher in males. Elevated in renal disease.
Calcium level	9-11 mg/dL	Provides the matrix for bone and is important in muscle contraction, neurotransmission, and clotting; in chronic renal failure, low levels of calcium lead to renal osteodystrophy.
Urinalysis		Obtain first-voided specimen in the morning. Presence of protein, WBC, RBC, glucose, bacteria, and hyaline casts indicate problems. Dipstick urinalysis is initially performed to determine levels of nitrites and leukocyte esterase related to infections.
Urine culture and sensitivity		Colony count of at least 100,000 colonies/mL of urine indicates infection.
Urine specific gravity	Adults: 1.003-1.030 Children: 1.001-1.030	May be increased when the client is dehydrated and with glomerulonephritis. A decrease is associated with decreased tubular absorption. In renal failure it may be fixed at 1.000 to 1.012. Proteinuria will increase the specific gravity.

Laboratory Diagnostics

Procedure	Clinical and Nursing Implications
KUB x-ray exam: A flat plate x-ray film of the abdomen and pelvis.	Bowel preparation may or may not be indicated.
Intravenous urography (IVP or excretory urogram): IV injection of radiopaque dye to visualize the urinary tract system.	1. Client's status is NPO for 8 hours before procedure. 2. Cathartic or enema given the evening before procedure. 3. Radiocontrast medium may cause an allergic (hypersensitivity) reaction in iodine-sensitive clients. 4. Instruct client that he or she will need to lie still on table while serial x-ray films are taken. 5. Evaluate for iodine reaction after test and force fluids after test to flush out the dye. 6. Be sure the older adult client is not dehydrated before the procedure; the contrast medium is nephrotoxic and can precipitate renal failure.
Retrograde pyelogram: An x-ray study of the urinary tract conducted during a cystoscopic exam; ureteral catheters are inserted into the renal pelvis, and dye is injected (retrograde) into the catheters.	1. Client's status is NPO for 8 hours before test. 2. Assess for sensitivity to iodine. 3. Explain that there may be discomfort on insertion of the cystoscope. 4. General anesthesia may be indicated for procedure.

Continued

Appendix 18-1   DIAGNOSTICS OF THE URINARY-RENAL SYSTEM —cont'd.

Procedure	Clinical and Nursing Implications
Renogram (renal scan): An IV injection of a radioactive nuclide (isotope) followed by use of a scanning device to detect radioactive emissions from the kidney(s); identifies renal blood flow, tubular functions, and renal excretion.	1. No specific activity or dietary restrictions. 2. Explain procedure to client.
Cystoscopy: A direct method to visualize the urethra and bladder by use of a tubular lighted scope (cystoscope). Scope may be inserted via the urethra or percutaneously.	1. Force fluids or administer fluids intravenously. 2. Explain lithotomy position that will be used. 3. Client may have general anesthesia or conscious sedation. 4. Preoperative medication is given. 5. Evaluate urine output after procedure; check for frequency, pink-tinged urine, and burning on urination (these are expected effects and will decrease with time). 6. Evaluate for orthostatic hypotension and thrombus formation after the procedure. 7. Provide warm sitz baths and mild analgesics to alleviate urethral discomfort.
Bladder scan: A portable ultrasound scanner used to estimate residual urine in the bladder.	1. No specific preparation. 2. After client voids, apply gel to the suprapubic area, and use scanner to visualize bladder and possible retained urine. 3. Make certain that the crosshairs on the aiming icon on the scanner are centered on or over the bladder, if crosshairs are offset then the reading may not be accurate.
Urodynamic studies **Cystometrogram (CMG):** A procedure to determine the pressure exerted against the bladder wall by inserting a catheter and instilling water or saline solution; used to evaluate bladder capacity, bladder pressure, and voiding reflexes. **Urethral pressure profile or urethral pressure profilometry (UPP):** Evaluates for urinary incontinence and retention by recording variations of pressure in the urethra. **Urine stream testing:** Evaluates pelvic floor muscle strength.	1. Assess and evaluate for UTI after procedure. 2. Tests are often indicated for clients having difficulty with urinary control (e.g., those with spinal cord traumatic injuries, stroke, etc.).
Renal biopsy: A percutaneous needle biopsy to evaluate renal disease by obtaining a specimen of renal tissue for pathologic examination. Rarely done if client has only one kidney.	1. Results of blood coagulation studies should be available on the chart before the biopsy procedure. 2. Results of IVP or ultrasound studies should be available before the biopsy. 3. Immediately after the procedure, pressure dressing is applied to biopsy site and checked frequently for bleeding. Right kidney is the usual biopsy site. 4. Assess for gross hematuria, flank pain, or a rise or fall in blood pressure. 5. Report pain radiating from the flank area to the abdomen. 6. Encourage intake of fluids: 3000 mL per day unless the client has renal insufficiency. 7. Assess for complication of hemorrhage; may necessitate emergency surgical drainage or nephrectomy.
Renal ultrasound exam: A noninvasive procedure in which ultrasound waves are used, with the aid of a computer, to record images related to tissue density.	1. Encourage fluids, as test requires a full bladder. 2. Placed in prone position. 3. Skin care to remove sonographic gel after procedure.

BUN, Blood urea nitrogen; *GFR,* glomerular filtration rate; *IV,* intravenous; *IVP,* intravenous pyelogram; *KUB,* kidneys, ureters, and bladder; *NPO,* nothing by mouth; *UTI,* urinary tract infection.

Appendix 18-2   RENAL MEDICATIONS

General Nursing Implications

- Encourage intake of 2000-3000 mL of fluid per day during treatment.
- Continue medication therapy until all medication has been taken.
- Most medications are better absorbed on an empty stomach; however, if GI distress occurs, they may be taken with food.
- Monitor intake and output, as well as symptoms of increasing renal problems.
- Check drug package insert for interactions with anticoagulants.
- See Appendix 5-10 for sulfonamide medications for UTI.

Medications	Side Effects	Nursing Implications
Urinary Tract Antiseptics: These drugs concentrate in the urine and are active against common urinary tract pathogens; they do not affect infections in blood or tissue.		
Nitrofurantoin **(Furadantin, Macrodantin, APO-Nitrofurantoin, Nitrofan):** PO, IM	GI upset, blood dyscrasia, pulmonary reactions	1. Requires adequate renal function to concentrate medication in urine.
Urinary Analgesics: Pain relievers typically used on urinary tract mucosa.		
Phenazopyridine hydrochloride **(AZO-Standard, Pyridium, Urodine, Urogesic):** PO Available OTC	Headache, GI disturbances	1. Contraindicated in renal and liver dysfunction. 2. Advise client to report any yellow discoloration of skin or eyes. 3. Urine will turn orange. 4. Administer with caution in clients with impaired renal function. 5. Can alter dipstick urine results.
Bladder Relaxants: Suppress detrusor contractions and enhance bladder storage (drugs with anticholinergic activity.		
Oxybutynin **(Ditropan, Ditropan XL):** PO, transdermal	Drowsiness, dizziness, weakness, blurred vision, dry mouth, constipation	1. Contraindicated in glaucoma, myasthenia gravis, or GI obstruction. 2. Used cautiously in older adults. 3. Can relieve bladder spasms in surgical clients. 4. Monitor intraocular pressure.
Tolterodine **(Detrol, Detrol LA):** PO Solifenacin succinate **(Vesicare):** PO	Fatigue, headache, dry mouth, dry eyes, constipation	1. Grapefruit juice can increase blood levels. 2. Caution client to avoid use of alcohol or OTC antihistamines.
Glycoprotein Hormones: Stimulate bone marrow production of RBCs.		
Epoetin alfa **(Epogen, Procrit):** IV, subQ	Hypertension, thromboembolic problems, headaches, GI disturbances	1. Closely evaluate hemodialysis access ports for clotting. 2. Evaluate client for adequate serum iron level, hematocrit, and blood pressure; adequate levels are required for medication to be effective. 3. *Uses:* maintain hemoglobin and hematocrit values in client with renal failure and those who are HIV+ or on chemotherapy. Do not administer if Hgb is 12 or greater.

GI, Gastrointestinal; *HIV+,* human immunodeficiency virus–positive; *IV,* intravenously; *PO,* by mouth (orally); *subQ,* subcutaneously; *UTI,* urinary tract infection.

| Appendix 18-3 | IMMUNOSUPPRESSIVE MEDICATIONS | |

General Nursing Implications

- Avoid exposure to infection; wash hands frequently.
- Wear protective clothing; use sunscreen.
- Report any sore throat, fever, or other signs of infection to health care provider.
- Take medication at the same time each day to maintain consistent blood levels.
- No live virus vaccines or immunity-conferring agents should be administered while client is immunosuppressed.
- Depending on level of immunosuppression, client may need protective isolation.

Medications	Side Effects	Nursing Implications
Immunosuppressive Medications: Inhibit the immunologic response.		
Azathioprine (**Imuran**): PO, IV	Dose- and duration-dependent. Bone marrow suppression: leukopenia, thrombocytopenia, anemia. Nausea, vomiting, anorexia. Alopecia, rash.	1. Interacts with allopurinol, causing an increase in **Imuran** toxicity. 2. Avoid use in pregnancy. 3. Take with food or milk to decrease GI upset. 4. Should not be given to client with active infection. 5. Follow-up CBCs should be done at least monthly while client is taking medication. 6. Closely monitor client for development of infections.
Cyclosporine (**Sandimmune, Neoral**): PO, IV Methotrexate (**Mexate**) Cyclophosphamide (**Cytoxan**)	Dose- and duration-dependent Infections, nephrotoxicity, hepatotoxicity, hypertension, hirsutism, gum hyperplasia, tremors.	1. Monitor renal function because nephrotoxicity occurs frequently. 2. Avoid use in pregnancy. 3. Use the pipette supplied by manufacturer to measure dose; mix with 4-8 oz. of water, milk, or juice. 4. Evaluate blood pressure and report elevations (especially occurs with heart transplants). 5. Monitor liver function studies. 6. Good oral hygiene should be practiced to reduce gum problems. 7. Teach client that he/she should not stop taking the medication or change dosage without physician's order. 8. Serum blood levels are monitored at regular intervals. 9. Hirsutism that occurs is reversible.
Antilymphocyte globulin (**ALG**): IV Murine monoclonal anti-lymphocyte therapy (**OKT3**): IV Daclizumab (**Zenapax**): IV	Fever, chills, tachycardia, hypotension, bronchospasm. Aseptic meningitis (**OKT3**) GI toxicity (diarrhea, nausea, abdominal pain).	1. More than 50% of clients experience a fever. 2. Have epinephrine and supportive emergency care available, because an allergic reaction can occur at any time during therapy. 3. Administer slowly over 4-6 hr. 4. Client may be premedicated with acetaminophen, diphenhydramine HCl, or methylprednisolone.
Methylprednisolone sodium succinate (**Solu-Medrol**): IV	See Appendix 5-7	
Tacrolimus (**Prograf, FK506**): PO	Hepatotoxicity, nephrotoxicity, neurotoxicity, hyperglycemia, seizures, hypertension, GI effects.	1. Monitor blood pressure closely. 2. Increases risk for infection.
Mycophenolate mofetil (**CellCept**): PO, IV	Leukopenia, thrombocytopenia, GI (diarrhea, nausea, vomiting), UTI, hypertension, peripheral edema.	1. Usually used in combination with other medications. 2. Give on an empty stomach.

CBCs, Complete blood counts; *GI*, gastrointestinal; *IL-2*, interleukin 2; *IV*, intravenous; *PO*, by mouth (orally); *RA*, rheumatoid arthritis; *UTI*, urinary tract infection.

Appendix 18-4   URINARY DIVERSION

A urinary diversion is a means of diverting urinary output from the bladder to an external device or via a new avenue.

Temporary Urinary Diversion

Nephrostomy tubes (catheters): Insertion of catheters into the renal pelvis by surgical incision or percutaneous puncture. A small catheter is inserted into the renal pelvis and attached via connecting tubing to a closed-system drainage. Nephrostomy tubes may be temporary or permanent.

Nursing Implications
1. Catheter should never be clamped or irrigated (renal pelvis capacity is 3 to 5 mL).
2. Complications: Infection and secondary renal calculus formation; erosion of the duct by the catheter.

Ureteral catheters: Small, narrow catheters placed through the ureters into the renal pelvis; drain each renal pelvis individually. Often client also has a urinary retention catheter draining the urinary bladder. The catheter splints the ureters during healing and prevents edema from occluding the ureter.

Nursing Implications

1. Check frequently for placement of ureteral catheters; tension should be avoided.
2. Ureteral catheter should not be clamped or irrigated.
3. Maintain accurate intake and output records and label all catheters.

Permanent Urinary Diversion

Ileal conduit (ileal loop): Transplantation of ureters into a segment of ileum or colon, which is then brought to the abdomen; a stoma is then constructed.

Nursing Implications
1. Stoma site is marked before surgery, because a device must be worn continuously.
2. Mucus is present in the urine after surgery when ileum segment is used; encourage a high fluid intake to "flush the ileal conduit."
3. Maintain meticulous skin care and changing of appliances.
4. Provide discharge instructions in regard to symptoms of obstruction, infection, and care of the ostomy; client needs information relating to purchase of supplies, ostomy clubs, follow-up visits, enterostomal therapists, and the importance of not irrigating the ileal conduit.

Continued

Appendix 18-4	URINARY DIVERSION—cont'd.

Continent Urinary Diversion

Kock, Mainz, Indiana, or Florida pouch: A segment of the bowel is made into a reservoir; client is taught to use a catheter to drain the pouch and maintain continence. The main difference among the diversions is the segment of intestine utilized (ileum, ileocecal segment, or colon).

Nursing Implications
1. Client will not need to wear an appliance but will need to self-catheterize every 4 to 6 hours.
2. A small bandage/pouch may be worn to collect any mucus drainage or small leaks.
3. Continuous assessment of status of skin around stoma.
4. Client should understand how to care for the stoma before he or she leaves the hospital:
    *   Know how continent diversion functions and how to prevent complications.
    *   Increase fluid intake.
    *   Contact PCP if there are changes in the color of the stoma or if urine becomes dark and foul smelling.
5. A catheter will be inserted into the reservoir every 4 to 6 hours to drain urine.

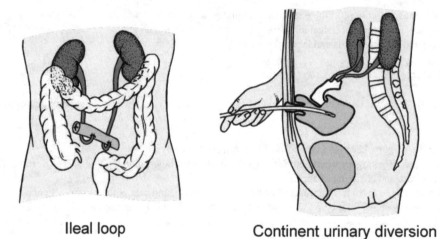

Ileal loop   Continent urinary diversion

FIGURE 18-3 Urinary Diversions. (From Potter P, Perry A: *Fundamentals of nursing,* ed 7, St Louis, 2008, Mosby.)

Appendix 18-5   NURSING PROCEDURE: URINE SPECIMEN COLLECTION

✔ KEY POINTS: Random Sample

- May be collected at any time.
- Client may be specifically ordered to collect first voided specimen or to collect sample on second voiding.

✔ KEY POINTS: Clean Catch and Midstream

- Specimen is collected for culture.
- Cleanse urinary meatus before specimen collection.
- For midstream collection, tell client to start the urinary stream and collect the specimen after voiding has begun. Regardless of how well the urinary meatus is cleansed, the specimen must be a midstream collection or the specimen will be contaminated with the bacteria in the urethra.

✔ KEY POINTS: Catheterized Specimen

- Straight in-and-out catheterization to obtain sample for culture.
- Procedure is discouraged because of introduction of bacteria and irritation producing a urinary tract infection. More common in infants and children and those unable to provide a midstream specimen.

✔ KEY POINTS: 12- to 24-Hour Collection

- When the collection time is started, have the client void, discard the urine, and start the collection with the next voiding.
- Mark the collection container and collect the urine over the prescribed time frame.
- When the time frame is completed, have the client void again, add it to the specimen collection, and send to lab for evaluation.

 TEST ALERT: Collection of urine specimens is a common nursing action; be sure to know why the sample is being obtained and the nursing management.

Appendix 18-6 NURSING PROCEDURE: URINARY CATHETERIZATION

✔ KEY POINTS: Insertion of a Retention Catheter

- A sterile procedure.
- Lubricate catheter with sterile lubricant provided in tray.
- Cleanse the meatus:

For a Female

1. Cleanse the meatus with sterile cotton ball held in forceps; use one downward stroke of the forceps.
2. Repeat at least three to four times using new sterile cotton ball each time.
3. Continue to hold the labia apart until you insert the catheter.
4. When urine appears, advance the catheter another 1 to 2 inches.

For a Male

1. Hold the penis upright. Hold the sides of the penis to prevent closing the urethra.
2. Cleanse the meatus in a circular motion from urinary meatus to glans with sterile cotton ball held in forceps; use one downward stroke of the forceps.
3. Repeat at least three to four times.
4. Continue to hold the penis until you insert the catheter.
5. Insert the catheter 1 to 2 inches beyond the point at which urine begins to flow. Inserting the catheter farther into the bladder ensures it is beyond the neck of the bladder.
6. Instill sterile water into balloon after catheter is inserted.

- Anchor the catheter.

  For a female: Anchor or tape catheter to the side of the leg.

  For a male: Anchor or tape catheter to the abdomen to prevent pressure on the penoscrotal angle.

- Attach drainage bag to bed frame (not side rails), so that it hangs freely, and below the level of the catheter.

✔ KEY POINTS: Providing Catheter Care

- Maintain external cleanliness around the catheter; wash thoroughly with mild soap and water when soiled—or at least once every 24 hours.
- Maintain closed system. Do not allow urine to flow from the bag or tubing back into the bladder.
- Encourage high fluid intake to maintain constant flow of urine. Increased flow of urine inhibits the upward movement of bacteria.

✔ KEY POINTS: Removal of a Catheter

- Clamp catheter.
- Do not cut the catheter with a scissors. Balloon may not totally deflate if cut.
- Withdraw fluid from balloon (usually 5 to 10 mL water in balloon).
- Pull gently on catheter to ensure balloon is deflated before attempting to remove. Damage to the urethra can occur if balloon is not totally deflated. If the catheter has been in place for longer than 10 days, reinflate the balloon after removal to assess for degradation.
- Record output on intake and output (I&O) bedside record.
- Wash perineum with soap and water. Dry thoroughly.
- Instruct client to drink fluids as tolerated and observe for signs and symptoms of urinary tract infection (burning, frequency, urgency).
- Offer bedpan or urinal at least every 2 to 4 hours after removing catheter, until voiding occurs. Keep accurate I&O record.

 TEST ALERT: Insert a urinary catheter.

Continued

Appendix 18-6	NURSING PROCEDURE: URINARY CATHETERIZATION—cont'd.

Clinical Tips for Problem Solving

1. If catheter is inserted in the vagina of female client:
    *   Leave the catheter in place so you do not reintroduce a new catheter into the vaginal area. Obtain a new catheter and sterile gloves.
    *   If sterile field has been contaminated, obtain a whole new kit.
2. If unable to insert catheter into male client:
    *   Obtain a new catheter kit.
        a. Hold penis vertical to the body.
        b. Insert catheter while applying slight traction by gently pulling upward on the shaft of the penis.
        c. If you encounter resistance, rotate the catheter, increase the traction, and change the angle of the penis slightly.
        d. When urine begins to flow, lower the penis.
3. If pain occurs during inflation of balloon:
    *   Remove any injected water and insert the catheter farther into the bladder.
4. If urine exceeds 1000 mL with catheterization:
    *   Clamp catheter for 20 to 30 minutes and then unclamp.
5. If catheter comes out with balloon still inserted:
    *   Assess client for signs of urethral trauma (i.e., bleeding, pain).
    *   Obtain a new catheter and repeat the catheterization procedure, making sure that the balloon is inflated with at least 10 mL water.
    *   Monitor urine output for bleeding.

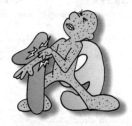

Integumentary System

PHYSIOLOGY OF THE SKIN

A. Structure
1. Epidermis – outermost layer.
2. Dermis – connective tissue below epidermis; vascular; assists in body temperature and blood pressure regulation.
3. Hypodermis (subcutaneous) – located below dermis; anchors the muscles and bones to the skin.
4. Nail.
   a. Consists of a hard, transparent plate of keratin.
   b. Grows from the root, which lies under a thin fold of skin called the cuticle.
5. Hair.
   a. Present over the entire body except for the palms of the hands and the soles of the feet.
   b. Piloerector response: contraction of the tiny erector muscles attached to the hair follicle that leads to hair "standing on end" or "gooseflesh."
6. Sebaceous glands: secrete sebum, which is an oily secretion that is emptied into the hair shaft.

B. Functions of the skin.
1. Protection: primary function.
2. Sensory: major receptor for general sensation.
3. Water balance.
   a. 600 to 900 mL of water is lost daily through insensible perspiration.
   b. Forms a barrier that prevents loss of water and electrolytes from the internal environment.
4. Temperature regulation.
5. Involved in the activation of vitamin D.
6. Involved in wheal-and-flare reaction.
   a. Wheal: swelling.
   b. Flare: diffused redness.
   c. These responses are due to local edema.

System Assessment

A. Health history (Box 19-1).
1. How long has the particular rash, lesion, or problem been present?
2. Is there any itching, burning, or discomfort associated with the problem?
3. Has the client been in contact with any irritants, sun, unusual cold, or unhygienic conditions?
4. Has anyone in the family ever had this same type of problem with his or her skin?
5. Is the client taking any medications?

6. What is the diet history? Does the client have any food allergies?

B. Physical assessment.
1. Inspection.
   a. Assess the skin for color: jaundice, cyanotic, flushed.
   b. Determine if there are areas of bruising, purpura, or petechiae.
   c. Determine if skin blanches on direct pressure.
   d. Assess lesions for type, color, size, distribution, and grouping; location and consistency.
   e. Assess for unusual odors, especially around lesions or areas (axilla, overhanging abdominal folds, and groin).
   f. Common dermatological lesions.
      (1) Macule: flat, circumscribed area of color change in the skin without surface elevation.
      (2) Papule: circumscribed, solid, and elevated lesion.
      (3) Nodule: raised, solid lesion that is larger and deeper than a papule.
      (4) Vesicle: small elevation in skin usually filled with serous fluid or blood; bulla: larger than a vesicle; pustule: vesicle or bulla filled with pus.
      (5) Wheal: elevation of the skin caused by edema of the dermis.
      (6) Cyst: mass of fluid-filled tissue that extends to the subcutaneous tissue or dermis.

BOX 19-1 | OLDER ADULT CARE FOCUS
Differences in Skin Assessment

Skin
- Increased wrinkling and sagging, redundant flesh around eyes, slowness of skin to flatten when pinched together (tenting)
- Dry, flaking skin: excoriation from scratching
- Decreased rate of wound healing
- Evidence of bruising

Hair
- Graying, thinning, baldness; dry, scaly scalp

Nails
- Thick, brittle nails with diminished growth; ridging
- Prolonged return of blood with blanching

2. Palpation.
   a. Determine temperature (use back of hand), skin turgor (on older adults pinch skin on abdomen or forehead), and mobility.
   b. Evaluate moisture and texture.

> **TEST ALERT:** *Assess skin integrity and use measures to maintain client skin integrity.*

 ## Acne Vulgaris

* **Acne is an inflammatory disorder of the sebaceous glands and their hair follicles.**

Data Collection

A. More common in teenagers; may persist into adulthood.
B. Under hormonal influence during puberty; affected by presence of androgen, which stimulates the sebaceous glands to secrete sebum.
C. Inflammatory lesions or pustules.
D. Cysts: deep nodules that may produce scarring.

Treatment

A. Medical: topical or systemic therapy.

Home Care

A. Instruct client to cleanse face twice daily but to avoid overcleansing.
B. May use a polyester sponge pad to cleanse, because it provides a mechanical removal of the epidermal layer.
C. Instruct client to keep hands away from face and to avoid any friction or trauma to the area; avoid propping hands against face, rubbing face, etc.
D. Emphasize the importance of a nutritious diet; encourage adequate food intake and use of vitamin A.
E. Avoid the use of cosmetics, shaving creams, and lotion, because they may exacerbate acne; if cosmetics are to be used, water-based make-up is preferable.
F. Instruct the client to administer medication appropriately: topical application; avoid sunlight while using medications, etc.

 ## Psoriasis

* **Psoriasis is a chronic inflammatory disorder characterized by rapid turnover of epidermal cells.**

Data Collection

A. Silvery scaling, plaques on the elbows, scalp, knees, palms, soles, and fingernails.
B. If scales are scraped away, a dark red base of the lesion is seen, which will produce multiple bleeding points.
C. May improve but often recurs throughout life.
D. Bilateral symmetry of symptoms is common.

Treatment

A. Medical.
   1. Topical therapy.
      a. Coal tar preparation (**Anthralin**).
      b. Corticosteroids.
   2. Photo chemotherapy (PUVA therapy): psoralen, ultraviolet A therapy (must wear protective eyewear during treatment and for 24 hours after therapy).
   3. Systemic therapy: antimetabolites (methotrexate); immunosuppressants.

Home Care

A. Encourage verbalization of anxiety regarding appearance.
B. Instruct client to use a soft brush to remove scales while bathing.
C. Assess client to determine factors that may trigger skin condition (e.g., emotional stress, trauma, seasonal changes).
D. Make sure client understands treatment and implications of care related to PUVA therapy

 ## Atopic Dermatitis

* **Atopic dermatitis (also called *eczema*) is a superficial, chronic inflammatory disorder associated with allergy with a hereditary tendency (atopy); condition usually occurs during infancy, usually between 2 and 6 months of age.**

Data Collection

A. Reddened lesions, occur on the cheeks, arms, and legs; antecubital and popliteal space in adults; may have oozing vesicles.
B. Intense itching (worse at night).
C. Infants with eczema are more likely to have allergies as children and adults and develop asthma.

Treatment

A. Pruritus is treated with Benadryl, topical steroids, and with immunomodulators.

Home Care

A. Teach parents about dietary restrictions; provide them with written guidelines.
B. Keep fingernails and toenails cut short.
C. Feed the child when he is well rested and is not itching.
D. Child should wear nonirritating clothing; wool and abrasive fabrics should be avoided.
E. Tepid bath with mild soap or a eumulsifying oil followed immediately by application of an emollient; cool compresses to decrease itching.

Contact Dermatitis

* *Contact dermatitis* is an inflammatory skin reaction that results because the skin has come in contact with a specific irritant - diaper dermatitis, prolonged contact with urine, feces, ointments, soaps, friction or an allergen (allergic contact dermatitis, which is usually a symptom of delayed hypersensitivity).

Data Collection

A. Pruritus; hive-like papules, vesicles, and plaques (more chronic).

B. Sharply circumscribed areas (with occasional vesicle formation) that crust and ooze.

Treatment

A. Medical.
1. Topical steroids; oral steroids for severe cases.
2. Antihistamines, antipruritic agents, and antifungals (diaper dermatitis).
3. Aveeno (oatmeal) baths and topical soaks.

Home Care

A. Teach importance of washing exposed skin with cool water and soap as soon as possible after exposure (within 15 minutes is best).

B. Provide cool, tepid bath; trim fingernails, and use measures to control itching.

C. Frequent diaper changes, keep skin dry, and use protective ointment (zinc oxide or petrolatum).

Pressure Ulcer

* A *pressure ulcer* (*decubitus ulcer, bedsore*) is localized injury to the skin and/or underlying tissue usually over a bony prominence, as a result of pressure, or pressure in combination with shear and/or friction.

> ✔ *NURSING PRIORITY: Identify potential for skin breakdown: a pressure ulcer can be and should be prevented. Identify those clients at increased risk for ulcer development and begin preventative care as soon as possible. Do not wait for the reddened area to occur before preventative measures are initiated.*

Assessment

A. Risk factors/etiology.
1. Prolonged pressure caused by immobility.
2. Malnutrition, hypoproteinemia, vitamin deficiency.
3. Infection, advancing age.
4. Skin dryness, maceration, excessive skin moisture.
5. Equipment such as casts, restraints, traction devices, etc.

Figure 19-1: Stages of Pressure Ulcers

Suspected Deep Tissue Injury: Purple or maroon localized area of discolored intact skin or blood-filled blister due to damage of underlying soft tissue from pressure and/or shear. The area may be preceded by tissue that is painful, firm, mushy, boggy, warmer or cooler as compared to adjacent tissue.

Further description: Deep tissue injury may be difficult to detect in individuals with dark skin tones. Evolution may include a thin blister over a dark wound bed. The wound may further evolve and become covered by thin eschar. Evolution may be rapid exposing additional layers of tissue even with optimal treatment.

Stage I: Intact skin with non-blanchable redness of a localized area usually over a bony prominence. Darkly pigmented skin may not have visible blanching; its color may differ from the surrounding area.

Further description: The area may be painful, firm, soft, warmer or cooler as compared to adjacent tissue. Stage I may be difficult to detect in individuals with dark skin tones. May indicate "at risk" persons (a heralding sign of risk)

Stage II: Partial thickness loss of dermis presenting as a shallow open ulcer with a red pink wound bed, without slough. May also present as an intact or open/ruptured serum-filled blister.

Further description: Presents as a shiny or dry shallow ulcer without slough or bruising.* This stage should not be used to describe skin tears, tape burns, perineal dermatitis, maceration or excoriation.

*Bruising indicates suspected deep tissue injury

Stage III: Full thickness tissue loss. Subcutaneous fat may be visible but bone, tendon or muscle are not exposed. Slough may be present but does not obscure the depth of tissue loss. May include undermining and tunneling.

Further description: The depth of a stage III pressure ulcer varies by anatomical location. The bridge of the nose, ear, occiput and malleolus do not have subcutaneous tissue and stage III ulcers can be shallow. In contrast, areas of significant adiposity can develop extremely deep stage III pressure ulcers. Bone/tendon is not visible or directly palpable.

Stage IV: Full thickness tissue loss with exposed bone, tendon or muscle. Slough or eschar may be present on some parts of the wound bed. Often include undermining and tunneling.

Further description: The depth of a stage IV pressure ulcer varies by anatomical location. The bridge of the nose, ear, occiput and malleolus do not have subcutaneous tissue and these ulcers can be shallow. Stage IV ulcers can extend into muscle and/or supporting structures (e.g., fascia, tendon or joint capsule) making osteomyelitis possible. Exposed bone/tendon is visible or directly palpable.

Unstageable: Full thickness tissue loss in which the base of the ulcer is covered by slough (yellow, tan, gray, green or brown) and/or eschar (tan, brown or black) in the wound bed.

Further description: Until enough slough and/or eschar is removed to expose the base of the wound, the true depth, and therefore stage, cannot be determined. Stable (dry, adherent, intact without erythema or fluctuance) eschar on the heels serves as "the body's natural (biological) cover" and should not be removed.

FIGURE 19-1 Stages of Pressure Ulcers — Reprinted with permission: National Pressure Ulcer Advisory Panel. (2007). *Pressure Ulcer Stages Revised by NPUAP*. Retrieved July 31, 2008 from http://www.npuap.org/resources.htm

B. Clinical manifestations – see Figure 19-1.

Treatment

A. Medical and surgical.
1. Debridement (initial care is to remove moist, devitalized tissue).
a. Sharp debridement: use of a scalpel or other instrument; used primarily, especially with cellulitis or sepsis.

b. Mechanical debridement: wet-to-dry dressings, hydrotherapy, wound irrigation, and dextranomers (small beads poured over secreting wounds to absorb exudate).

c. Enzymatic and autolytic debridement: use of enzymes or synthetic dressings that cover wound and self-digest devitalized tissue by the action of enzymes that are present in wound fluids.

2. Wound cleansing (use normal saline solution for most cases).

a. Use minimal mechanical force when cleansing to avoid trauma to the wound bed.

b. Avoid the use of antiseptics (e.g., Dakin's solution, iodine, hydrogen peroxide).

3. Dressings (should protect wound, be biocompatible, and hydrate).

a. Moistened gauze.

b. Film (transparent).

c. Hydrocolloid (moisture and oxygen retaining).

✓ **NURSING PRIORITY:** *Keep the ulcer tissue moist and the surrounding intact skin dry.*

B. Dietary.
1. Increased carbohydrates and protein.
2. Increased vitamin C and zinc.

Nursing Intervention

❖ **Goal:** To prevent or relieve pressure and stimulate circulation.

A. Frequent change of position; turn client every 1 to 2 hours.

B. Special beds with mattresses that provide for a continuous change in pressure across the mattress.

C. Silicone gel pads placed under the buttocks of clients in wheelchairs.

D. Sheepskin pads to provide a soft surface to protect the skin from abrasion.

E. Eggcrate or foam mattress to allow circulation under the body and keep the area dry.

F. Active and passive exercises to promote circulation.

❖ **Goal:** To keep skin clean and healthy and prevent the occurrence of a pressure ulcer.

A. Wash skin with mild soap and blot completely dry with soft towel.
1. Avoid hot water and excessive rubbing.
2. Use lotion or protective moisturizer after bathing.

B. Inspect skin frequently, especially over bony prominences.

✓ **NURSING PRIORITY:** *Avoid massage over bony prominences. When the side-lying position is used in bed, avoid positioning client directly on the trochanter use the 30° lateral inclined position. Do not use donut-type devices. Maintain the head of the bed at or below 30° or at the lowest degree of elevation. Encourage chair-bound persons, who are able, to shift weight every 15 minutes.*

C. Remove any foreign material from the bed, because it may serve as a source of irritation; keep sheets tightly stretched on bed to prevent wrinkles.

❖ **Goal:** To promote healing of pressure ulcer.

A. Use methods discussed to decrease the pressure on the area in which the pressure ulcer is found.
1. Air-fluidized beds - stage III or stage IV pressure ulcers.
2. Static support surfaces (use of a pressure reducing device, e.g., foam overlay, cushion) - not recommended for Stage III or IV.

B. Keep the ulcer area dry.
1. Minimize skin exposure to moisture caused by incontinence, perspiration, or wound drainage.
2. Use only underpads or briefs that are made of materials that absorb moisture and provide a quick-drying surface next to the skin.
3. Position the client with the ulcer exposed to air; may use light to increase drying and promote healing.

C. Use skin barriers to decrease contamination and increase healing of a noninfected ulcer.

D. Observe the ulcer for signs of infection. Infected ulcers will have to be debrided, if healing is to occur.

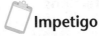 Impetigo

❋ **Impetigo is a bacterial skin infection caused by invasion of the epidermis by pathogenic *Staphylococcus aureus* and/or group A beta-hemolytic streptococci.**

Data Collection

A. Pustule-like lesions with moist honey-colored crusts surrounded by redness.

B. Pruritus; spreads to surrounding areas.

C. Appears more commonly on the face, especially around the mouth.

Treatment

A. Medical.
1. Local: topical treatment.
a. Gentle washing two to three times a day to remove crusts.
b. Topical mupirocin (**Bactroban**) antibiotic cream, if only a couple of lesions are found.
2. Systemic antibiotic therapy is the treatment of choice with extensive lesions.

Home Care

A. Teach the client and family the importance of good hand washing and that lesions heal without scarring.
B. Encourage adherence to therapeutic regimen, especially taking the full course of antibiotics.
C. Untreated impetigo may result in glomerulonephritis.

 Cellulitis

✳ *Cellulitis* **is an inflammation of the subcutaneous tissues often following a break in the skin caused by** *Staphylococcus aureus,* *Streptococcus,* **or** *Haemophilus influenzae.*

Data Collection

A. Intense redness, edema with diffuse border, and tenderness.
B. Chills, malaise, and fever.

Treatment

A. Medical.
   1. Moist heat, immobilization, and elevation of part.
   2. Systemic antibiotic therapy is the treatment of choice with extensive lesions.

 Home Care

A. Teach the client and family the importance of good hand washing.
B. Encourage adherence to therapeutic regimen, especially taking the full course of antibiotics.

 Fungal (Dermatophyte) Infections

Assessment

A. Types.
   1. Tinea corporis (ringworm): temporary hair loss, if scalp is affected.
   2. Tinea cruris ("jock itch"): small, red, scaly patches in the groin area.
   3. Tinea pedis (athlete's foot): scaling, maceration, erythema, blistering, and pruritus; usually found between the toes.
   4. Tinea unguium (onychomycosis): thickened, crumbling nails (usually toes) with yellowish discoloration.
   5. Candidiasis: caused by *Candida albicans*, known as moniliasis, may affect oral mucosa, groin, and moist areas; white plaques in mouth; diffuse red rash on skin.

Treatment

A. Topical antifungal cream (see Appendix 19-1).
B. Oral antifungal medication.
C. Systemic therapy: Griseofulvin; used primarily for extensive cases.

 Home Care

A. To prevent athlete's foot, client should be instructed to keep feet as dry as possible and wear socks made of absorbent cotton.
   1. Talcum powder or antifungal powder may be used; **Tinactin** may be applied twice daily.
   2. Encourage aeration of shoes to allow them to completely dry out.
B. Client should maintain hygienic measures to prevent the spread of fungal diseases, specifically ringworm of the scalp.
   1. Family members should avoid using the same comb.
   2. Scarves and hats should be washed thoroughly.
   3. Examine family and household pets frequently for symptoms of the disease.
C. Client should avoid infection.
   1. Any activity that allows heat, friction, and maceration to occur may lead to skin breakdown and infection.
   2. Loose-fitting clothing and cotton underwear are to be encouraged.

 Parasitic Infestations

A. Pediculosis.
   1. Types.
      a. *Pediculus humanus capitis:* head lice.
      b. *Pediculus humanus corporis:* body lice.
      c. *Phthirus pubis:* pubic lice or crabs.
   2. Clinical manifestations.
      a. Intense pruritus, which may lead to secondary excoriation and infection.
      b. Tiny, red, noninflammatory lesions.
      c. Eggs (nits) of both head and body lice are often attached to the hair shafts.
      d. Pubic lice are often spread by sexual contact.
B. Scabies: an infestation of the skin by itch mites.
   1. Intense itching, especially at night.
   2. Burrows are seen, especially between fingers, on the surfaces of wrists, and in axillary folds.
   3. Redness, swelling, and vesicular formation may be noted.

Treatment

A. Pediculosis.
   1. Permethrin 1% liquid (**Nix**): effective against nits and lice with just one application; shampoo hair first, leave Nix on hair for 10 minutes, rinse off; may repeat in 7 days.
   2. Pyrethrin compounds (e.g., **Rid**) for pubic and head lice.
B. Scabies: Permethrin 5% cream (**Elimite**). Cream is applied to the skin from head to soles of feet and left on for 8 to 14 hours, then washed off; only one application needed.

Home Care

A. All family members and close contacts need to be treated for parasitic disorders; lice can survive up to 48 hours; nits can hatch in 7-10 days when shed in the environment.

B. Bedding and clothing that may have lice or nits should be washed or dry cleaned; furniture and rugs should be vacuumed or treated.

C. Nurses should wear gloves when examining scalp to prevent spread to others.

D. When shampooing hair, use a fine-tooth comb or tweezers to remove remaining nits.

Viral Infections

A. Herpes simplex virus (fever blister, cold sore): herpes virus type 1 (HSV-1).
  1. Painful, local reaction consisting of vesicles with an erythematous base; most often appears around the mouth.
  2. Contagious by direct contact; is recurrent (lesions appear in same place); there is no immunity.
  3. Not to be confused with HSV-2, which primarily occurs below the waist (genital herpes).
  4. It is possible for the HSV-1 to cause genital lesions and for HSV-2 to cause oral lesions (see Sexually Transmitted Diseases in Chapter 17).

B. Herpes zoster (shingles).
  1. Related to the chicken pox virus: varicella.
  2. Contagious to anyone who has not had chicken pox or who may be immunosuppressed.
  3. Linear patches of vesicles with an erythematous base are located along spinal and cranial nerve tracts.
  4. Often unilateral and appears on the trunk; however, may also appear on the face.
  5. Pain, burning, and neuralgia occur at the site before outbreak of vesicles.
  6. Often precipitated by the same factors as herpes simplex infection.

C. Herpetic whitlow: occurs on fingertips and around nail cuticles; often seen in medical personnel.

Treatment

A. Usually symptomatic; application of soothing moist compresses.

B. Analgesics; gabapentin (**Neurontin**) for postherpetic neuralgia.

C. Antiviral agents (see Appendix 19-1).

D. Zoster vaccine is recommended for adults over 60 years.

Home Care

A. Alleviate pain by administering analgesics.

B. Antihistamines may be administered to control the itching.

C. Usually, lesions heal without complications; herpes simplex usually heals without scarring, whereas herpes zoster may cause scarring.

D. If hospitalized, establish contact precautions for herpes zoster.

Malignant Melanoma

Data Collection

A. Risk factors
1. Chronic UV exposure without protection or overexposure to artificial light (tanning bed).
2. Fair skin, genetic (first degree relative).
3. Has the highest mortality rate of any form of skin cancer.
   a. Often appears in preexisting moles in the skin.
   b. Common sites include back and legs (women); trunk, head, and neck (men).
   c. Sudden or progressive change or increase in size, color, or shape of a mole.
4. Symptoms (Box 19-2).

BOX 19-2   MALIGNANT MELANOMA

Melanomas tend to have:
A Asymmetry
B Border Irregularity
C Color Variegation
D Diameter great than 6 mm
E Evolving or changing in some way

Treatment

A. Surgical.
  1. Excisional surgery; laser treatment.
  2. Cryosurgery.
  3. Electrodesiccation and curettage.

B. Medical.
  1. Radiation therapy.
  2. Chemotherapy and biologic therapy.

Home Care

A. Teach the importance of avoiding unnecessary exposure to sunlight.

B. Apply protective sunscreen when outside.

C. Teach the warning signs of cancer.

Burns

A. Types of burns – thermal, electrical, chemical, smoke and inhalation.
B. Fluid shift considerations.
  1. Fluid shift and edema formation occur within 24 to 48 hours after burn injury.
  2. Fluid mobilization occurs within approximately 18 to 36 hours after burn injury.

Data Collection

A. Criteria suggesting pulmonary damage.
  1. History of burn injury occurring within a confined area.
  2. Burns around the face, neck or mouth or in the oral mucosa.
B. Circulatory status.
  1. Tachycardia and hypotension may occur early.
  2. Evaluate urine output.
C. Identify when client ate last; check gastrointestinal function.
D. Evaluate response to fluid therapy.
E. Evaluate circulatory status of the extremities.

> ✓ **NURSING PRIORITY:** *The client with burn injury is often awake, mentally alert, and cooperative at first. The level of consciousness may change as respiratory status changes or as the fluid shift occurs, precipitating hypovolemia. If the client is unconscious or confused, assess him or her for the possibility of a head injury.*

F. Determine the severity of the burn injury (Box 19-3 and Figure 19-2).
  1. Neck and face burns may lead to mechanical occlusion of the airway due to edema.
  2. Circumferential burns (burns surrounding an entire extremity) may lead to impaired circulation from edema formation and lack of elasticity of the eschar, leading to compartmental syndrome.

BOX 19-3   DEPTH OF BURNS

- Superficial or first-degree burn: Area is reddened and blanches with pressure; no edema present; area is generally painful to touch.
- Partial-thickness or second-degree burn: Dermis and epidermis are affected; formation of large, thick-walled blisters; underlying skin is erythematous.
- Full-thickness or third and fourth-degree burn: All of the skin is destroyed; may have damage to the subcutaneous tissue and muscle; usually has a dry appearance, may be white or charred; will require skin grafting to cover area; underlying structures (fascia, tendons, and bones) are severely damaged, usually blackened.

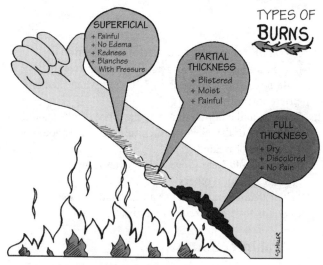

FIGURE 19-2 **Degree of Burn by Tissue Layer** — (From Zerwekh J, Claborn J, Miller CJ: *Memory notebook of nursing, vol 1*, ed 4, Ingram, 2008, Nursing Education Consultants.)

  3. Age.
    a. Infants have an immature immune system and poor body defense.
    b. Older adult clients heal slowly; more likely to have wound infection problems and pulmonary complications.
  4. Presence of other health problems:
    a. Diabetes and peripheral vascular disease delay wound healing.
    b. Poor nutritional state.
    c. Chronic conditions that compromise immune system.

Treatment

A. Stabilization of airway, breathing, and circulation.
B. If the burn area is small, apply cold compresses or immerse injured area in cool water to decrease heat; ice should not be directly applied to the burn area.
C. Administer tetanus injection.
D. Fluid resuscitation; IV fluids.
E. NPO; may need a nasogastric tube.
F. Analgesics are given intravenously; intramuscularly, subcutaneously, orally administered medications may not be absorbed effectively.
G. Methods of wound care (area is cleaned and debrided of necrotic burned tissue).
  1. Open method (exposure): Burn is covered with a topical antibiotic cream, and no dressing is applied.
  2. Closed method of dressing: Fine mesh is used to cover the burned surface; may be impregnated with antibiotic ointment or ointment may be applied before the dressing is applied.
  3. Escharotomy: Procedure involves excision through the eschar to increase circulation to an extremity with circumferential burns.
    a. Enzymatic debriders: **Collagenase**, fibrinolysin, and **Accuzyme** may be used.

4. Wound grafting: As eschar is debrided and granulation tissue begins to form, grafts are used to protect the wound and to promote healing.

H. Nutritional support.
   1. Diet is high in calories and protein.
   2. In clients who have large burn surface areas, supplemental gastric tube feedings or parenteral nutrition may be used.

I. Clients with a burn surface area less than 20% usually do not experience serious fluid shifts and fluid loss.

Nursing Intervention

❖ **Goal:** To maintain patent airway and prevent hypoxia.
A. Assess circumstances surrounding the burn.
   1. Monitor for cardiac irregularities, if electrical burn.
   2. Rinse skin with water, if a chemical burn.
   3. Inhalation burns: immediate priority is airway.
B. As edema phase begins, evaluate respiratory status.
C. Endotracheal intubation or tracheotomy may be necessary.
D. Anticipate transfer to burn unit if burns cover more than 20% of body surface area.
E. *Report to primary care provider (PCP) any significant changes in respiratory status.*

❖ **Goal:** To evaluate fluid and circulatory status and adequacy of fluid replacement.
A. Obtain client's weight on admission.
B. Assess status and time frame of fluid resuscitation.
C. Evaluate urine output.
D. Correlate vital signs with previous readings.
E. Monitor signs of adequate hydration.

❖ **Goal:** To prevent or decrease infection.
A. Implement infection control procedures to protect the client (e.g., sterile linen, gloves, cap, mask, and gown).
B. After eschar sloughs or is removed, assess wound for infection. Infection may be difficult to identify before eschar sloughs.

❖ **Goal:** To maintain comfort and homeostasis..
A. Maintain client's body temperature as close to normal as possible; keep room temperature warm.

B. Pressure under dressing should be evenly distributed; elastic tubular netting may be used to maintain stability of the dressing; perform circulatory checks every 2 to 3 hours.

❖ **Goal:** To maintain nutrition and promote positive nitrogen balance for healing.
A. Work with dietitian to maintain nutritional intake.
B. Provide tube feedings as indicated.
C. Monitor response to total parenteral nutrition.
D. Record daily weight.

❖ **Goal:** To prevent contractures and scarring.
A. Assist client to attempt mobilization and ambulation as soon as possible.
B. Passive and active range of motion should be initiated from the beginning of burn therapy and throughout therapy.
C. Position client to prevent flexion contractures; position of comfort for the client may increase contracture formation.
D. Use splints and exercises to prevent flexion contractures.
E. Use pressure dressings and garments to contour healing burn area to keep scars flat and prevent elevation and enlargement above the original burn injury area.

❖ **Goal:** To promote acceptance and adaptation to alterations in body image.
A. Maintain open communication and encourage expression of feelings.
B. Anticipate depression as a normal consequence of burn trauma; it should decrease as condition improves.

> ✔ **NURSING PRIORITY:** *It is important to recognize that the client's anger is not a direct attack on the care provider; it is an expression of grief and sorrow.*

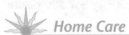 Home Care

A. Physical therapy.
B. Continue high-calorie, high-protein diet.
C. Wound care management.
D. Avoid exposure of burn area to direct sunlight.

Study Questions: Integumentary System

1. The nurse understands that pressure ulcers are most commonly caused by what problem?
   1 Muscles that are not being used in passive exercises.
   2 Poor nutrition, resulting in inadequate protein intake.
   3 Irritation of a bony prominence that is covered by infected skin.
   4 Pressure cutting off blood supply to the affected area of the skin.
2. In report, the nurse is told the client has a stage 1 pressure ulcer. What would the nurse expect to find on assessment of the area?
   1 A area of erythema that does not blanch with digital pressure.
   2 A moist area where the skin has sloughed.
   3 A well-circumscribed area that has a center crater in subcutaneous tissue.
   4 A reddened area of irritation and scaly plaques on the skin.
3. A client has a pressure ulcer that has necrosis in the subcutaneous level of tissue. There is undermining of the surrounding tissue. What is the nursing care for this stage of a pressure ulcer?
   1 Carefully clean the area with hydrogen peroxide and apply a dry dressing.
   2 Gently massage the area around the necrosis to stimulate healing.
   3 Apply a clean dressing and encourage an increased fluid intake.
   4 Keep pressure off the area and anticipate procedure for debridement.
4. Which of the following nursing interventions will assist in reducing pressure points that may lead to pressure ulcers?
   Select all that apply:
   1 Position the client directly on the trochanter when side-lying.
   2 Avoid the use of donut devices.
   3 Massage bony prominences.
   4 Elevate the head of the bed as little as possible.
   5 When side-lying use the 30° lateral inclined position.
   6 Avoid uninterrupted sitting in any chair or wheelchair.
5. What would the nurse teach an older adult client regarding how to care for her dry, itchy skin?
   1 Use a moisturizer on all dry skin areas.
   2 Wear clothes with 80% or more of cotton fibers.
   3 Shower twice a day with mild soap.
   4 Wear protective pads on dry skin areas.
6. A client has a third-degree circumferential burn on his left upper arm. Eschar has formed on the burn area. What is most important for the nurse to assess?
   1 Evaluate around the eschar for presence of infection.
   2 Status of circulation in the left hand.
   3 Presence of bilateral breath sounds.
   4 Status of urinary output and hydration.
7. What will be important for the nurse to tell the parents of a child who has a problem with head lice?
   1 Wash the child's hair with a coal tar–based shampoo and rinse thoroughly.
   2 Thoroughly wash all of the child's bedding and clothes.
   3 Use an anti-itch cream, but make sure the irritated areas do not get infected.
   4 Use an antibiotic ointment after shampooing with Permethrin 1% (**Nix**).
8. An older adult client in a long-term care facility has been diagnosed with herpes zoster. What is important nursing management for this client?
   1 Daily application of an antifungal cream to affected areas.
   2 Maintain client on standard precautions.
   3 Apply warm soaks to area of vesicles.
   4 Assist the client to deal with the neuralgia.
9. A client has been diagnosed with basal cell carcinoma and the area has been excised. What will be important for the nurse to explain to this patient?
   1 Pain, burning, and neuralgia may occur in the affected area.
   2 It is very important to use sunscreen any time you go outside.
   3 Use an antiinflammatory ointment to prevent a secondary infection in the area.
   4 Once the area has been excised, there should be no further problems.
10. A client has been diagnosed with psoriasis. What would be important for the nurse to discuss with this client?
   1 The use of topical steroids and ultraviolet light will help to control the problem.
   2 The area should be cleansed, scales removed, and then the antibiotic ointment applied.
   3 Warm, moist packs can be applied to the area to assist in the debriding of the lesion.
   4 The problem usually goes away with treatment, but the area may remain tender to the touch.
11. A child has scabies. What should the nurse explain to the mother?
   1 Carefully remove nits from area and then wash with alcohol.
   2 Spread **Elimite** cream all over body, leave on for 8 to 12 hours, and then wash off.
   3 Apply moist soaks of antifungal medication on burrowed skin lesions for 1 to 2 hours, then rinse.
   4 Encourage exposure to sunlight to dry the area and apply antibiotic ointment.

Answers and rationales to these questions are in the section at the end of the book titled Chapter Study Questions: Answers and Rationales.

Appendix 19-1 SKIN DIAGNOSTIC STUDIES

Skin testing

Purpose: confirm sensitivity to a specific allergen by placing antigen on or directly below skin (intradermal) to check for presence of antibodies.

1. Two methods –
   Allergen applied under the skin of the arms or back.
   - Cutaneous scratch test (also known as a *tine* or *prick test*)
   - Intracutaneous injection - high risk of severe allergic reaction
   Patch test – used to determine if client is allergic to testing material (small amount applied on back) – returns in 48 hours for evaluation.
2. Interpreting results.
   - *Immediate* reaction: appears within minutes after the injection; marked by erythema and a wheal; denotes a positive reaction.
   - *Positive* reaction: local wheal-and-flare response occurs.
   - *Negative* reaction: inconclusive; may indicate that antibodies have not formed yet or that antigen was deposited too deeply in skin (not an intradermal injection); may also indicate immunosuppression.
3. Complications: range from minor itching to anaphylaxis (see Chapter 5).

> ✔ *NURSING PRIORITY: Never leave client alone during skin testing due to risk of anaphylaxis. If a severe reaction occurs, anticipate antiinflammatory topical cream applied to skin site (scratch test) or a tourniquet applied to the arm (intracutaneous test) and possible epinephrine injection.*

Biopsy

Types: punch, excisional, incisional, shave
1. Verify if informed consent is needed.
2. Apply dressing and give postprocedure instructions – watch for bleeding.

Skin Culture

Purpose: identify fungal, bacterial, and viral organisms.
1. Scrape or swab affected area; label specimen and send to lab.

Appendix 19-2 | MEDICATIONS USED IN SKIN DISORDERS

GENERAL NURSING IMPLICATIONS
- Topical medications are used primarily for local effects when systemic absorption is undesirable.
- For topical application:
  - ✦ Apply after shower or bath for best absorption, because skin is hydrated.
  - ✦ Apply small amount of medication and rub in well.

Medications	Side Effects	Nursing Implications
ANTIFUNGAL: Inhibits or damages fungal cell membrane, either altering permeability or disrupting cell mitosis.		
Clotrimazole (**Lotrimin**): topical Nystatin (**Mycolog**): topical Ketoconazole (**Nizoral**): PO, topical Griseofulvin (**Fulvicin**): PO	Nausea, vomiting, abdominal pain. Hypersensitivity reaction: rash, urticaria, pruritus. Hepatotoxicity. Gynecomastia (ketoconazole).	1. Monitor hepatic function (when oral medication is given). 2. Avoid alcohol because of potential liver problems. 3. Check for local burning, irritation, or itching with topical application. 4. Prolonged therapy (weeks or months) is usually necessary, especially with griseofulvin (**Fulvicin**). 5. Take griseofulvin (**Fulvicin**) with foods high in fat (e.g., milk, ice cream) to decrease GI upset and assist in absorption. 6. *Uses:* tinea infections, fungal infections, candidiasis, diaper dermatitis.
ANTIVIRAL: Reduces viral shedding, pain, and time to heal.		
Acyclovir (**Zovirax**): topical, PO, IV. Penciclovir (**Denavir**): topical Vidarabine (**Ara-A, Vir-A**): IV, ophthalmic	IV: phlebitis, rash, hives. PO: nausea, vomiting. Topical: burning, stinging, pruritus. Anorexia, nausea, vomiting. Ophthalmic: burning, itching.	1. Apply topically to affected area six times per day. 2. Avoid auto-inoculation; wash hands frequently; apply with gloved hand. 3. Avoid sexual intercourse while genital lesions are present. 4. Drink adequate fluids. 5. Infuse IV preparations over 1 hour; use an infusion pump for accurate delivery. 6. *Uses:* herpes infections.
ANTIINFLAMMATORY: Decreases the inflammatory response.		
Triamcinolone acetonide (**Aristocort**): topical	Skin thinning, superficial dilated blood vessels (telangiectasis), acne-like eruptions, adrenal suppression.	1. Triamcinolone and hydrocortisone creams come in various strengths. Watch the percent strength. 2. Applied 2-3 times a day. 3. Use an occlusive dressing only if ordered. 4. Encourage client to use the least amount possible and for the shortest period of time.
IMMUNOSUPPRESANT: Suppresses T cells and decreases relaease of inflammatory mediators; alternative to glucocorticoids		
Pimecrolimus cream (**Elidel**): topical Tacrolimus ointment (**Protopic**): topical	Erythema, pruritus Burning sensaton at application site	1. Teach clients to use sunscreen, as makes client sensitized to UV light. 2. Long term effects can lead to skin cancer and lymphoma.

GI, Gastrointestinal; *IV,* intravenously; *PO,* by mouth (orally).

Appendix 19-3 TOPICAL ANTIBIOTICS FOR BURN TREATMENT

Medications	Side Effects	Nursing Implications
TOPICAL ANTIBIOTICS: Prevent and treat infection at the burn site.		
Silver sulfadiazine (**Silvadene**)	Hypersensitivity: rash, itching, or burning sensation in unburned skin	1. Liberal amounts are spread topically with a sterile, gloved hand or on impregnated gauze rolls over the burned surface. 2. If discoloration occurs in the **Silvadene** cream, do not use. 3. A thin layer of cream is spread evenly over the entire burn surface area; reapplication is done every 12 hours. 4. Client should be bathed or "tubbed" daily to aid in debridement. 5. Medication does not penetrate eschar. 6. For clients with extensive burns, monitor urine output and renal function; a significant amount of sulfa may be absorbed.
Mafenide acetate (**Sulfamylon 10%**)	Pain, burning, or stinging at application sites; excessive loss of body water; excoriation of new tissue; may be systemically absorbed and cause metabolic acidosis.	1. Bacteriostatic medication diffuses rapidly through burned skin and eschar and is effective against bacteria under the eschar. 2. Dressings are not required but are frequently used. A thin layer of cream is spread evenly over the entire burn surface. 3. Monitor renal function and possible acidosis, because medication is rapidly absorbed from the burn surface and eliminated via the kidneys. 4. Pain occurs on application. 5. Watch for hyperventilation, as a compensatory mechanism when acidosis occurs.

Maternal Care

Areas to Review: Normal prenatal, labor, postpartum care. The physiological changes.

CONTRACEPTION

* **Contraception is the voluntary prevention of pregnancy. Two important factors influence the selection of the particular type of contraceptive method: acceptability and effectiveness.**

Data Collection

A. Types of contraception.
   1. Temporary methods used to delay or avoid pregnancy.
   2. Permanent: voluntary sterilization.
B. Contraceptive methods (see Appendix 20-1).

NORMAL PREGNANCY CYCLE: PHYSIOLOGICAL CHANGES

Uterus

A. Increase in size as a result of the stimulating influence of estrogen and the distention caused by the growing fetus.
B. Irregular, painless uterine contractions (Braxton Hicks) begin in the early weeks of pregnancy; contraction and relaxation assist in accommodating the growing fetus.
C. Softening of the lower uterine segment (Hegar's sign).
D. Cervical changes.
   1. Softening of the cervix (Goodell's sign).
   2. Formation of the mucous plug to prevent bacterial contamination from the vagina.

Vagina

A. An increase in vaginal secretions.
B. A blue-purple hue of the vaginal walls is seen very early (Chadwick's sign).
C. Vaginal secretions: thickish white and acidic (pH is 3.5 to 6.0).

Breasts

A. Increase in breast size accompanied by feelings of fullness, tingling, and heaviness.
B. Superficial veins prominent; nipples erect; darkening and increase in diameter of the areola.
C. Thin, watery secretion (precursor to colostrum) may be expressed from the nipples by the end of the tenth week.

Cardiovascular System

A. Increased blood volume (40% to 50%).
B. Increase in heart rate (by 10 beats per minute) by the end of the first trimester.
C. Increase in cardiac output (30% to 50%).
D. Cardiac enlargement and systolic murmurs.
E. Hematocrit (Hct) decreases by 7%: physiological anemia.
F. Blood pressure (BP) will decrease slightly in the second trimester.

Respiratory System

A. Diaphragm is elevated; change from abdominal to thoracic breathing around the twenty-fourth week.
B. Breathes deeper; only slightly increased respiratory rate.
C. Common complaints of nasal stuffiness and epistaxis due to estrogen influence on nasal mucosa.
D. Increased oxygen consumption.

Urinary/Renal Systems

A. Ureter and renal pelvis dilate (especially on the right side) as a result of the growing uterus.
B. Increased frequency of urination (first and last trimesters).
C. Decreased bladder tone (due to effect of progesterone); bladder capacity increases: 1300 to 1500 mL.
D. Frequent spilling of glucose in urine (glycosuria).

Gastrointestinal System

A. Pregnancy gingivitis: gums reddened, swollen, and bleed easily.
B. Nausea and vomiting due to elevated level of human chorionic gonadotropin (HCG).
C. Decreased tone and motility of smooth muscles; decreased emptying time of stomach; slowed peristalsis leads to complaints of bloating, heartburn, and constipation.

Musculoskeletal System

A. Increase in the normal lumbosacral curve leads to backward tilt of the torso.
B. Center of gravity is changed, which often leads to leg and back strain and predisposition to falling.
C. Pelvis relaxes due to the effects of the hormone relaxin; leads to the characteristic "duck waddling" gait.
D. Abdominal wall stretches and loses tone.

Integumentary System

A. Increased skin pigmentation in various areas of the body.
   1. Facial: mask of pregnancy (chloasma).
   2. Abdomen: striae (reddish purple stretch marks) and linea nigra (darkened vertical line from umbilicus to symphysis pubis).
B. Appearance of vascular spider nevi, especially on the neck, arms, and legs.
C. Acne vulgaris, dermatitis, and psoriasis usually improve during pregnancy.

Placenta

A. Functions include transport of nutrients and removal of waste products from the fetus.
B. Produces human chorionic gonadotropin (HCG) and human placental lactogen (HPL).
C. Produces estrogen and progesterone after 2 months of gestation.
D. Production of posterior pituitary hormone oxytocin, which promotes uterine contractility and stimulation of milk let-down reflex.

Metabolism

A. Weight gain - determined by prepregnancy weight for height calculated by using the body mass index (BMI), which 19.8 to 26 is considered normal.
B. Normal weight gain: recommended 11.5-16kg; (average, 26-28 lb).
   1. Underweight: 12.5-18 kg.
   2. Overweight: 7-11 kg.
   3. Multiple gestations: 21-28 kg.

> ✓ **NURSING PRIORITY:** *The pattern of weight gain is important. Approximately 0.4kg per week for normal weight; 0.5kg/week for underweight; 0.3kg/week for overweight. Inadequate weight gain for a normal weight woman would be less than 1kg/month. Excessive weight gain is considered more than 3kg/month and should be evaluated, as it can indicate preeclampsia if it occurs after the 20th week of gestation.*

C. There are variations of recommended weight gain based on whether the woman is overweight, underweight, or carrying twins. An inadequate weight gain is associated with a higher risk for intrauterine growth retardation (IUGR).

PRENATAL CARE

Data Collection

A. Initial visit.
   1. Complete history and physical.
   2. Obstetrical history.
      a. Past pregnancies (date, course of pregnancy, labor and postpartum; information about infant and neonatal course).
      b. Present pregnancy.
B. Subsequent assessment data follow-up.
   1. Vital signs.
   2. Urinalysis: check for protein and glucose.
   3. Monitor weight.
   4. Measurement of height of uterine fundus.
   5. Auscultation of fetal heart rate (FHR).
C. Definition of Common Terms (Table 20-1).

TABLE 20-1	DEFINITION OF COMMON TERMS
COMMON TERM	**DEFINITION**
Gravida*	A pregnancy regardless of duration; includes present pregnancy
Para*	Refers to past pregnancies that continue to period of viability (legal definition: 24 to 28 weeks of gestational age; 20 weeks in some states)
Primigravida	Woman who is pregnant for first time
Multigravida	Woman who is pregnant for second or subsequent time
Nullipara (para 0)	Woman who has not had children
Primipara (para 1)	Woman who has carried a pregnancy to viability; term is often used interchangeably with primigravida
Multipara (para II, para III, para IV, etc.)	Woman who has given birth to two or more children
Parturient	A woman in labor

*The terms *gravida* and *para* refer to the number of pregnancies, not the number of fetuses. The woman who delivers twins on her first pregnancy remains a para 1, in spite of having two infants. She also is a para 1 if the fetus was stillborn or died soon after birth.

  Another system used to describe reproductive status is the five-digit identification system characterized by the acronym GTPAL:

G = total number of pregnancies
T = number of term infants (37 weeks of gestation)
P = number of preterm infants (before 37 weeks of gestation)
A = number of spontaneous or therapeutic abortions
L = number of living children

TABLE 20-2	SIGNS AND SYMPTOMS OF PREGNANCY

PRESUMPTIVE/SUBJECTIVE	PROBABLE/OBJECTIVE	POSITIVE/DIAGNOSTIC
1. Amenorrhea. 2. Nausea and vomiting. 3. Excessive fatigue. 4. Urinary frequency. 5. Breast changes: tenderness, fullness, increased pigmentation of areola, pre-colostrum discharge. 6. Quickening: active movements of the fetus felt by the mother. 7. Increased pigmentation of skin and abdominal striae.	1. Positive pregnancy test result. 2. Enlarged abdomen. 3. Hegar's sign: softening of lower uterine segment. 4. Chadwick's sign: bluish discoloration of vagina. 5. Goodell's sign: softening of cervical lip. 6. Ballottement: pushing on fetus (fourth to fifth month) and feeling it rebound back. 7. Fetal outline distinguished by palpation. 8. Braxton-Hicks contractions.	1. Fetal heart rate: tenth to twelfth week—doppler ultrasonography; eighteenth to twentieth week—fetal stethoscope. 2. Fetal movements. 3. Fetal skeleton on x-ray film (not used often). 4. Fetal sonography (after sixteenth week).

> 💡 **TEST ALERT:** *Be sure you are able to differentiate between presumptive, probable, and positive signs.*

D. Signs and Symptoms of Pregnancy (Table 20-2).
E. Summary of Nursing Management During the Antepartum Period (Table 20-3).

Diagnostics

A. Pregnancy tests: all tests including OTC "home pregnancy" tests are based upon the presence of hCG as the biologic marker. A false negative test may be due to testing too early. Whenever there is doubt about the results, further evaluation or retesting in a few days may be appropriate.
B. Laboratory tests.
   1. Urinalysis.
   2. Complete blood count (CBC), electrolytes, BUN, creatinine.
   3. Venereal Disease Research Laboratory (VDRL), rapid plasmin reagin (RPR), or fluorescent treponemal antibody-absorption (FTA-ABS) - serological screening for syphilis.
   4. Vaginal cultures for gonorrhea and chlamydia in high-risk populations.
   5. Antibody titers for HIV infection, rubella, and hepatitis B (HBsAg), tuberculin skin testing, maternal serum alpha-fetoprotein (MSAFP) at 15-22 weeks.
   6. Blood type and Rh; if Rh is negative, client will receive RhoGam.
   7. If mother is of African or Mediterranean descent, sickle cell screening.
C. Pelvic examination.
   1. Papanicolaou smear of the cervix (Pap smear).
   2. Pelvic measurements (pelvimetry).
D. Calculation of estimated date of birth (EDB).
   1. Nägele's rule: count back 3 calendar months from the first day of the last menstrual period (LMP) and add 7 days.

   2. Examples:
      a. LMP: April 10, 2009; EDC: January 17, 2010.
      b. LMP: October 25, 2009; EDC: July 2, 2010.

Nursing Interventions

❖ **Goal:** To educate families regarding general health practices.
A. Hygiene: tub baths permitted until the last trimester, when balance is altered due to change in center of gravity; no douching, no hot tubs.
B. Clothing: loose, comfortable clothing with good supporting brassiere; low-heeled shoes.
C. Employment: no severe physical straining, heavy lifting, or prolonged periods of sitting or standing.
D. Travel: avoid during the last month of pregnancy; when traveling by car or airplane, frequent walking and stretching is advised; use seat belts (both lap and shoulder), positioning the lap belt under the abdomen.
E. Rest and exercise: adequate amounts of exercise (e.g., walking, swimming); client should stop exercising when she begins to feel tired; *moderation* is the key word.
F. Smoking: not advised; associated with infants who are small for gestational age (SGA).
G. Alcohol: recommended not to consume any alcohol; the more consumed, the greater the risk for fetal alcohol syndrome (FAS).
H. Medications: client advised to avoid over-the-counter (OTC) medications, especially during the first trimester. She should consult with her primary care provider (PCP) before taking any medications.
❖ **Goal:** To promote relief of common discomforts through client education of Home Care measures (Table 20-4).
❖ **Goal:** To promote adequate nutrition.
A. Assess normal food intake.
B. Dietary instructions and nutrient requirements.

TABLE 20-3	SUMMARY OF NURSING MANAGEMENT DURING THE ANTEPARTUM PERIOD

Weeks of Gestation	Physical Signs and Symptoms	Characteristic Behaviors	Nursing Interventions
0-16	Amenorrhea Fatigue Nausea, vomiting Increased breast size and tenderness Urinary frequency Increased appetite	Ambivalence with mood swings. Anxiety related to confirmation of pregnancy. Tells selected close persons of pregnancy. *Couvade syndrome* refers to the presence of physical discomforts in the father during the pregnancy that mimic his partner's symptoms.	1. Obtain complete history, including gynecological and obstetrical histories. 2. Ascertain any maternal high-risk problems such as maternal age (greater than 35 years or less than 16 years), heart disease, diabetes or potential neonatal high-risk problems such as history of congenital defects, premature births, etc. (See complete discussion in this chapter on high-risk problems.) 3. Identify maternal nutritional status by assessing height, weight and compare with BMI chart. 4. Complete a diet history and instruction. Important to teach about necessary changes, rather than all the concepts of good nutrition. 5. Food cravings are usually benign and may be indulged, providing a well-balanced diet is maintained. Pica is an abnormal eating pattern and requires treatment. 6. Encourage client to express feelings or ambivalence about pregnancy. 7. Anticipatory guidance/teaching (including family) related to: OTC drugs, normal signs and symptoms of pregnancy, as well as reportable signs of possible complications, and the normality of her mood swings.
16-30	Quickening "Pregnant figure" Increased energy Feeling of well-being Round ligament pain	Wears maternity clothes. Tells the world she's pregnant; begins to notice other pregnant women. Interested in learning about birth and babies: reads books, seeks out and questions friends and family, attends classes. Increased dependency as time goes on. Promote father's involvement by allowing him to watch and feel fetal movement. Father needs to confront and resolve his own conflicts about the fathering he received as a child. Father will decide on what he does and does not want to imitate from his father role model.	1. Ongoing assessment of maternal/fetal status: FHR; vital signs; fundal height. Urine test for glucose (mild glycosuria is usually benign), and protein. Finger stick for hemoglobin analysis (12-14 g/dl normal). Balanced diet. 2. Prevent or minimize activity intolerance and promote adequate rest by: • Encouraging 8 hours sleep each day, plus one nap. • Scheduling rest periods at place of employment. • Napping at home while other small children are sleeping. • Using left lateral position while resting or sleeping. 3. Promote adequate exercise (e.g., Kegel, pelvic rocking, modified sit ups), sitting tailor-fashion (lotus position). 4. Anticipatory guidance/teaching (including family) related to: libido changes, mood swings, increasing dependency, introversion, and reportable signs of possible complications.

Continued

TABLE 20-3	SUMMARY OF NURSING MANAGEMENT DURING THE ANTEPARTUM PERIOD—cont'd.		
Weeks of Gestation	**Physical Signs and Symptoms**	**Characteristic Behaviors**	**Nursing Interventions**
30-40	Dependent edema Pressure in lower abdomen Frequent urination Round ligament pain Backache Insomnia Clumsiness Fatigue	Introversion. Increased dependency (craves attention and tenderness). Altered responsiveness and spontaneity, as well as abdominal bulk and fatigue, may decrease interest in genital sex. Intensifies study of labor and delivery. Increasingly feeling more vulnerable. Prepares nursery; buys baby things. Decides on feeding method for baby.	1. Ongoing continued physical assessment at more frequent intervals. 2. Reassure: provide emotional support related to attractiveness and self-worth. 3. Anticipatory guidance/teaching (including family) related to: Signs and symptoms of labor, environmental modification for coming infant, and providing rest for mother, teaching associated with either breast or bottle feeding, advising client concerning birthing and anesthesia options, promoting the developing parent/child attachment (encourage family to verbalize mental picture of infant and concepts of selves as parents).

> **TEST ALERT:** *Plan anticipatory guidance for developmental transitions. Pregnancy is considered a normal maturational crisis and developmental stage for the expectant couple.*

1. Increase calories for pregnancy (an additional 300 calories per day).
2. Increase calories for lactation (an additional 500 calories per day greater than prepregnant intake).
3. Increase protein (an additional 10 gm per day for pregnancy; an additional 5 gm per day for lactation).
4. Increase vitamins (generally all vitamin intake is increased, especially folic acid).
5. Increase amount of minerals (especially iron, calcium, and phosphorus).
6. Additional calories and protein may be recommended for the pregnant adolescent.

❖ **Goal:** To educate expectant family with regard to danger signs and symptoms requiring immediate attention (Box 20-1).

FETUS

Multifetal Pregnancy

A. Fraternal twins: can be either the same sex or a different sex.
B. Identical twins: same sex; resemble each other in appearance and structure.
C. Steady rise in multifetal pregnancies due to delayed childbearing and use of ovulation enhancing drugs.

Placenta

A. Transfer of oxygen, nutrients, and metabolites.
B. Elimination of waste products from the fetus.

BOX 20-1	DANGER SIGNS OF PREGNANCY

- Vaginal discharge of bloody or amniotic fluid
- Visual disturbances
- Swelling of face or fingers
- Fever and chills
- Severe continuous headache
- Pain in the abdomen
- Persistent vomiting
- Absence of fetal movement

C. Production of hormones: human chorionic gonadotropin (hCG), human placental lactogen (HPL), estrogen (estriol), and progesterone.
D. Fetal surface is shiny and slightly grayish: Schultze position.
E. Maternal side is rough and beefy red: Duncan's position.
F. Maternal and fetal bloodstreams are in close proximity to each other, but the circulations do not mix.

Fetal Circulation

A. Fetal lungs do not participate in respiratory gas exchange.
B. There are special fetal structures to bypass blood supply to the lungs.

FETAL AND MATERNAL ASSESSMENT TESTING

Amniocentesis

✳ **An invasive procedure performed on the mother to obtain amniotic fluid.**

A. An outpatient procedure performed at 14 to 16 weeks of pregnancy.

B. Procedure: Placenta is located by ultrasound examination; a needle is inserted through the abdomen (puncture site has been anesthetized); amniotic fluid is aspirated and sent to the laboratory for testing.

> ✔ *NURSING PRIORITY: The fetal heart rate (FHR) is assessed before and after amniocentesis.*

Ultrasonography

✳ **Ultrasonography is a noninvasive technique in which high-frequency pulse sound waves are transmitted by a transducer applied directly to the woman's abdomen or transvaginally.**

A. Purpose.
1. Identifies placental location for amniocentesis or to determine placenta previa.
2. Determines gestational age, detects fetal anomalies, and multiple gestations.
3. Monitors fetal growth, evaluates volume of amniotic fluid.

B. Procedure (abdominal).
1. Procedure is best done at 16 to 20 weeks' gestation when fetal structures have completed development.
2. Sometimes performed with a full bladder during the second trimester.
3. Client may be advised to drink 1 quart of water 2 hours before sonogram.
4. Requires approximately 20 to 30 minutes to perform; client must lie flat on back, which may be uncomfortable; transvaginal better tolerated as client is in lithotomy position and full bladder is not required.

C. Maturity studies.
1. Lecithin/sphingomyelin (L/S) ratio: the components of phospholipid protein substance that comprise surfactant; L/S ratio of 2:1 or greater is indicative of sufficient surfactant (occurs around 35 weeks' gestation).

Chorionic Villus Sampling

✳ **Chorionic villus sampling is a method of obtaining fetal tissue for genetic testing.**

A. Purpose: to obtain fetal tissue to establish a genetic profile as a first trimester alternative to amniocentesis; use is declining due to noninvasive screening techniques.

B. Procedure.
1. An invasive procedure performed with the use of ultrasound guidance between 10 and 12 weeks' ges-

TABLE 20-4	SUMMARY OF COMMON DISCOMFORTS AND RELIEF MEASURES
Discomfort	**Relief Measures**
First Trimester	
Nausea and vomiting (morning sickness)	Frequent small meals; avoid empty stomach; between meals eat crackers without fluid; take vitamin B_6 supplement.
Urinary frequency and urgency	Void frequently; decrease fluids before bedtime; avoid caffeinated or carbonated beverages; use perineal pads for leakage; perform Kegel exercises; report any pain or burning.
Breast tenderness	Well-fitting support bra; altering sleep positions; avoid using soap on the nipple and areola area.
Increased vaginal discharge	Good hygiene; use perineal or panty liner pads; cotton underwear; no douching unless prescribed; report if any pruritus, foul odor, or change in character or color.
Second and Third Trimesters	
Heartburn (pyrosis or acid indigestion)	Avoid fat and fried, spicy foods; eat small, frequent meals; maintain good posture; sit upright.
Ankle edema	Need ample fluid intake; avoid prolonged sitting or standing; support stockings should be applied before rising; elevate feet while sitting.
Varicose veins	Avoid prolonged periods of standing; apply support hose before rising; elevate feet while sitting; do not cross legs at knees.
Hemorrhoids	Avoid constipation, do not strain; use ointments, bulk-producing laxatives, anesthetic suppositories as prescribed.
Constipation	Increase fluid intake (6 to 8 glasses/day); eat food and fruits high in roughage; exercise moderately; use bulk-producing laxatives as prescribed.
Backache	Correct posture; low-heeled shoes; pelvic tilt exercise.
Leg cramps	Stretch affected muscle and hold till it subsides; warm packs; maintain adequate calcium intake.
Faintness	Sit or lie down; avoid sudden changes in position; and avoid prolonged standing.
Shortness of breath	Good posture; sleep with head elevated by several pillows.

 TEST ALERT: Instruct client on antepartal care.

tation; technique may be transcervically or transabdominal.
2. Administer RhoGam to Rh negative mothers because of possiblity of fetomaternal hemorrhage.

Percutaneous Umbilical Blood Sampling (PUBS)

✳ **An invasive procedure, also called cordocentesis, is obtaining fetal blood sampling during the second and third trimester.**
A. Purpose: Most widely used method for fetal blood sampling and transfusion.
B. Procedure.
 1. Insertion of a needle directly into a fetal umbilical vessel under ultrasound guidance.
 2. Continuous FHR monitoring for up to an hour and a repeated ultrasound an hour later to ensure that bleeding or hematoma formation did not occur.

Daily Fetal Movement Count

✳ **A simple activity performed by the mother is to count daily fetal movement, also called "kick counts."**
A. Purpose: to monitor the fetus when there may be complications affecting fetal oxygenation – e.g., preclampsia, diabetes.
B. Procedure.
 1. Count all fetal movements with a 12 hour period until a minimum of 10 movements are counted or count fetal activity 2-3 times daily (after meals and before bed) for 2 hours until 10 movements are counted.
 2. Any change in fetal activity, either an increase or a decrease, should be reported to the health care provider.
 3. Fetal alarm signal – no fetal movements during a 12 hour period.

✔ **NURSING PRIORITY:** *Alcohol, depressant medications, and smoking temporarily reduce fetal movement and obesity decreases the woman's ability to assess fetal movement. Fetal movement is not felt during fetal sleep cycle and the movements do not decrease as the woman nears term.*

Nonstress Test

A. Purpose: to observe the response of the FHR to the stress of activity.
B. Procedure.
 1. Requires approximately 20 minutes; client is placed in semi-Fowler's position; external monitor is applied to document fetal activity; mother activates the "mark button" on the electronic fetal monitor when she feels fetal movement.

2. If no fetal movement is detected, client may gently rub or palpate abdomen to stimulate movement or may be asked to eat a light meal, because an increased blood sugar level increases fetal activity.
C. Interpretation.
 1. Reactive: shows two or more fetal heart rate accelerations of 15 beats/min or more lasting at least 15 seconds for each acceleration within 20 minutes of beginning the test; indicates a healthy fetus. Test may be rescheduled, as indicated by condition. The 15 by 15 (15x15) criteria is for a fetus at least 32 weeks gestation.
 2. Nonreactive: Reactive criteria are not met. The accelerations are less than two in number, the accelerations are less than 15 beats/min, or there are no accelerations. If nonreactive, then the test is extended another 20 minutes; if the tracing becomes reactive, the NST is concluded. If the NST is still nonreactive after a second 20-minute trial (total of 40 minutes), then additional testing, such as a biophysical profile is considered. If gestation is near term, a contraction stress test (CST) may be done.

✔ **NURSING PRIORITY:** *Appearance of any decelerations of the FHR during an NST should be immediately evaluated by the physician.*

D. Advantages of NST.
 1. Simple; easy to perform.
 2. Does not require hospitalization.
 3. Has no contraindications.

Biophysical Profile

✳ **Noninvasive dynamic assessment of a fetus that is based on acute and chronic markers of fetal disease. Is an accurate indicator of impending fetal death.**
A. First choice for follow-up fetal evaluation.
B. Assesses five fetal variables: breathing movement, fetal body movement (FBM), muscle tone, amniotic fluid volume (AFV), and FHR. The first four are assessed by ultrasonography; the fifth is assessed by NST.
C. Each area has a possible score of 2: maximum score of 10. A score of 4 or below indicates need for immediate delivery.

Contraction Stress Test or Oxytocin Challenge Test and the Breast Self-Stimulation Contraction Stress Test

A. Purpose: To observe the response of FHR to the stress of oxytocin-induced uterine contractions; means of evaluating respiratory function (oxygen and carbon dioxide exchange) of the placenta as an indicator of fetal health.

> ✔ **NURSING PRIORITY:** *Many facilities now use the breast self-stimulation contraction stress test, because endogenous oxytocin is produced in response to stimulation of the breasts or nipples.*

> ✔ **NURSING PRIORITY:** *If the CST result is positive and there is no acceleration of FHR with fetal movement (nonreactive NST result), the positive CST result is an ominous sign, often indicating late fetal hypoxia. A negative CST result with a reactive NST result is desirable.*

B. Indications.
  1. Preexisting maternal medical conditions: diabetes mellitus, heart disease, hypertension, sickle cell disease, hyperthyroidism, renal disease.
  2. Postmaturity, intrauterine growth retardation, nonreactive NST results, preeclampsia.
C. Contraindications.
  1. Third-trimester bleeding.
  2. Previous cesarean delivery.
  3. Risk of preterm labor because of premature rupture of the membranes, incompetent cervical os, or multiple gestation.
D. Procedure: breast self-stimulation contraction stress test.
  1. Semi-Fowler's position, with fetal monitor in place.
  2. Nipple stimulation begins with woman brushing her palm across one nipple through her shirt or gown for 2 to 3 minutes. If contractions start, nipple stimulation should stop. If contractions do not occur, one nipple is massaged for 10 minutes.
  3. Advantages: takes less time to perform, is less expensive, and causes less discomfort because no intravenous line is used.
E. Procedure: oxytocin challenge test.
  1. Client must be NPO (receiving nothing by mouth) and be closely observed, either hospitalized or as an outpatient.
  2. Place client in semi-Fowler's to avoid supine hypotension.
  3. Intravenous (IV) administration of oxytocin stimulates uterine contractions; uterine activity and FHR are recorded by means of external monitoring.
  4. Hypoxia is reflected in late deceleration on monitor, which indicates a diminished fetal-placental reserve.
  5. IV oxytocin is delivered at a rate of 0.5 mU/min with the rate increased every 15-30 minutes until contractions occur at a rate of three per 10 minutes; then oxytocin is discontinued, and the woman is observed until contractions stop.
F. Interpretation: oxytocin challenge test.
  1. Negative (reassuring): shows no late decelerations after any contraction; implies that placental support is adequate.
  2. Positive (nonreassuring; abnormal): shows late decelerations with at least two of the three contractions; may indicate the possibility of insufficient placental respiratory reserve.

COMPLICATIONS ASSOCIATED WITH PREGNANCY

Abortion

✳ **An abortion is the termination of pregnancy before 20 weeks of gestation. Abortions can be spontaneous (miscarriage) or induced (therapeutic or elective); approximately 75% to 80% of all spontaneous abortions occur during the second and third months of gestation.**

Data Collection

A. Risk factors.
  1. Maternal: chronic infections, fibroid tumors, structural uterine anomalies.
  2. Acute infection.
B. Clinical manifestations (types of spontaneous abortions).
  1. Threatened abortion: slight bleeding, mild back and lower abdominal cramping, no cervical dilation, no passage of the products of conception.
  2. Inevitable abortion: moderate amount of bleeding and cramping, internal cervical os dilates, and membranes may rupture.
  3. Incomplete abortion: only part of the products of conception is expelled.
  4. Complete abortion: all the products of conception are expelled.
  5. Missed abortion: fetus dies in utero.
  6. Habitual or recurrent abortion: three or more successive, spontaneous abortions.

Treatment

Treatment varies according to type of abortion.
A. Threatened abortion: bed rest, sedation, and avoidance of stress and sexual intercourse.
B. Inevitable and incomplete abortion.
  1. Fluid replacement: IVs; type and cross-match for possible blood transfusion.
  2. Administration of oxytocin.
  3. Dilation and curettage (D&C) or suction evacuation to remove products of conception.
C. Missed abortion: If abortion does not occur spontaneously after 4 weeks, suction evacuation or D&C will be done to avoid risk of disseminated intravascular coagulation (DIC) or hemorrhage.
D. Habitual or recurrent abortion: determination of cause, then specific therapy to correct.
E. Administration of **RhoGAM** if mother is Rh negative (given within 72 hours). Given after every pregnancy.

Nursing Interventions

❖ **Goal:** To assess or control hemorrhage.
A. Monitor vital signs.
B. Ensure accurate counting of pads to assess bleeding.
C. *Report any signs of increased bleeding to RN.*
❖ **Goal:** To prevent complications.
A. Observe for shock.
B. Prevent isoimmunization by administration of **RhoGAM** for Rh- client.
C. Assess for elevated temperature.
❖ **Goal:** To provide emotional support to the couple experiencing the loss of pregnancy.
A. Encourage verbalization of feelings.
B. Be available and actively listen.

 Home Care

A. Report any increased bleeding.
B. Do not use tampons; use only peri-pads.
C. Check temperature every 8 hours for 3 days.
D. Do not resume sexual activity until PCP approves (usually after bleeding stops).

 Ectopic Pregnancy

✱ **Any pregnancy that develops outside the uterus (extrauterine) is an ectopic pregnancy. The majority of ectopic preg-nancies are tubal; more common on the right side.**

Data Collection

A. If tube ruptures, sudden excruciating pain in the lower abdomen, usually over the mass.
B. Possible referred shoulder pain as blood fills the abdomen.
C. Vaginal bleeding, hemorrhagic shock.
D. May be initially identified as undiagnosed abdominal pain (see Chapter 13).

Surgical Treatment

A. Laparoscopy, laparotomy, salpingectomy.

Nursing Interventions

❖ **Goal:** To prevent and detect early complications.
A. Provide nursing care for shock as indicated.
B. Prepare for surgery (e.g., IVs, oxygen, blood).
C. Administer **RhoGAM**, if indicated.
❖ **Goal:** To provide emotional support (loss of pregnancy and possibly reproductive organ).

 Hyperemesis Gravidarum

✱ **This disorder is characterized by excessive vomiting during pregnancy that results in weight loss of at least 5% of prepregnancy weight.**

Data Collection

A. Severe, persistent vomiting that is different from morning sickness.
B. If untreated, ketoacidosis (from loss of intestinal juices), hypovolemia, hypokalemia, elevated transaminase and bilirubin levels.
C. Decreased urine output.

Treatment

A. Medical: stop the vomiting; administer IV fluids, electrolytes, and vitamin B6 (pyridoxine), along with an antiemetic.
B. Dietary: NPO for first 48 hours; then begin small feedings alternated with liquid nourishment every 1 to 2-hours; if vomiting re-occurs, NPO and IV fluids restarted.

Nursing Interventions

❖ **Goal:** To assist with medical and dietary management.
A. Maintain accurate intake and output (I&O) records.
B. Perform daily weight checks and maintenance of intake and output measurements.
C. Desired urine output is 1000 mL in 24 hours; usually administration of IVs at 3000 mL in first 24 hours after admission to correct hypovolemia.
D. Follow oral hygiene measures.
E. Client should be NPO for first 48 hours, then clear liquids with gradual progression to small meals that are low-fat and high protein.
F. Stress may contribute to condition; provide emotional support.

 Hypertensive Disorders

✱ **Hypertensive disorders (preeclampsia and eclampsia) are a medical complication of pregnancy occuring in about 6-8% of pregnancies and the second leading cause of maternal and perinatal morbidity and mortality. Cause is unknown.**

Data Collection

A. Risk factors.
1. Diabetes mellitus, chronic hypertension.
2. Chronic renal disease, multiple gestations.
3. Age (younger than 20 or older than 40).
4. Primigravida.
B. Clinical manifestations of preeclampsia (Table 20-5).

> ✔ *NURSING PRIORITY:* The common symptoms of preclampsia are hypertension and proteinuria.

Treatment

A. Medical.
   1. Mild preeclampsia: bed rest in lateral recumbent position.
   2. Severe preeclampsia: absolute bed rest, sedatives, antihypertensives, anticonvulsants (see Appendix 20-2).
   3. Eclampsia: seizure precautions (vital signs, oxygen, suction, positioning), anticonvulsants.
B. Dietary: high-protein diet, no added salt intake, and fluid intake of 6 to 8 glasses of water per day.

Nursing Interventions

❖ **Goal:** (mild preeclampsia): To initiate preventative measures.

A. Instruction for home care: encourage bed rest, provide dietary instruction, and encourage regular prenatal checkups.
B. Tests to evaluate fetal status (e.g., fetal movement record, ultrasound, NST, estriol and creatinine levels).
C. Goals and nursing interventions for severely preeclamptic and eclamptic clients are outlined in Box 20-2.

LABOR AND DELIVERY

Maternal Data Collection

A. Signs and symptoms *before* true labor.
   1. Lightening: descent of the fetal head into the pelvis, experienced as "dropping" of the baby.
   2. Increased vaginal mucus discharge.
   3. Softening of the cervix.
   4. Braxton Hicks contractions may become uncomfortable, especially at night; discomfort is usually located in the abdomen.
   5. Sudden burst of energy approximately 24 to 48 hours before labor.
   6. Weight loss of 1 to 3 pounds; sometimes diarrhea, indigestion, nausea, and vomiting.
   7. Rupture of membranes.
      a. If rupture occurs before onset of labor, it is called premature rupture of the membrane.
      b. Delivery should occur within 24 hours to decrease incidence of infection.
      c. Test with phenaphthazine (nitrazine) paper; amniotic fluid is alkaline; nitrazine paper turns blue; normal vaginal and urinary secretions are acidic.
      d. Check for decreased FHR after rupture of membranes.
B. Signs and symptoms of *true* labor.
   1. Cervical dilation and effacement (Figure 20-1).
   2. Contractions occur at regular intervals and increase in duration and intensity; intensity usually increases with walking (Figure 20-2).
   3. Pain in the back that radiates around to the abdomen.
   4. Bloody show: expulsion of the mucus plug; labor begins 24 to 48 hours after bloody show, or bloody show may be observed at the onset of labor.
C. Stages of labor.
   1. First stage (stage of cervical dilation): begins with onset of regular contractions and ends with complete cervical dilation and effacement; divided into phases: latent, active, transition.
   2. Second stage (stage of expulsion): begins with complete cervical dilation and ends with delivery of the fetus.
   3. Third stage (placental stage): begins immediately after the fetus is born and ends when the placenta is delivered.
      a. Signs of placental separation: discoid to globular shape of uterus, gush of blood, lengthening of umbilical cord, and rise of uterine fundus.

TABLE 20-5	CLINICAL MANIFESTATIONS OF PREECLAMPSIA and ECLAMPSIA	
Mild Preeclampsia	**Sever Preeclampsia**	**Eclampsia**
Elevated BP: systolic increase to 140 mm Hg and diastolic increase of 90 mm Hg ×2 readings, 4-6 hr apart, no more than 1 week apart. Proteinuria: greater than 0.3 g/24 hr (1+ proteinuria).	Increased hypertension: systolic at 160 mm Hg; diastolic at 110 mm Hg or more on 2 separate occasions. Proteinuria: greater than 2 g/24 hr (3+ to 4+ proteinuria). Elevated BUN, serum creatinine, uric acid levels, LDH, ALT, AST. Oliguria: less than 500 mL/ 24 hr. Cerebral or visual disturbances. Severe headache. Vomiting. Epigastric pain (due to edema of liver capsule, usually indicative of impending seizure).	Convulsions appear suddenly and without warning. Increased hypertension and tonic contraction of all body muscles (arms flexed, hands clenched, legs inverted) precede the tonic-clonic convulsions. Hypotension follows and then coma. Nystagmus and muscular twitching persist for a time. Coma (lasts from few minutes to several hours).

BP, Blood pressure; *BUN*, blood urea nitrogen.

BOX 20-2   NURSING MANAGEMENT OF CLIENTS WITH GESTATIONAL HYPERTENSION AND PREECLAMPSIA

❖ **Goal:** To recognize the early signs of gestational hypertension and increased BP.
1. Check BP and record Korotkoff phase V (disappearance of sound) for diastolic reading. Take BP in left lateral recumbent position or seated. Allow 10 minutes of quiet rest before taking BP to encourage relaxation. No caffeine or nicotine use 30 minutes prior to taking BP.
2. Monitor urine for proteinuria.
3. Monitor for nondependent pathological edema (e.g., periorbital area and hands).

> ✔ **NURSING PRIORITY:** *Systolic increase of 30 mm Hg and a diastolic BP increase of 15 mm Hg warrant close observation if the BP elevation occurs with proteinuria.*

❖ **Goal:** To recognize progression of gestational hypertension symptoms and minimize or control their sequelae.
1. Institute weight controls. Check for sudden increases of 2 lb/wk or 6 lb/month.
2. Increase protein intake in the diet. Maintain normal sodium intake; avoid use of diuretics.
3. Institute bed rest.
4. Monitor for ominous signs of deteriorating condition: headache, visual disturbances, hyperreflexia, markedly decreased urine output, epigastric or right upper quadrant pain, dyspnea, vaginal bleeding (abruptio placentae), or any change in fetal activity.
5. Administer antihypertensives, as ordered, check maternal BP, pulse and fetal heart rate.
❖ **Goal:** To prevent or control seizures.
1. IV administration of $MgSO_4$ by the RN. (Have calcium gluconate available as antidote for possible respiratory/neurological depression).
2. Have emergency items readily available (e.g., oxygen, suction, airway, sedatives).
3. Modify environment to ensure rest and quiet.
   a. Eliminate noise, bright lights, and other harsh stimuli.
   b. Minimize number of personnel giving care.
   c. Initiate painful and/or intrusive procedures after sedation.
   d. Promote comfort and total bed rest.
4. Monitor I&O, edema and weight for evidence of vasodilation and increased tissue perfusion.
❖ **Goal:** To recognize alterations in fetal well-being and promote safe delivery of the infant.
1. Auscultate and record FHR pattern, noting presence of variability or accelerations, and report decelerations.
2. Instruct and support client during amniocentesis.
3. Collect specimen for estriol determination.
4. Assist with NST and/or oxytocin challenge test.
5. Give instructions about induction of labor and electronic FHR monitoring.

BP, Blood pressure; *FHR*, fetal heart rate; *IV*, intravenous; *MgSO₄*, magnesium sulfate; *NST*, nonstress test; *OCT*, oxytocin challenge test.

4. Fourth stage (maternal homeostatic stabilization stage): begins after the delivery of the placenta and continues for 1 to 4 hours after delivery.

Fetal Heart Rate Monitoring

A. Intermittent Auscultation (IA).
   1. Very common, inexpensive, easy-to-use method using either a DeLee-Hillis fetoscope or ultrasound fetoscope by counting the FHR for 30-60 seconds between contractions to obtain the baseline rate.
   2. Auscultate the FHR during a contraction and for 30 seconds after a contraction to identify any increases or decreases in FHR in response to the contraction.
   3. If ultrasound device is used, FHR can be heard as early as 10 to 12 weeks.
B. Electronic Fetal Monitoring (EFM).
   1. External monitoring: a noninvasive procedure which uses two external transducers placed on the maternal abdomen, which the ultrasound transducer uses high-frequency sound waves to detect FHR and the tocotransducer monitors frequency and duration of contractions by a pressure-sensing device.
      a. Advantage is its noninvasiveness.
      b. Does not require rupture of the membranes or cervical dilation.
   2. Internal monitoring: invasive, but provides accurate, continuous information through use of a spiral electrode applied to the fetal presenting part to assess FHR and an intrauterine pressure catheter (IUPC) to assess uterine activity (frequency, duration, and intensity of contractions) and pressure.
      a. Spiral electrode picks up electrical impulses from the fetal ECG.
      b. Membranes must be ruptured and cervix sufficiently dilated.

NURSING INTERVENTIONS DURING LABOR AND DELIVERY

Maternal

❖ **Goal:** To monitor changes during each stage of labor (Table 20-6).
❖ **Goal:** To provide relief from pain and discomfort.
A. Administer analgesic medication.
B. Do not administer PO or IM analgesic medication within 2 hours of delivery. Medication may depress neonate.
C. Monitor pain control with epidural analgesia or anesthesia.

Fetal

❖ **Goal:** To monitor fetal status and detect early complications.

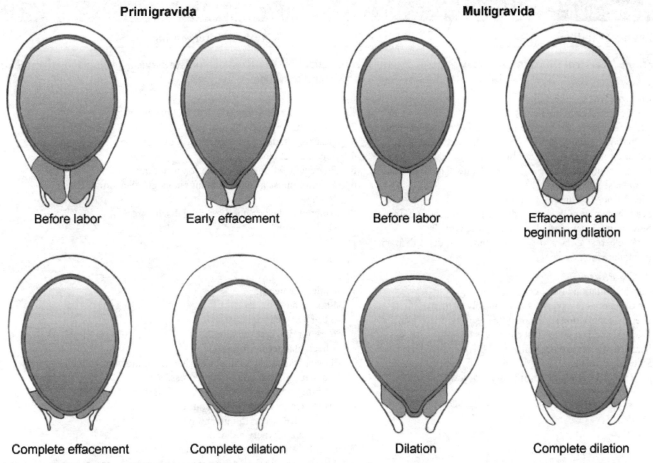

Primigravida

Before labor   Early effacement

Complete effacement   Complete dilation

Multigravida

Before labor   Effacement and beginning dilation

Dilation   Complete dilation

FIGURE 20-1 **Cervical Dilation and Effacement.** (From McKinney ES et al: *Maternal-child nursing*, ed 3, St Louis, 2009, Saunders.)

❖ Goal: To provide immediate care to the normal newborn.

A. Airway: clear air passages to establish respirations.

B. Body temperature: maintain warmth.

C. Apgar scoring: immediate appraisal of newborn's condition taken at 1 minute and again at 5 minutes (Table 20-7).

D. Care of the umbilical cord: clamped after pulsation ceases; examine for number of vessels (two arterial and one venous) and record (one umbilical artery may indicate increased incidence of congenital anomalies, especially renal and genitourinary); no dressing is applied to cord.

E. Care of the eyes: prophylaxis against ophthalmia neonatorum: ophthalmic antibiotic ointment.

F. Identification: wristbands fastened to both infant and mother and appropriate footprints taken before leaving delivery area.

G. Administration of vitamin K (**AquaMEPHYTON**): 0.5 mg to 1 mg IM injected into the upper outer aspect of the thigh for prevention of neonatal hemorrhagic disease, due to lack of *Escherichia coli* necessary for the synthesis of vitamin K in the intestines.

H. Inspection for gross abnormalities (e.g., clubfoot, imperforate anus, birthmarks).

I. Attachment: provide contact of newborn with mother as soon as possible after birth.

OPERATIVE OBSTETRICS

 ## Episiotomy

✳ **An episiotomy is an incision in the perineum to facilitate delivery by enlarging the vaginal outlet. Once done routinely, the practice is less common today. It is being replaced in many settings by manually supporting the perineum during birth and allowing small perineum tears rather than incising the perineum. Healing after a tear is faster and is less painful.**

Data Collection

A. Observe perineal site for bleeding, swelling, redness, or any discharge.

B. *Evaluate for pain and discomfort. Increased pain should be reported to RN.*

TABLE 20-6	SUMMARY OF OBSERVATIONS AND NURSING CARE DURING LABOR
Physical Findings	**Nursing Interventions**

Stage 1 Cervical Dilation: begins with onset of regular contractions and ends with complete cervical dilation and effacement; divided into phases—latent, active, and transition.

Physical Findings	Nursing Interventions
Latent Phase Cervical dilation: 0 to 3 cm. Cervical effacement in primipara is usually complete before dilation; in multipara, it occurs with dilation. Duration of latent phase: 6-8 hr. Uterine contractions are mild to moderate, 5 to 30 min apart, and last 30 to 45 sec. Membranes ruptured or intact. Scant brown or pink vaginal discharge or mucous plug. Station: primipara, usually 0; multipara, 0 to –2. FHR: clearest at level of or below umbilicus, dependent on fetal position.	1. Orient to hospital environment and personnel. 2. Assess history and physical status. 3. Assess attitudes, past experiences, expectations. 4. Teach about labor. 5. Practice breathing and relaxation techniques. 6. Monitor physical status: obtain vital signs including FHR. 7. Voiding. 8. Amount and character of vaginal discharge. 9. Oral hygiene.
Active Phase Cervical dilation: 4 to 7 cm. Duration of active phase: approximately 3- 6 hr Uterine contractions are moderate to strong, 3 to 5 min apart, and last 40 to 70 sec. Scant to moderate bloody mucus. Station: +1 to +2. FHR: heard slightly below umbilicus or lower abdomen.	1. Anticipate needs: Sponge face. Keep bed clean and dry. Care for dry, cracked mouth. Check bladder for fullness. 2. Stay at bedside, working through each contraction with client; praise woman's efforts; point out progress. 3. Reinforce supportive efforts of the father. 4. Use touch to soothe, relax, comfort. 5. Check FHR every 15 min and BP every 30 min. 6. Observe for hyperventilation. 7. Client may need analgesia to enhance coping. 8. Monitor IV and fluid status: increased risk of hypervolemia as a result of fluid retention. 9. Encourage ambulation if membranes intact. Lateral position preferred when in bed as it increases uteroplacental blood flow.
Transition Phase Cervical dilation: 8 to 10 cm. Duration of transition phase: 1 to 2 hr. Uterine contractions of transition phase: strong, 2 to 3 min apart, and last 45 to 90 sec. Copious bloody mucus. Station: +2 to +3. FHR: clearest directly above symphysis pubis.	1. Continue physical and supportive care. 2. Use palpation or uterine contraction monitor to help client define contractions and rest periods. 3. Observe perineum for bulging.

Stage 2 Expulsion of Fetus: begins with complete cervical dilation and ends with delivery of the fetus.

Physical Findings	Nursing Interventions
Cervical dilation complete at 10 cm. Cervical effacement 100%. Duration of stage 2: 20 to 50 min. Uterine contractions are strong, 2 to 3 min apart and last 60 to 90 sec; fetal bradycardia may occur during contraction. Membranes may rupture; copious bloody mucus. Station: fetal descent continues at a rate of 1 cm/hr in primiparas and 2 cm/hr or more in multiparas until perineal floor is reached. Urge to push begins. Perineum flattens, bulges. Crowning occurs. Infant is born.	1. Direct pushing efforts with father for each contraction. 2. Provide comfort measures and facilitate rest between contractions: Apply cool cloth to face. Keep perineum clean and dry. 3. Encourage efforts; point out progress. 4. Explain preparations being made for delivery. 5. Check FHR with each contraction. 6. Help with panting for delivery of head and shoulders.

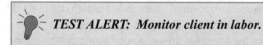
TEST ALERT: *Monitor client in labor.*

Continued

TABLE 20-6	SUMMARY OF OBSERVATIONS AND NURSING CARE DURING LABOR—cont'd.
Physical Findings	**Nursing Interventions**

Stage 3 Expulsion of Placenta: begins immediately after the infant is delivered and ends when the placenta is delivered.

Usually within 5 to 10 min of delivery. Uterine shape globular, usually firmer; fundus rises. Dark vaginal bleeding: gush or trickle. Umbilical cord protrudes further from introitus. Placenta intact: shiny presentation of fetal side of placental separation occurs from inner to outer margins (Schultze mechanism); rough presentation of maternal side of placental separation occurs from outer margins inward (Duncan mechanism).	1. Congratulate. 2. Initiate maternal contact with infant. 3. Coach in relaxation for delivery of placenta and perineal repair. 4. Watch for signs of placental separation: discoid to globular shape of uterus, gush of blood, lengthening of umbilical cord, and rise of uterine fundus. 5. May administer oxytocics after placenta has been delivered (see Appendix 20-3).

Stage 4 Maternal Homeostatic Stabilization: begins after the delivery of the placenta and continues for 1 to 4 hours after delivery.

Fundus firm or becomes firm when massaged, in midline at level of umbilicus. Moderate lochia rubra. Episiotomy or laceration repair clean without ecchymosis or discharge, minimal edema; tenderness commensurate with analgesia, usually mild; edges well approximated. Possible extrusion of hemorrhoids.	1. Facilitation of attachment: ensure that parents have time with newborn; mother may initiate breast-feeding. 2. Ongoing assessment (every 15 min for 1 hr, then every 30 min for 2 hr) of vital signs, fundus, lochia, episiotomy, and bladder function. 3. Encourage rest for both parents.

BP, Blood pressure; *FHR*, fetal heart rate.

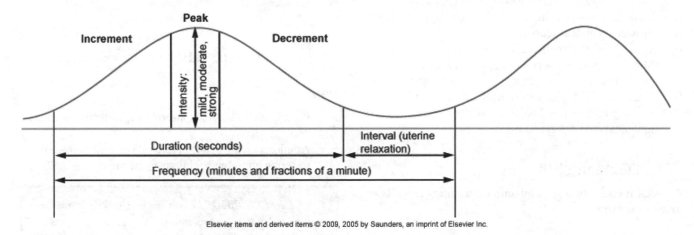

FIGURE 20-2   **Labor Contraction Cycle.** (From McKinney ES et al: *Maternal-child nursing*, ed 3, St Louis, 2009, Saunders.)

TABLE 20-7	APGAR SCORING SYSTEM

Sign	0	1	2
Heart rate	Not detectable	Slow (below 100 beats/min)	Greater than 100 beats/min
Respiratory effort	Absent	Slow, irregular	Good crying
Muscle tone	Flaccid, limp	Some flexion of extremities	Active motion
Reflex irritability	No response	Grimace	Cough, sneeze, or cry
Color	Blue, pale	Body pink, extremities pale	Completely pink

Nursing Interventions

❖   **Goal:** To alleviate pain and swelling and promote comfort.

A.   Ice pack (first 2 hours, then PRN for pain relief); later followed by sitz baths, application of dry heat lamp treatment for 20 minutes, three to four times per day.

B.   Analgesic sprays, ointments, or foam, as ordered.

C.   Teach importance of perineal cleansing (i.e., use of the squeeze spray bottle; direct flow from front to back; and change perineal pad after each elimination – apply peripad from front to back to avoid contamination).

 ## Forceps Delivery

✳   **A forceps delivery is the use of an instrument to extract the fetal head during delivery.**

Data Collection

A.   Criteria for forceps delivery.
1.   Head fully engaged.
2.   Complete dilation of the cervix.
3.   Membranes have ruptured.

B.   Monitor fetal heart rate, as forceps may compress umbilical cord.

Nursing Interventions

❖   **Goal:** To briefly explain procedure to couple.
A.   Monitor fetal heart rate.
B.   Provide emotional support.

❖   **Goal:** To detect complications for forceps application.
A.   Maternal: possible lacerations to birth canal and perineum.
B.   Fetal: possible cephalhematoma, lacerations and bruising to face, facial paralysis, skull fracture, umbilical cord compression.

 ## Cesarean Birth

✳   **An incision into the abdominal and uterine walls to deliver the fetus.**

Types

A.   Low-segment transverse incision.
1.   Preferred and most common method.
2.   Decreased blood loss; less chance of uterine rupture with subsequent pregnancy as incision is made into lower uterine segment.
3.   Fewer complications, such as peritonitis and postoperative adhesions.

B.   Classic cesarean incision.
1.   Used in cases of placenta previa when there are adhesions in the lower uterine segment, or in transverse fetal lie.
2.   Vertical incision is made between the umbilicus and symphysis pubis.

Common Indications

A.   Maternal.
1.   Uterine dystocia.
2.   Cephalopelvic disproportion (CPD).
3.   Severe preeclampsia and eclampsia.
4.   Previous cesarean birth or surgery on the uterus.
5.   Placenta previa and abruptio placentae.

B.   Fetal.
1.   Fetal distress.
2.   Prolapsed cord.

Data Collection

A.   Assess for possible indication for cesarean delivery.

B.   Trend is that once a cesarean birth occurs, it is highly likely that subsequent births will also be cesarean.

C.   Cesarean delivery may be planned for a specific date or may occur as an emergency procedure; common elective reasons are previous cesarean delivery, breech presentation, and cephalopelvic disproportion, along with medical risk factors of hypertension, active genital herpes, positive HIV status, and diabetes.

Nursing Interventions

❖   **Goal:** To provide preoperative preparation.
A.   Preparation is similar to that for any abdominal surgery.

❖   **Goal:** To provide postoperative care.
A.   Cesarean birth includes both normal abdominal postoperative care and postpartum care.

 ## Induction of Labor

Procedure

A.   Prostaglandin E2 gel is inserted vaginally to soften the cervix.

B.   Amniotomy: artificial rupture of membranes (bag of water); labor often begins spontaneously.

✔ ***NURSING PRIORITY:*** *FHR is assessed before and immediately after an amniotomy.*

C.   Oxytocin (**Pitocin**) is administered intravenously with a physician in attendance and a physician order. ***High Alert Medication.***
1.   Oxytocin is always piggybacked and hooked up to an infusion pump along with a primary intravenous (IV) line in case it needs to be discontinued.
2.   Nursing management and information regarding Pitocin is covered in Appendix 20-3.

Data Collection

A.   Careful assessment of uterine contractions is priority; tetanic contractions could result in uterine rupture, premature separation of placenta, and fetal hypoxia.

B.   Fetal heart rate (FHR) check every 15 minutes along with mother's vital signs.

Nursing Interventions

❖   **Goal:** To monitor and evaluate uterine response and fetal response to induction.

A.   Perform frequent vital sign checks and FHR checks (every 15 minutes); indirect or direct fetal monitoring may be used.

B.   *Report any of the following findings to the RN:*
   1.   Contractions are more frequent than every 2 minutes.
   2.   Contraction duration exceeds 75 to 90 seconds.
   3.   Uterus does not relax; remains contracted and tetanic.

COMPLICATIONS ASSOCIATED WITH LABOR AND DELIVERY

Preterm Labor

❋   **Preterm labor is defined as cervical changes and uterine contractions occurring between 20 and 37 weeks' gestation.**

Data Collection

A.   Contractions occurring in increasing frequency and intensity.

B.   Premature rupture of the membranes.

Treatment

A.   Tocolytic medications (see Appendix 20-4).
   1.   Tocolytics.
   2.   Prostaglandin synthetase inhibitors (NSAIDS) – Indomethacin (**Indocin**).
   3.   Antenatal corticosteroids.

Nursing Interventions

❖   **Goal:** To assist in delivery if maternal complications are present.

A.   Maternal complications: diabetes, preeclampsia, hemorrhage.

❖   **Goal:** To provide emotional support.

A.   Encourage expression of feelings related to anxiety and guilt.

B.   Identify and support coping mechanisms for couple.

❖   **Goal:** To minimize fetal complications.

A.   Promote fetal oxygenation.
   1.   Avoid supine position during labor: risk of supine hypotensive syndrome.

2.   Avoid maternal hyperventilation because it can lead to decreased oxygen to the fetus.

3.   Anticipate the administration of betamethasone (**Celestone**) or dexamethasone (**Decadron**) to minimize/prevent respiratory distress syndrome in the newborn.

Dystocia

❋   **Dystocia is a long, difficult, or abnormal labor.**

Data Collection

A.   Dysfunctional Labor.
   1.   Hypotonic contractions: slow, infrequent, weak contractions occurring more than 3 minutes apart and lasting less than 40 seconds.
   2   Hypertonic contractions: frequent, strong, painful contractions occurring 2 to 3 minutes apart, lasting 60 seconds or more.

B.   Abnormal Labor Patterns.
   1.   Cephalopelvic disproportion (CPD): also called fetopelvic disproportion (FPD) and is related to excessive fetal size (greater than 4000g or more).
   2.   Abnormal fetal presentation - breech, most common.
   3.   Prolonged or arrested labor: labor lasting for more than 24 hours after onset of regular contractions.
   4.   Precipitous delivery: a very rapid, intense labor of 2 to 4 hours' duration.

Treatment

A.   Mechanical dystocia relating to CPD, or faulty presentation, is treated by a cesarean delivery.

B.   Hypotonic uterine contractions or prolonged labor is treated by administration of **Pitocin** IV.

C.   Hypertonic uterine contractions are treated by sedation and rest.

Nursing Interventions

❖   **Goal:** To monitor level of fatigue and ability to cope with pain.

A.   Provide basic comfort measures, such as back rubs, change of position, clean dry linen.

B.   Provide emotional support to mother and significant other.

C.   Give reassurance and stay with client continually.

❖   **Goal:** To assist in the medical management of dystocia.

A.   Explain procedures needed to determine cause of dystocia (e.g., sonogram, x-ray studies).

B.   Monitor **Pitocin** levels if indicated for hypotonic dysfunction or prolonged labor.

C.   Prepare client for cesarean delivery (indicated in CPD and unfavorable presentation).

D.   Administer broad-spectrum antibiotics to decrease incidence of infection.

E. Maintain hydration, monitor intake and output, and administer oxygen if indicated.

❖ **Goal:** To detect early complications associated with dystocia.

A. Monitor maternal vital signs.

B. Assess mother for signs of exhaustion, dehydration, and increasing temperature, and report to PCP.

C. Assess fetal heart rate frequently through fetal electronic monitoring.

Supine Hypotensive Syndrome (Vena Caval Syndrome)

✳ **Shock-like symptoms seen when pregnant woman assumes a supine position. (The weight of the uterus causes partial occlusion of the vena cava, leading to decreased venous return to the heart.)**

Data Collection

A. Decreased BP; increased pulse rate.

B. Client feels faint; pale.

C. Decreased FHR.

Nursing Interventions

❖ **Goal:** To decrease supine hypotensive syndrome episode.

A. Educate mother to turn to left or right side; preferred position because pressure is removed from vena cava.

B. Administer oxygen via face mask.

C. *Assess fetal heart rates and report any changes to RN or PCP.*

Abnormal Fetal Position

Data Collection

A. Breech presentation.
    1. FHR usually auscultated above the umbilicus.
    2. Passage of meconium often occurs.
    3. Increased risk of prolapsed umbilical cord.

B. Transverse lie (shoulder presentation): dysfunctional labor patterns are seen.

Treatment

A. Cesarean delivery is most often performed.

Nursing Interventions

❖ **Goal:** To provide reassurance and explanations of procedures as indicated.

A. Provide explanation of possible cesarean delivery.

B. Assess for complications relating to prolonged labor and possible infection (e.g., temperature, fatigue).

Hemorrhage in the Pregnant Client

Nursing management of hemorrhage in the pregnant client is discussed in Table 20-8 and Figure 20-3.

Multifetal Pregnancy

Data Collection

A. Increased incidence of PIH, abruptio placentae, placenta previa, and hydramnios.

B. Auscultation of two FHRs.

C. Measurement of fundal height exceeds gestational age.

D. Increased experience of more physical discomfort (e.g.,-shortness of breath, dyspnea on exertion, backaches, and leg edema, due to excessive size of uterus).

Treatment

A. Medical.
    1. Bed rest in lateral position to treat hypertension.
    2. Antiemetic for nausea and vomiting past the first trimester.

B. Dietary: increase of 300 calories along with increased protein, iron, folic acid, and vitamin supplements.

Nursing Interventions

❖ **Goal:** To provide anticipatory guidance during the antepartal period.

A. Second trimester: prenatal visits every 2 weeks.

B. Third trimester: weekly visits if there are no complications.

C. Discourage travel, as labor may begin without warning.

❖ **Goal:** To provide psychological support.

A. Provide assistance and advice regarding care of twins at-home.

B. Because the twins are likely to be small, anticipate nursing care for a preterm neonate.

C. *Assess for maternal complications (e.g., postpartal hemorrhage) and report to RN.*

D. Ensure correct identification, such as Baby A and Baby B.

Prolapsed Cord

✳ **A prolapsed cord is the presence of the cord below the presenting part of the fetus.**

Data Collection

A. Commonly occurs following rupture of the membranes.

B. Cord is washed through the birth canal with a gush of amniotic fluid.

C. Visualization of the cord.

D. FHR is decreased.

TABLE 20-8   NURSING MANAGEMENT OF HEMORRHAGE IN THE PREGNANT CLIENT

Causes and Sources	Symptoms	Nursing Interventions
ANTEPARTAL PERIOD		
Abortion	Vaginal bleeding Intermittent uterine contractions Rupture of the membranes	1. Obtain history of onset, duration, amount of bleeding, and associated symptoms. 2. Observe perineal pads for amount of bleeding (blood loss can be measured by weighing perineal pads, approximately 1 g = 1 mL of blood).
Placenta previa	Painless vaginal bleeding	3. Monitor vital signs of mother and fetus (frequency is determined by severity of clinical symptoms).
Abruptio placentae	Vaginal bleeding Extreme tenderness in abdomen Rigid, board-like abdomen Increase in size of abdomen	

 TEST ALERT: *Recognize the occurrence of hemorrhage and assess mother for complications.*

Causes and Sources	Symptoms	Nursing Interventions
INTRAPARTAL PERIOD		
Placenta previa	Painless bright red vaginal bleeding	1. RN will place an IV access to provide volume replacement. 2. Request type and crossmatch for blood.
Abruptio placentae	Bright red vaginal bleeding, may be painful	3. Monitor administration of fluids and blood as prescribed. 4. Monitor intake and output.
Uterine atony in stage 3	Bright red vaginal bleeding due to ineffectual contractility	5. Minimize chances for further bleeding 6. *NO* vaginal or rectal exams. 7. Bed rest in position of comfort. 8. Anticipate delivery by cesarean section.
POSTPARTAL PERIOD		
Uterine atony	Boggy uterus	1. Massage fundus of uterus and anticipate administration of oxytocin for client with uterine atony.
Retained placental fragments	Dark vaginal bleeding Presence of clots	2. Reduce anxiety. 3. Keep woman and family advised of treatment plan. 4. Record amount of bleeding in a specific amount of time.
Lacerations of cervix or vagina	Firm uterus Bright red blood	5. Monitor vital signs: Overt hypotension and shock will not be seen until the woman has lost almost one third of her blood volume (1500-2000 mL); watch for tachycardia and orthostatic BP changes first.

✔ **NURSING PRIORITY:** *Frequent, accurate assessment and documentation of blood loss is a priority in postpartum care; two thirds of cases of postpartum hemorrhage occur without any predisposing risk factors.*

BP, Blood pressure; *IV,* Intravenous.

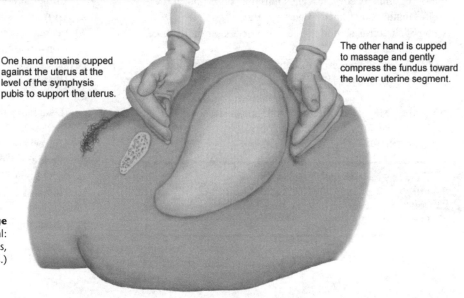

One hand remains cupped against the uterus at the level of the symphysis pubis to support the uterus.

The other hand is cupped to massage and gently compress the fundus toward the lower uterine segment.

FIGURE 20-3 Fundal Massage Technique. (From McKinney ES, et al: *Maternal-child nursing,* ed 3, St Louis, 2009, Saunders.)

Treatment

A. Medical.
    1. Insert gloved hand into the vagina and hold the fetal head off the cord to relieve the pressure.
    2. Administer oxygen to the mother.
    3. Positioning.
        a. Place mother in modified Sims'position, knee-chest position or in Trendelenburg position (head of bed or table is lowered); *administer oxygen to the mother and call for help.*
B. Surgical.
    1. If incomplete dilation, cesarean delivery necessary.
    2. Occasionally, if dilation is complete, vaginal delivery possible.

Nursing Interventions

❖   **Goal:** To maintain fetal oxygenation and assist with immediate delivery.

A. Provide continuing assessment of FHR.
B. Maintain woman in one of the positions described previously to alleviate compression of the cord and call for help.
C. Offer emotional support to the couple.

POSTPARTAL DATA COLLECTION

✳   **The postpartum period is the time spanning the first 6 weeks following delivery. It is often referred to as the "fourth trimester."**

Physiological Changes

A. Uterus.
    1. Uterine involution: process by which the uterus returns to its normal prepregnant condition.
    2. Immediately after delivery, top of fundus is several finger breadths above the umbilicus.
    3. Twelve hours after delivery, fundus of uterus is one finger breadth above umbilicus.
    4. Fundus recedes/descends into the pelvis approximately one finger breadth per day.
    5. The uterus should not be palpable abdominally after 2 weeks.
    6. Afterpains: alternate contractions and relaxations of the uterine muscle.
        a. Occur primarily in multiparas.
        b. May be severe, requiring analgesics.
        c. Usually subside in 48 hours.
    7. Lochia.

> ✔ **NURSING PRIORITY:** *Always check for a change in the lochia. Chart the amount first, followed by the character (e.g., moderate amount of lochia rubra).*

    a. Lochia rubra: dark red discharge; occurs the first 3 days.
    b. Lochia serosa: pinkish, serosanguineous discharge; lasts approximately 3 to 10 days.
    c. Lochia alba: creamy or yellowish discharge; occurs after the tenth day and may last a week or two.
    d. When lochia subsides, uterus is considered closed; postpartal infection is less likely.
B. Cervix.
    1. May be stretched and swollen.
    2. Small lacerations may be apparent.
    3. External os closes slowly; at end of first week, the opening is fingertip size.
C. Vagina/perineum.
    1. May be bruised and tender.
    2. Pelvic floor and ligaments are stretched.
    3. Muscle tone is improved by Kegel exercises.
D. Ovulation and menstruation.
    1. Non–breast-feeding women.
        a. Menstruation resumes in 6 weeks.
        b. Ovulation: 50% of women may ovulate during the first cycle.
    2. Lactating women.
        a. Ovulation and menstrual period varies.
        b. 45% resume menstruation within 12 weeks after delivery.
E. Abdomen.
    1. Soft and flabby.
    2. Muscle tone can be improved/restored within 2 to 3-months with exercise.
F. Breasts.
    1. Anterior pituitary releases prolactin, which stimulates production and secretion of milk.
    2. Engorgement may occur approximately 36 to 48 hours after delivery.
    3. Colostrum released: thin, yellowish fluid that contains antibodies and large amounts of vitamins.
G. Gastrointestinal (GI) system.
    1. Immediately after delivery, hunger is common.
    2. GI tract is sluggish and hypoactive, due to decreased muscle tone and peristalsis.
    3. Constipation may initially be a problem.
H. Urinary tract.
    1. Bladder is edematous and hyperemic.
    2. May be bruising and swelling due to trauma around the urinary meatus.
    3. Increased bladder capacity and urinary retention.
    4. Diuresis occurs during the first 2 days postpartum.
    5. Bladder distention may displace the uterus, leading to a "boggy" uterus and increased bleeding.
    6. Hematuria may occur after delivery.
I. Integumentary system
    1. Cholasma usually disappears at end of pregnancy.
    2. Spider nevi, darker pigmentation of arolae and linea nigra may persist.

3. Fingernails return to normal.
4. Profuse diaphoresis occurs immediate postpartum.
J. Vital signs.
1. Temperature may be slightly elevated (100.4° F) after a long labor; should return to normal within 24-hours. *Report any elevated temperature to the RN.*
2. Blood pressure may be slightly decreased after delivery; however, should remain stable.
3. Pulse rate slow after delivery.
K. Blood values.
1. Abnormal white blood cell (WBC) count (20,000/mm3 to 25,000/mm3).
2. Hemoglobin, hematocrit, and red blood cell (RBC) counts return to normal within 2 to 6 weeks.
3. Increased risk of development of thrombophlebitis and thromboembolism.
L. Weight loss.
1. Initial 10- to 12-lb loss occurs due to the weight of the infant, placenta, and amniotic fluid.
2. Diuresis leads to an additional 5-lb weight loss.
3. At 6 to 8 weeks postpartum: return to prepregnant weight if an average of 25 to 30 lb was gained.

Attachment: Psychosocial Response

A. Phases.
1. Taking-in phase.
   a. First few days postpartum.
   b. Characterized by passiveness and dependency.
   c. Preoccupied with own self-needs: food, attention, and physical comforts and care.
   d. Talkative.
2. Taking-hold phase.
   a. Occurs about 2 to 3 days postpartum; characterized by increase in own physical well-being.
   b. Emphasis on the present; woman takes hold of the task of mothering; requires reassurance.
   c. Very receptive to teaching.
B. Attachment behaviors.
1. Exploration and identification pattern.
   a. Touch: begins by stroking the extremities and the outline of the head with the fingertips; gradually moves toward using the entire surface of the hand; touches and observes first at arm's length, then on lap, or slightly away from the body; finally enfolds infant close to body with both arms.
   b. Eye-to-eye contact: *en face position* (gazing into the eyes of the infant).
C. Postpartum blues.
1. Transient period of depression (occurring during the puerperium).
2. Complaints of anorexia, insomnia, tearfulness, and a general let-down, sad feeling.
3. Thought to be caused by fatigue, discomfort,

sensory overload or deprivation, and hormonal changes.
4. Woman needs support and reassurance that it is usually transient and self-limiting experience.
5. Assess mental health status and report concerns to RN.
6. Educate the woman and her family about postpartum depression. Offer post discharge resources if "transient blues" become more serious. Stress the importance of seeking help for self and infant.

Nursing Interventions

❖ **Goal:** To initiate routine postpartum data collection.
A. General observations of mood, activity level, and feelings of wellness; routine vital sign data collection.
B. Inspection of breasts: check for beginning engorgement and presence of cracks in nipples, any pain or tenderness, and progress of breast-feeding.
C. Check uterine fundus: determine height of fundus in relation to umbilicus; should feel firm and globular and be midline; perform fundal massage if bleeding increases (see Figure 20-3).
D. Assess for bladder distention, especially during the first 24 to 48 hours, and *report to RN or PCP if client is distended.*
E. Perineal area.
1. Observe episiotomy site for hematoma.
2. Apply anesthetic sprays or ointments to decrease pain.
3. Determine presence of hemorrhoids and provide relief measures.
F. Lochia: record color, odor, and amount of discharge.
1. *Report any significant increase in amount or foul odor of lochia to the charge nurse or the PCP.*
2. Change perineal pads frequently.
G. Abdomen and perineum.
1. Initiate strengthening exercises for both abdominal wall and perineum (e.g., isometric Kegel exercises for strengthening pelvic floor, leg raises).
2. Kegel exercise – practice trying to stop the passing of gas or the flow of urine midstream, which replicates the sensation of the pelvic muscles drawing upward and inward.
❖ **Goal:** To provide comfort and relief of pain.
A. Episiotomy: use ice packs for first few hours, followed by dry heat light or sitz baths.
B. Perineal care: use of "peri bottles" to squirt over perineum (front to back) to prevent contamination; avoid use of toilet tissue.
C. Afterpain: use of analgesics (preferably 1 hour before feeding, especially for breast-feeding mothers).
D. Hemorrhoidal pain.
1. Sitz baths, anesthetic ointments, rectal suppositories, Tucks.
2. Encourage lying on side and avoiding prolonged sitting.

3. Stool softeners or laxatives may be indicated; usually normal bowel movement by second or third day after delivery.
E. Breast engorgement: well-fitting bra to provide support.
❖ Goal: To promote maternal-infant attachment and facilitate integration of the newborn into the family unit.
A. Use infant's name when talking about him or her.
B. Encourage parents to provide as much care as possible to the infant while still hospitalized.
C. Accept parents' emotions and encourage expression of feelings.
D. Help parents understand sibling behavior and to plan for the arrival of the new family member.
❖ Goal: To establish successful infant feeding patterns.
A. Lactation suppression.
1. Provide supportive bra, binder, or ice pack to decrease engorgement, application of fresh cabbage leaves inside of bra.
2. Explain proper position for feeding.
3. Formulas: ready-to-feed in disposable bottles often with disposable nipples.
B. Lactating mothers (lactation promotion).
1. Cleanse breast before infant nursing and afterwards.
2. Air-dry nipples at least 15 minutes after breast-feeding.
3. *Assess breasts for engorgement, nipple inversion, cracking, inflammation, or pain and report to RN.*
4. If mother experiences uterine contractions during breast-feeding, administer analgesics before breast-feeding.
❖ Goal: To prepare and plan for discharge.
A. Determine if mother will need household help (especially important if birth is twins).
B. *Assist the RN to teach the following infant care skills:*
1. Infant feeding. Always hold infant for feeding.
   a. Hold bottle so that air does not get into nipple.
   b. Method of cleaning bottles and making formula.
   c. Positioning and feeding for lactating mothers.
   d. How to break the infant's suction on the breast.
   e. Positioning for burping and bubbling.
2. Diapering.
   a. Frequent changing to prevent diaper rash.
   b. Vaseline or Desitin ointment to prevent irritation.
   c. Keep diaper below the umbilical cord.
3. Bathing.
   a. Use of a mild soap.
   b. Kitchen sink is often a good place to bathe infant.
   c. Lotions can be applied; best advice is to avoid use of powders.
4. Umbilical cord.
   a. Apply alcohol or wash with warm soap and water daily and after every diaper change, allow to dry.
   b. Stump usually falls off in 1 week to 10 days.
   c. Do not immerse abdomen during bathing until cord stump falls off.
5. Pacifiers.
   a. May be used to meet infant's sucking need.
   b. Usually discontinued around 4 to 6 months due to infant's lack of interest.
6. Sleeping.
   a. Usually sleeps through the night at around 2 to 3 months of age.
   b. Encourage mother to sleep while infant is sleeping, to avoid sleep deprivation.
7. Illness.
   a. Common behavior changes are irritability, crying, loss of appetite, and fever.
   b. Explain how to take an infant's temperature.
8. Taking the infant outside.
   a. Dress infant as you would dress yourself.
   b. Traveling: use a car seat.
9. Explain importance of follow-up well-baby checkup visits with health care provider.

COMPLICATIONS OF THE POSTPARTUM

Postpartum Infection

❋ **Puerperal infection is any clinical infection of the genital canal that occurs within 28 days after miscarriage, abortion, or childbirth.**

Data Collection

A. Predisposing factors.
1. Antepartal infection.
2. Premature rupture of the membranes.
3. Prolonged labor.
4. Laceration.
5. Anemia; postpartum hemorrhage.
6. Poor aseptic technique.
B. Clinical manifestations.
1. Temperature elevation 38° C (100.4° F), if taken at least four times daily on any 2 of the first 10 postpartum days, with the exception of the first 24 hours.
2. Symptoms vary according to system involved.
3. Area of involvement characterized by five cardinal symptoms of inflammation.
4. Tachycardia, chills, abdominal tenderness common.
5. Headache, malaise, deep pelvic pain.
6. Profuse, foul-smelling lochia.
C. Area involved.
1. Uterus is most often affected: endometritis.
2. May have localized infection of the perineum, vulva, and vagina.
3. Urinary system.
   a. Pyelitis.
   b. Cystitis.

Treatment

A. Medications.
1. Antibiotics.
2. Antipyretics.
B. Dietary.
1. High-protein, high-calorie, high-vitamin diet.
2. Encourage 3000 to 4000 mL of fluid per 24 hours.

Nursing Interventions

❖   **Goal:** To prevent postpartum infection.
A. Maintain meticulous aseptic technique during labor and delivery.
B. Assess and treat antepartal infection.
C. Prevent anemia: hemoglobin and hematocrit should be checked during prenatal visits and/or before delivery. *Report any significant decrease to PCP.*
❖   **Goal:** To promote mother's resistance to infection.
A. Administer antibiotic and antipyretic medications.
B. Encourage good nutrition.
C. Use semi-Fowler's position to promote free drainage of lochia and prevent upward extension of infection into pelvis.

 ## Mastitis

*   **Mastitis is the invasion of the breast tissue by pathogenic organisms.**

Data Collection

A. Predisposing factors.
1. Fissured nipples.
2. Erosion of the areola.
3. Causative agent is most frequently *Staphylococcus*, which is transmitted from the nasopharynx of the nursing infant.
B. Clinical manifestations.
1. Occurs most often between the first and fourth weeks of the postpartal period.
2. Chills and tachycardia.
3. Red, swollen, painful breast. Most often unilateral.
4. Fever.

Treatment

A. Medication.
1. Antibiotics.
2. Antipyretics.
3. Analgesics.

Nursing Interventions

❖   **Goal:** To prevent the complication of mastitis.
A. Teach mother how to cleanse breasts and nipples.
B. Explain importance of wearing a support bra.

❖   **Goal:** To promote comfort and maintain lactation if desired.
A. Apply ice to breasts to decrease pain.
B. May continue to breast-feed.
C. Encourage good nutrition and adequate rest.
D. Administer antibiotics as ordered.

 ## Thrombophlebitis

There is an increased risk (five times) for *thrombophlebitis* and *pulmonary* embolism during the postpartum. The reason for the increased incidence is a change in blood coagulation during pregnancy, along with engorgement of the veins of the lower extremities and pelvis, leading to pooling of blood and venous stasis. Data collection and nursing interventions are discussed in Chapter 16.

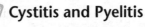 ## Cystitis and Pyelitis

*   **Cystitis and *pyelitis* occur as a result of bladder distention and incomplete emptying of urine postpartum; three common predisposing factors are trauma to the bladder mucosa, the temporary loss of bladder tone, and an increased bladder capacity (see Chapter 18).**

 ## Parental Reaction to Premature Infant or Infant with Special Needs

Data Collection

A. Period of disorganization.
1. Grief reaction characterized by guilt, anger, and sorrow.
2. Feelings of exhaustion, emptiness, and frequent crying.
B. Period of information-seeking and resource utilization.
1. Anxiety decreases; problem-solving begins.
2. Begins to resolve the crisis.
3. Often information-seeking leads to further anger and sorrow followed then by a period of denial or disbelief.
C. Resolution of the crisis situation.
1. Development of new coping strategies.
2. Acceptance and coming to terms with the situation.

Nursing Interventions

❖   **Goal:** To provide emotional support to the parents.
A. Encourage verbalization of feelings and expression of grief.
B. Promote parent-infant contact; point out normal characteristics.
C. Encourage parents to visit, touch, and care for their infant as much as possible.

Study Questions: Maternal Care

1. While discussing nutrition, the nurse explains the best way for a primigravida client to meet her increasing iron needs is to:
    1   Add an extra serving of red meat to her daily diet.
    2   Include at least two eggs in her daily diet.
    3   Increase her daily intake of spinach.
    4   Take an iron supplement with orange juice.

2. When teaching clients in a prenatal clinic, the nurse in cludes all of the following areas. What is the most important area of discussion for clients in their first trimester?
    1   Diet to promote fetal development and maternal well-being.
    2   Postpartal care with emphasis on hygiene and breast care.
    3   Anticipation and points on how to deal with sibling rivalry.
    4   Signs of beginning labor and instructions to come to the hospital as soon as the membranes rupture.

3. The nurse understands that the following finding is con sidered a positive sign of pregnancy?
    1   Nausea and vomiting.
    2   Changes in breasts.
    3   Fetal outline on ultrasound.
    4   Presence of quickening.

4. A young pregnant woman comes to the clinic and com plains of nausea and vomiting. What would the nurse suggest to assist in alleviating this problem?
    1   Take 3 tablespoons of bismuth subsalicylate (**Pepto-Bismol**) before eating.
    2   Increase fluids to 4000 mL per day.
    3   Increase protein in diet.
    4   Eat five or more small meals a day.

5. What is important for the nurse to teach a client regarding how to prevent venous stasis and varicose veins during pregnancy?
    1   Elevate feet and take frequent rest breaks.
    2   Wear loose shoes and clothes to help circulation.
    3   Decrease salt in the diet and increase fluids.
    4   Wear thigh-high TED hose throughout the night.

6. The nurse is checking a postpartum client the day after her delivery and notes the lochia has a foul smell. What is the best nursing intervention?
    1   Report the foul-smelling lochia to the supervisor.
    2   Do nothing; this is normal during the first few days after delivery.
    3   Begin vaginal irrigations to decrease the odor and increase client comfort.
    4   Stop the use of perineal pads for the next few days.

7. During the postpartum assessment, the nurse notes a blood pressure of 98/68 mm Hg, pulse rate of 110 beats per minute, respira-tions of 28 breaths per minute, and profuse lochia rubra. What is the priority nursing action?

    1   Immediately advise the charge nurse.
    2   Massage the mother's fundus.
    3   Check her urinary output.
    4   Change her perineal pad.

8. The nurse understands that the following is considered a sign of true labor:
    1   Effacement and cervical dilation.
    2   Uterine contractions 8 minutes apart.
    3   Braxton Hicks contractions every 4 minutes.
    4   Bloody show with contraction every 30 minutes.

9. How does the nurse measure the duration of a contraction?
    1   From the beginning of the contraction to the end of the contraction.
    2   From the beginning of one contraction to the end of the next contraction.
    3   From the point of maximal intensity until the contraction subsides.
    4   From the beginning of one contraction to the start of the next contraction.

10. In order for a pregnant woman to fulfill her daily need for folic acid, what would the nurse suggest adding to or increasing in her diet?
    1   Beef and chicken.
    2   Milk, yogurt, cheese.
    3   Green, leafy vegetables.
    4   Whole-grain breads.

11. A postpartum client complains of abdominal cramping following breastfeeding. What is the best nursing interpretation of this information?
    1   All women experience abdominal discomfort during the postpartal period.
    2   Breast-feeding causes the release of oxytocin, which acts on the uterus.
    3   Abdominal pain is not normal and may indicate problems of involution.
    4   Abdominal discomfort may be an indication of problems with peristalsis.

12. Considering a woman is of normal weight, the nurse would reinforce teaching related to the average recommended weight gain during pregnancy, which is:
    1   15 to 20 pounds.
    2   20 to 40 pounds.
    3   25 to 35 pounds.
    4   40 to 45 pounds.

13. While assessing a prenatal client, the nurse would be alert to symptoms of preeclampsia, which include:
    1   Oliguria, hypotension, proteinuria.
    2   Hypertension, tachycardia, tachypnea.
    3   Edema, tachycardia, nausea.
    4   Hypertension, edema, proteinuria.

14. Which condition would the nurse identify as contributing to the complication of intrapartal bleeding?
    1   Placenta previa.
    2   Third-degree laceration.
    3   Vena caval syndrome.
    4   Retained placental fragments.

15. What is the best position for the nurse to place a client in during labor?
    1   Position of comfort.
    2   Right Sims'.
    3   Supine.
    4   Left lateral.

16. The nurse is asked to complete an Apgar assessment:
    1   Within 2 hours of birth.
    2   At 1 minute and 5 minutes after birth.
    3   At 5 minutes and 10 minutes after birth.
    4   Within the first hour of birth.

17. The primigravida client is experiencing Braxton Hicks contractions. The nurse understands the following about the characteristics of this type of contraction:
    1   Contractions increase with ambulation.
    2   Do not increase in intensity or frequency.
    3   Cause a rapid dilation and effacement.
    4   Do not occur with the second pregnancy.

18. A young woman has been prescribed oral contraceptives. What is the priority information to teach her?
    1   Call the clinic if you have nausea, vomiting, or diarrhea.
    2   Take the pill with a glass of milk to increase the effectiveness.
    3   If you forget to take a pill, discontinue taking them until the next month.
    4   Call the clinic if you have a sudden headache or severe leg pain.

19. The nurse would anticipate which medication to be used to suppress contractions?
    1   Oxytocin (**Pitocin**).
    2   Conjugated estrogen (**Premarin**).
    3   Terbutaline (**Brethine**).
    4   Ergot alkaloid (**Cafergot**).

20. The client is in her last trimester and is concerned about the presence of "stretch marks" on her abdomen and breasts. What is the best nursing response?
    1   They cannot be prevented and occur in all pregnancies.
    2   Application of cocoa butter or vitamin E oil will decrease formation of scars.
    3   After delivery the reddish marks will gradually fade.
    4   There is nothing that can be done to prevent them.

Answers and rationales to these questions are in the section at the end of the book titled Chapter Study Questions: Answers and Rationales.

Appendix 20-1   CONTRACEPTIVE METHODS

Methods/Description	Nursing Implications/Client Teaching

FAMILY AWARENESS METHODS

Calendar (rhythm)
Basal Body Temperature (BBT)
Ovulation (Billings)
Cervical mucus
Symptothermal

Client Teaching
1. Calendar (rhythm) method: calculate the days of fertility; considered to be days 10 to 17 of a 28-day menstrual cycle.
2. BBT method: a slight decrease then an increase of about 0.4° to 0.8° in temperature when ovulation occurs; fertile period ends 3 days after temperature elevation. Need a special BBT thermometer.
3. Cervical mucus method: before ovulation, mucus becomes clear and stringy; nonfertile period occurs when mucus becomes thick, cloudy, and sticky or when no mucus is apparent.
4. Symptothermal method: combines two methods, usually cervical mucus and BBT.

IUD

Progesterone (**Progestasert**) IUD;
Copper T380A (**ParaGard**) IUD

Client Teaching
1. Discuss the technique and the experience of IUD insertion and removal.
2. Emphasize the need for yearly Pap smears; failure rate is less than 1%.
3. Encourage client to check IUD string, especially after each period.
4. Make sure the woman understands which type of IUD she has and when to return to have it checked or replaced. Copper IUD is approved for 10 years; progesterone IUD effective for up to 5 years and uterine cramping and bleeding is diminished as compared to the copper one.
5. Review common side effects, serious complications, and reports of any of the following symptoms (**PAIN**):
   P – period late, abnormal spotting or bleeding, **A** – abdominal pain, pain with intercourse, **I** – infection exposure, abnormal vaginal discharge, **N** – not feeling well, fever or chills, **S** – string missing; shorter or longer.

HORMONAL METHODS

Combined Oral Contraceptive: pill is a combination of estrogen and progestin
Progestin only (minipill): norethindrone; medroxyprogesterone
Transdermal Contraceptive Patch: applied once a week; has both hormones.
Vaginal Contraceptive Ring: a ring is inserted into the vagina for 3 weeks; removed for 1 week, then new ring inserted.

Client Teaching
1. Instruct as to correct use of medication, the need for followup checkup in 3 mo, and importance of taking the pill at same time each day; effectiveness is close to 100% when used correctly.
2. Explain if a pill is forgotten one day, she should take it when she remembers, then take the next pill as scheduled the following day.
3. If two pills are missed, she should take them as above and use some other form of contraception for the remainder of the month.
4. Review common side effects, serious complications, and reports of any of the following symptoms: **A**bdominal pain, **C**hest pain or shortness of breath, **H**eadaches, **E**ye problems, and **S**evere leg pain (**ACHES**).

> ✔ ***NURSING PRIORITY:*** *OTC medications, herbal supplements (St. John's Wort), phenytoin (Dilantin), rifampin, ritonavir, tetracyclines, and ampicillin can reduce the effectiveness of the pill.*

5. Progestin only pill causes more menstrual irregularity (breakthrough bleeding, variation in blood flow, etc.)

INJECTABLE/IMPLANTABLE PROGESTINS

Injectable (**DMPA, Depo-Provera**)

Client Teaching
1. Requires injections only 4 times per year (every 11-13 weeks).

> ✔ ***NURSING PRIORITY:*** *Do not massage the site after the injection because it may speed up absorption and decrease duration of effectiveness; effectiveness rate is comparable to that of oral contraceptives.*

2. Disadvantages include weight gain, prolonged amenorrhea, and breakthrough uterine bleeding. Long-term use may decrease bone density; need to encourage calcium intake and exercise.

Implantable: single rod implant (**Implanon**)

1. Requires a small incision in the inner aspect of the nondominant upper arm with a local anesthetic; provides up to 3 years of contraception.
2. The most common side effect is irregular menstrual bleeding.

Continued

Appendix 20-1	CONTRACEPTIVE METHODS—cont'd.

Methods/Description	Nursing Implications/Client Teaching

BARRIER METHODS

Diaphragm: a dome-shaped rubber device that fits over the cervix.

Client Teaching
1. Should be refitted after every pregnancy or when there is a weight gain or loss of 20 lb; failure rate in the first year of use may be 20%.
2. Instruct client to use spermicidal jelly or cream around diaphragm rim and in the dome.
3. Instruct client to leave diaphragm in place 6 to 8 hr after intercourse.
4. Explain the proper method for cleansing (use mild nonperfumed soap only), storing (dry thoroughly and dust with cornstarch, not baby powder), and checking for defects or holes in the diaphragm.
5. Allow for sufficient practice of insertion/removal techniques and use with a spermicide, such as nonoxynol-9 (N-9).

Condoms: "rubbers" are thin sheaths of rubber that fit over an erect penis.

1. Advise client to apply condom to erect penis by rolling the sheath along the entire shaft and leaving enough slack at the end of the penis to receive the semen.
2. Explain importance of holding the condom in place while withdrawing the penis to prevent emptying of sperm into the vagina.
3. Condom should be applied before any penetration because the pre-ejaculatory seminal fluid may contain sperm.
4. Ask client about allergy to latex.

> ✔ **NURSING PRIORITY:** *Use of nonoxynol-9 with diaphragms or condoms is not recommended for preventing STD's or HIV.*

UNRELIABLE PRACTICES

Withdrawal (coitus interruptus): withdrawal of penis before ejaculation.

Nursing Implications
1. Requires absolute cooperation and control of partner.
2. Good choice for couples who do not have other contraceptive methods available.
3. Douching may actually move the sperm upward in the vagina.

Client Teaching
1. Encourage use of a more reliable contraceptive practice.

Douching: the act of cleansing, washing the semen out of the vagina.

EMERGENCY CONTRACEPTION

Plan B: 2 doses of progestin.

Client Teaching
1. Available without a prescription; prescription required if under age 18.
2. Should be taken within 120 hours of unprotected intercourse.
3. Is ineffective if the woman is pregnant, since pills do not disturb an implanted pregnancy.

PERMANENT STERILIZATION

Tubal ligation (minilaprotomy)

Client Teaching
1. Discuss the permanence of the sterilization procedure with the couple – informed consent required for all procedures.
2. Explain that she may experience sensation of tugging, but not pain during procedure which is carried out via local anesthetic.

Essure System

1. Insertion of an occulsive agent (small metallic implants) into the uterine tubes, which stimulate scar tissue formation that occlude the tubes.
2. Procedure does not provide immediate contraception – need to use another form of contraception until tubal blockage is proven, which may take up to 3 months.

Vasectomy: surgical ligation and resection bilaterally of the vas deferens.

Client Teaching
1. Discuss with couple the permanence of vasectomy (informed consent required); even if the vas deferens is reconnected, the fertility varies between 5% and 60%.
2. Activity level should be moderate for 2 days; skin sutures are usually removed within a week.
3. Encourage the use of a scrotal support and application of ice for pain or swelling.
4. Follow-up visit for sperm sample is usually done in 4 to 6 wk.
5. Advise couple to use another form of birth control until two ejaculate sperm counts contains no sperm.

BBT, Basal body temperature; CO_2, carbon dioxide; *IUD*, intrauterine device.

Appendix 20-2 MAGNESIUM SULFATE

Medications	Side Effects	Nursing Implications

ANTICONVULSANT

Medications	Side Effects	Nursing Implications

Magnesium sulfate:
IV: Given via an IV pump, piggybacked to primary infusion. A bolus dose (4–6 g over 15–20 min) is routinely given, followed by a maintenance infusion (1-4 g/hr).
	Maternal: sweating, flushing, muscle weakness, depressed or absent reflexes, oliguria, respiratory paralysis.
	Fetal: crosses placenta; lethargy, hypotonia, and weakness.
	Contraindications: maternal—impaired renal function.
		1. Criteria for continuing administration:
		  a. Respirations: greater than 12 breaths/min.
		  b. Presence of patellar knee-jerk movement.
		  c. Urinary output: greater than 30 mL/hr.
		2. Check BP frequently for symptoms of hypotension.
		3. Antidote for magnesium sulfate is *calcium gluconate*; should be available at bedside in case of respiratory paralysis.
		4. Monitor FHR.
		5. Administration magnesium sulfate is continued at least 24 hrs after delivery to reduce risk of seizure activity.
		6. May be used as a tocolytic agent.
		7. *Uses:* prevention or control of eclampsia.

BP, Blood pressure; *FHR*, fetal heart rate; *IV*, intravenous.

Appendix 20-3 OXYTOCIC MEDICATIONS AND PROSTAGLANDINS TO CAUSE UTERINE CONTRACTIONS

Medications	Side Effects	Nursing Implications

OXYTOCIC MEDICATIONS: Stimulate contraction of uterine muscle fibers; have a mild antidiuretic effect; stimulate postpartum milk flow but do not affect amount.

Medications	Side Effects	Nursing Implications

Oxytocin (**Pitocin**): IM, IV, intranasal **High Alert Medication**
Ergonovine (**Ergotrate**): PO, IM, IV
Methylergonovine (**Methergine**): PO, IM, IV
	Maternal: tetanic uterine contractions, hypertension, tachycardia.
	Fetal: hypoxia, irregularity and decrease in FHR, possible hyperbilirubinemia.
	Contraindications: Severe pre-eclampsia or eclampsia. Predisposition to uterine rupture or CPD. Preterm infant or presence of fetal distress.
		1. Apply fetal monitor: assess FHR pattern throughout oxytocin administration.
		2. Assess maternal vital signs before increasing oxytocin infusion rate.
		3. Discontinue IV oxytocin and turn on primary IV solution, and *notify the charge nurse if any of the following occur*:
		  a. Non-reassuring fetal heart rate pattern; absent variability; abnormal baseline rate.
		  b. Sustained uterine contractions lasting greater than 90 secs.
		  c. Insufficient relaxation of the uterus between contractions.
		  d. Contractions occurring more often than every 2 minutes.
		  e. Repeated late decelerations or prolonged decelerations.
		4. **Pitocin** is the only oxytocic used to induce labor; others (**Ergotrate** and **Methergine**) are used after delivery to control bleeding.
		5. *Uses:* uterine dystocia; induction of labor, control of hemorrhage and uterine atony: uterine involution.

Prostaglandin F2a (**Hemabate**): IM	*Contraindications:* Asthma	1. Used to contract the uterus in situations of postpartum hemorrhage.

CPD, Cephalopelvic disproportion; *FHR*, fetal heart rate; *IM*, intramuscularly; *IV*, intravenously; *PO*, by mouth (orally).

Appendix 20-4   TOCOLYTIC AGENTS TO SUPPRESS LABOR

Medications	Side Effects	Nursing Implications
TOCOLYTIC AGENTS: Relax myometrial cells of the uterus leading to inhibition of labor. Also result in bronchial dilation and cardiac output.		
Ritodrine: IV, PO	**Maternal:** altered pulse and BP (dose-related), widening pulse pressure, tachycardia, hypotension, nausea and vomiting, hyperglycemia, nervousness and tremors, skin rash. **Fetal:** altered FHR (dose-related), increased serum glucose, acidosis, hypoxia, and hypotension at birth. **Contraindications:** Severe pre eclampsia, hypovolemia, cardiac disease; used with caution in diabetic mothers.	1. Obtain baseline maternal EKG 2. Assess maternal (especially pulse) and fetal vital signs frequently; fetal monitoring is necessary; notify physician if maternal pulse is greater than 120 beats/min or FHR is *greater than 180 beats/min.* 3. Strict I & O, daily weight. 4. Encourage lateral position (Sims') to decrease hypotension and increase placental perfusion. 5. IV: Use a pump for continuous infusion; infusion is continued for 12 hr after labor has stopped. 6. Watch for signs of pulmonary edema, assess blood glucose with IV Ritodrine administration and do not give in presence of an infection. 7. *Use:* premature labor.
Calcium channel blockers Nifedipine (**Procardia**): PO, sublingual	**Maternal:** facial flushing, mild hypotension, reflex tachycardia, headache, nausea.	1. No reported fetal side effects. 2. Not in common use as a tocolytic agent. 3. Monitor blood pressure for hypotension.
Prostaglandin synthesis inhibitors	**Maternal:** Nausea, vomiting, dyspepsia.	1. Used when other methods fail and gestational age is less than 30 weeks. 2. Administer for 48-72 hr or less as may close the fetal patent ductus. 3. Administer with food or use rectal route to decrease gastrointestinal distress.
Indomethacin (**Indocin**): PO or rectally	**Fetal:** oligohydramnios, premature closure of the ductus arteriosus in utero.	
NSAIDs	**Maternal:** promotes relaxation of smooth muscles.	1. ***Most commonly used tocolytic agent,*** because maternal and fetal/neonatal adverse reactions are less common than with the other tocolytic agents, especially the beta-adrenergic agonists (ritodrine and terbutaline).

BP, Blood pressure; *FHR*, fetal heart rate; *I & O*, intake and output; *IM*, intramuscularly; *IV*, intravenously; *NSAIDs*, nonsteroidal anti-inflammatory drugs; *PO*, by mouth (orally); *SQ*, subcutaneously.

Appendix 20-5   RhoGAM

Medication	Side Effects	Nursing Implications
IMMUNE GLOBULIN HUMAN Rh$_o$(D): Prevents Rho(D) sensitization in nonsensitized Rh-negative mothers following pregnancy or accidental transfusion; "tricks" the body into thinking it has already made antibodies.		
RhoGAM: IM	Pain and soreness at injection site	1. Is administered twice, at 28 weeks gestation and within 72 hours of delivery, or after an abortion, miscarriage, or transfusion. 2. Do not administer this to the infant. 3. *Uses:* prevention of hemolytic disease of the newborn. 4. *Contraindications:* sensitized Rh-negative woman.

Notes

Newborn

NORMAL NEWBORN

Biological Adaptations in the Neonatal Period

Data Collection

A. Respiratory system.
1. Respirations are usually established within 1 minute after birth, often within the first few seconds.
2. Lusty cry usually accompanies good respiratory effort.
3. Newborn respiration should be quiet; no dyspnea or cyanosis.
4. Cyanosis may be apparent in the hands and feet (acrocyanosis); circumoral cyanosis (around the mouth) may persist for an hour or two after birth but should subside.
5. Average respiratory rate: 30 to 60 breaths/min.
6. Respiratory movements: Diaphragmatic and abdominal muscles are used; very little thoracic movement.
7. Neonate breathes through the nose (obligate nose-breather); consequently, nasal obstruction with mucus will lead to respiratory distress.

B. Circulatory system.
1. Closure of the ductus arteriosus, the foramen ovale, and the ductus venosus.
2. Circulatory changes are not always immediate and complete: usually complete in a few days; often this period is called *transitional circulation.*
3. Pulse rate: 100-160 beats/min.
4. Normal BP is systolic 60-80 mm Hg and diastolic 40-50 mm Hg measured using Doppler ultrasonography– need correctly sized cuff.

C. Body temperature and heat production.
1. Body temperature may drop to 94° F (34.4° C) or even as low as 92° F (33.3° C) after birth unless the infant is adequately protected.

> ✔ **NURSING PRIORITY:** *Excessive heat loss occurs from radiation and convection because of the newborn's larger surface area as compared with body weight. It is important to remember that conduction loss occurs as a result of the marked difference between core body temperature and skin temperature.*

2. Heat is generated immediately by shivering; infant *shivering* is characterized by increased muscular activity, restlessness, and crying.
3. Metabolism of brown fat (brown adipose tissue) functions to produce heat under the stress of cooling.
4. Effect of chilling on the neonate.
   a. Increased heat production leads to increased oxygen consumption, which leads to increased metabolism of glucose and brown fat.
   b. When heat production is high, caloric need is high.
   c. Tendency to develop metabolic acidosis occurs.
   d. Production of surfactant is inhibited by cooling, and respiratory distress syndrome may occur.
   e. Increased risk with smaller neonates.

D. Length.
1. Average body length of term neonate: 45 to 55 cm (18 to 22 inches).
2. Infant is measured by being placed flat on the back on paper and determining the distance from head to heel; a pencil is used to mark the locations of head and heels, and the distance between locations is measured when the infant is removed.

E. Weight.
1. Average birth weight for a term neonate: 3400 gm (7 lb 8 oz).
2. Weight loss: between 5% and 10% of birth weight within the first few days of life; infant usually regains weight within 10 to 14 days.

F. Head.
1. Molding.
   a. Head may appear elongated at birth; molding usually disappears within 24 to 48 hours.
   b. Occurs as a result of abnormal fetal posture in utero and pressure during passage through the birth canal.
2. Caput succedaneum (Figure 21-1).
   a. Edema of the scalp caused by the pressure occurring at the time of delivery.
   b. Disappears within 3 to 4 days.
   c. Edema goes across the cranial suture lines.
3. Cephalhematoma.
   a. A collection of blood between the periosteum and the skull.
   b. Usually results from trauma during labor and delivery.

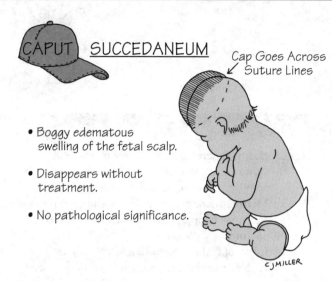

CAPUT SUCCEDANEUM
Cap Goes Across Suture Lines

- Boggy edematous swelling of the fetal scalp.
- Disappears without treatment.
- No pathological significance.

FIGURE 26-1 **Caput succedaneum.** (From Zerwekh J, Claborn J, Miller CJ: *Memory notebook of nursing,* vol 2, ed 3, Ingram, 2007, Nursing Education Consultants.)

   c. Absorbed in a few weeks; does not cross cranial suture lines.
4. Head measurement.
   a. Average head circumference of the term neonate: 34.2 cm; usual variation ranges from 33 to 35 cm (13 to 14 inches).
   b. Head circumference is approximately 2 to 3 cm greater than the chest circumference; extremes in size may indicate microcephaly, hydrocephaly, or increased intracranial pressure.

 TEST ALERT: Compare physical development of newborn with identified norms

5. Fontanels (anterior and posterior).
   a. Palpate for size and tension.
   b. Increase in tension may indicate tumor, hemorrhage, infection, or congenital anomaly.
   c. Decrease in tension (sunken fontanel) may indicate dehydration.
   d. Anterior will close in about 12 to 18 months; posterior will close in 2 to 3 months.
G. Umbilical cord.
1. Determine number of blood vessels; there should be two arteries and one vein surrounded by Wharton's jelly.
2. Cord atrophies and sloughs off by day 10 to 14.
H. Nervous system.
1. Nervous system is relatively immature and characterized by the following:
   a. Poor nervous control; easily startled.
   b. Quivering chin.
   c. Tremors of the lower extremities of short duration.
   d. Sleep and awake states.

   (1) Newborn sleeps an average of 16 to 20 hours a day during the first 2 weeks of life, with an average of 4 hours at a time.
   (2) May vary from a drowsy or semi-dozing state to an alert state to a crying state.
2. Presence of positive Babinski sign.
   a. Normal finding until the age of 1 year.
   b. Dorsiflexion of big toe and fanning of the other toes.
3. Neonatal reflexes (Table 21-1).

✔ *NURSING PRIORITY: Intactness of the neonate's nervous system is indicated by the state of alertness, resting posture, cry, and quality of muscle tone and motor activity.*

I. Hematological system.
1. *Physiological* jaundice; increased incidence in breast-fed infants; occurs on the second or third day of life as a result of an increase in the serum bilirubin level.
2. *Pathological* jaundice occurs within 24 hours of birth (see hemolytic disease of the newborn).
3. Transitory coagulation defects.
   a. Result from the lack of intestinal synthesis of vitamin K because of insufficient bacterial flora in the GI tract.
   b. Vitamin K (0.5 to 1.0 mg) is administered intramuscularly in the vastus lateralis to prevent complications.
J. GI tract.
1. Stools.

✔ *NURSING PRIORITY: Monitor the passage of the first meconium stool.*

   a. Meconium: sticky, black, odorless, sterile stool that is passed within the first 24 to 48 hours after birth; if no stool is passed, further assessment is needed.
   b. Stools change according to type and amount of feedings.
   (1) Transitional stools: occurs during period between second and fourth day; consist of meconium and milk; greenish brown or greenish yellow; loose and often contain mucus.
   (2) Milk stools: usually occur by the fourth day; stools of formula-fed infant are drier, more formed, paler, and occur once or twice daily or 1 stool every 2-3 days
   (3) Stools of breast-fed infants are golden yellow, have a pasty consistency, and occur more frequently than stools of formula-fed infants, 3-4 stools in 24 hours.

TABLE 21-1	MAJOR NEONATAL REFLEXES		
Reflex	Disappears	How to Elicit	Response
Rooting	3 to 4 mo; may persist during sleep until 7 to 8 mo	Stroke cheek.	Head turns toward side that is touched.
Babinski	1 yr	Lightly stroke lateral side of foot from heel to toe across the foot.	Infant's toes fan, with dorsiflexion of great toe.
Sucking	10 to 12 mo	Touch or stroke lips.	Infant sucks.
Moro (startle)	3 to 4 mo	Make a loud noise or suddenly disturb infant's equilibrium.	Infant stiffens, briskly abducts, and extends arms with hands open and fingers extended to C shape. Infant's legs flex and abduct, and arms return to an embracing posture. Crying is usual.
Grasp Palmar	3 to 4 mo	Press a finger against infant's palm.	Infant's fingers momentarily close around object.
Asymmetric tonic neck (fencer's position)	3 to 4 mo	Turn supine infant's head over the shoulder to one side.	Infant's arm and leg partially or completely extend on side to which head is turned; opposite arm and leg flex.

K. Genitourinary system.
 1. Thirty to 60 mL is voided per day during the first 2 days of life; followed by 200 mL per day by the end of the first week.
 2. Frequency of voiding: average of two to six times per day, increasing up to 10 to 15 times per day.

> ✔ **NURSING PRIORITY:** *Most newborns void within the first 24 to 48 hours after birth. Weigh dry diaper before applying, then weigh wet diaper after infant voiding. Each gram of added weight equals 1mL of urine.*

L. Integumentary system.
 1. Vernix caseosa: a white cheesy-like material covers the skin at birth, particularly noted in the folds and creases.
 2. Petechiae: pinpoint bluish discolorations primarily on the skin and face as a result of pressure from delivery; bruising of tissues may be seen.
 3. Lanugo: downy, fine covering of hair that may be present on the shoulders, back, earlobes, and forehead; disappears during the first week.
 4. Milia: pinpoint white bumps seen over the bridge of the nose and on the cheeks during the first 2 weeks of life.
 5. Erythema toxicum: splotchy pink papular rash appearing anywhere on the body; disappears within the first few days of life; no treatment is necessary.

 6. Mongolian spots: bluish darkened pigmented areas seen on the back or buttocks of dark-skinned infants (African American and Asian American infants and those of Mediterranean descent); usually disappears by school age.
M. Sensory system.
 1. Eyes appear large, and pupils appear small.
 2. Tears do not develop until 2 to 4 weeks of age.
 3. Sudden loud noises may elicit startle response.
 4. Differentiates between pleasant and unpleasant tastes.
 5. Most sensitive area is around the mouth.
 6. Searches for food when cheek is touched or begins sucking movement when lips are touched.
O. Musculoskeletal system.
 1. Assumes the position of comfort, which is usually the position assumed in utero.
 2. Normal palmar crease is present (simian crease is indicative of Down syndrome).
 3. Spine is straight and flat when in prone position.

Nursing Intervention

> **TEST ALERT:** *Provide physical care for a newborn.*

❖ **Goal:** To establish and maintain a patent airway and promote oxygenation.

A. Position infant with head slightly lower than chest; may use postural drainage or side-lying position.

B. Suction nostrils and oropharynx with bulb syringe.

C. *Observe for apnea, cyanosis, and mucus collection and if noted report to RN.*

> ✔ **NURSING PRIORITY:** *During first 4 hours after birth, the priority nursing goals are to maintain a clear airway, maintain a neutral thermal environment, and prevent hemorrhage and infection. Bathing will be initiated when infant's temperature is stabilized; feeding may begin immediately if infant is interested.*

❖ **Goal:** To protect against heat loss.

A. Immediately after birth, wrap infant in warm blanket and dry off amniotic fluid.

B. Replace wet blanket with warm dry blanket.

C. Cover wet hair and head with a blanket or cap.

D. Give infant to mother to cuddle; place infant on a warm padded surface, preferably under a radiant heater or in an incubator; or provide for skin-to-skin contact with the mother.

❖ **Goal:** To collect data and assess physical condition and behavior.

A. Determine Apgar score at 1 minute and again at 5 minutes (see Table 20-7 for Apgar scoring).

> ✔ **NURSING PRIORITY:** *The APGAR score at 1 minute evaluates the neonate's intrauterine oxygenation; at 5 minutes it evaluates the status of the neonate's cardiorespiratory adaptation after birth.*

B. Monitor vital signs every 15 minutes to 1 hour until infant's temperature stabilizes (usually in about 4 hours) and record incubator temperature.

C. Weigh and measure infant.

❖ **Goal:** To assess periods of reactivity.

A. First period of reactivity - newborn is alert, awake, and usually hungry.

B. Sleep phase - sleep usually occurs an average of 3 to 4 hours after birth and may last from a few minutes to several hours. Newborn is difficult to awaken during this phase.

C. Second period of reactivity.
1. Infant is alert and awake.
2. Lasts approximately 4 to 6 hours.

> ✔ **NURSING PRIORITY:** *It is important to monitor the infant closely because apnea, decreased heart rate, gagging, choking, and regurgitation may occur and require nursing intervention.*

❖ **Goal:** To protect against infection.

A. Follow guidelines for proper hand hygiene before and between handling infants.

B. Prevent ophthalmia neonatorum.
1. Administer prophylactic treatment to eyes soon after birth.
2. Place ophthalmic ointment in the lower conjunctival sac.

C. Avoid exposure to people with possible upper respiratory tract, skin, or GI infections.

D. Hepatitis B vaccination recommended at birth and routine HIV screening.

❖ **Goal:** To prevent bleeding problems (hypofibrinogenemia).

A. Administer 0.5 to 1.0 mg of vitamin K, intramuscularly into the upper third of the lateral aspect of the thigh (vastus lateralis).

❖ **Goal:** To properly identify infant.

A. Secure identification bands to wrist or ankle of infant and wrist of mother in the delivery room.

B. Prints of infant's foot, palms, or fingers may be obtained according to hospital policy; mother's palm prints or fingerprints may also be obtained.

C. Advise parents not to release the infant to anyone who does not have proper unit identification.

> **TEST ALERT:** *Promote newborn and family bonding.*

❖ **Goal:** To initiate feeding and to evaluate parents' ability to feed infant and provide nutrition.

A. Encourage breast feeding, if desired, immediately after delivery or in recovery area; breast milk is bacteriologically safe.

B. First formula feeding or test feeding: administer 10 to 15 mL of sterile water to assist GI tract patency followed by formula.

C. Considerations in infant feeding.
1. An infant should always be placed on the right side after feeding to avoid aspiration and prevent regurgitation and distention.
2. Infant will require more frequent feedings initially; will generally establish a routine of feeding every 3 to 4 hours.

❖ **Goal:** To provide daily general care.

A. Care of the umbilical cord stump.
1. Hospital protocol directs routine cord care, which may include using a drying solution of alcohol and triple dye that is applied to the cord.
2. Clean the umbilical cord stump several times a day with soap and water, especially after infant voids (for a male infant).
3. To encourage drying of the cord, expose umbilical area to air frequently and position diaper below umbilicus.
4. Observe for bleeding, oozing, or foul odor.

B. Circumcision care.
1. Keep area clean; change diaper frequently.

2. Observe for bleeding – check site hourly for 12 hours postprocedure.
3. A small sterile petrolatum gauze dressing may be applied to the area during the first 2 to 3 days (Gomco and Mogen clamp).
4. If a PlastiBell was used, keep area clean; application of petrolatum jelly is not necessary; plastic ring will dislodge when area has healed (5-7 days).

✔ *NURSING PRIORITY: Teach the parents that a whitish-yellow exudate around the glans is granulation tissue and is normal and not indicative of infection. It may be observed for 2 to 3 days and should not be removed.*

C. Neonate's bath.
1. Bath is delayed until vital signs and temperature stabilize.
2. Warm water is used for the first 4 days; do not immerse infant in water until umbilical cord stump has been released.
3. When bathing neonate, apply principles of clean-to-dirty areas; wash areas in the following order: eyes, face, ears, head, body, genitals, buttocks.
4. Head is an area of significant heat loss; keep it covered.
D. Determine weight loss over first 24 hours after birth – monitor wet diapers.
E. Assess stools.
1. Meconium stools.
2. Transitional stools.
❖ Goal: To detect complications and provide early treatment.
A. Newborn screening test after first 24 hours for a formula-fed infant or neonate; if mother is breast-feeding, explain importance of returning when infant is 1 week old to obtain blood sample; newborns are screened for the following disorders: galactosemia, hypothyroidism, and sickle cell anemia.
B. Administration of first hepatitis B vaccine before discharge; also, hepatitis B immune globulin is given intramuscularly, if mother is a hepatitis B carrier.
1. Encourage follow-up visits for second and third doses of hepatitis B vaccine and other immunizations.

✔ *NURSING PRIORITY: Explain to parents the importance of returning for a well-baby check when the infant is 2 to 4 weeks old.*

❖ Goal: To promote infant feeding.
B. Breast-feeding.
1. First feeding should occur immediately or within a few hours after birth.
2. Frequent feedings are important initially to establish milk production, often every 1½ to 2 hours.

C. Bottle-feeding.
1. It is not necessary to sterilize the water used to reconstitute infant's formula.
2. The infant should be placed in a semi-upright position for feeding.
3. Never prop the bottle, and always hold the infant.
4. Do not warm bottles or any food for infants in the microwave.

✔ *NURSING PRIORITY: Proportions of formula must not be altered, teach mother to not dilute or expand the amount of formula or concentrate it to provide more calories.*

☀ HOME CARE

❖ Goal: To teach about home phototherapy for mild to moderate jaundice.
A. Place nude infant under bili-lights, exposing all areas to the light except for eyes and genitalia; cover infant's eyes with an opaque mask or eye patch and cover genitalia with a diaper or a disposable face mask (string bikini to expose more skin).
1. Reposition infant every 2 hours to expose as much body surface as possible.
2. Chart pertinent information relating to time phototherapy was started and stopped, maintenance of shielding of the eyes from bili-light, type and intensity of lamp used, distance of light from infant, whether used in combination with an isolette or an open bassinet, and any side effects.

✔ *NURSING PRIORITY: If a face mask is used to cover genitalia, remove the metal nose strip to prevent burning the infant. If a fiberoptic blanket is used, infant's eyes do not need to be covered;*

B. If a fiberoptic blanket is used, should have a covering pad between the infant's skin and the fiberoptic blanket; with this method, the infant may remain in the room with the mother.

HIGH-RISK NEWBORN

Gestational Age Variation

Data Collection

A. Respiratory parameters.
1. Observe respiratory rate, rhythm, and depth.
   a. Initially, rate increases without a change in rhythm.
   b. Flaring of nares and expiratory grunting are early signs of respiratory distress.
2. Increase in apical pulse rate.

3. Subcostal and xiphoid retractions progress to intercostal, substernal, and clavicular retractions.
4. Color.
    a. Progresses from pink to circumoral pallor to circumoral cyanosis to generalized cyanosis.
    b. Increased intensity of acrocyanosis.
5. Progressive respiratory distress.
    a. Chin tug (chin pulled down and in with mouth opening wider—auxiliary muscles of respiration are used).
    b. Abdominal seesaw breathing patterns.
    c. Distinguish between apneic episodes (15 seconds or longer) and irregular breathing (cessation of breathing for 5 to 10 seconds).
6. Falling body temperature.
7. Progressing anoxia leading to cardiac decompensation and failure.
8. Increased muscle flaccidity: frog-like position.

B. Nutrition.
1. Assess readiness and ability to feed: swallowing, gag reflexes.
2. Screen for hypoglycemia.
3. Observe for congenital dysfunction and anomalies related to tracheoesophageal fistula, anal atresia, and metabolic disorders.
4. Check amount and frequency of elimination.
5. Assess for vomiting or regurgitation; a preterm infant's stomach capacity is small, and overfeeding can occur.
6. Check mucous membranes, urine output, and skin turgor to identify fluid and electrolyte imbalances.
    a. Skin turgor over abdomen and inner thighs.
    b. Sunken fontanel.
    c. Urinary output of less than 30 mL/day.

C. Temperature regulation.
1. Assess infant's temperature: frequently done with a skin probe for continuous monitoring of temperature in infants at high risk for complications.
2. Check coolness or warmth of body and extremities.
3. Detect early signs of cold stress.
    a. Increased physical activity and crying.
    b. Increased respiratory rate.
    c. Increased acrocyanosis or generalized cyanosis along with mottling of the skin (cutis marmorata).
    d. Male with descended testes: presence of cremasteric reflex (testes are pulled back up into the inguinal canal on exposure to cold).
4. Monitor infant's temperature.
    a. Axillary temperature: 36.5° C (97.7° F).
    b. Place a temperature skin probe on infant while he or she is in the radiant warmer or isolette.

Nursing Intervention for the High-Risk Newborn

Disorders Acquired During and After Birth (Table 21-2)

❖ **Goal:** To maintain respiratory functioning.
A. Provide gentle physical stimulation to remind infant to breathe.
1. Gently rub the infant's back.
2. Lightly tap the infant's feet.
B. Ensure patency of respiratory tract.
1. Maintain open airway by means of nasal, oral, or pharyngeal suctioning.
2. Position to promote oxygenation.
    a. Elevate head 10 degrees with neck slightly extended by placement of a small folded towel under the shoulders.
    b. Flex and abduct infant's arms and place at sides.
    c. Avoid diapers or adhere them loosely.
    d. Turn side to side every 1 to 2 hours.
    e. Do not place in prone position.
C. Assist infant's respiratory efforts.
1. Monitor oxygen pressure. Avoid high concentrations of oxygen for prolonged periods: leads to complications of bronchopulmonary dysplasia.
2. Continuous positive airway pressure (CPAP) counteracts the tendency of the alveoli to collapse by providing continuous distending airway pressure and is administered either by endotracheal tube or nasal prongs.

❖ **Goal:** To provide adequate nutrition.
A. Detect hypoglycemia and treat immediately: Administer 5% dextrose in water intravenously if infant is unable to tolerate oral feeding.
B. Oral feeding: initial feeding.
1. Use sterile water: 1 to 2 mL for a small infant.
2. Use preemie nipple to conserve infant's energy.
3. Because of small size of infant's stomach, feedings are small in amount and increased in frequency.
C. Orogastric tube feedings.
1. Usually administered by continuous flow of formula with an infusion pump (kangaroo pump) when the infant is:
    a. Having severe respiratory distress.
    b. Too immature and weak to suck.
    c. Tired and fatigues easily when a preemie nipple is used.
2. Placement and insertion of orogastric feeding tube.
    a. Position infant on the back or toward the right side with the head and chest slightly elevated.
    b. Measure correct length of insertion by marking on the catheter the distance from the tip of the nose to the ear lobe to the tip of the sternum.
    c. Lubricate tube with sterile water and slowly

insert catheter into mouth and down the esophagus into the stomach.

   d. Test for placement of the tube by aspirating stomach contents or injecting 0.5 to 1.0 mL of air for the premature infant (up to 5 mL for larger infants) and auscultating the abdomen for the sound.

   e. Before infusing a feeding by gravity into stomach, check for residual; this is done by aspirating and measuring amount left in stomach from previous feeding; often, the residual amount is subtracted from the current feeding so that overfeeding does not occur.

   f. If feeding is not continuous, remove tubing by pinching or clamping it and withdrawing it rapidly.

   g. Burp infant after feeding by turning head or positioning him or her on the right side.

D. Hyperalimentation (total parenteral nutrition) may be ordered to provide complete nutrition through an indwelling catheter threaded into the vena cava.

E. Detect complications that arise with feeding the preterm infant as a result of:

1. Weak or absent sucking and swallowing reflexes.
2. Necessity of high caloric content with a very small stomach capacity.
3. Poor gag reflex, leading to aspiration.
4. Increased incidence of vomiting and development of abdominal distention.
5. Inability to absorb essential nutrients.
6. Excessive loss of water through evaporation from the skin and respiratory tract.

❖ **Goal:** To maintain warmth and temperature control (see maintaining temperature of normal newborn).

A. Oxygen and air should be warmed and humidified.

B. Maintain abdominal skin temperature at 36.1° to 36.7° C (97° to 98° F); axillary temperature 36.5° C (97.8° F).

C. Monitor infant's temperature continuously; make sure that temperature probe is set on control panel, probe is in contact with infant's skin, and all safety precautions are maintained.

D. Prevent rapid warming or cooling; warming process is increased gradually over a period of 2 to 4 hours.

E. Infant may need extra clothing or need to be wrapped in an extra blanket for additional warmth.

TABLE 21-2	DISORDERS ACQUIRED DURING AND AFTER BIRTH		
	Trauma	**Peripheral Nerve Injuries**	**Neonatal Sepsis**
Assessment	Soft tissue injury. Caput succedaneum. Cephalhematoma. Injury to bone: Fractured clavicle is the most common; often occurs with a large-sized infant.	Temporary paralysis of the facial nerve is the most common. Affected side of the face is smooth. Eye may stay open. Mouth droops at the corner. Forehead cannot be wrinkled. Possible difficulty sucking. Brachial palsy: a partial or complete paralysis of the nerve fibers of the brachial plexus. Cannot elevate or abduct the arm. Abnormal arm position or diminished arm movements.	Apathy, lethargy, low-grade temperature. Poor feeding, abdominal distention, diarrhea. Cyanosis, irregular respirations, apnea. Hyperbilirubinemia. Infant often described as "not acting right" CBC, chest x-ray film, and viral studies **TORCH** blood screening.
Nursing Interventions	1. Place affected arm against chest wall with hand lying across chest. 2. Position is held by a figure-8 stockinette around the arm and chest. 3. Pick infant up carefully; shoulder should not be pressed toward middle of body. 4. Affected side should not be placed in gown or undershirt.	Facial nerve palsy: 1. Apply eye patch; may use artificial tears to prevent corneal irritation. 2. Provide support during feeding; infant may not latch on to nipple well. Brachial nerve palsy 1. Keep arm abducted and externally rotated with elbow flexed. 2. Arm is raised to shoulder height, and elbow is flexed 90 degrees.	1. Prenatal prevention, maternal screening for STDs, and assessment of rubella titers. 2. Maintenance of sterile technique. 3. Prophylactic antibiotic treatment. 4. Possible cesarean delivery for mother with genital herpes.

CBC, Complete blood count; *TORCH*, toxoplasmosis, other (congenital syphilis and viruses) rubella, cytomegalovirus, and herpes virus.

Respiratory Distress

❋ *Hyaline membrane disease* (HMD), also referred to as respiratory distress syndrome (RDS), occurs as a result of the deficiency of surfactant that lines the alveoli.

❋ *Meconium aspiration syndrome* occurs when the fetus passes meconium in utero and aspirates the meconium into the lungs, which leads to obstruction in the small airway passages.

Data Collection

A. Tachypnea: more than 60 breaths/min.
B. Apneic spells (in excess of 15 seconds).
C. Abnormal breath sounds: rales and rhonchi.
D. Chest retraction.
E. Chin tug: noticed on inspiration; mouth open, lips apart.
F. Flaring of the nares.
G. Expiratory grunting.
H. Meconium aspiration - meconium stained amniotic fluid.

> ✔ *NURSING PRIORITY: Grunting is an ominous sign and indicates impending need for respiratory assistance; most often, mucus needs to be cleared from airway.*

Complications

A. Hypoxia, acidosis caused by alveolar hypoventilation.
B. Bronchopulmonary dysplasia: chronic stiff, noncompliant lungs.

Treatment

A. Respiratory distress syndrome.
  1. CPAP is the primary treatment.
  2. Administration of surfactant through the airway into the infant's lungs.
B. Meconium aspiration.
  1. Administration of oxygen with humidification.
  2. Postural drainage and percussion; antibiotic therapy.
  3. Acid-base imbalance correction, if needed.

Nursing Intervention

❖ **Goal:** To promote oxygenation and respiratory functioning.
A. Administer a steroid (betamethasone) to mother at least 48 hours before delivery and administer surfactant to neonate after delivery to stimulate surfactant production.
B. Refer to nursing intervention for the high-risk newborn.

Cleft Lip and Cleft Palate

❋ *Cleft lip* is a fissure or split in the upper lip, which may vary from a slight notch to a complete separation extending into the nostril; may be unilateral or bilateral.

❋ *Cleft palate* is a fissure or a split in the roof of the mouth (palate).

Data Collection

A. Visible at birth on an incompletely formed lip.
B. Sucking difficulties and breathing problems with cleft palate.
C. Increased incidence of upper respiratory tract infection and otitis media.
D. Later problems related to speech and hearing difficulties with cleft palate.

Treatment

A. Surgical: closure of lip defect usually precedes treatment for a cleft palate (which is done in stages).
B. Long-term care management: speech therapy, orthodontics; frequent occurrences of otitis media.

Nursing Intervention

❖ **Goal:** To provide preoperative care.
A. Maintain nutrition.
  1. Use a large-holed nipple or a modified nipple to increase infant's ability to obtain milk without sucking.
  2. Feed slowly.
  3. Bubble and burp frequently (after every 15 to 30 mL).
  4. Rinse cleft with water after each feeding to help prevent infection.
  5. Do not place infant on pillow, elevate head of bed, or put the pillow under the mattress.
B. Prepare parents for newborn's surgery.
  1. Encourage parents to position infant flat on back or on side to accustom infant to the postoperative positioning.
  2. Encourage parents to place infant in arm restraints periodically before hospital admission, so they become familiar with restriction of arm motion after surgery.
  3. Encourage parents to feed infant with the same method that will be used after surgery.
❖ **Goal:** To provide postoperative care.
A. Prevent trauma to suture line.
  1. Position infant on back or side and elevate head (infant seat).
  2. Restrain arms with soft elbow restraints.
  3. Cleanse suture line gently after each feeding; use cotton-tipped applicator with prescribed solution and roll along the suture line; may apply antibiotic ointment.

4. Prevent any crust or scab formation on lip and suture line.
5. May use protective lip device.

B. Maintain a patent airway and facilitate breathing.
  1. Assess for respiratory distress.
  2. Observe for swelling of the nose, tongue, and lips.

C. Provide adequate nutrition.
  1. Feed in an upright, sitting position.
  2. Feed slowly and burp/bubble at frequent intervals.

D. Provide discharge teaching to parents.
  1. Encourage parents to cuddle and play with infant to decrease crying and prevent trauma to suture line.
  2. Teach feeding, cleansing, and restraining procedures.

Esophageal Atresia with Tracheoesophageal Fistula

✳ **Proximal end of esophagus ends in a blind pouch and the lower segment connects to the trachea.**

Data Collection

A. Characterized by the classic 3 Cs: *choking, coughing,* and *cyanosis.*
B. Excessive frothy saliva and constant drooling.
C. Aspiration is a complication, especially during feeding.

Nursing Intervention

> ✔ **NURSING PRIORITY:** *When there is any suspicion of possible esophageal problems, infant should receive nothing by mouth (have NPO status) until further evaluation can be done.*

❖ **Goal:** To provide preoperative care.
A. Maintain patent airway.
  1. Supine position with head elevated on an inclined plane of at least 30 degrees.
  2. Suction nasopharynx.
  3. Observe for symptoms of respiratory distress.
  4. Maintain NPO status.
B. Prepare parents for infant's surgery.
❖ **Goal:** To provide postoperative care.
A. Maintain respirations and prevent respiratory complications.
  1. Administer oxygen.
  2. Oral suction of secretions and position for optimum ventilation.
  3. Maintain care of chest tubes.
  4. Administer antibiotics.
  5. Place in warm, high-humidity isolette.
  6. Maintain nasogastric suctioning.
B. Provide adequate nutrition.
  1. Gastrostomy feedings may be started on the second or third postoperative day.

2. Oral feedings may be delayed until 2 weeks after surgery.
3. Meet oral sucking needs by offering infant a pacifier.

Imperforate Anus

✳ **An imperforate anus is an absence of the anal opening.**

Data Collection

A. Absence of meconium.
B. No anal opening.
C. Gradual increase in abdominal distention.

Nursing Intervention

❖ **Goal:** To identify anal malformation.
A. Detect increasing abdominal distention.
B. Inspect anal area for opening.

> ✔ **NURSING PRIORITY:** *Record the first passage of meconium stool. If infant does not pass stool within 24 hours, further assessment is required.*

❖ **Goal:** To provide postoperative care.
A. Prevent infection by maintaining good perineal care and keeping operative site clean and dry, especially after passage of stool and urine.
B. Do not take temperatures rectally.
C. Place infant in side-lying prone position.
D. May have a colostomy.

Neural Tube Defects

✳ **A neural tube defect (spina bifida) results in midline defects and closure of the spinal cord (may be noncystic or cystic); most common site is lumbosacral area.**

Data Collection

A. Types.
  1. Spina bifida occulta – bony defect (bone of spine does not cover spinal cord).
  2. Spina bifida cystica.
    a. Meningocele: a sac-like cyst of meninges filled with spinal fluid that protrudes through a defect in the bony part of the spine.
    b. Myelomeningocele: a sac-like cyst containing meninges, spinal fluid, and a portion of the spinal cord with its nerves that protrudes through a defect in the vertebral column; other defect most frequently associated with this is hydrocephalus.

Treatment

A. Surgical: closure of defect with 24 to 48 hours to decrease risk of infection, relieve pressure, repair sac, and possibly insert a shunt.

Nursing Intervention

> **NURSING PRIORITY:** *Correct positioning of the infant is critical in preventing damage to the sac, as well as in providing nursing care after surgery.*

❖ **Goal:** To provide preoperative care.
A. Prevent and protect sac from drying, rupturing, and infection.
1. Position infant prone on abdomen.
2. Avoid touching sac.
3. Provide meticulous skin care after voiding and bowel movements.
4. Often, sterile, normal saline soaks on a nonadherent dressing may be used to prevent drying.
B. Detect early development of hydrocephalus.
1. Measure head and check circumference frequently.
2. Check fontanels for bulging and separation of suture line.
C. Monitor elimination function.
1. Note whether urine is dripping or is retained.
2. Indwelling catheter may be inserted, intermittent catheterization may be done, or credé method may be used at regular intervals.
3. Assess for bowel function: Glycerin suppository may be ordered to stimulate meconium passage.
❖ **Goal:** To provide postoperative care.
A. Prevent trauma and infection at the surgical site.
1. Place infant in same position (prone on abdomen) as before surgery.
2. Continue to provide scrupulous skin care as described under preoperative goals.
B. Assess neurological status frequently for indications of increasing intracranial pressure, development of hydrocephalus, or early signs of infection.
1. Continue to measure head circumference daily.
2. Perform frequent neurological checks.
C. Provide parents with education in regard to positioning, feeding, skin care, elimination procedures, and range of motion exercises.
1. Encourage and facilitate parental bonding.
2. Refer to community and social agencies for financial and social support.
3. Encourage long-range planning and support of parents for long-term rehabilitation of infant.

Neonatal Sepsis

✳ **An infection in the neonate can be caused by maternal antepartal or intrapartal infection.**

Data Collection

A. Apathy, lethargy, poor temperature control.
B. Poor feeding, abdominal distention, diarrhea.
C. Cyanosis, irregular respirations, apnea.
D. Infant often described as "not acting right"; may be irritable

Nursing Intervention

❖ **Goal:** To prevent neonatal sepsis by prenatal prevention; maternal screening for sexually transmitted diseases and assessment of rubella titers.
A. TORCH (toxoplasmosis, other [congenital syphilis and viruses], rubella, cytomegalovirus, and herpes simplex virus) syndrome is discussed as it relates to the infant and adult in Chapter 17.

Isoimmune Hemolytic Disease of the Newborn

✳ **An antigen-antibody response causing destruction of fetal RBCs as a result of maternal sensitization of fetal RBC antigens and subsequent transfer of the resulting antibodies to the fetus.**

Data Collection

A. Clinical manifestations: ABO incompatibility.
1. Jaundice occurs in a cephalocaudal direction: It begins at the face, advances downward on the body to trunk and extremities, and finally to the palms and the soles of the feet.

> **NURSING PRIORITY:** *Press skin against a bony prominence (e.g., chin, nose) to detect early color change.*

2. Anemia.
B. Diagnostics.
1. Prenatal screening and prevention: Rh incompatibility.
a. Administration of $Rh_o(D)$ immune globulin to prevent Rh sensitization in first pregnancy of Rh-negative mother (see prenatal care).
b. Indirect Coombs' test: performed on the mother's serum.
c. Postdelivery detection (Rh incompatibility): direct Coombs' test on cord blood
d. $Rh_o(D)$ immune globulin is administered within 72 hours of an Rh-negative mother's delivery of an Rh-positive infant.

Nursing Intervention

❖ **Goal:** To recognize jaundice and distinguish the physiological type (which occurs within 48 to 72 hours) from the pathological type (which occurs within 24 hours).

A. Prenatal monitoring of maternal-fetal status.
B. Identify high-risk mother.
C. Monitor bilirubin levels in the newborn.

 ## Infant of a Diabetic Mother

Data Collection

A. Clinical manifestations
   1. Puffy, cushingoid appearance, with round cheeks and stocky neck.
   2. Enlarged heart, liver, and spleen.
   3. Rapid, irregular respirations.
   4. Increased Moro reflex and irritability on slight stimulation or lethargy at times.
B. Common complications.
   1. Hypoglycemia: blood glucose level of below 36 mg/dl within 1½ to 4 hours after birth.
      a. Lethargy, irritability, hypocalcemia.
      b. High-pitched cry.
      c. Twitching, jitteriness, seizures.
      d. Apneic spells and abdominal distention.

   2. Respiratory distress syndrome.
   3. Polycythemia.
   4. Birth trauma caused by excessive size.
   5. Congenital defects, specifically cardiac (patent ductus arteriosus is most common) and central nervous system defects (anencephaly, myelomeningocele, and hydrocephalus).

> ✓ **NURSING PRIORITY:** *Prolonged hypoglycemia can cause irreversible brain damage.*

Nursing Intervention

❖ **Goal:** To monitor glucose levels.
A. Frequently check blood glucose levels.
B. Minimize trauma to heel site by performing heel stick correctly.
   1. Warm heel for 5 to 10 minutes before sticking.
   2. Cleanse site with alcohol and dry before sticking.
   3. The lateral heel is the site of choice.

Study Questions: Newborn

1. What equipment should the nurse have available immediately after birth to assist the infant with the initial respiratory effort?
   1. Stethoscope and suction catheter.
   2. Heated crib and a stocking cap.
   3. Bulb syringe and oxygen.
   4. Oxygen and stethoscope.
2. The nurse is assessing a newborn for the presence of a caput succedaneum. What findings would confirm the presence of this condition?
   1. Swelling confined to the parietal areas of the skull.
   2. Diffuse edema under the scalp.
   3. A collection of blood under the scalp.
   4. Petechial hemorrhages in the conjunctivae.
3. What signs would a nurse observe in a newborn with respiratory distress?
   1. Flaring of the nares, grunting, and chest wall retractions.
   2. Lusty crying, heaving chest wall, and flailing arms.
   3. Respiratory rate of 50 breaths per minute, pulse rate of 166 beats per minute, and sneezing.
   4. Uncontrolled crying, acrocyanosis, and respiratory rate of 60 breaths per minute.
4. The nurse is assessing the newborn. What nursing assessment data would cause the most concern?
   1. Has loud crying with periods of light sleep.
   2. Has a blood glucose level of 75 mg/dl.
   3. Turns dusky and cyanotic when crying.
   4. Acrocyanosis is present 4 hours after birth.
5. The newborn is given vitamin K soon after birth. What is the purpose of this medication?

   1. Is used as a prophylactic measure because the newborn does not have an immediate supply.
   2. Assists with building iron stores in the blood of the newborn.
   3. Helps to stabilize the electrolytes in the newborn's system.
   4. Prevents jaundice by breaking down the newborn's bilirubin.
6. To meet the goal of promoting infant feeding in a breastfed baby, the nurse should teach the mother to: Select all that apply:
   _____ 1. Feed the baby on a 3- to 4-hour schedule.
   _____ 2. Alternate breast and formula for each feeding.
   _____ 3. Stop breast-feeding if her nipples get sore.
   _____ 4. Maintain demand breast-feeding for the first 4 weeks.
   _____ 5. Drink lots of fluids and get adequate rest.
   _____ 6. Offer a pacifier between feedings to meet sucking needs.
7. What is a characteristic finding when performing a nursing assessment on a newborn with hypoglycemia?
   1. Acrocyanosis.
   2. Respirations of 50 breaths per minute.
   3. Increased irritability.
   4. Decreased pulse rate.
8. What nursing measures are important to decrease the loss of body heat in a newborn?
   1. Keep the infant bundled with a stocking cap on the head.
   2. Regulate the room temperature between 68° F and 70° F.

3 Keep the infant in a warmer for the first 8 hours after birth.

4 Assess the core temperature and respirations every 3 hours.

9. What is a nursing measure to reduce the possibility of infection in the newborn?

1 Keep the cribs at least 3 feet apart in the nursery.

2 Wash hands before and after care delivered to each newborn.

3 Wash hands before diaper changes.

4 Decrease visiting times to only 1 hour and for groups of three people.

10. The nurse is observing a new mother breastfeed her infant. To decrease the amount of air the infant swallows, what would the nurse suggest to the mother?

1 Place the newborn on the back with the head turned to the left.

2 Offer the infant the pacifier after each feeding.

3 Burp or bubble the infant after the first few minutes of feeding.

4 Limit the infant to only 10 minutes of nursing at one feeding.

11. In which situation would the nurse anticipate $Rh_o(D)$ immune globulin human (Rh_oGAM) to be given?

1 When the mother is Rh positive.

2 Within 48 hours after delivery.

3 After a postpartal hemorrhage.

4 When the mother is Rh negative.

12. What laboratory test is important to obtain on the newborn in order to detect complications?

1 Alpha-fetoprotein.

2 Urinalysis.

3 Phenylketonuria (PKU).

4 Serum iron.

13. Which behavior exhibited by the mother with her newborn would the nurse identify as maladaptive regarding parent-infant attachment?

1 Cuddles newborn close to her breast.

2 Looks at the face of the newborn, while talking.

3 Explains to the nurse how the newborn is feeding.

4 Seldom looks at newborn when family is visiting.

14. The clinic nurse observes that a 3-day-old baby girl is jaundiced. A bilirubin level is drawn, and it is 11.4 mg/dl. What causes this bilirubin level?

1 Physiologic jaundice.

2 Hemolytic disease.

3 Erythroblastosis fetalis.

4 Sepsis.

15. The nurse assigned to the nursery understands the importance of keeping the newborn swaddled in a warm blanket in order to prevent heat loss because:

1 Chilling leads to increased heat production and greater oxygen needs.

2 The newborn's metabolic rate is decreased.

3 Evaporation will affect the newborn's ability to feed.

4 The newborn will sleep more comfortably.

16. The newborn's mother is concerned about the shape of the baby's head after delivery. She states that it looks like a "cone head." The most appropriate response by the nurse is the following:

1 "You don't need to worry about it. It is perfectly normal after birth."

2 "It is molding caused by the pressure during birth and will disappear in a few days."

3 "I will report it to the health care provider and he will order a diagnostic scan."

4 "It is a collection of blood related to the trauma of delivery and will absorb in a few weeks."

17. The nurse is responsible for documenting the first meconium stool the newborn passes. If the newborn does not have a stool in the first 24 hours of life, the nurse should first:

1 Insert a rectal thermometer to facilitate the process.

2 Inspect the anal area for an opening.

3 Monitor the vital signs for an increase in temperature.

4 Increase oral feeding to stimulate passage of stool.

18. The best way for the nurse to maintain the safety of the newborn in the hospital is to:

1 Have the mother come to the nursery to pick up the baby for feedings.

2 Take the baby to the mother's room for rooming-in.

3 Ask the mother her name and social security number.

4 Compare the name band information of the mother and baby.

19. A newborn has a Plastibell circumcision. In reinforcing the teaching with the parents, which instructions would you give the parents for care of the circumcised penis? Select all that apply:

_____1 Remove any exudates that form during the first 24 hours.

_____2 Wash penis gently during diaper change to remove urine and feces.

_____3 Apply sterile petroleum gauze to the penis for first 24 hours.

_____4 Clean the glans with alcohol to promote healing.

_____5 Avoid positioning the infant on the abdomen during the healing process.

_____6 Report any edema; purulent, malodorous discharge; increased temperature.

20. The nurse understands that meconium is:

1 Well formed and dark in color.

2 Often passed in the first 4 hours of life.

3 Light in color and loose.

4 Passed within the first 2 days of life.

Answers and rationales to these questions are in the section at the end of the book titled Chapter Study Questions: Answers and Rationales.

Chapter Study Questions: Answers and Rationales

CHAPTER 2: HEALTH IMPLICATIONS ACROSS THE LIFE SPAN

1. ① If there is dislodgement of a radiation implant, there should always be a lead container and tongs in the room to place the radiation source. Getting the client away from the radiation source is most important to prevent skin irradiation. The room does not need to be evacuated. If gloves are ever used, they must be lead-lined.

2. ② DPT, polio, and hepatitis B as well as the influenza vaccination are required immunizations by age 6 months. Varicella and MMR are not given until the infant is 1-year-old.

3. ④ Recommendations are for the infant to be kept on formula until age 6 months, if tolerated. This decreases the incidence of allergies. Rice cereal should be the first solid offered.

4. ① A 9-month-old infant should be able to sit alone without support. The other options—shows no interest in walking, anterior fontanel remains open, and does not respond to name—are expected at this stage of growth.

5. ③ The primary difference between benign and malignant tumors is the ability of the malignant tumor to invade adjacent tissues and metastasize. Benign tumors tend to be encapsulated, and both types of tumors can lead to death; benign tumors can expand and affect normal organ function.

6. ②, ③, ⑤, ⑥ Adverse effects of antineoplastic drugs can be classified as acute, delayed, or chronic. Acute toxicity includes anorexia, nausea, vomiting, dysrhythmias, and allergic reactions. Delayed side effects include stomatitis, alopecia, and bone marrow depression. Chronic toxicity involves organ damage. Urinary problems are often cystitis and nephrotoxicity. Drugs do no commonly cause problems with peripheral edema or change the specific gravity of the urine.

7. ② The skin in the area of radiation is sensitive to sunlight; it is important to leave the markings on the skin so the radiologist will know the boundaries of the treatment. There is no dietary implications after radiation therapy.

8. ① Physiological needs must be addressed first. The other options may be used for this client; however, the vomiting and dehydration must be addressed first. The daily weight and small meals are appropriate; however, the nausea and vomiting have to be addressed first.

9. ③ Recognition of familiar faces begins around age 4 months, especially recognition of the mother's face.

10. ② The fluid balance needs to be carefully monitored in order to determine changes in output as well as fluid retention. Baseline fluid balance should be determined when the client is started on chemotherapy.

11. ② The client should be encouraged to eat fresh fruits and vegetables (e.g., fresh fruits, fruit juices, tomatoes) to increase his potassium intake, because the diuretic causes loss of potassium.

12. ① The wound should be cleansed to prevent infection. After taking immediate care of the wound, the client needs to be evaluated regarding the need for a tetanus injection.

CHAPTER 3: NURSING CONCEPTS

1. ③ To avoid potential skin problems associated with immobility, it is important to make sure there is no pressure on bony prominences. A circulating air mattress would provide this relief, and/or an egg crate mattress would assist to prevent this pressure. The client does not need to be bathed twice a day. Indwelling catheters should be inserted only when accurate measurement of urine is necessary or when the client cannot void. Bed rest is not an indication for an indwelling catheter. Activity schedules will be developed when the client becomes mobile—ambulating twice a day, physical therapy, etc.

2. ③ Errors in charting on a paper chart should never be obliterated, recopied, or covered with correction fluid. When the erroneous information is not legible, it raises questions as to what the person was trying to cover up.

3. ② If the client is nauseated and vomiting, he or she should not be offered any further fluids by mouth until the cause of the vomiting has been identified or the nausea has subsided. The client should be placed in either semi-Fowler's position or on his or her side and the RN should be notified.

4. ① This is the best descriptor of the event without including opinions. The nurse does not know that the client fell out of bed; he was on the floor at the side of the bed. It is important to not place blame regarding the incident.

5. ① Constipation and urinary retention are common side

effects, especially in older adult clients. The client should be advised to increase the intake of fiber and possibly use a stool softener to prevent problems with constipation. The hydrocodone is a combination drug that contains acetaminophen, additional acetaminophen should not be used. There is no need to return to the clinic to determine toxic levels. The medication does not cause changes in the skin or increased bruising.

6. ③ Since the client does not have control of their body needs during surgery, basic needs need to be addressed prior to and during the surgery. This will prevent over distention of the bladder and or incontinence during surgery.

7. ①, ④, ⑤   Frequent assessments of basic needs are required at least every two hours. Continuation of restraints requires a physician order every twenty-four hours (not every shift). Restraints should never be tied to the side rails, because doing so can cause injury to the client if the side rail is lowered without untying the restraint. Restraints should be tied with a knot that can be quickly released. Frequent assessment and documentation should be completed to determine whether the client's condition has improved enough to remove the restraints.

8. ④ If there is too much strain on the suture line, the area will pull apart, which is dehiscence. Evisceration is extrusion of the intestine through the incision, which may occur after the dehiscence.

9. ③ It is important to relieve pain around the clock and before the client experiences severe pain. If the nurse depends on it to be PRN, frequently the client is already in severe pain before they call to request the medication.

10. ② Healing by first intention is when the wound edges are well approximated and are healing well. Secondary intention is when the wound heals from the inside out by formation of granulation tissue.

11. ④ If an incision is dehisced or open, there is an increased risk of an evisceration, or extrusion of intestine. Placing the client on bed rest will help to prevent further pressure on the incision. The RN should be notified immediately.

12. ① The primary purpose of turn, cough, and deep breath is to prevent respiratory complications.

13. ④ The informed consent means that the client was provided information regarding the surgery and understands the surgery and the risk involved. It is the doctor's responsibility to initially discuss with the client the surgery and the risk involved. The nurse should validate the client understands the risk involved prior to witnessing the client's signature on the consent form.

14. ① The older adult client has decreased respiratory re-

serve and does not breath as deeply as younger adults.

15. ③ The knee and the anterior iliac spine will be areas of pressure when the client is prone, or on his abdomen. This position may be utilized for clients who have had an amputation or who are recovering or healing from a pressure area on the coccyx.

CHAPTER 4: PHARMACOLOGY

1. ① Frequently, the older adult client is receiving several different medications. The client does not excrete them differently. Medications are still primarily metabolized and excreted by the liver and the kidneys; however, these organs may not work as efficiently as in the younger client.

2. ③ The client will receive two tablets in the morning and two at noon for a total of four tablets for the day.

3. ③ If the order is for 300 mg and 500 mg is on hand, then divide 300 by 500, which equals 0.6 mL.

4. ① If there is 40 mg/mL and the desired dose is 60 mg, divide 60 by 40, which equals 1.5 mL or 1 1/2 vials.

5. ③ It is important to make sure the medication administration record and the primary health care provider's order correlate. Checking the client's ID band verifies that you have the correct client.

6. ③ The dose should be recorded as "not taken" and the nurse should waste the poured dose. If the dose is a controlled substance, the wasted dose must be witnessed by another nurse. Checking the medication order for changes before accessing the medication helps to eliminate waste.

7. ② Liquid oral medications are already in solution and are thus absorbed more rapidly.

8. ④ Medications are absorbed. Elimination is when the body excretes the medication.

9. ④ The medication administration record should be reviewed for current physician's orders. Medication administration records are routinely reviewed to determine currency of medication orders. The client's name and hospital number are checked to validate client identification prior to administration of the medication. The nurse should check the medication for the expiration date when she prepares the medication, and the physician will order the route of administration.

10. ② Only one antibiotic should be administered at a time, therefore if the medications are given on the same hour the IV tubing will need to be flushed between the medication administration. Both drugs should be administered at the time ordered.

11. ① Intradermal is under the skin; if it is injected further, it becomes a subcutaneous injection. A 25- to 28- gauge needle is used.

12. ④ The tip of the applicator should not touch the eye, and

the medication should be placed in the middle of the lower conjunctival sac. The client should open and close his or her eye after the medication is instilled.

CHAPTER 5: HOMEOSTASIS

1. ③ When a client is taking any corticosteroid, it is important for the client to continue the medication schedule, and the medication should be taken with food. The body is dependent on the level of steroid intake to maintain homeostasis and discontinuing the medication could have very serious side effects. A side effect is fluid retention, therefore the client needs to watch his fluid intake.

2. ① An anaphylactic reaction is the most severe type of reaction, whether it is to a medication such as penicillin, or to an insect bite. It can be fatal if medication, antihistamines or epinephrine is not available to reverse the reaction.

3. ② Autoimmune is the term used for diseases that alter the body's immune system where the body has difficulty recognizing itself. Therefore, these diseases are called autoimmune diseases. Option 1 refers to an anaphylactic reaction, option 3 is diseases that affect the normal function of the immune system, as in clients with AIDS. Option 4 is the normal response of the body to an immunization – MMR, etc.

4. ① All corticosteroids are anti-inflammatory medications. These medications decrease the ability of the body to fight infection. Corticosteriods do not affect coagulation and do not play a roll in anaphylaxis. Clients are generally on decreased fluids because steroids increase body retention of fluid.

5. ④ Active acquired is a vaccination. Natural active is when the client has the disease. An example of passive immunity is the immunity that is transferred from the mother to the infant.

6. ④ The body produces antibodies in response to an invasion of pathological organisms or antigens. When a child receives a vaccination, antibodies are produced that recognize the antigen the next time the child is exposed and prevents the development of the disease (measles, chicken pox).

7. ③ Dehydration frequently precedes the development of fluid deficit. Orthostatic hypotension is an early sign of problems with fluid deficit. Peripheral edema, weight gain are indications of retention of fluid. Dilute urine in normal amounts indicates adequate fluid balance. When fluid deficit occurs, hypovolemia may develop and there is an increased risk of the client developing low blood pressure and consequences of poor cardiac output.

8. ② The best way to determine the adequacy of body fluids is to measure the daily weight at the same time each day. Sudden increases or loss of body weight is most often due to fluid loss or retention.

9. ④ 1+ edema is lowest level, with 4+ being severe pitting edema.

10. ① The kidney is responsible for maintaining the fluid and electrolyte balance in the body.

11. ① Fever increases the body's loss of fluid, therefore it is important to encourage fluids in the client who has a fever. Tachycardia would be more of an issue than bradycardia. The question states the client has a fever and does not provide further information, therefore the client would not be at risk for fluid retention but for fluid loss.

12. ③ Dry, flushed skin is typically of a client who is experiencing a fever and fluid loss, which may be the beginning of dehydration.

13. ③ Dry mucous membranes and confusion are cardinal signs of dehydration in an older adult client. The nurse should further evaluate the client regarding a problem with fluid deficit. If a problem with fluid balance identified, then it would be important to evaluate the client's serum lab values for electrolyte balance.

14. ② The very young and the older adult (over 65 years) are more susceptible to fluid changes. These two clients frequently do not have adequate compensatory mechanisms to deal with sudden changes in fluid balance. The older adult client frequently has chronic conditions that affect the ability to compensate for sudden changes in fluid status.

15. ④ Anytime there is a risk of body fluids being splattered, the nurse should wear protective eye gear. A mask but not protective eye ware is required of the client with droplet precautions. Droplet precautions are used when the organism is transmitted via respiratory droplets.

16. ④ Respiratory acidosis is most often the result of inadequate ventilation. There is an increase in the retention of carbon dioxide. Oxygen does not play a factor in respiratory acidosis; the initial problem is the carbon dioxide. Stimulating the postoperative client to cough and deep breath will increases the loss of carbon dioxide and improve ventilation.

17. ① The human immunodeficiency virus is most often transmitted via unprotected sexual contact. The other options are methods of transfer, however, the most common is via sexual transmission.

18. ② A priority problem with an immunocompromised client is the development of infections. The client does not have an intact immune system to resist the infection. The other options are important, but not as important as preventing infection.

19. ④ The aminoglycoside classification of antibiotics causes neurotoxicity resulting in ototoxicity, as well as nephrotoxicity resulting in renal problems. It will be important for the nurse to observe the client's

response and interactions to determine if the client is experiencing any problem with hearing.

20. ①, ②, ⑤ Contact precautions would require the nurse to:

1. _✓_ Wear clean gloves to remove the old dressing.

2. _✓_ Put on a gown when entering the room.

5. _✓_ Leave all extra dressing supplies in the room.

A face shield is not necessary unless splattering of fluids is anticipated. The gown and mask should be disposed of in the client's room; they should not be removed from the room. The stethoscope and scissors should not be taken into the client's room.

CHAPTER 6: PSYCHIATRIC NURSING CONCEPTS AND CARE

1. ① Physiological needs must be taken care of first; it is important to determine the extent of client injuries, check vital signs, and establish if the client is stable or unstable. The client is exhibiting symptoms of elder abuse, but assessment data must be obtained before further action can be taken.

2. ② Physiological needs are a priority for a confused client. They often will forget to eat and not remember when and where to eat or bathe, for example. After the physiological needs are met, then safety and security would be the next level.

3. ① An interpreter is preferred over family members. A father might not feel comfortable discussing his symptoms if his daughter is interpreting. Spiritual and comfort needs will be addressed after the physiological needs are met.

4. ② The client's background and history of drug abuse raise historical issues in the nurse's past that she may not have dealt with. The derogatory comments are a defense mechanism to help her avoid her unresolved family issues.

5. ③ It is very important to be direct and honest but not too overly friendly with a paranoid client. Touching should be avoided because it may be misinterpreted as a threat (delusion of persecution).

6. ① It is important to determine the source of the anxiety and then intervene to prevent it from escalating, which means not leaving the client alone. Administration of medications would occur after you have evaluated the situation. If you restrain the client at this point, the client's anxiety may escalate.

7. ①, ②, ③ The client is demonstrating paranoid behavior, which necessitates an approach that is matter-of-fact, accepting of the client's statements in a nonjudgmental way, and listening attentively to the issue. Options 4, 5, and 6 do not help the paranoid client gain trust to talk with the nurse.

8. ② During a depressive episode, there is a general slowing down of body systems and behavior (e.g., anorexia, sad affect, psychomotor retardation, lack of social interaction, and poor grooming).

9. ③ It is important to maintain consistency in the staff caring for a client at the end of life. This helps to prevent feelings of abandonment and maintains continuity of care and communication with family members.

10. ① Classic symptoms of schizophrenia include disturbances in perception, which are characterized by hallucinations, delusions, and illusions. Other symptoms include inappropriate affect, thought disorder, difficulty relating to others, and disorganized purposeless activity.

11. ③ Symptoms of Parkinson's disease (e.g., shuffling gait, cogwheel rigidity, pill-rolling tremor) are characteristic of some of the extrapyramidal side effects of antipsychotic medications, such as chlorpromazine (Thorazine).

12. ② Safety is a concern when a client experiences an auditory hallucination, as he may hear a voice that tells him to do something harmful or inappropriate.

13. ③ Do not offer advice or false reassurance. The nurse can encourage the family to share experiences and memories. Encourage family members to hold the client's hand and talk with her. The imminent death should not be discussed in the client's presence. Sympathizing and giving of advice are not appropriate.

14. ③ It is helpful and supportive to the family who may feel overwhelmed with the care of a family member with Alzheimer's disease. Prioritizing care and supporting them for their efforts along with providing respite care are important nursing measures. Option 4 is important for safety but would be inclusive in option 3.

15. ④ Safety and security are enhanced with a familiar environment characterized by routine, repetition, and reinforcement.

16. ④ Careful documentation and reporting to proper authorities are the legal responsibility of the practical nurse when child or elder abuse is suspected. This should be done through the chain of command at the agency. If the supervisor does not report the incident, then the practical nurse should report the incident to child protective services.

CHAPTER 7: SENSORY SYSTEM

1. ② Before cataract surgery, a mydriatic (or a cycloplegic medication) is administered to promote pupil dilation. This is necessary to obtain access to the lens for removal. The eye may feel irritated and the client will be light sensitive, however these are not the desired effects of the medication. Remember, mydriatic has a "D" in it so it DILATES the pupil.

2. ④ Clients with glaucoma experience an increase in intraocular pressure that is controlled by miotic eye medications, such as Timoptic. Peripheral vision is affected by glaucoma, but it cannot be reversed after it occurs. Visual acuity, the ability to see well, is not a primary problem of glaucoma but is often a problem with aging. Prevention of infection is appropriate for all clients.

3. ① Ménière's disease is characterized by vertigo, tinnitus, and sensorineural hearing loss. Attacks may occur that last from 10 minutes up to several hours. There is no pain or loss of consciousness. The client is at risk for falls.

4. ① Miotic (remember, little o in miotic is little pupil) eye medications cause pupillary constriction; these are commonly used in the care of the glaucoma client. The medication does not increase visual acuity, it does not cause dilation of the pupil and it does not relieve any irritation.

5. ④ It is important to decrease the risk of otitis media recurrence by preventing milk from pooling around the eustachian tube by holding or elevating the infant's head while feeding. The bottle should not be propped. Encourage water before sleeping.

6. ② The medication should be placed in the lower conjunctival sac. Asepsis should be maintained on the applicator tip. There is no need for the client to blow his nose. The client should be in the supine position, but prevent solution from flowing into opposite eye.

7. ② Glaucoma is a condition characterized by an increase in intraocular pressure and progressive loss of peripheral vision. It is a chronic disease and a leading cause of blindness.

8. ③ Penicillin and cephalosporin medications are not ototoxic. Aminoglycosides are ototoxic. Rubella and high intensity sound waves have been linked to hearing loss. The question asks for conditions that would not increase risk for hearing loss.

9. ① Because the hearing impaired depend readily on their hearing aids, it is important to teach them to have an extra set of batteries on hand. The hearing aids should not be soaked in alcohol and should be turned off when not in the client's ear. It is not necessary to wear the hearing aid while sleeping and may in fact be uncomfortable for the client.

10. ① Mydriatic medications, such as atropine (**Atropisol**), are contraindicated in the care of the glaucoma client. Pilocarpine (**Pilocar**) is a miotic and is used to reduce intraocular pressure. Meperidine (**Demerol**) and fentanyl (**Duragesic**) can be administered to a glaucoma client.

11. ② The use of an ophthalmic anesthetic agent in the eye would necessitate the nurse to teach the client not to rub his eye until the "feeling" has returned (usually in 30 minutes) to avoid injury to the eye.

12. ② The use of warm normal saline irrigation along with instillation of mineral oil would soften the wax to assist in the removal of the cerumen from the ear canal.

13. ③ It is not necessary to use short sentences with frequent pauses for the hearing impaired. Helpful strategies are to stand in front of the client at eye level, to speak with light on your face (this helps with speech reading, i.e., reading lips), and to get the client's attention by raising your hand or arm. Do not walk back and forth in front of the client while speaking, and speak clearly and in an even tone; do not shout. The question asks for a nursing intervention that would be least effective.

14. ② The hearing aid amplifies sound, but does not change the overall ability to hear. It is used for conductive hearing loss clients. It will amplify all sound, not just the spoken voice.

CHAPTER 8: ENDOCRINE SYSTEM

1. ① Kussmaul's respirations, which are deep and rapid, are typically seen in ketoacidosis. This occurs when the client's blood glucose level is high. Cheyne-Stokes respirations are most often seen at the end of life. Rapid shallow respirations may cause respiratory alkalosis.

2. ④ A blood sugar less than 60mg/mL is considererd hypoglycemia; therefore the client will need glucagon. This is a high concentration of glucose that can be given IV. In severe cases of hypoglycemia, oral intake is not sufficient to increase the glucose level rapidly enough. The other options are all types of insulin, and the blood sugar is already too low.

3. ② Regular insulin is the only type that is given with sliding scale dosing.

4. ① The fruity breath is a symptom of high blood glucose levels (hyperglycemia); the blood glucose level should be checked immediately. The urine could possibly test positive for ketones, but the priority is obtaining the blood glucose level. Urine output and BUN may be ordered to evaluate renal function.

5. ① Glycosylated hemoglobin (HbA1c) reflects the level of blood glucose control over the past 120 days. Fasting blood glucose is the measurement of the current blood glucose level. There is no blood test that determines the level of insulin; only the serum glucose levels are determined.

6. ④ Increased activity, difficulty sleeping, and weight loss are common findings with hyperthyroidism. Weight gain, bradycardia, decreased blood pressure, and dry skin are symptoms associated with hypothyroidism.

7. ①, ③, ⑤, ⑥ A high-calcium diet will not be of benefit at this time; if the client needs calcium replacement, it will be done IV. The client should not have range of

motion of the neck—this would increase tension on the suture line. All of the other options are correct for the care of a client post thyroidectomy.

8. ② The Cushing's syndrome client will be at increased risk for infection due to the decreased inflammatory response. The client will tend to retain fluid, gain weight, and have hyperglycemia. These clients are most often on a low-sodium diet, and their hydration is carefully evaluated.

9. ① The client with Addison's disease has difficulty maintaining a stable blood pressure. The client may have a significant decrease in blood pressure with activity. The other options are not common complications associated with Addison's disease.

10. ④ Rapid and deep ventilations, tachycardia, and confusion occur in diabetic ketoacidosis. Cool, clammy skin with normal respirations and lethargy occurs with low blood sugar.

11. ④ Adult-onset diabetes may be controlled with diet, exercise, and frequently oral hypoglycemics. Insulindependent diabetes most often has an onset before age 15 years. These clients require insulin.

12. ② Airway is critical post thyroidectomy. A tracheotomy set should be easily available in case of respiratory distress. If swelling occurs at the operative site, an oral airway will not be effective.

CHAPTER 9: HEMATOLOGIC SYSTEM

1. ④ The abnormal white blood cells from the leukemia affect the ability of the immune system to protect the body from infection. Infections are most often the cause of death.

2. ①, ③, ⑥ Aplastic anemia is commonly seen in the chemotherapy or cancer client. The client should be kept warm and should be evaluated for respiratory distress and tachycardia. He should be encouraged to be active, but only to a level of tolerance. Ambulating three times a day may be too much for him. Increasing his iron intake will not necessarily improve his anemia problem, and vitamin K intake is not a factor in care of this client.

3. ③ Prevention of infection is a primary goal—all fruits and vegetables should be thoroughly washed, peeled, or cooked to eliminate bacteria. A temperature above 100° F should be reported; joints should have cold compresses applied to them, not warm packs. There is no specific diet; it should be well balanced with adequate protein.

4. ③ Aplastic anemia is the anemia that results as a serious side effect to some medications. This frequently occurs with treatment of a malignancy. Poor dietary intake results in iron-deficiency anemia, hemorrhage is loss of blood, and pernicious anemia is caused by lack of the intrinsic factor in the stomach.

5. ① Pain management is an important priority for a child in a sickle cell crisis. Temperature elevation is not a characteristic problem. Swollen, bleeding joints frequently are the source of the pain, but pain control will be priority to application of pressure and cold packs on the affected joints. Decreased bowel sounds are not characteristics of a sickling crisis.

6. ④ The client is going to be at risk for bleeding due to low platelets, especially skin and gum bleeding. Standard precautions are adequate. Increasing fluid intake is good but not specific to the question. If the client has joint hemorrhage, then cold packs would be appropriate; however, that was indicated.

7. ② The characteristics of hemophilia are those of bleeding, irrespective of whether the bleeding is internal or external. The large joints of the body are a common area of bleeding.

8. ④ The primary use of epoetin alfa (**Epogen**) is to stimulate bone marrow to increase production of red blood cells, regardless of the cause of the decreased cell production. It is commonly used in the renal failure client and in the client on chemotherapy for malignancy.

9. ② The client has a low hemoglobin level; therefore activity should be limited. The client frequently is cold, and tachycardia is not an uncommon problem.

10. ① One of the primary measures to prevent another sickle cell crisis is to maintain adequate hydration. Normal growth and development and routine immunizations are encouraged.

11. ③ Toddlers who have a high milk intake are prone to development of an iron-deficiency anemia. The other clients listed may be prone to other types of anemias, but not to a problem with iron deficiency.

12. ② Pressure at the site is the first step to stop bleeding. The ice bag can be obtained after the pressure has been applied, and pressure should be applied to the radial artery.

13. ② Soft toothbrushes, no flossing, and frequent mouth rinses are encouraged for oral hygiene. Generally, daily coagulation studies are not done. The client should not be catheterized because trauma to the urinary tract should be avoided; increased intake of iron may be healthy, but it does not address bleeding precautions.

14. ④ If bleeding is active, it is important to keep the joints immobilized. The client should not be up walking, and the nurse should not perform range-of-motion exercises. (RICE: rest, ice, compression, elevation.)

15. ① Pernicious anemia is treated with injections of vitamin B12; it is not effective taken orally. The other options are not nursing implications for vitamin B12.

16. ① The first action to stop the bleeding is to apply pressure. The client should lean forward so he will not swallow

the blood and become nauseous. Ice packs to the nose will help, but pressure should be applied while the ice pack is being obtained.

CHAPTER 10: RESPIRATORY SYSTEM

1. ② Pulse oximetry does not require any invasive procedure, it is a clip that is placed on the client's finger or ear lobe and is an estimate of the oxygen concentration in the blood (SpO₂). Spirometry measures capacity of the lungs, it does not measure the oxygen levels; arterial blood is drawn for arterial blood gas analysis; and pulmonary lung scan involves injecting a dye and a scan of the lung.

2. ③ The COPD client is dependent on his lower level of oxygen saturation for his stimulus to breath, to increase his oxygen level too much will decrease his stimulus to breath and he will begin to hypoventilate with a decreased respiratory rate and depth of respirations. Apnea can develop. Sputum production and irritability are not necessarily indicative of problems with increased inspired levels of oxygen.

3. ② The client needs to be in an upright position leaning over a bedside table for easier access to the thoracic cavity. An alternative position may be with the client on his side with the head of the bed elevated and his knees drawn up toward this chest.

4. ① Regardless of the precipitating cause of pneumonia, there is a decrease in breath sounds over the area of consolidation. The use of accessory muscles indicates difficulty breathing, not necessarily pneumonia. The cough is usually productive and the client has increased respiratory rate.

5. ② Expectorants liquefy respiratory secretions to stimulate coughing and to make the mucus easier to cough up. Antihistamines and decongestants dry up the mucus and make it difficult to remove by coughing. A bronchodilator will decrease difficulty breathing by opening the airways.

6. ③ Most decongestants cause vasoconstriction which will cause an increase in the blood pressure. This will increase the difficulty in maintaining control of the client's hypertension. A headache may occur, but this is not the reason for caution in a client with hypertension.

7. ① The respiratory rate is within normal limits. The increased pulse rate and the low oximetry levels correlate with respiratory difficulty and are not indicative of an improvement in the client. Secretions should mobilize as client improves.

8. ④ Pulmonary embolus is the common complication of immobility (venous pooling of blood), deep vein thrombosis (increased incidence of venous pooling and clot formation). Pulmonary emboli is secondary to venous pooling, which most often occurs from immobility. The only client listed that is immobilized

is the client with the fractured femur.

9. ③ Dyspnea and fatigue are characteristic in the progression of chronic pulmonary disorders. Corpulonale (right side heart failure) commonly occurs as the condition progresses. Production of sputum and cough are common and not indicative of progression of the disease. Temperature and headache may be indicative of an infection. An infection would be a complication, not progression of the condition.

10. ① Hypoxemia is the condition of decreased oxygen in the blood. Septicemia is a systemic infection, hypercapnia is the increase of carbon dioxide in the blood, and hyperventilation is rapid respirations.

11. ② In a total laryngectomy the client will have a permanent tracheotomy and will have lost his normal voice. The tracheotomy should be suctioned as necessary, however, not every hour. He may or may not experience respiratory fatigue with activity. His lungs were not the site of the malignancy, it was in his throat or larynx.

12. ① Three days after surgery the lung should be expanded, which means there will be a minimum amount of dark drainage and no fluctuation of the fluid level in the tubing. 300 mL of serosanguineous drainage would be expected on the operative, as well as the first postoperative day. There should be no bubbling in the collection chamber. There should not be any bright red blood at this time.

13. ③ The wheezing is due to bronchospasm, edema and narrowing of the airways. The mucus plugs the airways and causes trapping of distal air. Tachypnea and bradycardia do not affect the characteristics of the lung sounds.

14. ④ The catheter is advanced till slight resistance is met, and suction is applied intermittently on withdrawal of the catheter. Suctioning on withdrawal will help to decrease trauma during suctioning. Suction is applied only about 15-20 seconds to prevent precipitation of hypoxia. Suction is not applied during insertion of the catheter.

15. ③ The chest collection bottle should always be kept below the level of the chest to prevent drainage from going back into the pleural cavity. The chest tube should not be clamped and the chest tubes are not disconnected.

16. ② The ineffective clearing of secretions with resultant pooling can lead to an increased risk of infection. Their appetite is usually decreased and they have an increased A-P diameter of the chest. Immobility would contribute to the pooling of the secretions, dehydration would make the secretions thick and it would be difficult for the client to cough them up.

17. ① Symptoms of tuberculosis include fatigue, cough, low grade fever, night sweats, shortness of breath, and weight loss. They usually do not have problems

with rash, pleural edema, or oliguria. Respiratory precautions with a room that is specially ventilated would be required.

18. ④ When interpreting a tuberculosis skin test for a non-high risk individual a 15mm raised area (induration) indicates the person has been exposed to the TB bacillus. A 16mm induration is positive and he should have a chest x-ray, and possibly follow up with a sputum study.

19. ① On the first postoperative day, the fluid level in the chest tubes should be fluctuating with each ventilation due to the pressure changes in the thoracic cavity. If the lungs are re-expanded breath sounds should be present, and there should be no fluctuation. It is too early postoperative to expect the lungs to be reexpanded. Bloody drainage should be present, however it does not reflect the functioning of the chest tubes in reestablishing a negative pressure within the pleural cavity.

20. ② The ability of the client to speak indicts air is moving past the endotracheal tube (ET) and into the area of the larynx. Increased swallowing efforts would indicate an irritation in the throat from the ET tube. An increase in the peak pressure of the ventilator is indicative of the amount of pressure the ventilator must deliver to achieve a preset tidal volume.

CHAPTER 11: VASCULAR SYSTEM

1. ④ After ambulation, it is important to determine the quality of the peripheral pulses to assess the integrity of the graft. The pulse rate and blood pressure are important to evaluate if there is any indication of difficulty with the activity/ambulation. The temperature of the affected extremity is another method to determine adequacy of circulation, however pulse checks are priority.

2. ②, ③ The healing of venous stasis ulcers is dependent on relief of the venous congestion in the extremity. Compression devices and elevation of the extremity are the most effective methods. Claudication pain is characteristic of arterial disease. Cool packs are not used; warm packs may be used. Dressings should be changed as frequently as necessary because there may be excessive drainage.

3. ① The nurse should allow the client to sit at the side of the bed before standing. Orthostatic hypotension occurs when the client has been lying down and suddenly assumes an upright position. This commonly occurs in clients who are starting antihypertensive medications, who are hypovolemic, or who have severe bradycardia. To validate the hypotension, the blood pressure would be assessed with the client lying down and then with the client standing at the bedside.

4. ④ The medication is injected subcutaneously with the

smallest gauge needle, and the area is not rubbed after the injection. The activated partial thromboplastin (APTT) time is checked before the administration of heparin. Whether or not the lab work is checked before administration of the heparin depends on how much medication is being administered, and for what purpose. Prophylactically administered heparin and a maintenance dose heparin do not require lab work to be evaluated before every dose.

5. ④ These are considered to be modifiable risk factors for the development of atherosclerosis, which predisposes a client to the development of cardiac disease and hypertension. Remember, on the testing strategies, if any part of the option is incorrect, the entire option is incorrect.

6. ③ To maintain effective control, the hypertensive client is frequently on medication indefinitely. If the client begins a regular exercise routine and loses excess weight, it will impact the medication dosage and it could be decreased or reevaluated.

7. ①, ③, ⑤, ⑥ Long-term impairment of venous return leads to chronic venous insufficiency that is characterized by leathery, brawny appearance from erythrocyte extravasation to the extremity, persistent peripheral edema, stasis dermatitis, and pruritus. Venous stasis ulcers characteristically form near the ankle on the medial aspect, with wound margins that are irregularly shaped with tissue that is a ruddy color. Gangrenous wounds and diminished peripheral pulses are associated with arterial occlusive disease.

8. ① With arterial occlusion, there is a decrease in quality of the pulse, and the feet are frequently pale and cool to touch. Healing ability is significantly diminished. Edema is associated with venous problems. The pedal pulses are significantly diminished or absent prior to the changes in the color of the feet.

9. ① The surgery puts the client at an increased risk for renal complications because an aortic aneurysm is commonly in the area of the renal arteries. A normal urinary output should be around 30mL per hour. A urinary output of 80 mL over 4 hours is too low, and the physician should be contacted immediately. If the feet are cool, a blanket should be placed over them and they can be checked again at a later time.

10. ③ The client would be on bed rest to prevent the dislodgement of a thrombus. The client will also be on an anticoagulant. Active range of motion would not be done on the affected extremity. Any contraction and flexion of muscles in the leg should be avoided to prevent pressure on the area of the DVT.

11. ④ The affected area will be warm, inflamed, and tender. Thrombophlebitis is a problem of the venous system. The peripheral pulses should be normal because the arterial circulation is not usually affected.

12. ④ Intermittent claudication is the term used to describe

pain in the legs that is relieved by resting the muscle. The other options are not characteristic of intermittent claudication. Pain in the leg at rest is indicative of advanced arterial disease. Analgesics are usually not necessary as pain decreases significantly or goes away when client is at rest.

13. ① Peripheral vascular disease is a complication of diabetes. The 76-year-old with a history of diabetes and hypertension puts this client at higher risk of developing the problem than any of the other clients listed.

14. ④ The typical symptoms of deep vein thrombosis are venous pooling, pain on dorsiflexion of the foot, and swelling, warmth, and tenderness over the affected area. The condition is most often not bilateral; redness and swelling only occur on the affected extremity.

15. ② Warfarin sodium (**Coumadin**) may be taken by mouth; it is the most common oral anticoagulant. Heparin cannot be taken by mouth, but both medications will still require monitoring of the coagulation studies. Heparin is a very rapid acting, short term medication. Coumadin is longer acting and easier for the client to manage.

16. ① The only option that indicates a decrease in tissue perfusion is the decrease in urine output. Jugular vein distention is present with an increase in venous pressure. The chest tube output is expected, and the vital signs can be a result of anxiety or stress. The urine output should be at least 30mL per hour. Urine output is a critical indicator of the adequacy of renal perfusion.

17. ③ Caffeine, amphetamines, and nicotine all cause an increase in blood pressure and would affect the control of the client's blood pressure. This option is more of a risk then the option with chocolate, tea, and caffeine. Testing strategy: all of the options must be correct if it is the answer.

18. ① Most diuretics increase the excretion of potassium. Fruits are usually high in potassium, especially dried fruits. It is important for the client who is taking diuretics to maintain an adequate intake of potassium.

19. ② The classic indications of arterial insufficiency include intermittent claudication; decreased or absent pulses; paresthesia or numbness and tingling in the extremity; thin, shiny, hairless skin; thick, ridged, toenails; cool skin temperature; pallor when leg is elevated; and dependent rubor (reactive hyperemia or redness of the foot when in a dependent position).

20. ③ All responses are correct but cessation of smoking is of most importance because the disease process is thought to be triggered by smoking. All other responses are appropriate but will not be of as much benefit, especially if the client continues to smoke.

CHAPTER 12: CARDIAC SYSTEM

1. ① After a cardiac catheterization, the client will be required to lie flat. The client is usually awake and alert, and pain should not be a problem. The client will not be allowed out of bed for several hours; however, a urinary catheter is not used, unless he cannot void from a supine position.

2. ③ An allergy to shellfish may be indicative of an allergy to iodine. The dye used in the catheterization may be an iodine-based dye. An allergy to milk products, eggs and penicillin are of concern, but not for a cardiac catheterization.

3. ① The isoenzymes are indicative of cardiac tissue damage. The isoenzyme CPK-MB is a specific indicator of damage to the cardiac muscle. Troponin is also a myocardial protein that is released into the circulation after myocardial injury. This test does not determine cardiac contractility or a specific area of myocardial damage.

4. ② The apex of the heart is located at the fifth intercostal space in the mid-clavicular line on the left side. This is the point of maximum impulse (PMI) and is the best area to count an apical pulse rate. Apical pulse rate should be counted when an irregular pulse rate is present or before administering digitalis medications.

5. ③ With bacterial endocarditis, the client will be on antibiotics for an extended period of time. It is very important that he maintain the dosing schedule, missed doses of the antibiotic may increase bacterial resistance to the antibiotic. Increased fruit juice is not a specific need, and the client will not need to return for weekly ECG evaluation. The client will begin exercise based on his activity tolerance.

6. ① Sodium increases the client's retention of fluid (where goes the sodium, so goes the water). An increase in fluid retention increases the preload and puts an increased workload on the heart. Therefore when there is a decreased sodium intake, less fluid will be retained and it will assist to improve cardiac function. There is no specific correlation between sodium restriction and potassium. Myocardial contractility is not dependent on sodium levels.

7. ④ The primary action of nitroglycerin is vasodilation of the arteries. This may precipitate a headache as the cerebral arteries are dilated as well as the coronary arteries. The other options are not characteristic of nitroglycerin.

8. ④ High-Fowler's position with the legs dependent will assist to decrease venous return; this will decrease the workload of the heart and increase cardiac efficiency. Increasing cardiac efficiency will assist to improve the quality of ventilation. Oxygen should be started immediately as well. Dyspnea and tachycardia are indications the CHF is progressing. When he last

had his medications is not a priority at this time. A supine position with the feet elevated will increase the cardiac workload, increase the venous return, and also increase the dyspnea.

9. ④ Nitroglycerin should be taken at the first sign of any chest pain; if the pain is not relieved within 5 minutes, then another tablet should be taken and emergency assistance (EMS) should be called. If the client continues to experience chest pain prior to the arrival of assistance, another SL nitroglycerine should be taken. Medication should be stored in a dark container, and should be allowed to dissolve under the tongue. It does have a rapid onset, but it is most important to tell the client to take it at the first indication of chest pain.

10. ① The action of digitalis is to strengthen and slow the heart rate, which will improve cardiac output. As cardiac output is improved, so is renal perfusion, which increases urinary output. The other options listed are not the desired or therapeutic responses to digitalis.

11. ①, ③, ⑥ The client's apical pulse rate should be determined before being given any digitalis preparations, as well as when the client has an irregular pulse rate. With an irregular pulse rate, it is easy to miss beats at the radial artery. The apical rate is easier and more reliable on an infant. Hypertensive clients and MI clients do not require an apical pulse rate to determine an accurate pulse rate, providing they have a regular pulse. Orthostatic hypotension is transient; the pulse should be easily palpable after the client lies down.

12. ④ As edema is reduced, the fluid moves back into the vascular system. With increased vascular volume, the kidneys will excrete more water, thereby increasing the urinary output. The nurse should also expect to observe a more effective breathing pattern as well.

13. ③ Right-sided heart failure causes an increase in pressure within the right ventricle, thus causing an increase in pressure in the venous system. The increased venous pressure causes jugular vein distention. Pulmonary congestion would be associated with a pulmonary problem. Right-sided heart failure causes venous congestion and there is difficulty pumping blood into the lungs. There may or may not be a decrease in urinary output; this is dependent on the blood pressure and renal perfusion.

14. ④ Tachycardia in the client with cardiac disease increases cardiac workload and oxygen use. An irregular rhythm is indicative of a dysrhythmia. Dysrhythmias are a common complication and cause of death after an MI. Jugular vein distention in the supine position is normal; it is abnormal when the client is sitting; urine output cannot be evaluated if the intake is not known.

15. ④ Increasing irritation and confusion are early indications of hypoxia. The blood pressure and pulse are within expected levels. Peripheral edema of 1+ is not unusual

with the CHF, but the confusion and irritability are priority concerns.

16. ② When a client states he has chest pain, he/she should immediately be returned to the bed and oxygen should be started. After this is done, assessment of the chest pain and possibly administration of nitroglycerine can be accomplished. The charge nurse should be notified immediately and the health care provider can be notified after further assessment of the client. What the client last ate is not immediately relevant to the situation.

17. ③ The dietary intake is the only one that the client can control. Nonmodifiable risk factors are the ones in which the client has no control.

18. ② When a client experiences problems with a permanent pacemaker, the pacemaker is most often not capturing or pacing the client's heart rate. This puts the client at an increased risk for severe bradycardia which can produce syncope and increase the risk of falling. Normal fluid intake should be encouraged, the client should remain in bed or out of bed only with assistance due to the possible syncope. Hypoxia is not a common problem unless there are other chronic conditions present.

19. ③ The right arm needs to remain abducted to prevent the inadvertent movement of the pacemaker wires that were inserted via the right subclavian vein. Checking the radial pulse does not determine if the pacemaker is functioning or if the client is maintaining his own rhythm. There are no external wires on a permanent pacemaker, and the current status of the incision is not of high importance in preventing immediate complications.

20. ① During CPR, the heart is compressed between the sternum and the spine to push the blood out of the ventricles. It is this pumping motion that produces cardiac output. Compressions should be done on a hard surface to be most effective.

CHAPTER 13:
GASTROINTESTINAL SYSTEM

1. ② A solution of 1/2 strength peroxide, normal saline, or a weak bicarbonate solution is nonirritating to the suture line in the mouth. The sutures should be rinsed off every time the client eats. Commercial antiseptic mouthwashes should not be used. If the client is eating, then cool or warm foods are allowed, but there should be no temperature extremes. Glycerin swabs are not appropriate after surgery.

2. ① Nasogastric tubes are put into the stomach to decrease the gastric distention in the client with a bowel obstruction. It will not eliminate nausea and vomiting; however, it will make vomiting less likely.

3. ④ The lower in the colon the colostomy is performed, the more formed the stool will be. Black and bloody stools are indicative of a disease process. An ileostomy client will have a liquid stool.

4. ② Provide oral hygiene immediately after removing the nasogastric tube. The client is most often offered clear liquid initially. Abdominal distention and bowel sounds will need to be evaluated later to determine client's tolerance of removal of the tube. Removal of the tube will not immediately change bowel sounds; bowel sounds should be evaluated before the removal of the tube.

5. ③ This is only the day after surgery; therefore the area around the stoma has not had time to heal. There will be some capillary bleeding. The stoma should be pinkish red and moist, and often there is some swelling present. There should be no edema, sloughing around the stoma, or discoloration of the stoma.

6. ② It is important to know if the client is experiencing problems with weight loss along with vomiting, diarrhea, and constipation. These have implications on the client's fluid and electrolyte balance and may need to be addressed immediately.

7. ① Sometimes it is difficult to hear bowel sounds, especially in the postoperative client after abdominal surgery. The nurse should listen for at least 1 minute in each abdominal quadrant before noting that bowel sounds are not heard.

8. ③ It is the client's right to refuse treatment or to refuse to have a diagnostic procedure done. The physician should be notified.

9. ③ Before an appendectomy, the client is usually maintained in a position of comfort and kept NPO, and no heat is applied to the abdomen. Narcotics are used sparingly. It is important to be able to identify changes in the character of the client's pain.

10. ④ It is most important to maintain patency and drainage of the nasogastric tube postoperatively. The nasogastric tube should not be repositioned on this client. The tube should not be irrigated until patency is determined. The tube should not be clamped, especially when the client is complaining of nausea. The gastric output is most often measured at the end of the shift, even if it appears to be excessive. Measuring the output would not take precedent over evaluating for patency.

11. ④ Concentrated formula given too rapidly will cause problems with cramping, distention, and diarrhea. When administered via a bolus and gravity flow, there is increased incidence of intolerance. The optimal method of tube feeding is the continuous drip method. Intermittent via a drip rate is the next preferred method.

12. ④ Clients who experience problems with GERD should not lie down after they eat, or eat within 3 hours of going to bed. They should rest in the sitting position

after eating, and maintain an adequate amount of fluid intake with their meals. Antacids will not relieve the problem.

13. ③ Positioning the client on his side will facilitate the client spitting out the vomitus. High-Fowler's position is also a good position to assist in preventing aspiration.

14. ④ The histamine antagonist medications actually decrease the production of gastric acid. Antacids such as Maalox and Mylanta coat the stomach to neutralize the acid that is present.

15. ② Old blood that has been disintegrated by the digestive juices has the appearance of coffee grounds. This does not reflect any active bleeding; however, the old blood is probably a result of the recent surgery. Vital signs should be assessed, the drainage monitored, and the RN notified as to the status of the drainage. Coffee ground appearance does not reflect whether any bile is present or absent.

16. ② Peritonitis, or an inflammation of the lining of the peritoneal cavity, occurs if the appendix ruptures before removal. Symptoms include those associated with an acute infection, plus rigid guarding of the abdomen, shallow respirations, and absent bowel sounds.

17. ① can. The order is for 55 mL per hour of half-strength formula; half-strength would require administering 27.5 mL of formula with 27.5 mL of water per hour: 27.5 mL × 8 = 220 mL of formula or 1 can.

18. ② Bulk laxatives that contain psyllium or methylcellulose increase the bulk and moisture in the stool and should be recommended over those laxatives that are irritable in nature. The question states that dietary modifications are not working; therefore changes in the diet are not the best answer. Enemas should not be recommended.

CHAPTER 14: HEPATIC AND BILIARY SYSTEM

1. ④ The primary method of transmitting hepatitis A is via contamination of food and poor hygiene. Shellfish caught in contaminated water, improper handling of food, improper hygiene practices, and crowded living conditions are the primary methods of transmission.

2. ④ Direct contact of blood with mucous membranes carries a higher risk than the other options listed.

3. ① Acetaminophen products are hepatotoxic. Any client with liver problems should not take products that contain acetaminophen. The vitamins are okay, and there is usually no problem with cough medications.

4. ① Vaccination for hepatitis B is strongly recommended for all health care workers. HBV is transmitted via blood and is more severe than HAV. There are no vaccinations for HIV, and varicella is a childhood vaccination that should be obtained during childhood,

but it is not a health hazard in the hospital if a person is not immunized.

5. ① There are many medications that are detoxified by the liver. If the liver is not functioning normally, these toxins are not eliminated from the body and become hepatotoxic. The liver does inactivate or break down medications, but this is the normal response. The diseased liver will not increase the action of the medications, and the client will not need to take larger doses.

6. ① The client with liver disease will have problems with bruising, petechiae, and spider angiomas. There is a characteristic yellowing or jaundice color of the skin due to the increased bilirubin level. There should not be a problem with hypoxia or changes in LOC until the final stages of the disease.

7. ④ When the bilirubin levels increase in the client with liver problems, a yellowish tinge occurs in the skin and sclerae of the eyes. This is known as jaundice and is commonly seen in clients with liver disease.

8. ③ Fresh fruits and vegetables have the lowest sodium content. The client should avoid breads, pastries, dairy products, and all processed meats.

9. ④ The client with liver disease has a problem with portal hypertension that causes the problem of ascites—a collection of fluid in the abdominal cavity. Melena or bloody stool may occur with bleeding problems; there is usually no problem with urinary output, or maintaining normal blood pressure levels.

10. ① Postoperative laparoscopic cholecystectomy clients frequently have diaphragm irritation from the carbon dioxide. This position will promote the movement of the CO_2 from the area of the diaphragm to decrease the irritation.

11. ② The increased blood ammonia will cross the blood-brain barrier and cause problems such as altered or decreased levels of consciousness. The other options are common in clients with liver problems, but are not due to the blood ammonia level.

12. ① The client with liver problems will also have problems with the utilization of vitamin K, which is necessary for normal clotting factors. Supplemental vitamin K preoperatively will help decrease postoperative bleeding problems.

13. ① It is important to report any bile drainage; this could cause problems of peritonitis. There is no need to return for lab work; vitamin K is not necessary. Steatorrhea stools tend to occur in clients with pancreatitis or cystic fibrosis.

14. ① Hepatitis is sexually transmitted. Even if a client has a monogamous sexual partner, a condom should still be used to prevent transmission of hepatitis. The client should not consume any alcohol. Green, leafy vegetables are good for a balanced diet, but there is no

specific indication for them. Acetaminophen should be avoided because it is hepatotoxic.

15. ② Problems occur with esophageal varices if bleeding begins. Increasing portal hypertension will continue to cause increased esophageal pressure, and frequently the varices will begin to bleed. The client usually does not have problems with swallowing, or with the gag reflex. Anorexia is a common problem with cirrhosis, but not with varices.

16. ① There are four small incisions made where the scope was passed into the abdomen; they are often covered with large Band-Aids or a very light dressing. A urinary catheter is not routine, and the client is allowed fluids and a light diet, if tolerated, the evening of surgery. The pain is most often in the right upper quadrant or the right shoulder due to diaphragm irritation.

17. ① Protein causes an increase in the client's blood ammonia level, which contributes to the client's encephalopathy. Protein restriction is based on the client's current blood ammonia levels and mental status.

18. ① The client is most often more comfortable in the semi–Fowler's position due to the fluid in the abdomen. Dyspnea can be a problem, and the semi–Fowler's position helps to relieve the pressure of the abdominal fluid on the diaphragm.

CHAPTER 15: NEUROLOGICAL SYSTEM

1. ① L-dopa is the most common medication used for treatment of Parkinson's disease. The desired effect is to reduce the tremors. These tremors most often occur in the upper extremities. They are usually present at rest and decrease with purposeful movement.

2. ② To promote safety, the client should always be assisted out of bed on the unaffected side. The wheelchair should be placed on the unaffected side. This option is specific to the situation. The client should be placed near the edge of the bed, but in the semi–Fowler's position to facilitate sitting up prior to standing.

3. ① It is dangerous to give a client anything to eat or drink if he does not have a gag reflex, which may occur after stroke. This is the first information to obtain when there is a question about the possibility of aspiration. After any diagnostic test when the throat has been anesthetized, it is important to determine the presence of a gag reflex.

4. ② The nurse should closely observe the client for any change in intracranial pressure; this may be indicated by unilateral change in the size and reaction of the pupils. Decreased bilateral breath sounds are not unusual postoperatively, and the nurse should encourage frequent deep-breathing. The urinary output is not unusual, but the nurse should observe for adequacy of hydration. Clients are frequently confused and disoriented after surgery. The nurse should

continue to reinforce orientation.

5. ② The spinal needle is inserted at L3-L4. If there is any oozing after the procedure, it could be spinal fluid. This would increase the risk of headache as well as infection. Headache is not uncommon; if the patient remains in the supine position, it should help prevent the headache. Weakness of the upper muscles is not relevant to the lumbar puncture, and many clients have difficulty voiding while on bed rest.

6. ④ The removal of cerebral spinal fluid can cause a headache. To decrease the likelihood of headache, the client is kept supine for 6 to 12 hours to prevent further leakage of spinal fluid. Oral fluids are encouraged during this time to assist in replacing the spinal fluid. Position the client on his side to administer oral fluids.

7. ④ It is important that the nurse remain with the client and prevent him from injuring himself by hitting his head or extremities on the bed or bed rails during the seizure activity. The airway cannot be adequately assessed during the seizure. After the seizure is over, the airway is assessed and patency is maintained.

8. ③ When a client has a CSF leak, he should be maintained on bedrest and low–Fowler's position until advised otherwise. The client is at increased risk for infection (meningitis). The ears and nose should not be cleaned; spinal fluid should be allowed to drain and be gently wiped if it is draining from the nose or the outer ear. The client should not be suctioned or encouraged to cough vigorously.

9. ③ The first sign of increasing intracranial pressure is a change in level of consciousness. This should be reported to the RN or PCP. The changes in blood pressure and pulse rate should be monitored, but they are not indicative of significant problems. With a decrease in breath sounds, the client should be encouraged to deep-breathe or to use an incentive spirometer.

10. ④ Reality checks assist the nurse to determine confusion and disorientation early. The other options do not determine the presence of confusion. Reality checks are more specific to the mental status than the level of consciousness. A person can be lethargic but oriented.

11. ③ With increased intracranial pressure, one eye may be larger and have a decreased or sluggish reaction as compared to the other eye. The dilation frequently occurs ipsilaterally, or on the same side as the lesion. As ICP becomes more severe, there is pressure on the optic nerve and both eyes will dilate with no reaction to direct light stimulus.

12. ① Encouraging mobility and providing plenty of fluids is the first step to preventing constipation. A diet high in fiber should also be encouraged. Enemas and laxatives should be discouraged. Glycerin suppositories may be used to stimulate defecation, but only after other measures have been unsuccessful.

13. ④ Immobility is a common complication for a stroke client. He should be encouraged to be as mobile as possible and deep-breathe to prevent respiratory complications (pneumonia). Bleeding problems and urinary output are not common problems with a stroke client. Performing neurological checks every hour is too often now that the client is recovering.

14. ④ Based on the Glasgow Coma Scale, this client is comatose with no response to verbal commands: eye opening may be a 1, verbal response would be a 1, and the best motor response could be a 2 if there is unintentional extension movement, for a total score of 4.

15. ① The client needs to be positioned so that the head and neck can be maintained in an extended state to maintain the open airway; this will also allow for drainage of oral secretions. The side-lying position best meets these needs. The semi–Fowler's position allows expansion of the chest wall for deep-breathing but does not prevent the tongue from obstructing the airway.

16. ② The airway is the most critical physiological need at this time. The other options are important to implement, but at a later time when life-threatening problems with the airway have been addressed.

17. ① Nursing activities include actions to prevent deformity of the extremities: active ROM on the unaffected side and passive ROM on the affected side. The client's affected side should be protected; he should not be positioned on the affected side the same length of time as the unaffected side. Injections should be given on the unaffected side; the muscle tone and vascular status are better on the unaffected side.

18. ② Importance is placed on the client remaining as still as possible for test accuracy in performing a CT scan. Iodine is not swallowed for the test; if a contrast medium is used, it is administered intravenously. A lumbar puncture would have the client remain flat (usually for at least 4 to 8 hours) after the procedure. An electroencephalogram (EEG) is the test in which electrodes are attached to the head.

19. ④ The term quadriplegia refers to an injury involving the cervical vertebrae and involves all four extremities. The severity of the damage depends on the cervical vertebrae affected, and determines what responses or movement the client will eventually be able to achieve. He will experience sustained weakness of the voluntary muscles in the upper extremities as well as paralysis of the lower extremities.

20. ④ Any time a client is immobilized, there is increased risk for skin breakdown. Spinal cord injury clients have also suffered damage to the nerves and cannot determine if there is pain in an area. These clients

should always be visually checked for redness and skin breakdown. It is not adequate to ask the client if the area is uncomfortable.

CHAPTER 16: MUSCULOSKELETAL SYSTEM

1. ③ Bright red bleeding should not be occurring this late after surgery. A small amount of bleeding may be expected immediately postoperatively. Serosanguineous drainage is normal; however, purulent drainage would be indicative of an infection.

2. ④ In any client in traction, a nursing priority is to make sure the feet are not touching the end of the bed. This eliminates the pull of the traction on the affected extremity. The weights must also be hanging freely for countertraction to be effective.

3. ② The normal capillary refill time is 2 to 3 seconds. Increased time may be due to poor peripheral circulation resulting from arterial constriction, edema, or cold temperature.

4. ③ The sensation of phantom limb pain is not uncommon in the amputee. The client feels the amputated extremity, and the nerve endings do not accurately reflect the area of the pain. The client needs to be medicated, and the pain is usually self-limiting.

5. ② The casted extremity should be supported on a pillow that will not absorb the moisture and keep the cast moist. The client needs to be turned frequently to allow for air circulation around the cast for drying. The cast should be handled with the palm of the hand to prevent indentations in the cast. Heat should not be applied; however, a fan will increase movement of air and accelerate drying of the cast.

6. ① When a pin is inserted, the periosteum of the bone is broken and there is an increased risk of infection. Skeletal traction and pin insertion help to maintain an effective realignment of the bone. There is no reason to suspect a flexion contraction. Compartment syndrome occurs when there is a circulatory problem, most often with a cast.

7. ② This amount of drainage is within normal limits immediately after surgery. The operative record will be of no benefit. It will not help to put pressure on the incisional area because the drainage is coming from deep within the wound.

8. ① The increase in pain and warmth over the cast are indicative of an infection under the cast. Capillary refill and decreased movement are problems with circulation or nerve compression. Itching and general discomfort are expected.

9. ② Increasing pain unrelieved by medication often is indicative of compartment syndrome. This is more likely to be the problem than a thrombosis. Compartment syndrome should always be considered when there is a significant increase in the level of pain.

10. ③ "Petaling" of the cast is done by taking pieces of tape and applying them around the edges of the cast to keep it from crumbling and to decrease skin irritation from the edges of the cast. It is important to assess the problem precipitating the discomfort and use other methods to relieve the pain as appropriate.

11. ② When joints are painful and swollen, they should be placed in a position of comfort and cold packs should be applied to reduce the swelling and inflammation. When the swelling and inflammation are reduced, the client may begin range-of-motion exercises and warm packs to facilitate the movement of the joints.

12. ② The client will most likely be placed in Buck's traction to maintain immobility and alignment of the fracture site. A temporary hip spica cast will not be used, and skin breakdown is not a priority at this time. Bryant's traction may be used to temporarily stabilize toddlers with a fractured femur.

13. ④ In the postoperative laminectomy client, it is important to assess for any indication of pressure against the spinal column. This may be caused by swelling or by a hematoma. Numbness and tingling, as well as inability to move the extremity, are common indicators of this problem. The surgery does not cause any circulatory compromise, and pain is to be expected immediately postoperative.

14. ④ Balanced suspension traction is a type of skeletal traction and does not use the boot for traction. Weights should not be removed, but the weights should always hang free on any type of traction.

15. ④ The crutch should not put any pressure on the axillary area. The axillary bar should be at least 2 fingers' width (2 inches) below the axillary area. The client's arms should be at a 30-degree angle in order to support the client's weight. When going up the stairs, the unaffected leg is advanced first.

16. ① The pain from a fracture is most often described as sharp and piercing.

CHAPTER 17: REPRODUCTIVE SYSTEM

1. ① A small amount of bleeding is expected after this surgery. A bladder irrigation system is usually not used following a suprapubic prostatectomy.

2. ② Hand washing is critical to prevent contamination of other areas of the body. Herpes virus type II is concentrated in the vesicles, and therefore the infection is highly contagious. The virus can be transferred to another area of the body by direct contact.

3. ② The Centers for Disease Control studies the profiles of STDs and develops programs to decrease the incidence, to identify areas of higher concentration of problems, and to establish protocols for treatment. Each state

has responsibility for establishing what conditions are reportable. Most states adhere to guidelines from the CDC.

4. ②, ⑤, ⑥ Important teaching to include in the discharge plan of care for a mastectomy client includes the avoidance of needlesticks in the arm on the side of the mastectomy and avoidance of blood pressure measurements on this arm. This is to avoid any type of trauma, which might lead to the development of lymphedema. Active exercises, such as pendulum swings and wall climbing, are started after the incision has healed. As the area heals, abduction and external rotation will help to improve the range of motion.

5. ① A painless sore is characteristic of the chancre lesion of syphilis. Gonorrhea is characterized by urethral discharge, and herpes simplex (HVH II) has a characteristic painful lesion. The human papillomavirus is a genital wart.

6. ④ It is important for the bladder to be empty. This will promote comfort for the client and make it easier for the physician to examine the pelvic contents. A cleansing enema is not done. The client may be any-where in her cycle; however, clients usually do not schedule an exam during their menstrual period. Pregnancy is a consideration; however, an empty bladder is more important immediately before the examination.

7. ③ It is important to observe the arm on the affected side of the client who has had a mastectomy. If the lymph drainage in the arm has been compromised, there is an increased risk of swelling and edema on the affected arm. The arm should be protected from tests such as needlesticks or blood pressure assessment. The temperature and slight increase in blood glucose level are normal for the first day postoperative.

8. ② The itching and burning may be caused by drying of the vaginal walls. The estrogen cream will help to decrease this problem. The client should not douche, and soap may further irritate the area. A water-based lubricant such as petroleum jelly may improve lubrication during sexual activity, but will not resolve the problem.

9. ② Frequency, urgency, difficulty starting the urinary stream, and hematuria are common findings with BPH. The bladder may have residual, but should not be distended. There may be a burning pain present if the client has a UTI.

10. ③ The physician or PCP will evaluate the client's prostate by doing a digital rectal examination. No special equipment is needed other than gloves and lubricant.

11. ① Clots in the urinary drainage system are common problems in the immediate postoperative period. The physician should be notified immediately if the nurse cannot easily reestablish catheter patency. The irrigation fluid should be stopped. The catheter placed postoperatively is an irrigation catheter that is specific for use with a bladder irrigation. If a new one is placed, the physician will do it.

CHAPTER 18: URINARY-RENAL SYSTEM

1. ③ The nurse should encourage the client to void whenever she feels the urge. Refraining from voiding increases the concentration of urine in the bladder and increases the irritation.

2. ④ Dysuria, or painful urination, is a common complaint of clients with UTI. Low back pain occurs with upper UTI, and painless hematuria is not a characteristic of lower UTI.

3. ② The first specimen is discarded, and then all urine is saved for the next 24 hours. The client is asked to void again, and that specimen is added to the container to complete the 24-hour collection.

4. ① To promote continence, a schedule for toileting should be established. Oral fluids should be encouraged, except immediately before bedtime. Assessing for distention is important; however, the question asks about methods to establish continence.

5. ③ The shunt should be lightly palpated for the presence of a "thrill" or vibration. The shunt may also be auscultated for bruits or sounds of blood passing through the shunt.

6. ② Circumcision is usually delayed until the repair of the urethral opening can be completed. This is usually somewhere between 3 and 6 months of age.

7. ③ Injections would actually be discouraged. All other options are important in preventing infections in the client who has a compromised immune system.

8. ① These are classic symptoms in the GI system that occur with the development of uremia. Other changes occur throughout the body and may include confusion, bleeding, hypertension, and an increase in serum potassium levels.

9. ① The most common cause of acute renal failure is the client who has experienced an episode of low blood pressure. Of all of these clients, the one with placenta previa is at highest risk for a period of low blood pressure. The diabetic client is at risk for development of chronic renal failure.

10. ② Erythropoietin is produced by the kidneys and is responsible for the production of red blood cells. Anemia is a common problem in the chronic renal failure client.

11. ④ The nephrostomy tube should not be clamped or irrigated. The position of the tube should not be changed. The collection container should be below the level of the client to ensure gravity drainage.

12. ① The pain is described as sharp and severe as the calculi or stone progresses down the ureter. It frequently will radiate down the leg or to the groin area.

13. ③ The perineal area should be cleansed from the front to back to avoid contaminating the urethra with Escherichia coli. All other options are encouraged.

14. ① This is the best description for the cystoscopy examination. The client is most often in lithotomy position and conscious sedation may be used. It is important to explain to the client that he should not experience severe pain.

15. ④ The skin is typically sallow yellow in color and dry, and frequently the client complains of itching. Uremic frost may be noted. The bruising occurs due to the effect of renal failure on coagulation.

16. ③ Increasing peripheral edema associated with the development of congestive heart failure is the only option listed that is associated with an increase in fluids. The other options may be associated with complications of renal failure, but they are not associated with the increase in fluid volume.

17. ④ The classic sign of oliguria is urine output between 100 and 400 mL over 24 hours. The potassium level is increased, hematuria is not common, and the specific gravity usually is at a fixed level.

18. ④ When urine is not present after catheterization, the most common reason is the catheter is not in the bladder. For a female, it is most often in the vagina.

CHAPTER 19: INTEGUMENTARY SYSTEM

1. ④ Most pressure ulcers, or decubitus ulcers, are caused from pressure on an area that interferes with adequate blood supply to that area. Poor nutrition slows healing, and also places the client at an increased risk, but it does not cause the pressure ulcer initially.

2. ① The first stage of a pressure ulcer is a reddened area that does not blanch with slight digital pressure. When this occurs, damage has already taken place in the capillary bed of the tissue under the skin. If the skin is broken and the area is moist, it is a stage 2 ulcer. Other options are not characteristic of pressure sores.

3. ④ Whenever there is necrosis in a pressure ulcer, the area must be debrided. This may be done with medication or by surgical excision of the area. Hydrogen peroxide should not be used to cleanse the ulcer. A sterile, moist dressing should be used to protect the tissue. Massaging around the pressure ulcer will not stimulate healing.

4. ②, ④, ⑤, ⑥ Elevating the head of the bed to 30° or less will decrease the chance of pressure ulcer development from shearing forces. When placing the client in sidelying position, use the 30° lateral inclined position. Do not place the client directly on the trochanter, which can create pressure over the bony prominence. Avoid the use of donut-shaped cushions because they reduce blood supply to the area, which can lead to extension of the area of ischemia. Bony prominences should not be massaged, as it increases the risk of capillary breakage and injury to underlying tissue leading to pressure ulcer formation.

5. ① There are many commercial moisture creams available. Showering will increase the dryness, and protective pads will not help decrease the problem. The cotton clothing h1elps, but frequently the problem occurs in areas not covered by clothing.

6. ② It is critical to assess the status of circulation when eschar forms on a circumferential burn. The swelling under the eschar can cause circulatory compromise. The client does not have any increased risk factors for respiratory problems, and the burn is not large enough for a severe hydration problem to exist. Infection cannot be accurately assessed until the eschar sloughs or is removed and the tissue underneath can be assessed.

7. ② It is very important to wash all of the bed linens and clothes, as well as to treat any other items the child has frequent contact with. Permethrin shampoo should be used, but it does not require use of an antibiotic ointment. A coal tar or dandruff shampoo will not be beneficial. If there are areas where the child has scratched, an antibiotic ointment should be used.

8. ④ Herpes zoster in older adults is accompanied by nerve pain (neuralgia). This may be reduced by medication or the recently released herpes zoster vaccine. Warm soaks and antifungal cream will not be effective. All clients should be maintained on standard precautions as a standard of care.

9. ② Prevention of further damage or occurrence is most important. The client should always use sunscreen and avoid any sun damage to the skin. The condition can recur, so the client should maintain regular checkups. Antiinflammatory ointment does not heal an infection. Once the area is excised, there should be minimal discomfort.

10. ① Steroid cream and ultraviolet (sun) light are frequently the first line of treatment for the psoriasis client. The condition is chronic and recurring. Warm packs are not effective, and the area may be very tender and begin to bleed if the scales are removed.

11. ② Topical application of a scabicide is the best way to kill the mite. Due to the tunneling effect of the mite and the burrowed eggs, it is important to leave the scabicide on for 8 to 12 hours before washing it off. All family members should be treated. Antibiotic ointment may help to prevent an infection in an irritated area, but it does not treat the problem. Moist soaks are not beneficial in killing the mite.

CHAPTER 20: MATERNAL CARE

1. ④ Iron needs during pregnancy can most readily be met by taking iron supplements. Iron supplements

should be taken with additional vitamin C to increase absorption.

2. ① Ideally, counseling about nutrition begins at the first prenatal visit, starting with the assessment of dietary intake. Labor and postpartal needs are appropriate teaching for the third trimester.

3. ③ Positive signs of pregnancy are those that are diagnostic. These signs demonstrate without a doubt there is a fetus in the uterus. Quickening, nausea, vomiting, and changes in the breast are presumptive or subjective signs.

4. ④ Suggest to the woman that she eat smaller meals. Fluids and protein are good to increase in the pregnancy, but will not assist in decreasing the nausea and vomiting. Over-the-counter medications should not be recommended.

5. ① Elevating the feet and legs assists to decrease venous stasis. When the client is standing, the pregnant uterus exerts increased pressure on the large pelvic veins. It is not recommended that the pregnant client restrict sodium intake, and an increased fluid intake is okay; however, it does not assist to decrease venous stasis.

6. ① Foul odor may indicate the presence of an infection and should be reported to the RN or the PCP. The PCP will probably start antibiotics.

7. ② The postpartum vital signs are indicative of hemorrhage. The quickest way to stop uterine hemorrhage in a postpartum client is to massage the uterus (fundus). The nurse should stay with the client, perform measures to keep the fundus firm, and have someone else call the physician.

8. ① Regardless of the length of the contractions, whether the membranes have ruptured, or if a bloody show is present, if the woman is not having any effacement or dilation she is not considered to truly be in labor.

9. ① The duration of the contraction is the length of the contraction from the beginning of the contraction to the end of it. The frequency of contractions is from the beginning of one contraction to the beginning of another.

10. ③ Green, leafy vegetables; citrus fruits; and yeast products are good sources of folic acid. Folic acid is necessary for DNA synthesis.

11. ② The release of oxytocin from the posterior pituitary during the infant's suckling increases the contractions of the uterus and leads to afterpains.

12. ③ The recommended weight gain during pregnancy for a woman of average weight is 25 to 35 pounds. There is considerable variation, but this is the average amount that is consistently recommended.

13. ④ Weight gain, edema, proteinuria, and increased blood pressure are the classic indications of the development of early problems with pregnancy-induced hypertension.

14. ① During labor and delivery (intrapartum period), placenta previa would cause problems with bleeding and potentially severe hemorrhage. This is the only condition listed that is associated with severe bleeding problems during the intrapartum period.

15. ④ Left lateral position increases the delivery of blood to the placenta, as well as preventing the problems of vena caval syndrome.

16. ② The Apgar score is completed at 1 minute to assist in identifying any intrauterine problems and to evaluate the current status. The Apgar score is performed again at 5 minutes to determine any problems in the transition to extrauterine life.

17. ② Braxton Hicks or false labor contractions usually decrease when walking, are not concentrated in one part of the uterus, and do not increase in intensity and frequency. These contractions do not result in cervical effacement and dilation.

18. ④ The serious side effects of oral birth control pills include problems with hypertension and clotting. If the woman develops a headache or leg pain, she needs to report it to the physician immediately.

19. ③ Terbutaline (Brethine) may be used to suppress contractions. Another medication used to suppress contractions is magnesium sulfate.

20. ③ Stretch marks cannot be prevented with any type of lotions or oils. They will gradually fade and become silvery streaks during the months after delivery. There is nothing that can be done to prevent them; however, a positive answer that they will fade is a better approach.

CHAPTER 21: NEWBORN

1. ③ Immediately after birth the infant frequently has mucus in the upper airway. The airway needs to be suctioned and occasionally the infant will need additional oxygen. A bulb syringe to suction the upper airways should be kept in the infant's crib.

2. ② This is the characteristic description of the caput. It is a collection of fluid under the scalp and it crosses the suture line on the cranium. It will gradually be absorbed and does not require treatment.

3. ① These three factors—grunting, flaring nares, and sternal retractions—are classic symptoms of respiratory distress in infants. A lusty cry, heaving chest wall, flailing arms, respiratory rate of 30 to 60 breaths/min, pulse rate of 110 to 160 beats/min, sneezing, crying, and acrocyanosis are normal findings in the newborn.

4. ③ There is frequently a concern with cardiac output when the infant turns dusky with crying. The other options are within the normal range of findings for a newborn.

5. ① E. coli is necessary for the utilization of vitamin K. Since the newborn's bowels are sterile at birth, he has

difficulty with the synthesis of vitamin K. An injection is given to provide enough vitamin K until his system begins to function.

6. ④, ⑤, ⑥ The mother should be taught to feed the baby on demand for at least the first 4 weeks, until lactation is well established. Feeding only breast milk frequently stimulates milk production. Nipple soreness is one of the most common problems; however, the use of a cream to soften the nipples is often helpful as well as offering a pacifier to meet sucking needs of the newborn. Adequate rest and good fluid intake help promote milk production.

7. ③ Problems with hypoglycemia may range from increased irritability to generalized seizures. Acrocyanosis is normal in a newborn. The respiratory rate is around 40 to 60 immediately after birth and levels off to 30 to 50 after the first 24 hours.

8. ① Keep the head covered to decrease convection heat loss. It is important to promote bonding during the first 8 hours; therefore the infant is not kept in the warmer. Bathing is delayed until the infant's vital signs have stabilized.

9. ② Hand washing between care of clients is just as critical in the nursery as it is in other patient care units. This is the most effective way to decrease the transmission of infection.

10. ③ The infant should be burped or bubbled after the first few minutes of feeding. The first few minutes of feeding is when air is more likely to enter the infant's stomach. If the air is not removed, the infant tends to "burp up" a large amount of feeding. This occurs in breast-fed and bottle-fed infants.

11. ④ **RhoGAM** is administered when the mother is Rh negative. If she is carrying an Rh-positive infant, she will begin to build up antibodies that will affect the next pregnancy. **RhoGAM** prevents the buildup of the antibodies.

12. ③ The PKU test can be done from the blood on a heel stick. It will identify a complication in the ability of the infant to convert phenylalanine. It can be handled by dietary management.

13. ④ Some inappropriate or maladaptive behaviors that are considered postpartum danger signs for parentnewborn relationships include the following: passive reaction by parents in which they do not hold or examine newborn or speak to the newborn in affectionate terms or tones; lack of eye contact; disappointment over sex of the newborn; hostile reaction, either verbal or nonverbal; and nonsupportive interactions between the parents.

14. ① Approximately 40% to 60% of all full-term babies develop jaundice between the second and fourth days of life. In the absence of disease or specific cause, this is referred to as physiological jaundice. Hemolytic jaundice and erythroblastosis fetalis usually occur during the first 24 hours of life.

15. ① The priority is to prevent chilling, which leads to greater oxygen consumption, increased use of glucose and brown fat, higher caloric needs, decreased surfactant production, and a tendency to develop acidosis. The metabolic rate is actually high; evaporation occurs when the newborn is wet with amniotic fluid.

16. ② This option provides the most appropriate response. The nurse reassures the mother that it is molding, which will disappear in a few days and is related to the pressure of the delivery. The nurse should not tell a concerned mother not to worry, it does not require a diagnostic scan, and response 4 is the definition of a cephalohematoma.

17. ② The lack of passage of a meconium stool requires further assessment; it may be a sign of imperforate anus. The first assessment the nurse should perform is to visually inspect the anal area for an opening. Inserting a rectal thermometer could tear the anal mucosa, and if an imperforate anus is present, all oral feedings will be stopped.

18. ④ The mother and baby have identification bands secured to their wrist or ankle in the delivery room. These should be compared by the nurse every time the baby is returned to the mother and when the infant is prepared for discharge. The other responses are incomplete and will not ensure the safety of the baby.

19. ②, ⑤, ⑥ If a Plastibell circumcision is performed, there is no need for petroleum gauze, because the plastic bell that covers the glans will not stick to the diaper. Good hygiene using warm water and soap to remove urine and feces is appropriate during a diaper change. The dried yellow exudate that forms in 24 hours and persists for 2 to 3 days is part of the healing process and should not be removed. It is recommended not to position the infant on the abdomen for the first 24 hours after the procedure, but this is also good practice for any newborn, especially after feeding.

20. ② The meconium stool is often passed within the first few hours after birth. It is thick, greenish black, and sticky. It will gradually become lighter and more of a stool consistency.

Index

Page numbers followed by *b, t* and *f* indicate boxes, tables, and figures, respectively.